Biology

of the

Periodontium

Biology

of the

Periodontium

Edited by

A. H. MELCHER
W. H. BOWEN

Royal College of Surgeons of England,
Lincoln's Inn Fields, London, England

Academic Press
LONDON · NEW YORK
1969

ACADEMIC PRESS INC. (LONDON) LTD
Berkeley Square House
Berkeley Square,
London, W1X 6BA

U.S. Edition published by
ACADEMIC PRESS INC.
111 Fifth Avenue,
New York, New York 10003

Library of Congress Catalog Card Number: 70–82393
Standard Book Number: 12–489550–6

PRINTED IN GREAT BRITAIN BY
ABERDEEN UNIVERSITY PRESS LTD

Contributors

D. J. ANDERSON   Department of Oral Biology, The University of Bristol, Bristol, England

W. H. BOWEN   Department of Dental Science, Royal College of Surgeons of England, London, England

J. E. EASTOE   Department of Dental Science, Royal College of Surgeons of England, London, England

H. W. FERGUSON   School of Dental Surgery, University of Liverpool, Liverpool, England

G. M. HODGES   Imperial Cancer Research Fund, London, England

A. H. MELCHER   Department of Dental Science, Royal College of Surgeons of England, London, England*

H. W. NOBLE   Department of Dental Anatomy, Dental School, University of Glasgow, Glasgow, Scotland

D. C. A. PICTON   Department of Dentistry, University College Hospital Medical School, London, England

C. J. SMITH   Department of Dental Science, Royal College of Surgeons of England, London, England

A. R. TEN CATE   Unit of Anatomy in Relation to Dentistry, Anatomy Department, Guy's Hospital Medical School, London, England*

J. P. WATERHOUSE   Department of Oral Pathology, College of Dentistry, University of Illinois, Chicago, Illinois, U.S.A.

* Present Address: Faculty of Dentistry, University of Toronto, Toronto, Canada

Preface

The periodontium comprises epithelia and connective tissues which largely resemble those found elsewhere in the body, but which are modified to perform particular roles in a special environment. In planning this book it therefore seemed to us that a general understanding of the biology of epithelia and connective tissues is a prerequisite to a full appreciation of the structure and function of the periodontium; and furthermore, that the basic properties of epithelia and particularly connective tissues, and their interactions with one another, should be described in addition to those with which we are concerned particularly.

The material has been assembled with the needs of the graduate in mind. It is hoped that it will be of use to people with a special interest in the periodontium such as research workers, clinicians, especially periodontists and orthodontists, graduate students of dentistry, and dental teachers, and that it may be of some value as a reference book to undergraduates. Study of the periodontium and its constituent tissues has attracted the attention of both dentists and scientists trained primarily in other disciplines. It became apparent early in the preparation of the book that if basic scientific facts were provided for the former and fundamental dental information for the latter, much that is elementary would have to be written. Nevertheless, elementary material has been included in what is intended to be an advanced text in the belief that this will enhance its value to a readership drawn from many disciplines. Consequently, we hope that when the reader encounters that which appears to be simple and familiar, he will pass over it quickly and tolerantly in the knowledge that it was written for people trained in other fields.

We would not like to complete this preface without mentioning our appreciation of the considerable assistance and cooperation that we have received throughout from our publishers.

JUNE 1969

A. H. MELCHER
W. H. BOWEN

Contents

1*

9 | Effect of Nutrition on the Periodontium

H. W. FERGUSON

10 | Effects of Endocrine Secretions on the Periodontium and its Constituent Tissues

J. P. WATERHOUSE

11 | The Gingival Environment

W. H. BOWEN

12 | Healing of Wounds in the Periodontium

A. H. MELCHER

1 | The Evolution of the Mammalian Periodontium

HENRY W. NOBLE

Department of Dental Anatomy, Dental School, Glasgow, Scotland

I. Introduction

The socketed attachment of teeth is but one of many important modifications which took place during the period some 200 million years ago when the earliest mammals were evolving from their reptilian predecessors. The success of this modification is indicated by the fact that it appears to have been rapidly adopted throughout the many different groups of emerging mammalia. This method of tooth attachment also occurred in primitive birds which evolved from reptilian ancestors which possessed dentitions. Of the present-day reptilia the members of the crocodile order demonstrate Thecondont Gomphosis (see page 9) which, although differing in many important respects from mammalian gomphosis, is nevertheless an attempt to achieve the same end though the tissues involved were less readily adaptable.

The evolution of the mammalian periodontium is largely a story of the changing and developing relationship between tooth and bone of jaw, or more specifically, between dentine and bone. The complete story is unlikely to be elucidated by the examination of present-day descendants of lower forms of vertebrate animals, although they exhibit many interesting variations of the specialized tissues concerned. Instead, bone and dentine in earlier fossil examples must be examined, as this allows observations to be made on the developing relationships between these tissues as tooth roots and bony sockets make their appearance.

Primitive bone and dentine were both present in the earliest vertebrates, Archodus and Palaeodus from the Early Ordovician of Russia, approximately 400 million years ago. Although a primitive form of bone was present, these earliest vertebrates were jawless and it is interesting to note that primitive tooth-like structures preceded jaws in development. An early example of the combination of jaws and teeth is to be found in the Acanthodii, which are members of the Gnathostomata (Denison, 1963).

Text-book descriptions of the various forms of tooth attachment in vertebrates have varied only slightly over a long period (Tomes, 1898; Widdowson, 1906; Aitchison, 1940; Scott and Symons, 1964). There has been, however, a decline in the assurance with which statements concerning the evolution and homology of the tissues have been made. This reflects firstly, the changing outlook upon the position and importance of the cartilaginous skeleton of the Elasmobranchii (Romer, 1942, 1964); and secondly, the realization that the facile equation of bone of attachment with alveolar bone cannot be maintained beside the clearer picture which is now available of the histology of some types of attachment (Gillette, 1955; Kerr, 1959; Parsons and Williams, 1962). A knowledge of the phylogenetic development of the periodontium is an important aspect of the background information upon which a correct understanding of its functions and structure must be based.

II. Types of Vertebrate Tooth Attachment

A. Fibrous Attachment

In this method of attachment, commonly found in the sharks, rays, skate and other members of the Elasmobranch class, the teeth are attached to the skeleton by a union of their basal portions with the fibrous tissue covering the cartilaginous jaws (Fig. 1). The teeth are composed of tubular dentine with a thin covering layer of vitro dentine. At their base they have a mass of irregular calcified tissue in which are embedded fibres from the fibrous layers covering the jaws. This basal portion is a continuation of the tubular dentine, but contains few tubules. The odontoblast layer is continuous on its inner

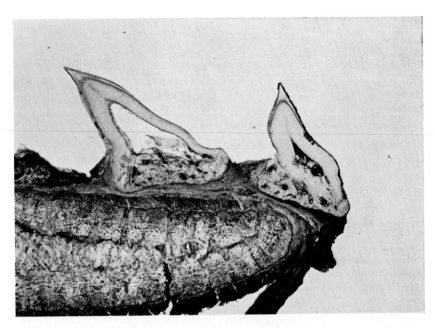

FIG. 1. Lower jaw of Shark showing teeth attached by their bases to fibrous membrane covering jaw composed of modified cartilage. The irregular mass of calcified tissue at the base of each tooth merges imperceptibly with the dentine and contains vascular spaces and the embedded Sharpey's fibres from the fibrous covering of the jaw.

aspect but many coarse collagen fibres are incorporated into its outer surface. A succession of such teeth is commonly present. These erupt from an area of development on the inner aspect of each jaw, known as the thecal fold. It is believed that tooth replacement in present-day members of this class does not occur with the same frequency as previously, but several dentitions still develop successively within the thecal fold. Erruption is thought to occur by means of a gradual movement, over the edges of each jaw, of the fibrous tissue to which the teeth are attached. This movement is generally attributed to growth of the jaws or to growth of the animal generally, resulting in the developing teeth on the inner aspect of each jaw being brought to a functional position at each jaw margin.

Cartilage was believed to be a more primitive tissue than bone, and it was thought that the presence of the cartilaginous skeleton in the present-day Elasmobranchii was an example of the retention of a more primitive type of skeleton by these fish. The attachment of the specialized placoid scales lining the oral cavity to the layer of fibrous tissue covering the cartilaginous skeleton was also regarded as an example of the persistence of a more primitive form of tooth attachment. Doubts concerning the antiquity of the cartilaginous skeleton suggest that fibrous attachment as observed in the present-day Elasmobranch may not be a primitive arrangement. (See page 11.)

B. ANCHYLOSIS

In the earliest vertebrates a calcified union existed between the tubercles of primitive dentine and the bone of the underlying skeleton. A similar form of rigid attachment unites the teeth to the bone of the jaws in most fish, amphibians and reptiles. This type of attachment is known as anchylosis. A certain amount of confusion about this method of attachment exists in the literature of comparative dental anatomy. A calcified union of the tooth with the underlying jaw bone is not present in every case normally included under this heading, for a variety of forms of attachment where a layer of fibrous tissue intervenes are also described. A good example of this type of attachment is to be seen in the teeth of the Python. Here the tubules of ortho-dentine mingle with the layers of the bone of attachment, which is in turn directly linked by calcification to the bone of the jaw. The weakest part of this attachment lies between the bone of attachment and the jaw bone. As a result, the accidental loss of a tooth leaves a saucer-shaped depression on the margins of the jaw bone where the bone of attachment existed. A succession of teeth erupt; consequently, a bony attachment must be formed at the base of each tooth following its eruption into a functional position. This type of calcified anchylosis is found in many members of the Teleostei where an outer row of anchylosed teeth surrounds an inner row or rows of hinged teeth (Fig. 2). Particularly large anchylosed teeth occur in the lower jaw of the Pike.

The term "acrodont anchylosis" has been used to describe the position of a tooth that is perched on top of the bone to which it is attached. This form of attachment has been described in the Eel and some amphibia. The tooth is attached by its base to a small cylindrical pedicel of bone, the bone of attachment, which is in turn attached by calcification to the bone of the jaw. A slight variation of the relationship between the base of the tooth and the upper surface of the bone of attachment has been described in the Haddock. Here the inner surface of the bone of attachment is slightly recessed to take a projection from the base of the tooth which is therefore half perched upon, and half situated within, the bone of attachment. In the Mackerel a further stage of development has been described. The lower part of each tooth is situated entirely within the cylindrical bone of attachment. This form of attachment is known as pleurodont anchylosis.

In Amphibia the pedicel bone of attachment often appears to be formed

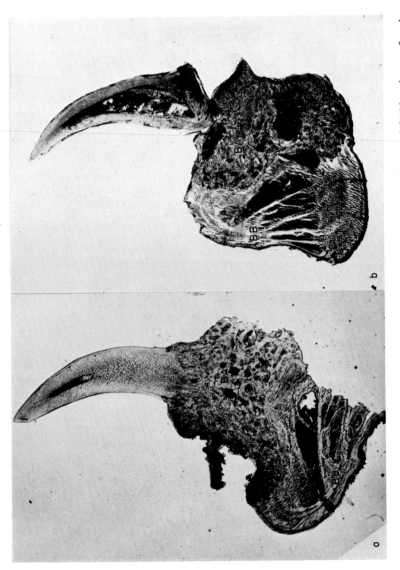

Fig. 2. Vertical sections through Cod jaw showing relative positions of (a) anchylosed and (b) hinged rows of teeth. The distinction between the regular architecture of the basal bone (BB) and the irregular arrangement of the bone of attachment (BA) can be clearly seen.

by the same layer of cells as form the dentine in the crown (Lawson, 1965).
The fibrous tissue between the tooth and the pedicel would thus appear to be
uncalcified dentine matrix. Kerr (1959) draws attention to the similarity
between this form of anchylosis and the early forms of hinge attachment. He
suggests that slight movements of a hinge-like nature are permitted in a
lingual direction because of the shape of the junction between the tooth and
the bone of attachment.

C. Hinged Attachment

In accounts of this type of attachment an uncalcified fibrous hinge has been
described between the tooth and the bone of attachment (Fig. 3). This hinge

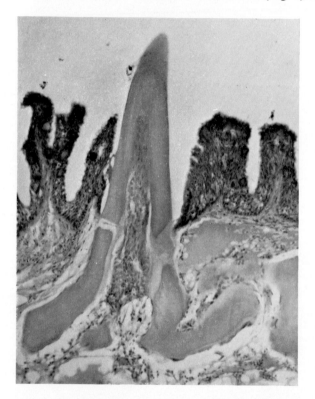

Fig. 3. Hinged attachment in the Goby fish. An uncalcified area of dentine matrix can be
seen to the right and a gap in the dentine on the left. Note that the epithelial attachment
doe not appear to expose the hinge attachment within the oral cavity.

in the Angler takes the form of a simple strip of fibrous tissue extending from
the distal surface of the tooth to the bone of attachment. In the Pike, the
posterior fibrous hinge is supplemented by more centrally placed uncalcified
trabeculae of osteodentine. These extend from the pulp cavity to the bone of

attachment, imparting elasticity and resilience to the hinged arrangement. The posterior part of the hinge in the Hake consists of a combination of uncalcified dentine and fibrous tissue. Anteriorly, and to either side of the midline, two restraining fibrous ligaments pass from the tooth to the bone of attachment, protecting the blood supply to the vascular dentine. Hinged attachment is an adaptive modification which, together with the recurved form of the tooth in these animals, greatly assists the swallowing of a slippery prey.

D. GOMPHOSIS

Gomphosis is the only form of tooth attachment present in mammals. Great variations exist in the size and position of the socket, but the suspensory function of the periodontal ligament, whereby biting or masticatory forces are transmitted to the bony walls of the socket, is a common factor in every case (Fig. 4).

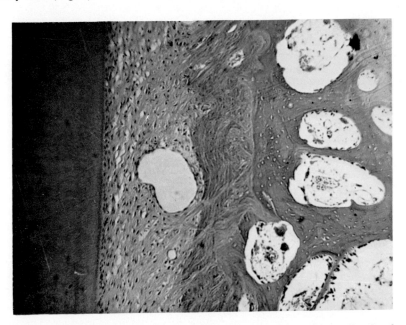

FIG. 4. The suspensory ligament in gomphosis. Fibres pass in an oblique direction from the cemental surface of the tooth to the lamina dura where they are embedded as Sharpey's fibres in the most recently formed layers.

Socketed attachment has been described in some fish. The teeth present on the rostral snout of Pristis are attached by fibres to the walls of sockets within the cartilaginous snout (Fig. 5). The anterior teeth in Sargus are also attached by a form of gomphosis (Beust, 1938). In reptiles, members of the

Crocodilia exhibit a form of socketed attachment of their polyphyodont dentitions. In this case, however, remodelling of the bone of the socket does not take place to suit each successional tooth. The sockets, once formed, persist and as each successional tooth erupts, it is attached by fibrous tissue to the walls of the socket. Miller (1967) examined serial sections from a group

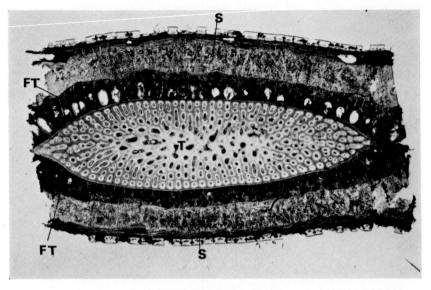

FIG. 5. Transverse section of embedded portion of tooth (T) from rostral snout of Pristis. The surface of the tooth is connected by fibrous tissue (FT) to the walls of the socket (S) in the cartilaginous snout.

of young Caiman sclerops, a small crocodilian reptile. He observed that a channel is formed by the outer and inner plates of bone in each jaw within which the polyphyodont dentition developed. Subdivision of this channel to form individual sockets commenced near the front of each jaw and progressed backwards, but in the oldest specimens the groove remained undivided in the most posterior part of each jaw. The innermost layer of cementum on each root was acellular, but this was followed by layers of cellular cementum attaching fibres from the fibrous follicle in an irregular manner. The bone lining each socket did not show evidence of additional layers formed to attach the fibres that support the tooth in the socket: nor was it adapted closely to the root of the tooth. By contrast, proliferation of cementum appeared to reduce the space between the cylindrical tooth and the tubular socket. Furthermore, in the posterior part of each jaw, where individual sockets were not present, the apposition of cementum produced roots which were oblong in cross section as they lay within the groove formed by the outer and inner plates of bone. This specialized form of attachment is known as Thecodont Gomphosis.

Observations made upon the different types of tooth attachment which occur in vertebrates have led to the development of the following ideas concerning the evolution of the attachment apparatus. It is thought that teeth were originally firmly attached to the bone of the jaw by an underlying area of bone, known as the bone of attachment. The fibrous membrane which developed between the tooth and the bone of attachment, as in the Eel, is regarded as the earliest development of the periodontal ligament, the bone of attachment later developing into the alveolar process. The different relationships between the teeth and the bones of attachment, as seen in the Haddock and Mackerel, are believed to represent the process whereby the tooth gradually developed a root portion which remained within the bone of attachment. Further differentiation of the crown from the root portion was accompanied by a redistribution of the dental tissues. The development of a dental follicle or sac around the tooth germ, and the appearance of cementum, are believed to be the transitional stages between pleurodont anchylosis and gomphosis in the course of the evolution of this higher method of attachment.

Hinged attachment is not regarded as occupying any place in the sequence of changes leading to Gomphosis. It is regarded as a specialized form of anchylosis which has developed to satisfy a particular need in fish (Kerr, 1959).

An alternative view of the evolutionary steps leading to the development of Gomphosis was taken by Hertwig (1874 and 1879), who believed that the bone of attachment is homologous with the cementum. Furthermore, he proposed that the periodontal membrane developed as a fibrous ligament between the bone of attachment and the basal bone, and that the fibrous membrane observed between the bone of attachment and the tooth in the anchylosed and hinged teeth of fish disappeared later.

III. Evolution of the Tissues of Tooth Attachment

A. BONE OF THE JAWS

1. Definition

Bone is a mineralized connective tissue consisting of a matrix composed of collagen fibres embedded in a mucopolysaccharide ground substance, and calcium salts principally in the form of hydroxyapatite. Some of the bone forming cells, or osteoblasts, are included in each layer of bone as it is deposited. The included cells are then known as osteocytes; the spaces which they occupy as lacunae (see Chapter 6). The enclosed cells are nourished through a system of canaliculi which connect neighbouring lacunae.

Bone is the principal component of the skeleton in most vertebrates and, in the earlier forms, took part in the formation of a protective outer covering (exoskeleton). Later it helped form rigid central supports for the limbs and the internal organs (endoskeleton). The bones of the jaws and the vault of the cranium are believed to be derived from the exo-skeleton.

2. Earliest Appearance

Bone is regarded as a primitive tissue associated with the dawn of vertebrate history (Romer, 1964). Small fragments of dermal calcification have been identified as belonging to fossil vertebrates from the Early Ordovician geological strata in Russia. Many specimens of a similar nature have been discovered in geological deposits of a slightly later period (Middle Ordovician) in the American mid-West (Denison, 1963). Histological investigation of these calcified fragments of exoskeleton showed a coarse-fibred type of bone without any osteocyte lacunae. This is called aspidin. True bone appears in the fossil record 50 million years later, in specimens from Late Silurian deposits. Lacunae and canaliculi similar to those in modern bone were arranged in layers around vascularized spaces. Although this bone was mainly developed within the exoskeleton, layers of bone were also found at this stage lining internal surfaces such as canals for blood vessels and nerves. Here the bone is presumed to have been forming upon the framework of a cartilaginous endoskeleton which has not been preserved. In later fossils, cancellated endo-chondral bone and calcified cartilage made their appearance. As the internal cartilaginous skeleton was gradually replaced by a bony one in successive species of early vertebrates, there appears to have been a concomitant gradual reduction in the exoskeleton.

The biological functions which the evolution of bone as a tissue originally filled is a matter for speculation. Its possible roles include: protection against water scorpions (eurypterids) and other marine predators (Romer, 1946); a waterproofing protection against salt loss by osmosis (Smith, 1939, 1953); a method of excreting excess phosphate (Berrill, 1955); storage of phosphate conveniently accessible for extensive muscular activity (Pautard, 1959, 1961, 1962). Tarlo (1964), having reviewed the available evidence, arrived at the conclusion that bone initially functioned as a storehouse of phosphates. Later it fulfilled a protective function, and finally succeeded to the mechanical role of a supporting skeletal framework.

There appears to be fairly general agreement that the so-called membrane bones are homologues of the scaly plates which appear to have arisen as a result of fragmentation of the calcified carapace. These bones do not have any direct connection with the surface, but are derived from membranous tissue within the deeper layers of the dermis.

3. Varieties

The acellular bone of the modern Teleostei appears to be derived from the cellular bone of more ancient fish. The earlier fossils do not exhibit acellular bone, and it thus appears unlikely that the presence of acellular bone in Teleostei can be an example of the persistence of a primitive trait.

4. Contribution of Cartilage

The importance of cartilage in the evolution of a bony skeleton is difficult to assess. The earliest occurrence of bone precedes that of cartilage in the fossil record. In Late Silurian Osteotraci, cartilage is presumed to have formed the bulk of the endocranium which supported, on its surfaces, the earliest perichondral layers of bone from which an endoskeleton developed. By this time, however, bone was well established as a tissue of the exoskeleton. Romer (1942) and Tarlo (1964) both insist that bone has evolved separately from cartilage. Romer (1942) recognizes the importance of cartilage as a biological adaptation which accomplishes the embryonic development of an internal skeleton. However, he regards its presence in the adult animal as neoteny, that is, the persistence of an embryonic stage of development; and he does not consider it as evidence of an earlier stage in evolution. Denison (1963) is less certain about the early history of cartilage. He believes that lack of preservation possibly explains why it does not appear in ancestral verte-brates before they acquired the ability to mineralize their skeletons.

5. History of Development

The histological appearance of dinosaur bone was investigated by Currey (1962). He found a degree of physiological specialization greater than that seen in living reptiles. Furthermore, dinosaur bone was similar in structure to that of recent mammals. It was even more vascular than that of modern artiodactyls, while many modern reptiles have bone that is almost avascular. Although modelling resorption of bone was observed in one species, this feature was not present in the majority of specimens of dinosaur bone. This investigation has shown some of the many modifications of tissues which went into the evolutionary melting-pot during the period when reptiles reached heights of specialization, and the earliest mammals made their appearance. Many of these modifications later disappeared from the reptiles, but some formed a basis for further development among the mammalia which tentatively had appeared at this time.

B. THE EVOLUTION OF DENTINE

1. Definition

Dentine is a highly elastic, mineralized, connective tissue composed of a matrix of collagen fibres lying within a mucopolysaccharide ground sub-stance. It is devoid of cells and blood vessels, but is permeated by tubules which radiate from its developing surface and which contain protoplasmic extensions of the odontoblast cells. These tubules are narrowed by continuing apposition of mineralized tissue on to their walls. Dentine is the most superficial of the calcified mesodermal tissues and was, in the earliest stages of its evolution, always related to the exoskeleton. It is usually connected to deeper cellular and vascular mineralized structures by calcified tissue or by fibrous tissue.

2. Earliest Appearance

Tubular dentine, strikingly similar to that which composes the bulk of each mammalian tooth, evolved as an outer layer of the carapace of the earliest vertebrates over four hundred million years ago (Bryant, 1936). Sections of fossils show tubercles of dentine closely associated with the surface layers of a calcified exoskeleton. In some cases, these tubercles are covered by a structureless layer resembling enamel (Fig. 6).

The tubular appearance of the earliest known dentine is extraordinarily similar to tubular orthodentine of the present day (Fig. 7). Although no soft tissues remain to explain the manner of development of this earliest dentine, its position suggests that it was formed initially by a surface layer of mesoderm in contact with a basal layer of epithelial cells.

3. Varieties of Dentine

Tubular orthodentine is the most primitive type of dentine to be found in the fossil record. Osteodentine and vasodentine are therefore modifications resulting from alterations in the dentine-forming mesoderm. Plicidentine is a complex infolding of the walls of a single central pulp cavity, the actual dentine being otherwise identical in structure to tubular orthodentine.

4. History of Development

The earliest vertebrates were jawless. The development of jaws was possibly accompanied by fragmentation of those parts of the surface layer which covered the jaws and extended into the mouth cavity. Extensive modification of the dentine tubercles upon the surface layer of the fragmented carapace led to the appearance of teeth. The small areas of calcified attachment tissue at the base of each placoid scale and each tooth in the elasmobranch fishes may represent a remnant of the dermal bone of the carapace.

C. DENTAL FOLLICLE

1. Definition

The developmental origins of the periodontal ligament are closely associated with the earliest appearance of the dental follicle. The dental follicle is that part of the tooth germ from which arises the cementum, the periodontal ligament and, perhaps, some of the alveolar bone. (See Chapter 3.) The

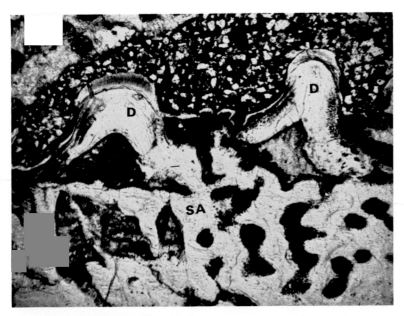

FIG. 6. Section through dermal denticles (D) attached to spongy aspidin (SA) from surface of Ostracoderm of Colorado Ordovician period some 500 million years ago. Note layer with appearance of enamel covering each denticle. Brit. Mus. Geol. Dept. Specimen P10624a.

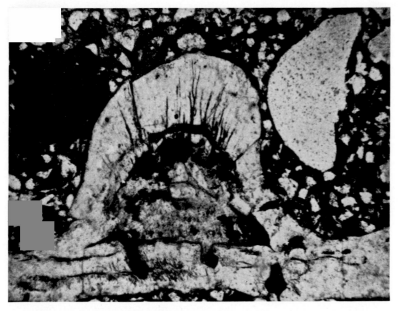

FIG. 7. Section of dermal denticle from same source as Fig. 6 showing irregular arrangement of dentinal tubules. Brit. Mus. Geol. Dept. Specimen P10624b.

dental follicle originates from the differentiating mesodermal tissue at the base of the dentine papilla. It has been described as spreading laterally, and towards the surface, from this base below the lower rim of the epithelial enamel organ eventually meeting the enamel organ's connection with the dental lamina (Mummery, 1920).

The dental follicle is believed to have many functions. It plays a part in protecting the developing tooth, and permits it to erupt into a functional position in the dental arch. In addition, its cells are responsible for formation of cementum on the surface of the roots and crowns of teeth (see Chapter 3), and they synthesize the suspensory fibres which extend from the cementum to the inner wall of the alveolar bone of the socket (see Chapter 6). It is impossible to distinguish between the tissue of the dental follicle and the periosteum which covers the inner surface of the crypt and later the tooth socket. Consequently, it is uncertain that the follicle contributes to the formation of bone on the inner surfaces of these cavities. (See the discussion of this topic in Chapter 3.) The existence of a follicle, and of the periodontal ligament which arises from it, provides a large measure of protection against harmful forces which is lacking in teeth attached by a calcified form of anchylosis.

2. Earliest Appearance

The earliest appearance of a follicle in present-day vertebrates is difficult to determine. Horny teeth, such as those in the Lamprey, which develop within the layers of the epithelium, possess no dental follicle. In Elasmobranchs, for example Dogfish, no investing sac or follicle extends from the base of the dentine papilla around the tooth germ. An irregular area of calcified fibrous tissue develops at the base of these teeth and, by reason of its continuity with the dentine and with the underlying fibrous tissue which is incorporated in its matrix, each tooth becomes attached to the fibrous membrane covering the jaw (Fig. 8). The cells which form the calcified tissue may have been stimulated to differentiate by the epithelium of the enamel organ, but the tissue to which they give rise is not formed in direct contact with an internal enamel epithelium (Fig. 9), as is the case with dentine.

3. History of Development

It is believed that the pedestal bone of attachment in those fish where the teeth have a hinged attachment is likewise developed from mesodermal tissue at the base of the dentine papilla. The mesodermal tissue is stimulated to differentiate by the enamel organ, although not initially formed in contact with the internal enamel epithelium.

The principal difference between the calcified tissue at the base of an anchylosed tooth, the pedestal-like bone of attachment in bony fish, and the cementum surrounding the roots of gomphosed teeth, is one of arrangement.

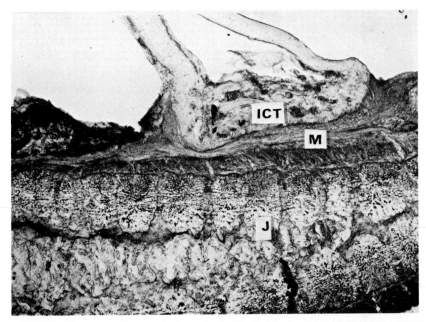

FIG. 8. Attachment by fibrous membrane in the Shark. The irregular calcified tissue (ICT) at the base of the tooth incorporates fibres from the membrane (M) covering the jaw (J).

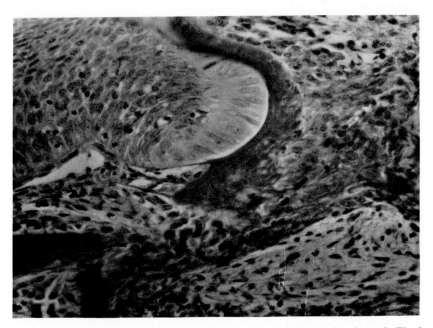

FIG. 9. Development of base of tooth in Dog-fish in area similar to that shown in Fig. 8. Tubular dentine is forming against epithelial layer at top of field while irregular tissue incorporating connective tissue fibres is forming at base of tooth but not in contact with organizing epithelial surface.

As a result of the dental follicle being formed by the spreading upwards of the tissue from the base of the dentine papilla around the sides of the developing tooth, the calcified tissue which eventually arises from this follicle is located around the sides of the roots and perhaps also on the crown of gomphosed teeth.

D. The Evolution of Cementum

1. Definition

Cementum is the least specialized of the calcified tooth tissues, and most closely resembles bone in its histology and composition (see Chapter 6). It is an integral part of the attachment apparatus in the gomphosed tooth, being mainly concerned with the attachment to the tooth surface of fibres which relate the teeth to the jaws. This function commences as the tooth erupts into its position in the arch. It is continued throughout the life of the tooth, permits variations in the forces applied to the tooth, and allows any further eruptive movements to take place.

2. Earliest Appearance

Cementum is present throughout the Mammalia as part of the attachment apparatus of gomphosed teeth. Although normally present on the roots of teeth, it is also found as a tissue on the crown of teeth of persistent growth and continuous eruption, such as those of the horse and other Ungulates. In the Herbivore's teeth of semi-persistent growth, it covers the enamel of the crown of the tooth. It thereby provides attachment for the supporting fibres of the periodontal ligament, since the roots of these teeth do not make their appearance until a much later stage in tooth development.

A tissue similar to cementum has been described on the roots of socketed teeth in those fish and reptiles which exhibit this mode of attachment. Otherwise, little attention has so far been paid to the investigation of the earlier forms of this tissue.

3. Variations

Cellular and acellular forms of this cementum occur in most species of Mammalia. The reason why two forms of cementum should occur has not yet been investigated fully. It has been suggested that the type of cementum formed may be related to the fact that some surfaces of a root are exposed to tension while others are exposed to pressure during the functional use of the tooth. It is also recognized that cellular cementum is deposited when a greater bulk of this tissue is required to be formed rapidly.

4. History of Development

A distinct layer of cementum cannot be observed in those teeth attached by anchylosis. Although the tissue of the bone of attachment is frequently quite different in structure from the bone of the remainder of the jaw, it is felt that this area of modified bone is comparable to the alveolar process of the gomphosed tooth. Cementum therefore probably made its appearance with the advent of the periodontal ligament, satisfying the demand of this tissue for attachment to the outer calcified surface of the dentine.

E. The Evolution of Alveolar Bone

1. Definition

Alveolar bone first appears around developing tooth germs to form the protective crypts. During the eruption of the teeth, the crypts are modified by further apposition of bone to form the sockets or alveoli which surround the roots of the functional teeth. The alveolar processes therefore surmount the basal bone of each jaw and transmit forces between the teeth and basal bone. Alveolar bone is indistinguishable from basal bone histologically and biochemically. There is reason to believe that it is very responsive to physiological forces transmitted from the teeth. Variations in the strength and direction of the forces transmitted by the teeth are reflected in the architecture of the alveolar process (see Chapter 6). It thus plays a very important part in the establishment and maintenance of occlusion.

2. Earliest Appearance

Alveolar bone is, by definition, only present when teeth develop within the bone of the jaw, erupt, and are then attached by gomphosis. Alveolar bone is therefore present in very few fish, but becomes quite a prominent part of the tooth-bearing portions of each jaw among reptilia and, in particular, the members of the Crocodilia. Because of its avascularity, however, this bone is not as vital a tissue as in the Mammalia. Resorption of the alveolar process following the loss of each tooth, and its regeneration accompanying the eruption of the successor, does not occur (thecodont gomphosis).

3. Variations

Considerable variations in the bulk and structure of the alveolar bone exist throughout the Mammalia. In the Carnivora and Insectivora the stationary positions of the teeth, once erupted, make little demand upon the powers of adaptation of the alveolar bone. In the Rodents and Herbivora, however, active eruption throughout the life of the tooth is accomplished only by means of continuous activity of alveolar bone. This is particularly so in the case of the molar teeth of the Elephant, where the alveolar process must resist considerable forces and must also maintain a constant physiological mesial drift. This drift is necessary to compensate for loss of occlusal tooth substance due to attrition, and to transport each succeeding molar from its developmental crypt towards the front of each jaw.

When the alveolar bone surrounding each tooth germ must develop entirely outwith the basal bone, as is the case of the posterior molar teeth in the upper jaw of the Pig, then a wafer-thin, balloon-like structure known as an alveolar bulb develops. The extra demands for support made by such teeth as the canine tusks of the Wild Boar and the Wart Hog, give rise to considerable increases in the thicknesses of the bone surrounding the sockets of these teeth. In every case, however, a close relationship can be seen to exist between the size, shape and number of the roots of a tooth, and the direction and strength of the demands for support transmitted from the tooth to the alveolar bone. This close relationship has led Baume (1956, 1961) to speak of the way in which the tooth and investing bone form a "developmental entity". Thomas (1934) insisted that tooth and alveolar bone were distinct developmentally, but he believed that the presence of teeth influences the growth of bone (see Chapters 2 and 3 for a discussion of this topic).

4. History of Development

The absence of information concerning the early stages in the evolution of gomphosis makes it difficult to discuss the early evolutionary history of alveolar bone. Many similarities exist between mammalian alveolar bone and the bone of attachment of anchylosed or hinged teeth in fish, amphibians and reptiles. The labial plate of alveolar bone is always first to develop and, because of the manner in which teeth in these species become attached by their sides to this bone, the term "labial pleurodontism" is used by Jacobshagen (1955). In each case this bone has the function of supporting the tooth and uniting it to the bone of the jaw.

F. EVOLUTION OF THE PERIODONTAL LIGAMENT

1. Definition

In the early fully functional tooth, the alveolar bone is closely adapted to the root surface, but is everywhere separated from it by a layer of connective tissue containing blood vessels, nerves and lymphatics. Microscopical examination of the orientation of this connective tissue suggests that the "membrane" should more correctly be referred to as a "ligament", since the majority of the fibres take part in the process of connecting these two surfaces rather than separating them as is more commonly the function of a membrane. The alveolo-dental ligament, as the periodontal ligament is sometimes known, has firstly the function of attaching each tooth to its investing alveolus and, secondly, the more important and complex function of receiving and transmitting the forces generated during mastication and other processes associated with the use of the dentition (see Chapters 6 and 8).

2. Earliest Appearance

The periodontal ligament is present throughout the Mammalia and occurs in a simpler form in those fish and reptiles which have gomphosed teeth. The presence of a fibrous ligament between the base of the tooth and the bone of attachment in certain anchylosed teeth, for example the Eel, has been cited as an early example of a periodontal ligament. However, as with cementum and alveolar bone, homologies are doubtful in these descendants of more primitive vertebrates, and a continuous chain of evolutionary evidence is lacking in this respect.

3. Variations

Since, among Mammalia, the periodontal ligament is associated not only with attachment and support of the tooth but also with degrees of active

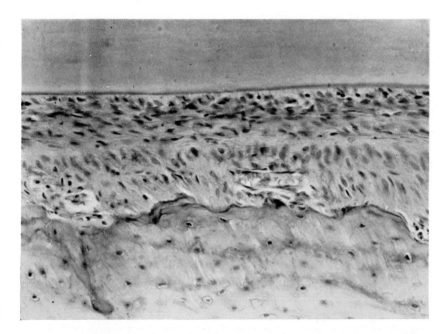

Fig. 10. Periodontal ligament from mouse incisor showing double arrangement of fibres and central intermediate plexus. Layer nearest tooth is more cellular while layer nearest bone is more vascular. Cell nuclei and fibres in each layer are almost at right angles to each other.

eruption during the functional period, which vary widely from species to species, the distribution and orientation of the periodontal fibres is not uniform. The most prominent variation is that seen in the ligament of continuously growing teeth such as the rodent incisor. The cells and fibres of the ligament are arranged in two distinct systems of preferential orientation. One is related to the cementum surface and the other to the alveolar bone, with an intermediate area where the two systems meet (Fig. 10). (See Chapters 3 and 6 for further discussion of the intermediate area.) It is believed that the continuous changes in the suspensory ligament, which are necessary to accommodate the continuous growth and eruption of the tooth, take place in the intermediate plexus (Sicher, 1964; Eccles, 1964).

4. History of Development

The periodontal ligament is an essential element in the attachment of teeth by gomphosis, a method of attachment which was not always as closely confined to Mammalia as is the case at the present day. This method of attachment was present in many of the advanced mammal-like reptiles which are now extinct. As a method of tooth attachment, gomphosis may be said to have evolved at least 120 million years before the appearance of the earliest mammals. Many of the Jurassic birds which lived 85 million years before mammals appeared are known to have possessed gomphosed dentitions. Since the periodontal ligament is a soft tissue, the possibility of obtaining a complete record of the various stages in its evolution from the examination of fossil material is unlikely. An indication of its presence or absence may, however, be deduced from examination of the relationships of teeth and bone and from the nature and extent of root development.

IV. Processes Associated with the Evolution of the Mammalian Periodontium

A. ROOT DEVELOPMENT

In the more primitive forms of tooth attachment the teeth were simply attached by their basal surfaces to the underlying tissues. Bone gradually developed around the base of the tooth (particularly on the labial side). This process continued until there was sufficient bone for the attachment of the tooth. Such a transition is exemplified by the acrodont type of anchylosis seen in the Eel, the intermediate stage seen in the Haddock, and the fully developed pleurodont type of anchylosis seen in the Mackerel. It is a logical supposition that earlier development of the bone associated with prolongation of the development of the base of the tooth led to the early examples of gomphosis as seen in some present-day fish and the crocodilian reptiles.

A key element in the evolution of a root is, of course, the epithelial root sheath of Hertwig which determines the surface contour of the root dentine. The root portions of the earliest gomphosed teeth were simply cylindrical extensions of the lowermost cross-section of the crown portion. There was no narrowing of the root at the apical foramen which was a wide funnel-shaped opening into the pulp cavity of the tooth. This type of root is however

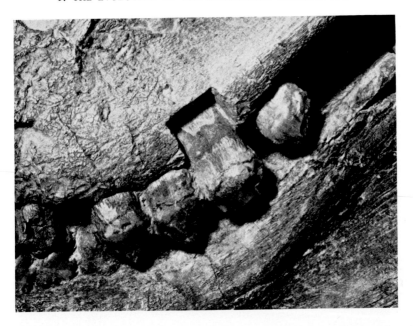

FIG. 11. *Cynognathus crateronotus*, a fossil reptile showing cheek tooth with tapered root, single but deeply grooved.

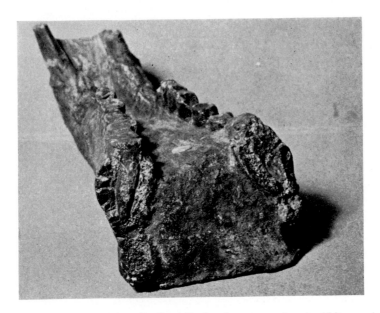

FIG. 12. *Diademodon browni*, a fossil reptile showing a tapered root within a socket at the fractured end of the specimen.

2

essential for the purposes of attachment of a polyphyodont dentition by a process of thecodont gomphosis.

The evolution of tapering roots, and later the evolution of divided roots, made greater demands upon the ability of the alveolar bone to mould itself

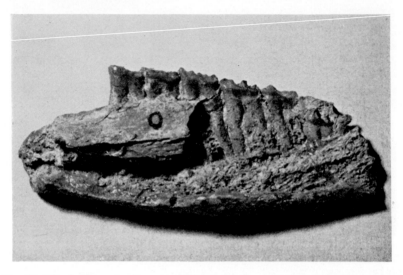

Fig. 13. *Oligokyphus*, a fossil mammal-like reptile about the size of a rabbit and having many of the characteristics of the first mammals. From Liassic age deposits in Somerset, England, it is about 180 million years old. The bunodont nature of the gomphosed, multi-rooted, cheek teeth can be clearly seen.

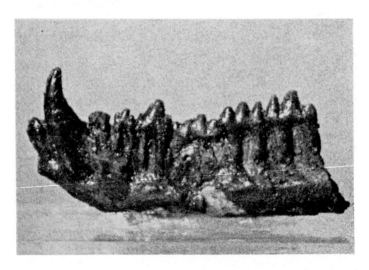

Fig. 14. *Triconodon mordex*, a primitive mammal, shows a heterodont dentition, and cheek teeth with a marked bifurcation and mesial and distal roots.

accurately to the root surface of each tooth. Examples of early stages in root development can be seen in the fossil exhibits of the Natural History Museum, London, England. The teeth of *Ichthyosaur* (a fish-eating lizard), which appear to consist of plicidentine, show evidence of narrowing to a root apex. *Cynognathus crateronotus* possesses a heterodont dentition consisting of incisors, canines, premolars and triconodont molars. This is illustrated in Fig. 11, where a small piece of bone has been removed to show that the roots of the triconodont molars are tapered and single, but deeply grooved. *Diademodon browni* has a well developed heterodont dentition and, at the fractured end of the specimen illustrated in Fig. 12, a well-formed root apex may be seen. *Oligokyphus* is a small mammal-like reptile whose cheek teeth have short crowns with cusps and ridges, and long roots with a deep bifurcation (Fig. 13). *Triconodon mordex* shows teeth with a large central cusp and mesial and distal cuspules. Each tooth has a mesial and a distal root, (Fig. 14).

The anchorage of a tooth whose root portion is other than a simple continuation of the widest part of the crown of the tooth implies a more advanced type of attachment than thecodont gomphosis. The above examples show that root development, the associated bone socket, and intervening membrane or ligament, were in existence at a time when the earliest mammals were making their appearance.

B. ERUPTION

Since the earliest teeth and placoid scales developed on, or just below, the surface epithelium, no great movement was required for these teeth to reach their functional position. In present-day Elasmobranchs, evidence exists of a form of eruption involving a movement across a surface to a position of optimal function. A protected area of development exists on the inner surface of each jaw, and "eruption" in this case means a movement over the surface of the jaw to a position on the margin. Here each tooth of the polyphyodont dentition can play an effective part in seizing prey, or crushing molluscs and crustaceans, according to the type of tooth and nature of the diet.

In the case of the hinged and anchylosed teeth of the bony fish, development commences below the surface. Eruption proceeds as the tooth develops in length, until the tooth reaches its full height and functional position, when anchylosis or the development of the hinged attachment occurs. The teeth of the polyphyodont dentition of reptiles erupt from intra-bony crypts into the sockets of their predecessors, and are anchored by supporting fibres at a suitable height. The persistent portion of the dental lamina remains lingual to each developing tooth which must first move in a buccal direction to line up with the long axis of the preformed socket. A notch at the base of each tooth develops to permit this early buccal movement on the part of its successor. The persistent socket, which gives the name of "thecodont gomphosis" to this form of attachment, appears to occur because reptilian bone is not sufficiently vital for the reconstructive activity to take place, which is necessary to accommodate this polyphyodont dentition in closely adapted sockets.

In most mammals, there are, in addition to the prefunctional eruption of each tooth, varying degrees of active eruption during the period that the tooth is actually in use. This movement is at its greatest in the constant formation and eruption of such teeth as the rodent incisor; is a factor of great importance in the case of teeth of semi-persistent growth such as herbivorous molars; is of some slight importance in the human dentition, particularly when attrition is severe; and finally, is of almost no consequence in the dentitions of Carnivora and Insectivora. It is to be expected, however, that histological examination would show a difference between periodontal ligaments which merely support and attach the tooth in constant position, and ligaments which, in addition, contrive to produce or permit a considerable degree of eruption at the same time. This difference has been detected, it is believed, in the form of the intermediate plexus so clearly seen in the periodontal ligament of the rodent incisor. This appearance has not, however, been detected convincingly in other situations such as herbivorous molars, where this arrangement might be expected to occur.

It is not known whether continuous eruption throughout the functional life of a tooth is a more primitive feature than a stationary form of attachment in a functional position. Certainly, earlier dentitions were polyphyodont, and the gradual reduction to two dentitions has been a trend followed by most Mammalia. Although anchylosed teeth were stationary in their functional position, it is uncertain whether the earliest gomphosed teeth in reptiles were also stationary, or were constantly erupting. Eruption is therefore a process of great importance when considering the evolution of the mammalian periodontium.

C. ROOT RESORPTION

Although resorption is not associated with bone development in fish and reptiles to as great an extent as in mammals, resorption of unwanted tooth substance has been observed in bony fish and has been described elsewhere in the case of Crocodilia. Shedding of teeth from a polyphyodont dentition could be necessary when succeeding teeth develop and seek a place in the dentition without prior loss of their predecessors. In the absence of some form of continuous eruption, resorption is the only method whereby the socketed root of a tooth belonging to an earlier dentition can be removed. Eruption of a succeeding tooth can then follow, with establishment of an efficient periodontal ligament to attach and support it.

D. Bone Reconstruction

Although a form of attachment by periodontal ligament is possible without extensive bone reconstruction, the tooth form must be simple and uniform. Correspondingly, greater demands are placed upon the fibrous attaching tissue. This form of attachment, as observed in the case of the Crocodile, is not a particularly effective mechanism; it is not one which would permit development of the diversity of sizes, shapes and multi-rooted teeth, which are found among Mammalia. Bone formation, coupled with modelling resorption, is the sensitive mechanism which has permitted the efficient, well organized periodontal ligament to evolve. By investing each root with an economical, but adequately strong layer of bone, refinements in the evolution of the periodontium have been made possible. These have resulted in a harmonious system of attachment and support.

E. Occlusion

The dentitions in opposing jaws of Fish, Amphibia and Reptiles do not usually occlude. Instead, they fit in with each other, or interdigitate. The exceptions include Fish, such as the Wolf Fish, where blunt-cusped teeth (composed of plicidentine and anchylosed to each jaw) meet. This facilitates the crushing of shell-fish. In general, occlusion is associated with evolution of the mammalian periodontium and the more complex mammalian temporo-mandibular articulation. The development of occlusion between the various cusps, facets, pits and fissures of the teeth in opposing jaws requires a sensitive mechanism for adjustment of tooth height and position. The periodontal ligament plays an important part in transmitting to the alveolar bone forces exerted upon the tooth crowns. The alveolar bone responds to these stresses (see Chapters 6 and 8).

F. Mastication

Crushing shell-fish may be regarded as a simple form of mastication. However, the role of the dentitions of Fish, Amphibians and Reptiles are normally limited, in the case of recurved and hinged teeth, to prehension and assistance in swallowing. The more elaborate preparation of food for digestion undertaken by the mammalian dentition is consequent upon the evolution of occlusion and attachment by gomphosis.

The periodontium exerts a cushioning effect (see Chapter 8). This, in many cases, protects the calcified dental tissues from accidental fracture. At the same time the proprioceptive innervation of the periodontal ligament reflexly guards against the exertion of excessive forces by the masticatory musculature (see Chapter 7).

References

Aitchison, J. (1940). "Dental Anatomy and Physiology for Students", 1st ed. Staples Press, London, England.

Baume, L. J. (1956). *Oral Surg.* **9**, 736.

Baume, L. J. (1961). *Am. J. Orthod.* **47**, 881–901.

Berrill, N. J. (1955). "The Origin of Vertebrates." Oxford.

Beust, T. B. (1938). *J. Am. dent. Ass.* **25**, 114–118.

Bryant, W. L. (1936). *Proc. Am. phil. Soc.* **76**, 409.

Currey, J. D. (1962). *Palaeontology* **5**, 238–246.

Denison, R. H. (1963). *Clin. Orthop.* **31**, 141–152.

Eccles, J. D. (1964). *Archs oral Biol.* **9**, 127.

Gillette, R. (1955). *Am. J. Anat.* **96**, 1–36.

Hertwig, O. (1874). *Jena Z. Naturw.* **8**, 331.

Hertwig, O. (1879). *Arch. mikrosk. Anat. EntwMech.* **11**, Suppl. 1.

Jacobshagen, E. (1955). *Anat. Anz.* **102**, 249–270.

Kerr, T. (1959). *Proc. zool. Soc. Lond.* **133**, 401–422.

Lawson, R. (1965). *Proc. zool. Soc. Lond.* **145**, 321–325.

Miller, W. A. (1967). I.A.D.R. Abstract. (In Press.)

Mummery, J. H. (1920). *Br. dent. J.* **41**, 49–60.

Parsons, T. S. and Williams, E. E. (1962). *J. Morph.* **110**, 375–390.

Pautard, F. (1959). *Proc. XVth Int. Congr. Zool., Lond.* 478–479.

Pautard, F. (1961). *New Scient.* **12**, 364–366.

Pautard, F. (1962). *Clin. Orthop.* **24**, 230–244.

Romer, A. S. (1942). *Am. Nat.* **76**, 394.

Romer, A. S. (1946). "Vertebrate Palaeontology." University of Chicago Press, Illinois, U.S.A.

Romer, A. S. (1964). *In* "Bone Biodynamics" (H. M. Frost, ed.), pp. 13–37. J. & A. Churchill Ltd., London, England.

Scott, J. H. and Symons, N. B. B. (1964). "Introduction to Dental Anatomy", 4th ed. E. & S. Livingstone Ltd., Edinburgh and London.

Sicher, H. (1964). *Periodontics* **2**, 144–145.

Smith, H. (1939). "Studies in the Physiology of the Kidney." Kansas, U.S.A.

Smith, H. (1953). "From Fish to Philosopher." Boston, U.S.A.

Tarlo, L. B. H. (1964). *In* "Bone and Tooth Symposium" (H. J. J. Blackwood, ed.), pp. 3–17. Pergamon Press, Oxford, England.

Thomas, J. A. M. (1934). *Qu. J. microsc. Sci.* **76**, 481.

Tomes, C. S. (1898). "A Manual of Dental Anatomy, Human and Comparative", 5th ed. J. & A. Churchill, London, England.

Widdowson, T. W. (1906). "Special or Dental Anatomy and Physiology and Dental Histology", Vol. 2. Staples Press Ltd., London, England.

2 Stromal-epithelial Interactions

GISELE M. HODGES

Imperial Cancer Research Fund, London, England

I. Introduction

Interactions between tissue components are an essential feature of normal embryonic development. The interactive processes between cells and tissues are important, not only for the initiation of differentiation, but probably also for the maintenance of differentiated organ systems.

The objectives of this chapter are three-fold: firstly, to review the pertinent facts concerning stromal-epithelial interactions in vertebrate organogenesis (avian and mammalian tissues); secondly, to examine the evidence for such interactions in the adult; and thirdly, to discuss the role of the "basement membrane".

II. Stromal-epithelial Interactions in Organogenesis

A. INTRODUCTION

Organogenesis is a complex, multi-step process, and the study of this problem at various levels has given rise to a very extensive literature, the analysis of which is outside the province of this chapter. More recent comprehensive reviews include Holtfreter and Hamburger (1955), Rudnick (1955), Dalcq (1960), Saxen and Toivonen (1962).

Tissue interdependence has long been recognized in the developing embryo, in particular from *in vivo* experiments and transplantation studies. The continued differentiation of one group of cells has been shown to be dependent upon the "inductive" influences of other proximal groups of cells of different types (Spemann, 1938; Rawles, 1955; Dalcq, 1960; Saxen and Toivonen, 1962; Sengel, 1965).

A more detailed study of these tissue inter-relationships has been made possible in recent years by the development of methods which allow the dissociation of embryonic organs into the constituent tissues or cells (Moscona, 1952; Grobstein, 1953a). A new field of research has developed since the 1950s in which the inductive relations of different tissues and, more especially, the stromal-epithelial interactions have been analysed at the morphological and, to a more limited extent, at the biochemical levels by *in vitro* culture methods.

There is very little data available relating to tissue inter-relationships in the periodontium (see Section IE). In this chapter the principle features of tissue interactions and the methods employed are described in the hope that further interest may be stimulated concerning the possible interactive influences that may be exerted by the different tissues of the periodontium.

B. METHODS

1. Tissue Dissociation

A variety of physical and chemical methods are available for the dissociation of tissues into their cellular components. (For discussions of procedures and principles see Rinaldini (1958), Moscona (1961b), Moscona *et al.* (1965), Curtis (1966), Weiss (1967).) The basis of all these methods is the alteration of the intercellular attachments so that the cells lose their connections and separate easily. However, the mechanism of cell attachment varies considerably according to the tissue, to the cell type, and to the age of the organism. The development of a general tissue dissociation procedure is therefore precluded and the choice of the method must depend on the type of tissue and the experimental objectives.

The most effective methods evolved to date for the dissociation of tissues into their epithelial and stromal components are based on enzymatic procedures. The modern development of enzymatic dissociation of tissues is due to the Mosconas (Moscona, 1952; Moscona and Moscona, 1952), and derives from earlier observations made by Rous and Jones (1916) on the release of cells from the outgrowth of plasma-clot cultures by crude trypsin.

Experimental Procedures		*Purpose*
Dissected embryonic organ		
↓		
Ca—Mg-free balanced salt solution (CMF) (based on Tyrode, Earles, Hanks or Dulbecco solutions).	1–5 min at 18°–20°C	Ca—Mg ions considered to increase cell surface cohesiveness. Therefore lowering of divalent cations content in tissues by soaking in CMF aids dissociation process.
↓		
Enzyme solution (1–3% trypsin; 3% trypsin-pancreatin; 0·05% collagenase).	20–45 min; 1–3 h at 3°–6°C 5–20 min at 20°C 5–15 min at 37°C	Enzyme solutions act probably by proteolytic activity. Chelating agents are thought to augment CMF influence.
or		
Chelating solution (0·02–0·4% disodium ethylene diaminetetraacetate (Versene)).		Precise information on mechanisms of action not available in either case.
↓		
CMF. Rinse tissues 1–3 times.		Diluting out of enzyme or chelating agents present in tissue.
↓		
Complete balanced salt solution (BSS).		
or		
BSS+serum (or other trypsin inhibitor).		Serum inactivates residual trypsin.
↓		
Culture medium—Organ culture.		Final separation of tissue carried out at this stage using microscalpels or needles.

FIG. 1. Outline of steps in the separation of embryonic rudiments into epithelial and stromal components.

Most embryonic rudiments and organs are amenable to tryptic action, and trypsin or trypsin plus pancreatin solutions are extensively employed in tissue dispersal techniques. Other enzymes have been tested but are not generally as effective (Moscona *et al.*, 1965; Rinaldini, 1959; Weiss, 1963).

It is observed that the epithelia of embryonic tissues tend, after immersion in enzyme solutions, to separate as intact sheets from the adjoining stroma before subsequently undergoing disaggregation into individual cells (Moscona, 1952). This differential susceptibility to dissociation agents shown by various cell types has been exploited in the development of epithelial-stromal separation techniques (Grobstein, 1953a). There are now a variety of methods for the dissociation of embryonic organs into their tissue components which are based upon the procedures of Grobstein (1955a, 1956) (Fig. 1) and employ

2*

enzymatic or chelating agents. References to these techniques are given in Section IC.

In general, the breakdown of older embryonic and of adult tissues is not readily achieved by the various methods indicated above. Medawar (1941) working with Thiersch grafts introduced the method of separating the epidermis from the dermis of adult skin using a dilute solution of trypsin at 37°C. It was found that both layers remained viable after separation and were suitable for grafting. Szabo (1955) showed that the two layers of skin could be separated with greater ease and still remain viable if treatment with trypsin was carried out at 4–6°C for a longer period of time.

No satisfactory procedure has yet been reported which allows adequate tissue components from adult organs to be obtained for *in vitro* investigations. Recent studies indicate, however, that adult mouse bladder can be separated into viable epithelial and stromal components after exposure to pronase, and may subsequently be maintained *in vitro* on a chemically defined medium for varying periods of time (Hodges, 1967).

2. Organ Culture

There are a number of comprehensive reviews on organ culture methods (Fell, 1953; Moscona *et al.*, 1965; Wolff, 1965). The salient feature of the organ type of culture is that it allows an integrated organized structure to be maintained *in vitro* away from the complex interacting factors which influence the tissue *in vivo*. The success of an organized culture depends on a number of factors and includes adequate gaseous exchange and the restriction of cellular outgrowth (Moscona *et al.*, 1965; Wolff, 1965).

The classical technique of organ culture devised by Fell and Robison (1929) is still extensively utilized either as such or in various modified forms (Chen, 1954; Trowell, 1954; Shaffer, 1956). In the original method of Fell and Robison (1929) the organ explants are placed on the surface of a plasma clot. The plasma clot is formed in an embryological watch-glass which itself rests on a pad of cotton wool in a Petri dish. The cotton wool is kept moist with distilled water to prevent excessive evaporation from the dish. The increasing use of liquid media (in particular of chemically defined media) has resulted in a number of modifications to this method. The explants may be placed on rafts formed from open-weave cellulose-acetate (rayon) fabric (Shaffer, 1956); or tea-bag paper (Jensen *et al.*, 1964); or membrane ("Millipore") filters (Grobstein, 1956). These rafts permit easy manipulation of the tissue without any actual disturbance of the tissue itself and can be positioned on stainless steel grids to ensure that the explants do not become immersed in the fluid medium (Trowell, 1954).

The "Millipore" membrane has been employed as a filter barrier in tissue interaction studies (Grobstein, 1956, 1957, 1965). Separate epithelial and mesenchymal components of organs are placed on either side of thin

("Millipore" TH *ca*. 20 μ thick) filter membrane assemblies. Such trans-filter systems allow more controlled analysis of "inductive" processes in organogenesis.

TABLE 1

Studies on epithelial-mesenchymal interaction in normal morphogenesis

Tissue	Animal	Reference
In vitro organ culture studies		
Feather, scale, beak, spur	Chick	Sengel, 1958, 1964; Rawles, 1963
Gonads	Duck	Haffen, 1960, 1961
		Wolff and Haffen, 1965
Kidney	Mouse	Grobstein, 1956; Torrey, 1965
Limb	Mouse	Milaire, 1965
Liver	Chick	Le Douarin, 1964, 1965
Lung	Chick	Dameron, 1961, 1962
		Sorokin, 1965
Lung	Mouse	Alescio and Cassini, 1962
Otic capsule	Chick	Benoit, 1960, 1964
Pancreas	Mouse	Golosow and Grobstein, 1962
		Kallman and Grobstein, 1964
		Rutter *et al.*, 1964
Ant. pituitary	Chick	Sobel, 1958
Proventriculus	Chick	Sigot, 1962
Salivary gland	Mouse	Grobstein, 1953a,b, 1956
Skin	Chick	Sengel, 1958, 1964; Rawles, 1963
		Wessells, 1962, 1965
Skin—hair, vibrissae	Mouse	Kollar, 1966
Thymus	Mouse	Auerbach, 1960a, 1965
Tooth	Mouse	Koch, 1965, 1967
		Dryburgh, 1967
Ureter	Mouse	Grobstein, 1955a,b
Ureter	Chick	Calame, 1961;
		Bishop-Calame, 1966
Uropygial gland	Duck	Gomot, 1959, 1961
In vivo extirpation and transplantation studies		
Chorion	Chick	Kato and Hayashi, 1963
Eye	Chick	Coulombre, 1965
Eye	Rat	Stroeva, 1960
Heart	Chick	DeHaan, 1965
Kidney	Chick, Mouse	Torry, 1965
Limb—wing	Chick	Saunders *et al.*, 1958
		Zwilling, 1956, 1961, 1964
		Amprino, 1965
Liver	Chick	Le Douarin, 1964
		Croisille and Le Douarin, 1965
Otic capsule	Chick	Benoit, 1960, 1961
Salivary gland	Mouse	Borghese, 1950
Skin—feather, scales, claws	Chick	Saunders and Weiss, 1950
		Cairns and Saunders, 1954

C. Survey of Epithelial-mesenchymal Interactions in
   Normal Morphogenesis

Many organs are formed from the confrontation of two primordial tissue components—ectoderm and mesoderm. One of the problems in experimental embryology has been to determine which component is responsible for the differentiation process and to know the role of each in the formation of an organ. It is possible to separate the two tissues by various dissociation procedures (see Section IB) and to follow the development of the two components by *in vitro* organ culture studies. Such investigations provide a sensitive analysis of tissue determinism, and in general have confirmed *in vivo* transplantation and extirpation studies.

Different recombination experiments and culture of the isolated tissue components have shown that the interaction of epithelium and mesenchyme is essential for the formation and proper differentiation of a number of embryonic organs, at least, for those so far studied (Table 1). It has been shown that in the course of development the two components may act one on the other by a series of reciprocal inductions (e.g. chick embryo skin, Sengel, 1958, 1964; mouse embryo metanephros, Grobstein, 1955a, b).

D. Special Aspects of Epithelial-mesenchymal Interactions

1. *Histogenesis of Isolated Epithelia and Mesenchyme*

Embryonic epithelial and stromal isolates do not appear to follow the normal ontogenetic pattern when cultured *in vitro*. Their behaviour varies according to the type and age of the tissue and on the substrate and culture conditions (Table 2).

In general, epithelia cultured on plasma clots in the absence of mesenchyme remain small, fail to develop, show no or very few mitoses, and die in a few days (references Table 2). The basal cells of the isolated chick embryo epidermis rapidly lose their columnar appearance when cultured on plasma clots, lens paper or membrane filters ("Millipore") in synthetic medium (Wessells, 1962). The thymidine-H^3 incorporation rate under these conditions is found to drop to almost zero after 12 hours *in vitro* (Wessells, 1963). Similarly, mouse pancreatic epithelium after 24 hours *in vitro* incorporates thymidine-H^3 at only one-half the rate observed in "epithelium plus mesenchyme" cultures (2·59 against 4·86 labelled nuclei per 1000 μ^2 on radioautographs) (Wessells, 1964a).

Dodson (1963, 1967a, b) has shown that the histogenesis of 12 day embryonic chick metatarsal epidermis varies according to the substrate (see Table 2). Frozen-killed dermis and collagen gels provide a suitable substrate when tissues are grown in natural media containing embryo extract. Membrane ("Millipore") filters are also effective but only if the concentration of embryo extract is increased. The epidermal basal cells can maintain columnar orientation, thymidine-H^3 incorporation and mitosis in synthetic media provided

In vitro culture characteristics of isolated embryonic epithelia and dermis

Epithelial isolates from:					
Animal	Tissue	Age	Medium/Substrate	Observations	References
Chick	Chorion	4–6 days	Natural medium, agar	Survives 5–6 days Cells lose orientation	Bonetti, 1959
Chick	Gastric	5 day	Natural medium, plasma clot	Spreads, secretes mucus, no mitosis Degenerates in 8–9 days	McLoughlin, 1961a
Chick	Limb epidermis	5 day	Natural medium, plasma clot	Very few mitoses Complete keratinization within 10 days	McLoughlin, 1961a Moscona, 1961a,b
Chick	Lung	5 day	Natural medium, agar	Spreads, no differentiation	Dameron, 1962
Chick	Metanephros	5½–6 days	Natural medium, agar	No development of epithelial element (ureter)	Calame, 1961 Bishop-Calame, 1966
Chick	Proventriculus	5 day	Natural medium, agar	Rounds up, no development	Sigot, 1962
Chick	Skin—dorsal	6–8 days	Natural medium, agar	Largely necrotic within 3–4 days No keratinization	Sengel, 1958
Chick	Skin—shank	10–11 days	Synthetic medium, lens paper or Millipore filter	Loses rapidly, columnar orientation of basal layer and ability to incorporate thymidine-H^3 No keratinization Necrotic by 3–4 days	Wessells, 1962, 1963
Chick	Skin—shank	12 day	Natural medium, plasma clot, heat-killed dermis, Alginate, fibrin gels, gel film, frozen-killed dermis, frozen-killed dermis—trypsinized collagen gel, "Millipore" filter,	Does not survive Does not survive Does not survive Does not survive Does not survive Survives and keratinizes Differentiates at first then degenerates Survives and keratinizes Survives but only in presence of increased concentration of embryo extract. Stratum corneum formed	Dodson, 1963, 1967a,b

[continued

TABLE 2—(continued)

Epithelial isolates from:

Animal	Tissue	Age	Medium/Substrate	Observations	References
Chick	Skin—shank	11 day	Synthetic medium, "Millipore" filter, collagen gel, frozen-killed dermis	Epidermal basal cells maintain columnar orientation; thymidine-H^3 incorporation and mitosis if macromolecular fraction of chick embryo extract present, otherwise no survival	Wessells, 1964b
			Lens paper, 100,000 g embryo fraction pellet homogenate	Does not maintain epithelium	
Duck	Gonad	5–10 days	Natural medium, agar	7½–9 day male germinal epithelium gives rise to 2 differentiated structures 5–7 day male germinal epithelium—no differentiation 7½–9 day female germinal epithelium differentiates to form ovarian cortex. 5–7 day female germinal epithelium forms ovarian cortex	Wolff & Haffen, 1959, 1965
Duck	Uropygial gland	8–10 day	Natural medium, agar	Rounds up, no development No keratinization	Gomot, 1959
Mouse	Pancreas	11 day	Natural medium, plasma clot Natural medium, collagen gel	Spreads, no differentiation Differentiates, but high level of embryo extract essential	Golosow and Grobstein, 1962 Wessells and Cohen, 1966
Mouse	Salivary gland	13 day	Natural medium, plasma clot	No differentiation	Grobstein, 1953a
Mouse	Skin	11–14 days	Natural medium, plasma clot	Almost complete keratinization within 5 days	Kollar, 1966
Mouse	Thymus	12½ days	Natural medium, plasma clot	Rounds up, no development	Auerbach, 1960a

Mouse	Tooth	16 days	Natural medium, membrane filter or collagen gel	Spreads, no differentiation	Koch, 1967
Mesenchymal isolates from:					
Chick	Lung	5 days	Natural medium, agar	Spreads, no histological differentiation	Dameron, 1962
Chick	Metanephros	5½–6 days	Natural medium, agar	Spreads, no histological differentiation	Calame, 1961
Chick	Skin—shank	12 day	Natural medium, rayon raft-plasma clot Synthetic medium, lens paper, "Millipore" filter	Spreads, no histological differentiation	Dodson, 1967a,b Wessells, 1962
Duck	Uropygial gland	8–10 days	Natural medium, agar	Spreads, no histological differentiation	Gomot, 1959
Mouse	Metanephros	11 day	Natural medium, plasma clot	Spreads, no histological differentiation	Grobstein, 1956
Mouse	Salivary gland	13 day	Natural medium, plasma clot	Spreads, no histological differentiation	Grobstein, 1953a
Mouse	Skin	11–14 days	Natural medium, plasma clot	Spreads, no histological differentiation	Kollar, 1966
Mouse	Thymus	12½ days	Natural medium, plasma clot	Spreads, no histological differentiation	Auerbach, 1960a

that an adequate physical substrate is available (frozen-killed dermis, collagen gel, membrane "Millipore" filter), and that whole or macromolecular fractions of chick embryo extract are present (Wessells, 1964b). Collagen can also serve as a substrate for mouse pancreatic epithelium, but again high levels of embryo extract are necessary for continued histogenesis *in vitro* (Wessells and Cohen, 1966). The stromal isolates are found to survive in culture but do not show histological differentiation (Table 2).

2. Specific and Non-specific Interactions of Epithelia and Mesenchyme

The morphological differentiation of a tissue can be profoundly modified according to the type of mesenchyme which is associated with the epithelial component. Studies on the influence of stroma on epithelial morphogenesis demonstrate that certain epithelia are dependent on specific mesenchymes for their continued normal differentiation. Thus the epithelia of mouse submandibular salivary gland (Grobstein, 1953a), duck uropygial gland (Gomot, 1959), chick proventriculus (Sigot, 1962), chick skin, feather, scale (Sengel, 1958), chick lung (Dameron, 1962), chick ureter (Bishop-Calame, 1966), differentiate normally in response only to their own specific stroma. Other epithelia exhibit, on the contrary, a non-specific mesenchyme dependence. Mouse pancreas (Golosow and Grobstein, 1962) and mouse thymus (Auerbach, 1960a, 1965) epithelia show normal differentiation in the presence of mesenchyme from a wide variety of sources.

The stroma can play a determinant role in the regional characterization of the epithelia, and this finding has been established in the chick embryo skin (Cairns and Saunders, 1954; Sengel, 1958; Rawles, 1963, 1965). The specific effects of epithelium on mesenchyme are less well documented. Chick embryo skin epidermis is responsible for the induction of the dermal pulp of the feather germ and for the orientation of the feather (Sengel, 1958, 1964). Dermal behaviour with regard to the site of appearance of intercellular materials has been shown to be influenced by the associated epithelium (see Herrmann, 1960). Heterogeneous combinations of epithelia and mesenchyme have now been investigated in a number of vertebrate rudiments. A different and characteristic alteration of tissue differentiation is obtained according to the type of mesenchyme with which the epithelium is associated (Table 3). The various observations suggest that the primary source of morphogenetic influence is mediated through the stroma and precedes epithelial effects on the mesenchyme. The spreading behaviour of epithelia observed in certain associations appears to be determined by the underlying mesenchyme (McLoughlin, 1961a, b; 1963). It has been suggested that this could be related to the (theoretically) different "basement membranes" that may be formed according to the epithelial-mesenchymal combination (but see Section **III**). Epithelial mitosis is influenced by the presence of mesenchyme (see Section

TABLE 3

Examples of modified epithelial differentiation in heterogenous recombinations of epithelium and mesenchyme

Animal	Stroma	Epithelium	Direction of epithelial differentiation	Reference
Chick	Proventriculus 5 day	Limb 5 day	Initially fails to keratinize and instead secretes mucus then reverts to normal differentiation and keratinizes	McLouglin 1961b
	Gizzard 5 day	Limb 5 day	Fails to keratinize, instead secretes mucus and may become ciliated	
	Heart 5 day (fibroblasts)	Limb 5 day	Keratinizes very rapidly and extensively	
	Heart 5 day (myoblasts)	Limb 5 day	Spreads as single layer of squamous cells that do not keratinize	
Chick	Gizzard 5 day	Proventriculus 5 day	Differentiates into a gizzard epithelium	Sigot, 1962
	Mesonephros 5 day	Proventriculus 5 day	Differentiates into a gizzard epithelium	
	Proventriculus 5 day	Gizzard 5 day	Differentiates into glandular structure typical of proventriculus	
Chick	Shank skin 11–13 days	Wing-dorsal 5–8½ days	Scales develop instead of feather germs	Sengel, 1958
	Wing-dorsal skin 5–15 days	Shank skin 5–15 days	Feather germs instead of scales	Rawles, 1963, 1965
Chick	Muscle 11 day	Shank skin 11 day	Fails to keratinize	Wessells, 1962
Chick	Skin dermis 7–13 days	Chorion 5–6 days	Transforms into integumentary epidermis	Bonetti, 1959
Chick	Metanephros 5 day	Bronchus 5 day	Epithelium cuboidal, similar to ureter	Dameron, 1966
	Dermis 6 day	Bronchus 5 day	Bronchial lobe develops with pseudostratified epithelium	
Chick	Lung 5 day	Ureter 5 day	Ureter differentiates into structure analogous to bronchial epithelium Secondary urinary tubes form in lung stroma	Bishop-Calame, 1966
Chick	Proventriculus 5 day	Ureter 5 day	Ureter forms large thickened tube with pseudostratified epithelium	Bishop-Calame, 1966
	Intestine 5 day	Ureter 5 day		
Duck	Uropygial gland 8 day	Oesophagus 10 day	Epithelium produces typical early uropygial gland	Gomot, 1961
Duck	Female gonad medulla 5–10 days	Male germinal epithelium 5–10 days	Male germinal epithelium transforms to ovarian cortex	Wolff and Haffen, 1959 Haffen, 1960

D*I*) but the extent of mitotic activity may also be modified by the type of stroma present (McLoughlin, 1963).

The quality or age of the mesenchyme can influence the "inductive" capacity of the dermis in the chick embryo skin (Wessells, 1962; Rawles, 1963) and the thymidine-H^3 incorporation rate (Wessells, 1963). The ability of the duck male germinal epithelium to differentiate into ovarian structure (that is, in a direction opposite to the normal) diminishes with age (Haffen, 1960). Studies by Sengel (1958) and Rawles (1963) show, however, that epidermal differentiation in the chick embryo skin can be modified to produce an alternative structure at relatively late developmental stages.

Direct contact between epithelium and mesenchyme is not necessary for tissue differentiation to occur. The influencing "factors" can traverse thin membrane filters (*ca.* 20 μ thickness) interposed between the two tissue components. Trans-filter effects have been demonstrated for a number of tissues including thymus (Auerbach, 1960a), salivary gland (Grobstein, 1953c), pancreas (Golosow and Grobstein, 1962), skin (Wessells, 1962), tooth (Koch, 1967).

The trans-filter system lends itself to investigations of the time required for "induction" influences to take effect. Studies on the mouse pancreas have shown that associated mesenchyme is necessary for pancreatic epithelial differentiation during the first 30 to 36 hours in culture but can be removed subsequently without any detrimental effect on the behaviour pattern of the epithelium (Grobstein, 1963; Kallman and Grobstein, 1964). Although little data is available, it could be supposed that the duration of the inductive stimulus may vary with each kind of tissue (see Grobstein, 1966).

There is evidence that a critical mass of cells of a common embryonic type must be attained before they can express their developmental capabilities (Zwilling, 1960), although the proportion of cells required seems to vary from tissue to tissue. Dameron (1961, 1962) and Alescio and Colombo Piperno (1967) have observed that in chick embryo lungs cultured *in vitro* tubule formation is in direct proportion to the amount of mesenchyme present relative to the epithelium. The intact embryonic mouse thymus has relatively few mesenchymal cells but these suffice to ensure normal morphogenesis *in vitro* (Auerbach, 1960b). Further data is required to assess the importance of critical cell mass in inductive phenomena.

3. *Possible Mechanisms of Mesenchymal and Epithelial Effects*

The precise mechanism of "interactive" effects between stromal-epithelial tissue components is not known.

The various studies indicated in the preceding sections suggest that epithelial histo-differentiation does not depend entirely on the continued metabolic activity of stromal cells. An important feature in the differentiation of epithelia appears to be the substratum, the nature of which must be such as to allow normal polarization of the basal cells. In the absence of "normal" orientation epithelial histogenesis is modified.

Orientation and mitotic activity of epithelia is apparently dependent upon whole or macromolecular fractions of chick embryo extract under the experimental conditions so far employed (Wessells, 1962). The nature of the factor involved is not known, but McLoughlin (1961a) has shown that isolated intercellular material, possibly a mucopolysaccharide, can control the orientation of epithelial cells, and Marin and Sigot (1963, 1965) have found that a lipoprotein (?) material can affect epithelial differentiation. There is evidence that each cell lies within its own microenvironment and the macromolecular materials synthesized by the cells (which may vary on the time scale and according to site) are important determinants of their behaviour and influence (Moscona, 1961a,b, 1965). Herrmann (1960) has drawn attention to the role which metabolic tissue interactions may play in the course of embryonic development, and has demonstrated in the cornea an obligatory interdependence related to the enzyme content of epithelium and stroma.

A number of investigations have implied that collagen may play an important role in the provision of an appropriate substratum in the stromal-epithelial junction region (Dodson, 1963, 1967a,b; Grobstein, 1965; Grobstein and Cohen, 1965; Wessells, 1964b). It has been found that collagen can serve as a substrate for certain epithelia if high levels of embryo extract are present (see Section A, Wessels, 1964b). Collagen has been implicated as an important factor in muscle cell mitosis and fusion (Hauschka and Konigsberg, 1966), and the possibility has been raised that collagen mediates or actively participates in the inductive tissue interactions. However, recent studies imply that stable surface-associated complexes (like collagen), which may be present in the chick embryo extract fractions, are not in fact the active agents of the embryo extract (Wessells and Cohen, 1966).

Transfilter radioautograph experiments employing tritiated proline indicate that tropocollagen may be synthesized by the mesenchyme and, after crossing the membrane filter in a "soluble" form, polymerizes as fibres at the epithelial surface (Kallman and Grobstein, 1965). Investigations employing tritiated glucosamine show that a mucopolysaccharide material localizes at the epithelial surface but, in contrast to the tritiated proline, does not extend beyond this tissue (Kallman and Grobstein, 1966). It is suggested that the epithelial surface may possess special polymerizing properties leading to collagen fibrogenesis, but it is not known whether this has any particular morphogenetic significance.

It has been postulated from such observations that epithelium and mesenchyme may each contribute particular materials that interact at the interfaces of the two tissues to produce new macromolecular complexes. Such new complexes may in turn modify the microenvironment of the cells which then affects the subsequent developmental behaviour of the cells (Grobstein, 1966).

E. GENERAL CONSIDERATIONS RELEVANT TO THE PERIODONTIUM

The periodontium, composed of the alveolar bone, the periodontal ligament, the cementum and the gingiva, forms a complex functional and anatomical unit, the developmental process and normal behaviour pattern of which has been ascertained essentially on morpho-histological evidence (see Chapter 3). No detailed analysis (comparable to the studies discussed in the preceding sections) on possible stromal-epithelial and inter-stromal influences in periodontal tissue formation has, however, been carried out to substantiate views, at times speculative, on certain aspects of periodontium development.

In vitro organ culture techniques have been used mainly to elucidate the mechanism of normal tooth development (reviewed by Glasstone, 1965). More recently Dryburgh (1967) has studied in detail the potentiality and significance of epithelium and mesenchyme in early tooth differentiation. However, *in vitro* investigations of the periodontal complex using the organ culture system are lacking, and the little experimental data available on tissue interactive influences comes from *in vivo* transplantation studies.

The possible formative influence of the tooth on the surrounding tissues has been studied by Hoffman (1960, 1966) in autotransplants of developing hamster molars. The enamel organ and dental papilla were removed from the dental sac (before root formation) and the tooth buds transplanted to the subcutaneous connective tissue and femurs of the host. Typical periodontal ligament and a shell of alveolar bone were found to develop in the surviving transplants. Hoffman postulates from this evidence the existence of an organizing factor probably emanating from the developing root (Hertwig's epithelial root sheath) which influences the host to form these periodontal tissues. (See Chapter 3 for further discussion of this topic.)

The interaction between transplanted tooth buds and bone tissue taken from different regions of the body has been investigated by Weinreb *et al.* (1967). Developing rat molars were autotransplanted into the dorsal connective tissue, either alone, with alveolar bone, or with a segment of tibia. Tooth development occurred only in the transplants with alveolar bone. This is thought to suggest that the inductive (?) properties related to tooth development of alveolar bone are different from those of tibial bone.

III. Stromal-epithelial Interactions in the Adult

A. A GENERAL REVIEW

The important role of tissue interactions has been demonstrated clearly in organogenesis in embryonic tissues. There is, however, little evidence that specific stimuli may be necessary for the continued maintenance of the differentiated state in adult tissue.

The possibility that stromal-epithelial interactions may continue in the adult system has been supported by the results of a number of investigations on normal and tumour tissue. It is thought that stromal cells may be essential for the normal growth and function of adult organs. Lasfargues (1957) has shown that *in vitro* cultures of the mouse breast epithelium alone could not form milk fat. An organized complex of epithelium, stroma and adipose tissue was necessary before normal secretion could occur. Franks and Barton (1960) observed differences between the normal epithelium of organ cultures of mouse ventral prostate and the sheets of unorganized epithelial cells which grew out from the explant edge. The cells within these sheets showed a general disorganization in ultrastructural pattern and a loss of responsiveness to testosterone. It was concluded that epithelium alone cannot form its characteristic secretion and a functional unit is constituted only when the epithelium is in its normal relationship to the supporting stroma and muscle (the epithelial-fibromuscular complex). Mechanically isolated epithelium from human adult prostate rarely grows *in vitro* although morphologically normal. However, a rapid outgrowth of epithelium occurs if explants of epithelia and stroma are made (Franks, 1963).

Different behaviour patterns according to culture conditions are reported for three hormone-dependent tumours from hamsters (Algard, 1963). The tumours can proliferate as monolayers in the absence of oestrogen, but in organotypic cultures these tumours can be maintained only when the medium is supplemented with this hormone. The retention of specific hormone dependency appears therefore to be related to the maintenance of tumour architecture, with the stromal component possibly mediating the endocrine stimulation. There are now a number of investigations which imply that tumour progression and responsiveness is governed by the supporting stroma (Lasfargues *et al.*, 1960; Van Scott and Reinertson, 1961; De Ome, 1962). Other studies indicate that tumour initiation may be associated with stromal changes (Gillman *et al.*, 1955; Orr, 1963).

Circumstantial evidence suggests that dermal structures affect the differentiation of the epidermal appendages. The presence of a dermal component in pelage and vibrissal hairs is considered necessary for the maintenance and regeneration of these structures in the adult (Crounse and Stengle, 1959; Cohen, 1961). Feather formation in the adult bird depends also on the dermal papilla, since regeneration of feathers does not occur in its absence (Lillie and Wang, 1944). Recent transplantation studies in the adult rat suggest that regional differences in the appendages depends initially on the local dermis (Cohen, 1965). It is postulated that the dermis maintains the regional character of its overlying epidermis and of the ectoderm of the appendage follicle associated with it. This follicular ectoderm then acts upon the dermal papillae. The dermis appears unable to act directly on the dermal papillae without the intervention of the follicular ectoderm. Oliver (1966) provides further evidence that follicular epidermis may influence the formation of new hair follicle papillae, and it is possible that this is regulated indirectly by the local dermis (Cohen, 1965).

The influence of mammalian dermis on the regional character of its over-lying epidermis has been investigated in a series of experiments by Billingham and Silvers (1963, 1965, 1967). Thin grafts of skin displaying distinctive regional characteristics were studied. Dermis of one integumentary type was combined with epidermis of another and the "recombinant" grafts trans-planted to compatible hosts. The dermis was found to determine the epidermal characteristics in recombinant grafts involving the ear, the sole of the foot and the trunk, but not in recombinants which included tongue, oesophagus or cheek pouch epithelia. A more critical *in vitro* analysis is required to establish the continued and specific influence of stroma on epithelial specificity.

B. Possible Tissue Interaction Sites in the Mature Periodontium

There are a number of situations in the mature periodontium where the maintenance of tissue characteristics may be the result of stimuli elicited by interacting influences between tissues. The precise and readily recognizable differences observed in the architecture of the adjoining epithelia of the attached epithelial cuff, the crevice, the marginal and attached gingiva, and the alveolar mucosa (see Chapter 5), and of the contiguous connective tissues of the attached gingiva and alveolar mucosa (see Chapter 6), are pertinent examples.

The epithelium of the attached epithelial cuff is bounded on one aspect by soft connective tissue and, on the other, by mineralized tissue of either mesodermal or ectodermal origin. The epithelium of the crevice, while bounded by similar structures, is contiguous only with soft connective tissue and is separated from mineralized tissue by a space. The epithelium of the marginal and attached gingiva, on the one hand, and that of the alveolar mucosa, on the other, are continuous with very different connective tissues; the former with dense fibrous connective tissue devoid of elastic fibres, the latter with a loose, elastic fibre-containing, connective tissue. The nature of the influences that dictate the development and maintenance of such differing adjacent soft connective tissues provides in itself a tantalizing problem.

It is remarkable that the periodontal space is maintained throughout life and is not colonized by alveolar bone and cementum. This is true whether the teeth are in function or not. It seems possible that this situation exists because of some interplay between soft and hard connective tissues, but in addition to this, the unknown role of the epithelial rests of Malassez should be borne in mind. The cells of the epithelial rests are separated from the connective tissue of the periodontal ligament by a "basement membrane" (Valderhaug and Nylen, 1966).

There is, unfortunately, no information which might provide insight into these problems. This is regrettable, in that their solution could contribute greatly to knowledge of the physiology and pathology of the periodontium.

IV. Role of the "Basement Membrane"

A. DEFINITION, ORIGIN AND NATURE

The region between the epithelium and the underlying stroma of a given tissue is traditionally considered to be the site of the "basement membrane". Recent studies show, however, that "basement membranes" may also form between two epithelial systems (Pierce *et al.*, 1962, 1963; Pierce, 1965) (see Chapter 5, page 116).

The term "basement membrane" has been employed to describe structures seen with both the optical and the electron microscope, but with different connotations, and this has led to confusion in terminology. At the optical microscope level the "basement membrane" usually is a well-defined extra-cellular layer of variable thickness depending on age and type of tissue. This extracellular layer characteristically gives a positive periodic acid-Schiff reaction (paS reaction), indicating 1 : 2 glycol groups of sugars (Pearse, 1961), and may demonstrate the presence of reticulin (and elastin) (see Chapter 6, page 276).

The boundary regions between normal epithelia and stroma show, at the electron microscope level, an extracellular electron-dense band, 200 to 700 Å thick as a rule, which may closely follow the plasma membrane of the basal epithelial cells. Within this zone, less electron-dense regions may be observed in certain old tissues (Rowlatt, 1967). The electron-dense band is generally separated from the cell membrane by a more electron-lucent zone, 100 to 450 Å in width (Fawcett, 1966). The thickness of both the electron-lucent and the electron-dense zones varies with species, age and tissue (see Chapter 5, page 117).

Numerous terms have been given to the electron-dense zone: basement membrane (Ottoson *et al.*, 1953); limiting membrane (Yamada, 1955); dermal membrane (Selby, 1955); adepidermal membrane (Salpeter and Singer, 1959); basement lamina or basal lamina (Fawcett, 1962).

Terminology employing the word "membrane" is not entirely satisfactory for, at the electron microscope level, "membrane" has come to denote a trilaminar structural lipoprotein component of the cell: two opaque layers separating a lighter interspace. These triple-layered membranes, referred to as "unit membranes" (Robertson, 1959, 1964, 1966), show an overall thickness of approximately 75 to 120 Å. The electron-dense zone does not conform to this unit membrane pattern and has variable dimensions. High magnification reveals that this zone is made up of an amorphous matrix in which are embedded numerous very fine filaments 30–50 Å in width

(Kurtz and McManus, 1960; Faarup and Christensen, 1965). Electron microscope studies of human gingiva and rat cheek (Stern, 1965), of human cervix (Younes *et al.*, 1965) and of human oral mucosa (Susi *et al.*, 1967) show the occurrence of fine filaments (20–60 Å in diameter). These pass from the stromal regions through the electron-dense and electron-lucent zones, and attach to the cell membrane of the basal epithelial cells. Aggregates of these filaments form fibrils beneath the electron-dense region. These are similar to the "anchoring fibrils" described by Palade and Farquhar (1965) in amphibian and rat skin, and in rat stomach and lingual mucosa, which appear to link the electron-dense zone to the underlying stroma.

A systematized nomenclature is needed to denote those structures which may be observed, at the present electron microscope level of resolution, in the epithelial—stroma boundary zone. The following terminology has been adopted throughout the ensuing chapters. The term of "lamina lucida" is given to the electron-lucent zone and the term of "lamina densa" is given to the electron-dense region (Hall, 1955; Stern, 1965). The term "basement membrane" is used only to describe the structure seen with the optical microscope. Immediately adjacent to the lamina densa may be observed a region of reticulin (see Chapter 6), the organization of which varies with age and species. This region in amphibians is termed the stratum reticulare by Hay (1964).

Extracellular electron-lucent and electron-dense zones are not restricted to the epithelia only, and may be observed surrounding cells of mesenchymal origin such as the endothelial cells of capillaries (Majno and Palade, 1961), smooth and striated muscle fibres and fibroblasts (Fawcett, 1964). Several terms have been given to this electron-dense investing layer: boundary membrane (Low and Burkel, 1965); glycocalyx (Bennett, 1963); external lamina (Fawcett, 1966). To obviate a proliferation of terms the nomenclature of lamina lucida and lamina densa is assigned to these two investing zones. This parallels the terminology applied to the extracellular structures of the basal surface of the epithelial cells in the epithelial—stromal boundary regions. It is implicit that the properties of the extraneous cell layers may vary according to cell type and histological situation. It would appear from the studies of Rambourg *et al.* (1966) and Rambourg and Leblond (1967a) that the lamina lucida may form part of the cell surface termed the "cell coat" located outside the plasma membrane.

The precise relationship between the various electron microscope layers of the epithelial—stroma junction and the paS positive zone of optical microscopy has not been fully determined. It has been suggested that the lamina densa is not involved in the paS reaction and that the paS positive reactive site is located on the dermal side of the lamina densa in the reticulin-rich region (Kobayasi, 1961; Swift and Saxton, 1967).

However, Rambourg and Leblond (1967b) consider that the cell coat (lamina lucida), "basement membrane" (lamina densa) and reticulin region are all stained by the paS technique, but that it is only the cell coat and the "basement membrane" which contribute to the continuous paS positive layer seen with the optical microscope.

The "basement membrane" has been regarded as a connective tissue derivative representing condensations of intercellular substances formed of a polymerized complex of acid mucopolysaccharides and reticular fibres (Gersh and Catchpole, 1949). However, recent studies (Hay and Revel, 1963; Pierce et al., 1962, 1963) indicate that the lamina densa, at least, is of epithelial origin. The radioautograph experiments of Hay and Revel (1963) on the regenerating *Ambystoma* limb show that tritiated proline incorporated by the epithelial cells is secreted into the region of the lamina densa and subsequently moves towards the underlying fibroblasts. The epidermal cells would appear therefore, to synthesize a proline-rich, possibly collagenous material and to contribute to the formation of collagen in the basement membrane of the regenerating amphibian skin. Pierce et al. (1962, 1963) have demonstrated by immunohistochemical techniques that a "basement membrane" of the mouse embryo, Reichert's membrane, which lies between two epithelial layers, is a secretion of parietal yolk sac epithelium and is formed in a situation devoid of connective tissue elements. The epithelial cell is implicated as the source of the lamina densa of differentiating epithelial organs (Pierce, 1966), of epithelium-derived tumours (Pierce, 1965) and of kidney glomeruli (Kurtz, 1964). This evidence suggests that stromal tissue may not be necessary for lamina densa formation.

Midgely and Pierce (1963), using an immunohistochemical technique, have shown that the antigens of the lamina densa are related, not to any antigens found in connective tissue, but to antigens that are present in epithelial cells. The production of the lamina densa material has been thought to be associated with the endoplasmic reticulum of cells (Pierce et al., 1963). Mukerjee et al. (1965) have shown that the lamina densa contains proline and hydroxyproline, but in proportions different to those in collagen. They conclude that tumour epithelial "basement membrane" of the mouse is chemically and immunologically distinct from collagen. The normal canine glomerular "basement membrane" is considered on the other hand to be a polymerized substance containing at least a glycoprotein, and a collagen-like protein (Kefalides and Winzler, 1966).

It has been suggested that the lamina densa represents a reaction precipitate between intercellular products of the epithelium and stroma (Mercer, 1961, 1964). It is postulated that since intercellular substances of different connective tissues and epithelia vary, the lamina densa for each given epithelial-stromal complex will show distinctive and unique characteristics. However, the immunohistochemical studies of Midgely and Pierce (1963) and Pierce (1966) indicate a common antigen for the laminae densae so far studied in the mouse, and suggest the probability that all are chemically similar to each other.

B. Enzymatic Products of Stromal and Epithelial Tissues

Studies on the modification of connective tissue of the tail fin of metamorphosing anuran tadpoles have demonstrated the production of enzymes by epithelial and stromal tissues. A collagenolytic enzyme and a hyaluronidase have been demonstrated in the medium of sterile cultures of tail fin tissues. The culture of separated tail fin epithelium and mesenchyme on collagen gels indicate that only the epithelial cells produce collagenase (Gross and Lapiere, 1962; Lapiere and Gross, 1963) and the mesenchymal cells are the source of hyaluronidase (Silbert *et al.*, 1965; Eisen and Gross, 1965). It is suggested that these enzymes are involved in remodelling of mesenchymal tissues during amphibian metamorphosis. Enzyme activity of this kind may play a role in more general morphogenetic mechanisms, enzyme production depending on interaction between epithelial and mesenchymal components.

C. Possible Functional Significance of the "Basement Membrane"

There is little data concerning the role of the "basement membrane" complex adjacent to epithelial cells in developing systems. It has been considered that a close association between epithelium and "basement membrane", and the proximity of mesenchyme (that is, of a source of extracellular materials), are important conditions for normal epithelial differentiation in embryonic tissues (Cohen, 1961; McLoughlin, 1963; Grobstein, 1961, 1965; Mercer, 1961, 1964, 1965; Dodson, 1967a, b). Recent studies suggest that the "basement membrane" (lamina densa and lamina lucida layers) may not be an essential requisite for epithelial cell orientation and mitotic activity in the chick embryo skin (Kallman *et al.*, 1967). Dodson (1967b) notes that it is not necessary for the "basement membrane" (lamina densa zone) to be present continuously for the survival and the subsequent development of the basal cells of isolated chick embryo metatarsal epidermis. The basement membrane can be absent for 24–30 hours without the basal cells undergoing irreversible changes; however, after this period, the cells lose their normal differentiation potentialities.

It has been postulated that the "basement membrane" is probably the principal protein filtration barrier in the renal glomerulus of the normal adult, and thickening of this "basement membrane" associated with disease is considered to be of great significance (Farquhar and Palade, 1961; Latta *et al.*, 1960; Kurtz, 1964).

Modifications in "basement membrane" integrity have been suggested to represent one mechanism by which tumour invasion may occur (Ozzello and Speer, 1958; Pierce, 1965; Fasske and Morgenroth, 1966; Tarin, 1967). Epithelial projections have been observed protruding through the "basement membrane" in naturally occurring and experimentally induced tumours (Frei, 1962; Ashworth *et al.*, 1961; Tarin, 1967); it is not known whether this is the result of epithelial enzymatic activity.

The preceding sections show that there is still little detailed information on the origin, nature and function of the "basement membrane". The evidence indicates that the "basement membrane" is a relatively "plastic", complex structure, important for the maintenance of normal tissue relationships. It has been suggested that the "basement membrane" forms a macromolecular "barrier" between epithelium and mesenchyme and may influence the interchange of molecules between the two tissues (Mercer, 1961, 1964, 1965). Intrinsic and extrinsic factors, by their action on epithelium or stroma, can modify the type of intercellular substance formed and may alter the nature of the materials polymerized at the lamina densa level. Modifications in the composition of the lamina densa could result in an alteration in the physicochemical properties of this region influencing the passage of molecules and thus the synthesis of certain substances in either epithelial or mesenchymal cells. Grobstein (1962, 1963, 1966) considers that interactive mechanisms of this type at the molecular level could be significant in induction processes in developing systems, whilst playing a "stabilizing" role in the adult. The "basement membrane" may therefore be a keystone in the sequence of events which lead to the differentiation of an organ and its maintenance in the adult.

References

Alescio, T. and Cassini, A. (1962). *J. exp. Zool.* **150**, 83–94.
Alescio, T. and Colombo Piperno, E. (1967). *J. Embryol. exp. Morph.* **17**, 213–227.
Algard, F. T. (1963). *Natn. Cancer Inst. Monogr.* **11**, 215–222.
Amprino, R. (1965). *In* "Organogenesis" (R. L. De Haan and H. Ursprung, eds.), pp. 255–281. Holt, Rinehart and Winston, New York, U.S.A.
Ashworth, C. T., Sternbridge, V. A. and Luibel, F. J. (1961). *Acta Cytol.* **5**, 369–384.
Auerbach, R. (1960a). *Devl. Biol.* **2**, 271–284.
Auerbach, R. (1960b). "The Organization and Reorganization of embryonic cells in self-organizing systems." Pergamon Press, New York, U.S.A.
Auerbach, R. (1965). *In* "Organogenesis" (R. L. De Haan and H. Ursprung, eds.), pp. 539–557. Holt, Rinehart and Winston, New York, U.S.A.
Bennett, H. S. (1963). *J. Histochem. Cytochem.* **11**, 14–23.
Benoit, J. A. A. (1960). *Ann. Sc. Nat. Zool.* **2**, 323–385.
Benoit, J. A. A. (1961). *C. r. hebd Séanc. Acad. Sci., Paris* **253**, 2257–2258.
Benoit, J. A. A. (1964). *C. r. hebd Séanc. Acad. Sci., Paris* **258**, 334–336.
Billingham, R. E. and Silvers, W. K. (1963). *New Engl. J. Med.* **268**, 477–480; 539–545.
Billingham, R. E. and Silvers, W. K. (1965). *In* "Biology of the skin and hair growth" (A. G. Lyne and B. F. Short, eds.), pp. 1–24. Angus and Robertson, Sydney, Australia.
Billingham, R. E. and Silvers, W. K. (1967). *J. exp. Med.* **125**, 429–446.

Bishop-Calame, S. (1966). *Archs Anat. microsc. Morph. exp.* **55,** Suppl. 215–309.

●Bonetti, D. (1959). *C. r. hebd Séanc. Acad. Sci., Paris* **429,** 1940–1941.

Borghese, E. (1950). *J. Anat. Lond.* **84,** 303–318.

Calame, S. (1961). *Archs Anat. microsc. Morph. exp.* **50,** 299–308.

Cairns, J. M. and Saunders, J. W. Jr. (1954). *J. exp. Zool.* **127,** 221–248.

Chen, J. M. (1954). *Expl. Cell Res.* **7,** 518–529.

Cohen, A. I. (1961). *Devl. Biol.* **3,** 297–316.

Cohen, J. (1965). *In* "Biology of the skin and hair growth" (A. G. Lyne and B. F. Short, eds.), pp. 183–199. Angus and Robertson, Sydney, Australia.

Coulombre, A. J. (1965). *In* "Organogenesis" (R. L. De Haan and H. Ursprung, eds.), pp. 219–251. Holt, Rinehart and Winston, New York, U.S.A.

Croisille, Y. and Le Douarin, N. (1965). *In* "Organogenesis" (R. L. De Haan and H. Ursprung, eds.), pp. 421–466. Holt, Rinehart and Winston, New York, U.S.A.

Crounse, R. G. and Stengle, J. M. (1959). *J. invest Derm.* **32,** 477–479.

Curtis, A. S. G. (1966). *Sci. Prog. Lond.* **54,** 61–86.

Dalcq, A. M. (1960). *In* "Fundamental aspects of Normal and Malignant Growth" (W. W. Nowinski, ed.), pp. 305–494. Elsevier, Amsterdam.

Dameron, Fl. (1961). *J. Embryol. exp. Morph.* **9,** 628–633.

‣Dameron, Fl. (1962). *Path. Biol.* **10,** 811–816.

Dameron, Fl. (1966). *C. r. hebd Séanc. Acad. Sci., Paris* **262,** 1642–1645.

De Haan, R. L. (1965). *In* "Organogenesis" (R. L. De Haan and H. Ursprung, eds.), pp. 377–419. Holt, Rinehart and Winston, New York, U.S.A.

De Ome, K. B. (1962). *Fedn. Proc. Fedn Am. Socs exp. Biol. Fd. Res.* **21,** 15–18.

Dodson, J. W. (1963). *Expl. Cell Res.* **31,** 233–235.

Dodson, J. W. (1967a). *J. Embryol. exp. Morph.* **17,** 83–105.

Dodson, J. W. (1967b). *J. Embryol. exp. Morph.* **17,** 107–117.

Dryburgh, L. (1967). *J. dent. Res.* **46,** 1265 (Abstract).

Eisen, A. Z. and Gross, J. (1965). *Fedn. Proc. Fedn Am. Socs exp. Biol.* **24,** 558.

Faarup, P. and Christensen, H. E. (1965). *Acta. path. microbiol. Scandinavica* **64,** 71–82.

Faaske, E. and Morgenroth, K. (1966). *Oncologia, Basle* **20,** 113–128.

Farquhar, M. G. and Palade, G. E. (1961). *J. exp. Med.* **114,** 699–716.

Fawcett, D. W. (1962). *Circulation* **26,** 1105–1125.

Fawcett, D. W. (1964). *In* "Modern Developments in Electron Microscopy" (B. M. Siegal, ed.), pp. 257–353. Academic Press, New York, U.S.A.

Fawcett, D. W. (1966). "The Cell. Its organelles and inclusions." W. B. Saunders, Philadelphia, U.S.A.

Fell, H. B. (1953). *Sci. Prog. Lond.* **162,** 212–231.

Fell, H. B. and Robison, R. (1929). *Biochem. J.* **23,** 767–784.

Franks, L. M. (1963). *Natn. Cancer Inst. Monogr.* **11,** 83–91.

Franks, L. M. and Barton, A. A. (1960). *Expl. Cell Res.* **19,** 35–50.

Frei, J. V. (1962). *J. Cell. Biol.* **15,** 335–342.

Gersh, I. and Catchpole, H. R. (1949). *Am. J. Anat.* **85,** 457–522.

Gillman, T., Penn, J., Bronks, D. and Roux, M. (1955). *Experientia* **11,** 493–494.

Glasstone, S. (1965). *In* "Cells and Tissues in Culture" (E. N. Willmer, ed.), Vol. 2, pp. 273–283. Academic Press, London, England.

Golosow, N. and Grobstein, C. (1962). *Devl. Biol.* **4,** 242–255.

● Gomot, L. (1959). *Archs Anat. microsc. Morphol. exp.* **48,** 63–141.

Gomot, L. (1961). *In* "La Culture Organotypique", Coll. int. CNRS No. 101 Paris, pp. 117–132.

Grobstein, C. (1953a). *J. exp. Zool.* **124**, 383–414.
Grobstein, C. (1953b). *J. Morph.* **93**, 19–43.
Grobstein, C. (1953c). *Nature* **172**, 869–871.
Grobstein, C. (1955a). *Expl. Cell Res.* **10**, 424–440.
Grobstein, C. (1955b). *J. exp. Zool.* **130**, 319–340.
Grobstein, C. (1956). *Adv. Cancer Res.* **4**, 187–236.
Grobstein, C. (1957). *Expl. Cell Res.* **13**, 575–587.
Grobstein, C. (1961). *Expl. Cell Res.* Suppl. 8, 234–245.
Grobstein, C. (1962). *J. cell comp. Physiol.* Suppl. **1, 60**, 35–48.
Grobstein, C. (1963). *In* "Cytodifferential and Macromolecular Synthesis". Academic Press, New York, U.S.A.
Grobstein, C. (1965). *In* "Cells and Tissues in Culture" (E. N. Willmer, ed.), Vol. I, pp. 463–488. Academic Press, London, England.
Grobstein, C. (1966). *Natn. Cancer Inst. Monogr.* **26**, 279–299.
Grobstein, C. and Cohen, J. (1965). *Science* **150**, 626–628.
Gross, J. and Lapiere, C. M. (1962). *Proc. natn. Acad. Sci. U.S.A.* **48**, 1014–1022.
Haffen, K. (1960). *J. Embryol. exp. Morph.* **8**, 414–424.
Haffen, K. (1961). *In* "La Culture Organotypique". Colloques Internationaux du Centre National de la Recherche Scientifique no. 101 (Paris), pp. 133–144.
Hall, B. V. (1955). *Proc. 6th Ann. Conf. on Nephrotic Syndrome*, pp. 1–39. New York, U.S.A.
Hauschka, S. D. and Konigsberg, I. R. (1966). *Proc. natn. Acad. Sci., U.S.A.* **55**, 119–126.
Hay, E. D. (1964). *In* "The Epidermis" (W. H. Montagna and W. C. Lobitz, Jr., eds.). Academic Press, New York, U.S.A.
Hay, E. D. and Revel, J. P. (1963). *Devl. Biol.* **7**, 152–168.
Herrmann, H. (1960). *Science*, **132**, 529–532.
Hodges, G. M. (1967). Unpublished results.
Hoffman, R. L. (1960). *J. dent. Res.* **39**, 781–798.
Hoffman, R. L. (1966). *Am. J. Anat.* **118**, 91–102.
Holtfreter, J. and Hamburger, V. (1955). *In* "Analysis of Development" (B. H. Willier, P. A. Weiss, V. Hamburger, eds.), pp. 230–296. W. B. Saunders Co., Philadelphia and London.
Jensen, F. C., Gwatkin, R. B. L. and Biggers, J. D. (1964). *Expl. Cell Res.* **34**, 440–497.
Kallman, F. and Grobstein, C. (1964). *J. Cell Biol.* **20**, 399–413.
Kallman, F. and Grobstein, C. (1965). *Devl. Biol.* **11**, 169–183.
Kallman, F. and Grobstein, C. (1966). *Devl. Biol.* **14**, 52–67.
Kallman, F., Evans, J. and Wessells, N. K. (1967). *J. Cell. Biol.* **32**, 231–236.
Kato, Y. and Hayashi, Y. (1963). *Expl. Cell Res.* **31**, 599–602.
Kefalides, N. A. and Winzler, R. J. (1966). *Biochemistry* **5**, 702–713.
Kobayasi, T. (1961). *Acta derm.-vener. Stockh.* **41**, 481–491.
Koch, W. E. (1965). *Anat. Rec.* **151**, 373.
Koch, W. E. (1967). *J. exp. Zool.* **165**, 155–170.
Kollar, E. J. (1966). *J. invest. Derm.* **46**, 254–262.
Kurtz, S. M. (1964). *In* "Electron Microscopic Anatomy" (S. M. Kurtz, ed.). Academic Press, New York, U.S.A.
Kurtz, S. M. and McManus, J. F. A. (1960). *J. Ultrastruct. Res.* **4**, 81–87.
Lapiere, C. M. and Gross, J. (1963). *In* "Mechanisms of Hard Tissue Destruction". Publ. No. 75, pp. 663–694, Am. Assoc. Advanc. Sci., Washington, D.C., U.S.A.

Lasfargues, E. Y. (1957). *Expl. Cell Res.* **13**, 553–562.
Lasfargues, E. Y., Murray, M. R. and Moore, D. H. (1960). *Natn. Cancer Inst. Monogr.* **4**, 151–166.
Latta, H., Maunsbach, A. B. and Madden, S. C. (1960). *J. Ultrastruct. Res.* **4**, 455–472.
Le Douarin, N. (1964). *J. Embryol. exp. Morph.* **12**, 141–160.
Le Douarin, N. (1965). *C. r. Séanc. Soc. Biol.* **159**, 90–96.
Lillie, F. R. and Wang, H. (1944). *Physiol. Zool.* **17**, 1–31.
Low, F. N. and Burkel, W. E. (1965). *Anat. Rec.* **151**, 489–490.
Majno, G. and Palade, G. E. (1961). *J. biophys. biochem. Cytol.* **11**, 571–605.
Marin, L. and Sigot, M. (1963). *C. r. hebd Séanc. Acad. Sci., Paris* **257**, 3475–3477.
Marin, L. and Sigot, M. (1965). *C. r. Séanc. Soc. Biol.* **159**, 98–101.
McLoughlin, C. B. (1961a). *J. Embryol. exp. Morph.* **9**, 370–384.
McLoughlin, C. B. (1961b). *J. Embryol. exp. Morph.* **9**, 385–409.
McLoughlin, C. B. (1963). *In* "Cell differentiation", Symp. Soc. Exp. Biol. University Press, Cambridge, **17**, 359–388.
Medawar, P. B. (1941). *Nature (Lond).* **148**, 783.
Mercer, E. H. (1961). "Keratin and Keratinization—An Essay in Molecular Biology." Pergamon Press, New York, U.S.A.
Mercer, E. H. (1964). *In* "The Epidermis" (W. Montagna and W. C. Lobitz, eds.), pp. 161–178. Academic Press, New York, U.S.A.
Mercer, E. H. (1965). *In* "Organogenesis" (R. L. De Haan and H. Ursprung, eds.), pp. 29–53, Holt, Rinehart and Winston, New York, U.S.A.
Midgley, A. R. Jr. and Pierce, G. B. Jr. (1963). *Am. J. Path.* **43**, 929–943.
Milaire, J. (1965). *In* "Organogenesis" (R. L. De Haan and H. Ursprung, eds.), pp. 283–300, Holt, Rinehart and Winston, New York, U.S.A.
Moscona, A. (1952). *Expl. Cell Res.* **3**, 535–539.
Moscona, A. (1961a). *In* "La Culture Organotypique", pp. 155–168. Coll. Inter. CNRS No. 101, Paris.
Moscona, A. (1961b). *Int. Rev. exp. Path.* **1**, 371–428.
Moscona, A. (1965). *In* "Cells and Tissues in Culture" (E. N. Willmer, ed.), Vol. I, pp. 489–529. Academic Press, London, England.
Moscona, A. and Moscona, H. (1952). *J. Anat.* **86**, 287–301.
Moscona, A., Trowell, O. A. and Willmer, E. N. (1965). *In* "Cells and Tissues in Culture" (E. N. Willmer, ed.), Vol. I, pp. 19–98. Academic Press, London and New York.
Mukerjee, H., Sri Ram, J. and Pierce, G. B. Jr. (1965). *Am. J. Path.* **46**, 49–57.
Oliver, R. F. (1966). *J. Embryol. exp. Morph.* **15**, 331–347.
Orr, J. W. (1963). *Natn. Cancer Inst. Monogr.* **10**, 531–537.
Ottoson, D., Sjöstrand, F. Stestrom, S. and Svaetichin, G. (1953). *Acta Physiol. Scand.* **29**, Suppl. 106, 611–624.
Ozzello, L. and Speer, F. D. (1958). *Am. J. Path.* **34**, 993–1009.
Palade, G. E. and Farquhar, M. G. (1965). *J. Cell Biol.* **27**, 215–222.
Pearse, A. G. E. (1961). "Histochemistry Theoretical and Applied", 2nd ed. J. & A. Churchill, London.
Pierce, G. B. Jr (1965). *Cancer Res.* **25**, 656–669.
Pierce, G. B. Jr. (1966). *Devl. Biol.* **13**, 231–249.
Pierce, G. B. Jr., Midgley, A. R. Jr., Sri Ram J. and Felman, J. D. (1962). *Am. J. Path.* **41**, 549–566.
Pierce, G. B. Jr., Midgley, A. R. Jr., and Sri Ram, J. (1963). *J. exp. Med.* **117**, 339–348.
Rambourg, A., Neutra, M. and Leblond, C. P. (1966). *Anat. Rec.* **154**, 41–72.

Rambourg, A. and Leblond, C. P. (1967a). *J. Cell Biol.* **32**, 27–53.
Rambourg, A. and Leblond, C. P. (1967b). *J. Ultrastruct. Res.* **20**, 306–309.
Rawles, M. E. (1955). *In* "Analysis of Development" (B. H. Willier, P. A. Weiss and V. Hamburger, eds.), pp. 499–519. Saunders, Philadelphia, U.S.A.
Rawles, M. E. (1963). *J. Embryol. exp. Morph.* **11**, 765–789.
Rawles, M. E. (1965). *In* "Biology of the skin and hair growth" (A. G. Lyne and B. F. Short, eds.), pp. 105–128 Angus and Robertson, Sydney, Australia.
Rinaldini, L. M. (1958). *Int. Rev. Cytol.* **7**, 587–647.
Rinaldini, L. M. (1959). *Expl. Cell Res.* **16**, 477–505.
Robertson, J. D. (1959). *Biochem. Soc. Symp.*, 16 (Cambridge, England), 3–43.
Robertson, J. D. (1964). *In* "Cellular Membranes in Development" (M. Locke, ed.), pp. 1–81. Academic Press, New York and London.
Robertson, J. D. (1966). *In* "Intracellular transport" (K. B. Warren, ed.), pp. 1–31. Academic Press, New York and London.
Rous, P. and Jones, F. S. (1916). *J. exp. Med.* **23**, 549–555.
Rowlatt, C. (1967). Personal communication.
Rudnick, D. (1955). *In* "Analysis of Development" (B. H. Willier, P. A. Weiss and V. Hamburger, eds.), pp. 297–314. W. B. Saunders Co., Philadelphia and London.
Rutter, W. J., Wessells, N. K. and Grobstein, C. (1964). *Natn Cancer Inst. Monogr.* **13**, 51–61.
Salpeter, M. M. and Singer, M. (1959). *J. biophys. biochem. Cytol.* **6**, 35–40.
Saunders, J. W. Jr. and Weiss, P. (1950). *Anat. Rec.* **108**, 581.
Saunders, J. W. Jr., Gasseling, M. T. and Gfeller, M. D. Jr. (1958). *J. exp. Zool.* **137**, 39–74.
Saxen, L. and Toivonen, S. (1962). "Primary Embryonic Induction." Logos Press. Academic Press, London.
Selby, C. C. (1955). *J. biophys. biochem. Cytol.* **1**, 429–444.
Sengel, P. (1958). *Ann. des. Sc. nat., Zool.* **20**, 431–514.
Sengel, P. (1964). *In* "The Epidermis" (W. Montagna and W. C. Lobitz, Jr., eds.), pp. 15–34. Academic Press, New York and London.
Sengel, P. (1965). *In* "Les Cultures Organotypiques" (J. Andre Thomas, ed.), pp. 283–336. Masson et Cie., Paris.
Shaffer, B. M. (1956). *Expl. Cell Res.* **11**, 244–248.
Sigot, M. (1962). *C. r. hebd Séanc. Acad. Sci., Paris* **254**, 2439–2441.
Silbert, J. E., Nagai, Y. and Gross, J. (1965). *J. biol. Chem.* **240**, 1509–1511.
Sobel, H. (1958). *J. Embryol. exp. Morph.* **6**, 518–526.
Sorokin, S. (1965). *In* "Organogenesis" (R. L. De Haan, and H. Ursprung, eds.), pp. 467–491. Holt, Rinehart and Winston, New York, U.S.A.
Spemann, H. (1938). "Embryonic Development and Induction." Yale University Press, New Haven, U.S.A.
Stern, I. B. (1965). *Periodontics* **3**, 224–238.
Stroeva, O. G. (1960). *J. Embryol. exp. Morph.* **8**, 349–368.
Susi, F. R., Belt, W. D. and Kelly, J. W. (1967). *J. Cell Biol.* **34**, 686–690.
Swift, J. A. and Saxton, C. A. (1967). *J. Ultrastruct. Res.* **17**, 23–33.
Szabo, G. (1955). *J. Path. Bact.* **70**, 545.
Tarin, D. (1967). *Int. J. Cancer* **2**, 195–211.
Torrey, T. W. (1965). *In* "Organogenesis" (R. L. De Haan and H. Ursprung, eds.), pp. 559–579, Holt, Rinehart and Winston, New York, U.S.A.
Trowell, O. A. (1954). *Expl. Cell Res.* **6**, 246–248.
Valderhaug, J. P. and Nylen, M. U. (1966). *J. Periodont. Res.* **1**, 69–78.
Van Scott, E. J. and Reinertson, R. P. (1961). *J. invest. Dermatol.* **36**, 109–131.
Weinreb, M. M., Sharav, Y. and Ickowicz, M. (1967). *Transplantation* **5**, 379–389.
Weiss, L. (1963). *Expl. Cell Res.* **30**, 509–520.

Weiss, L. (1967). "The cell periphery, metastasis and other contact phenomena." North-Holland Publishing Co., Amsterdam.

Wessells, N. K. (1962). *Devl. Biol.* **4,** 87–107.

Wessells, N. K. (1963). *Expl. Cell Res.* **30,** 36–55.

Wessells, N. K. (1964a). *J. Cell Biol.* **20,** 415–433.

Wessells, N. K. (1964b). *Proc. natn. Acad. Sci., U.S.A.* **52,** 252–259.

Wessells, N. K. (1965). *Devl. Biol.* **12,** 131–153.

Wessells, N. K. and Cohen, J. H. (1966). *Expl. Cell Res.* **43,** 680–684.

Wolff, E. (1965). *In* "Les Cultures Organotypiques" (J. Andre Thomas, ed.), pp. 1–13. Masson, Paris, France.

Wolff, E. and Haffen, K. (1959). *Archs Anat. microsc Morph. exp.* **48** bis, 331–345.

Wolff, E. and Haffen, K. (1965). *In* "Cells and Tissues in Culture" (E. N. Willmer, ed.), Vol. 2, pp. 697–743. Academic Press, London and New York.

Yamada, E. (1955). *J. biophys. biochem. Cytol.* **1,** 551–566.

Younes, M. S., Steele, H. D., Robertson, E. M. and Bencosme, S. A. (1965). *Am. J. Obstet. Gynecol.* **92,** 163–171.

Zwilling, E. (1956). *J. exp. Zool.* **132,** 173–187.

Zwilling, E. (1960). *Natn. Cancer Inst. Monogr.* **2,** 19–35.

Zwilling, E. (1961). *Adv. Morphogenesis.* **1,** 301–330.

Zwilling, E. (1964). *Devl. Biol.* **9,** 20–37.

3 | The Development of the Periodontium

*A. R. TEN CATE

*Unit of Anatomy in Relation to Dentistry, Anatomy Department,
Guy's Hospital Medical School, London, England*

I. Introduction

The existence of a periodontium around socketed teeth depends on the evolution of a dental follicle, or sac, around the tooth germ. This structure is considered by some to be characteristic of mammals, and its presence

* Present address: Faculty of Dentistry, University of Toronto, Toronto, Canada

3

separates the tooth from the bone of the jaw. The phylogenetic development of the follicle is discussed in Chapter 1 and will not be considered here. Correct interpretation of the genesis of the periodontium requires that the ontogenetic development of the follicle be considered in some detail. Before doing so, however, the terminology must be discussed as inaccuracies in interpretation have led to some confusion.

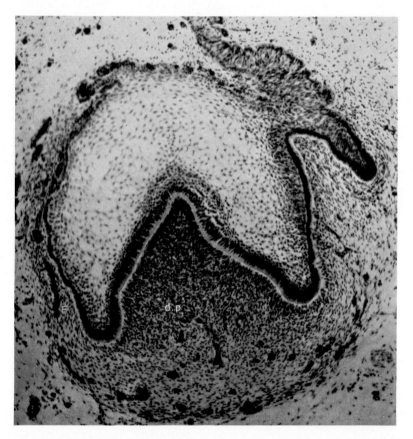

FIG. 1. Human tooth germ at the bell stage of development showing continuity between the cells of the dental papilla and the innermost layer of the "dental follicle" d.p. = dental papilla, F = Follicle. (H. & E. Photomicrograph kindly lent by E. B. Brain.)

Few would dispute that the periodontal ligament and the cementum are derived from the dental follicle. Confusion arises because the term *dental follicle* has been used with different connotations by different writers. For example, Scott and Symons (1964) consider the dental follicle to be the mesenchmyal condensation which is in contact with the outer surface of the external dental epithelium, and which is continuous with the dental papilla around the rim of the dental organ (Fig. 1). It is stated later in the same text that the tooth follicle is developmentally and morphologically part of the dental papilla. Although these statements appear contradictory they both imply that the dental follicle is that tissue immediately surrounding the tooth germ, with additional mesenchymal tissue between the follicle and the developing alveolar bone.

Orban's (1962) description of the dental follicle is imprecise, being defined as a condensation of mesenchyme around the tooth germ. No attempt is made to define its limits or origins. However, in the account of the development of the periodontal ligament, the follicle is described as consisting of three zones, an inner zone related to the tooth, an outer zone related to alveolar bone and, between the two, an intermediate zone. From this description it is evident that Orban considers all the tissue between the developing alveolar bone and the tooth germ as dental follicle.

In the recent literature concerning the nature of the dental follicle, a distinctive inner zone is clearly described. Fearnhead (1961) describes this zone as being closely applied to the outer dental epithelium and the base of the dental papilla. He also describes the tissue between this zone and the alveolar bone as follicle, and it must be taken that he considers the follicle to consist of two layers. Tonge (1963) also recognizes a distinct layer surrounding the tooth germ, and considers it to act as a limiting capsule separating the environment of the tooth germ from that of the adjacent potentially osteogenic tissue. Although Tonge hinted quite strongly at the distinctiveness of this inner layer, he still regards as follicle all the tissues between the tooth germ and the forming alveolar bone, because he later describes an outer layer of the follicle forming in relation to the alveolar bone.

Thus, the dental follicle has variously been described as a single mesenchymal layer immediately adjacent to the tooth germ (Scott and Symons); as the entire tissue between the developing tooth germ and forming alveolar bone, and consisting of two layers (Fearnhead); and finally, as the entire tissue between the tooth germ and the forming alveolar bone and consisting of three layers (Orban, Tonge).

II. The Ontogeny of the Tissue Surrounding Developing Teeth

When the ontogeny of the tissues surrounding the tooth germ is studied, it becomes evident that there is a good case for reserving the term dental follicle for that tissue immediately in contact with the tooth germ. The remaining tissue should be termed perifollicular mesenchyme. To avoid confusion at this stage, and to facilitate the presentation of the evidence, the tissue in immediate contact with the tooth germ is, for the time being, termed the investing layer.

A. The Origin of the Mesenchyme of the Jaws

1. Comparative Studies

The mesenchyme of the first branchial arch is derived from two sources; from the ectoderm of the neural crest, and from primitive streak mesoderm. This type of mesenchyme is usually collectively designated *ectomesenchyme* to indicate its neural crest component. Some authorities, however, reserve the term ectomesenchyme exclusively for those cells within mesenchyme of neural crest origin. A discussion of the correctness of either interpretation is not necessary here, except to point out that the latter definition is used in this text.

The literature dealing with the migration of neural crest tissues to the developing jaws has recently been reviewed extensively by Gaunt and Miles (1967), and there can be little doubt that ectomesenchyme contributes to the developing tooth. It has been established (Sellman, 1946) that removal of presumptive neural crest tissue results in failure of tooth development in amphibian embryos. Whilst experimental methods such as these are not possible in mammalian embryos, histochemical studies of mammalian embryonic material (Dalq, 1953; Milaire, 1959; Pourtois, 1961) have shown that ectomesenchymal cells can be distinguished from mesodermal mesenchymal cells by their glycogen, ribonucleic acid, and alkaline phosphatase content. Utilizing these histochemical characteristics the migration of neural crest into the mandibular and maxillary processes of the mouse embryo has been traced. The ectomesenchymal cells remain closely packed, and form a band beneath the oral epidermis at a stage in development preceding the thickening of epidermis in the presumptive dental regions of the jaw. Gaunt (1959) found that in the cat embryo this condensation of ectomesenchyme appears almost simultaneously with the thickening of the overlying epidermis in the region of the developing tooth band, thereby making determination of the exact sequence of events difficult. It is important to determine the exact sequence of events occurring at this time, so that the site where the inductive influence for tooth formation resides may be identified. However, the observation relevant to this discussion is that ectomesenchyme can be distinguished and shown to be involved in tooth formation.

Gaunt (1959) has termed this band of ectomesenchyme *perilaminar mesenchyme*. He describes it as being divided into two zones, an outer follicular zone and an inner pulpal zone. The cells of the pulpal zone are distinguished by virtue of their small nuclei, many of which show mitotic figures, and their lack of any preferred orientation. In the follicular zone the cells are larger, with elongated nuclei which are arranged in a circumferential manner. A great deal of fibrous material is present between the cells of the follicle zone.

With the attainment of the cap stage of development, further marked changes in the perilaminar mesenchyme were noted by Gaunt. The ecto-mesenchyme of the pulpal zone is now entirely confined within the concavity of the dental organ where it constitutes the primordium of the dental pulp. The follicular zone becomes more fibrous and, in addition, expands around the tooth germ to encapsulate it and form an investing layer.

2. Human Studies

Examination of comparable stages in human tooth development indicates a clear demarcation of cells in the region of the primary epithelial band

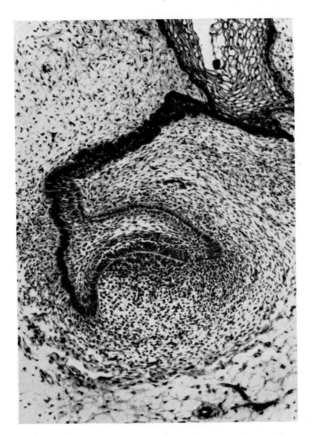

FIG. 2. Human tooth germ at the cap stage of development showing the condensation of mesenchyme surrounding the dental organ. (Mallory.)

which is similar to those found in the mouse and cat embryo, and it is reasonable to assume that these too are ectomesenchymal. At the cap stage of development it is relatively easy to distinguish a condensation of mesenchyme surrounding the dental organ. This is continuous with the mesenchyme of the papilla, which is distinct from the mesenchyme of the jaw (Figs. 1 and 2). Use of histochemical staining methods also help to differentiate this investing mesenchyme. Figure 3 illustrates the glycogen content of the tissues surrounding the developing human tooth at the cap stage of development. Glycogen, which is indicated by the black dots, appears at first glance to be concentrated

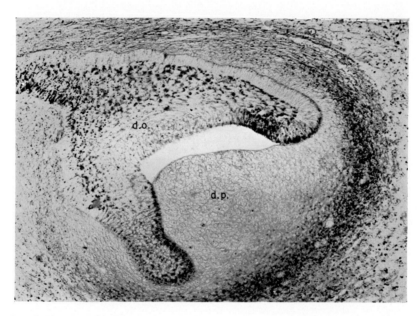

FIG. 3. Human tooth germ at the cap stage of development. The condensation of mesenchyme surrounding the dental organ and continuous with the papilla, can be distinguished by virtue of the absence of glycogen from these cells. Glycogen is seen in this photomicrograph as black particulate material p.a.S. d.o. = dental organ, d.p. = dental papilla. (Reproduced by kind permission of the Editors of the Archives Oral Biology.)

in the mesenchyme surrounding the developing tooth. However, a thin layer of glycogen-free cells, continuous with the glycogen-free cells of the dental papilla, invests the dental organ. This might seem a curious observation in view of the fact that the argument is being developed that the investing layer surrounding the tooth germ is of ectomesenchymal origin. It has already been stated that a distinctive feature of ectomesenchymal cells is their glycogen content but, according to Pourtois (1961), this biochemical feature is lost as the ectomesenchymal cells are diluted within the mesenchyme of the jaw.

Further evidence, suggestive of a distinctive investing layer around the developing tooth, is obtained when early tooth germs are dissected from embryonic jaws. This is not such a difficult procedure as might be imagined, for the tooth germs can be shelled out of their crypts like peas from a pod. When removed in this manner the tooth germ is spherical in shape. This suggests the presence of a retaining structure and, after sectioning, a thin fibro-cellular layer can be demonstrated histologically around the tooth germ (Fig. 4). It is also significant that, when sections of isolated tooth germs are examined, there is often separation between the tissue of the dental organ

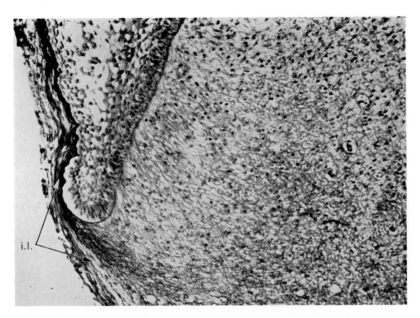

FIG. 4. Human tooth germ at the late bell stage dissected from its bony crypt. Note the investing layer (i.l.) around both the dental organ and papilla. (Gordon & Sweets.)

and the dental papilla. This implies a weak union between these two tissues; and further, were it not for the presence of an investing layer, separation of these two components of the tooth germ might occur during excision.

Thus, there is evidence from histological, histochemical, and experimental studies to suggest that the developing tooth germ is encapsulated by a distinctive fibro-cellular layer derived from neural crest tissue. Further supporting evidence comes from organ culture and organ transplantation studies, but the presentation of this evidence is delayed until the structure, function and fate of the investing layer has been discussed (see page 70).

B. THE INVESTING LAYER UP TO THE COMMENCEMENT OF ROOT
   FORMATION

The information presented in the following account is culled from the literature and from the author's own examination of human developing teeth, reinforced occasionally by reference to developing teeth of the monkey. Examination of histological sections of human tooth germs *in situ*, and also of complete germs removed from their bony crypts at early stages of development (prior to root formation), reveals that the tooth germ is surrounded by a fibro-cellular layer some three to four cells thick (Fig. 5). Where this layer is in contact with the external dental epithelium its innermost cells are fusiform, and exhibit prominent rounded nuclei. The outermost cells have a more

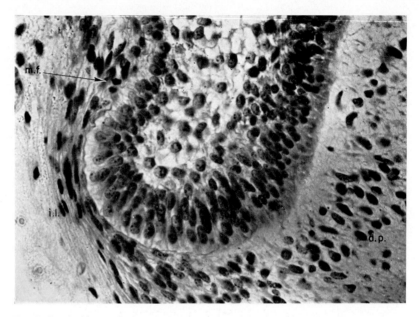

Fig. 5. Cervical loop of a human tooth germ at the bell stage of development. A mitotic figure (m.f.) can be seen in the investing layer. H. & E. i.l. = investing layer, d.p. = dental papilla.

accentuated spindle morphology, and their nuclei are thin and flattened. As the investing layer sweeps round the cervical loop to come into contact with the cells of the dental papilla, all its cells are spindle shaped with elongated nuclei. The investing layer again reverts to two layers after passing the cervical loop region. The cells of the investing layer which are closest to the dental papilla are squat, have rounded nuclei, and merge imperceptibly with the cells of the dental papilla. The outermost cells, on the other hand, retain their spindle shape and are orientated circumferentially around the base of the papilla. Mitotic Figures can be seen within the cells of the investing layer (Fig. 5).

The fibres of the investing layer are readily demonstrated by silver impregnation methods, but not by most of the stains which are used to demonstrate collagen fibres. These fibres have characteristics of young developing collagen fibres (Robb-Smith, 1957; see Chapter 6). Immediately external to the cuboidal cells of the external dental epithelium is a dense aggregation of argyrophilic fibres. External to this the fibres are somewhat finer and have a wavy course. However, in the region of the cervical loop, all fibres appear, in section, to run a straighter course. After passing the cervical loop the fibres

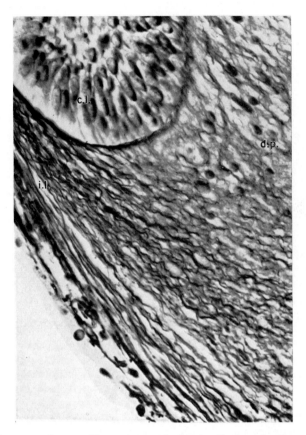

FIG. 6. Human tooth germ. Photomicrograph showing the investing layer as it passes from the dental organ on to the surface of the dental papilla. c.l. = cervical loop of dental organ, d.p. = dental papilla, i.l. = investing layer. (Gordon & Sweets.)

diverge; those in the outer part of the investing layer maintaining a straighter course, and those in the inner part reverting to a wavy configuration. At the same time, the innermost fibres fan out to merge with the fibres of the papilla (Fig. 6). Another feature of the investing layer is the many capillaries which lie against its outer surface.

With the onset of dentinogenesis changes occur in the configuration of the external dental epithelium. The epithelium folds to make a more intimate contact with the capillary network, whilst its cells lose their cuboidal shape and become squamous. These changes coincide with an apparent "collapse"

3*

of the dental organ. However, there is no evident alteration in the curvature of the investing layer (Fig. 7). This suggests two possibilities: that "collapse" is perhaps an erroneous term, and that it is the tip of the growing cusp pushing

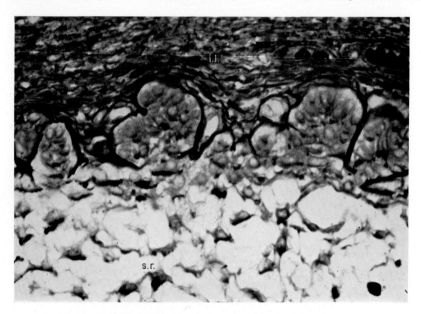

Fig. 7. Human tooth germ. Photomicrograph showing the investing layer surrounding the "collapsed" dental organ. s.r. = stellate reticulum, i.l. = investing layer. (Gordon & Sweets.)

upwards towards the external dental epithelium, coupled with shrinkage and displacement of the stellate reticulum, that creates this illusion; and that folding of the external dental epithelium, which results in ridge-like projections protruding into the investing layer, is a consequence of its intrinsic growth.

The character of the investing layer remains essentially unchanged during further development until root formation begins. Thus, it is still easy to distinguish the investing layer around tooth germs when amelogenesis is relatively well advanced, but where there is no evidence of root formation. Until the onset of root formation the developing germ is completely contained within the spherical investing layer. However, as the roots develop, the spherical form of the investing layer changes to accommodate them.

C. The Investing Layer in Relation to Root Formation

1. The Investing Layer in Relation to Hertwig's Root Sheath

Root formation commences with epithelial proliferation at the cervical loop of the dental organ. This leads to formation of Hertwig's epithelial root sheath. If the outer aspect of the forming root sheath is examined, a fibro-cellular layer can be distinguished. This layer is continuous with the investing layer around the forming crown. Its presence around the growing root sheath implies that it is growing. This view is reinforced by the occurrence of mitotic figures within its cells. In fact, there is strong evidence that the investing layer helps to determine the pathway of the advancing root sheath. Published figures showing the epithelial root sheath lying at right angles to the long axis of the forming root, in the manner of an epithelial diaphragm, are open to doubt. It is relatively difficult, in well prepared sections, to demonstrate the epithelial diaphragm lying at right angles to the long axis of the root; more frequently it is found to lie along the arc of a gentle curve. Moreover, where the root sheath can be demonstrated to lie at right angles to the long axis of the tooth, there is invariably present an artefactual space between the root sheath and the papilla cells, so that the layer of newly differentiated odontoblasts is distorted and the cells appear to be crowded together. This feature suggests that the root sheath has been "deflected coronally", possibly by shrinkage of the papilla during fixation and processing. The suggestion is further supported by the examination of poorly processed sections in which a great deal of shrinkage of the tissues is apparent: the epithelial diaphragm is seen to be inverted into the pulp chamber forming an acute angle with the long axis of the forming root.

2. The Investing Layer in Relation to the Apex of the Tooth

Macroscopic inspection of the open apical region of young, extracted, human teeth shows tissue of the papilla protruding beyond the forming root margin and presenting a smooth, rounded surface. If direct continuity existed between the tissue of the pulp and the periodontal tissue, the papilla would more likely present a torn and damaged surface. When this region is examined histologically, the presence of a limiting layer between the pulp and perio-dontal tissue can be demonstrated.

It must be pointed out, however, that the presence and nature of this limiting structure is still in dispute. Sicher (1942a,b) first described fibrous tissue stretching across the open aspect of the pulp chamber. He called this structure the "cushion hammock ligament" because he thought that it contains numerous spaces filled with mucoid substance, and that it is attached at either side to the bony walls of the alveolus. He ascribed to the cushion hammock ligament an important role in eruption, believing that it transmits forces derived from cellular proliferation in the pulp to the bone as a tensile force, thereby preventing bone resorption and causing axial movement of the tooth. This structure was described as present under the roots of single rooted teeth only. Scott (1953) supported Sicher's conclusions but, in addition, reported the presence of the ligament under the roots of all teeth. Eccles (1961) has described three zones of connective tissue in this area: a thin layer of periosteum adjacent to the alveolar bone; a broad zone of less dense fibrous tissue; and an inner zone, closely applied to the base of the pulp, consisting of a thin sheet of fibres which, centrally, turns inwards to the pulp. This inner zone, corresponding to the cushion hammock ligament, was found nearly always to be present, merging laterally with the periodontal ligament, not the alveolar bone.

Main (1965), in a comprehensive search for the cushion hammock ligament in several species, but not in man, found that a collagenous membrane exists under the roots of single rooted teeth of limited eruption, and that this membrane is attached laterally to the innermost layer of the periodontal ligament and not to alveolar bone. Because of its lateral attachments it could not have the function ascribed to it by Sicher and Scott, and therefore Main renamed this membrane the pulp limiting membrane. Main also found that this membrane was not demonstrable in the earlier stages of tooth development, collagen fibres being detectable only during the later stages of crown development. The staining methods he employed, however, were those for mature collagen. However, it has been pointed out above that a limiting membrane across the base of the papilla can be demonstrated, by silver impregnation, in the early stages of development of both single and multi-rooted teeth. Indeed, retrospectively, it is a little difficult to understand why Sicher reached the conclusion that the cushion-hammock ligament was attached at either extremity to alveolar bone for, if his original photo-micrograph is consulted, the ligament appears to converge towards the apical extremity of the forming root and to continue occlusally in contact with the surface of the newly formed dentine. Given, therefore, that the investing layer persists at the forming root margin delineating the pulp tissue from the perio-dontal tissue, it is now necessary to trace its fate between this point and the future cement-enamel junction as elongation of the root occurs.

3. The Investing Layer in Relation to the Sides of the Forming Root

(a) The fragmentation of Hertwig's root sheath. The initial formation of root dentine is accompanied by well-recorded changes in the tissues adjacent to it. The epithelial root sheath of Hertwig, its function of organizing the differ-entiation of odontoblasts completed, becomes slightly separated from the newly formed root surface and fragments to form the epithelial cell rests of Malassez. From the connective tissue collecting between the cell rests and the root surface the cementum-forming cells differentiate. Although these histo-logical changes are well known, their functional significance is still in doubt. Schour and Massler (1940) thought that the epithelial root sheath probably stimulates cells of the dental follicle to form cementum, after which they degenerate to form the epithelial cell rests of Malassez. On the other hand, Orban (1928) believed that the root sheath does not degenerate following the initiation of cementogenesis and, that after it becomes separated from the root surface, it continues to exert a stimulatory influence on the cementoblasts as the epithelial cell rests of Malassez.

Recently, several workers have enquired into the precise nature of the disruption of the root sheath. Selvig (1963) studied the disrupting root sheath in the mouse incisor with the aid of an electron microscope, and reported that the thickness of the root sheath gradually diminishes until it is only one cell thick. He noted a simultaneous diminution in the number of mitochondria, and the appearance of dense granules in the epithelial cells. The epithelial cells were found to separate from each other and to drift away from the dentine surface concurrent with the initiation of dentine mineralization. Collagen fibres appeared in the newly created intercellular spaces. A study of the electron micrographs reproduced in Selvig's paper fails to provide evidence of epithelial degeneration during the migration and disruption of the root sheath. In a histochemical study, Ten Cate (1965) demonstrated oxidative enzyme activity in human cell rests, thus showing that these structures were not degenerate. A further investigation in which the fragmenting human root sheath was examined electron microscopically and histochemically for evidence of cellular degeneration (Ten Cate, 1967), revealed the absence of fat deposits, increased hydrolytic enzyme activity and mitochondrial change. These features were taken as evidence indicating that the root sheath cells do not undergo degeneration as the sheath disrupts. However, Diab and Stallard (1965), in a radio-biological study of the root sheath of the developing rat molar, found that although there was a rapid turnover of root sheath cells as they organized the differentiation of root odontoblasts, in general no labelling was retained by the cells of the root sheath. This finding appears to suggest first, that the root sheath cells degenerate and do not contribute to the formation of epithelial cell rests and second, that cementum formation is dependent on neither the presence nor absence of the epithelial root sheath. Whilst the second suggestion, in the absence of any other evidence apart from histological evidence, could be correct, the first must be treated with some caution in view of conflicting electron microscopical and histochemical evidence. Whatever the role and fate of the root sheath at this time of tooth development, there is no doubt that connective tissue comes to lie in contact with the newly formed root dentine.

(b) *The connective tissue in contact with root dentine.* The origin of this connective tissue is uncertain. Selvig (1963) found that, at the apical end of the root sheath, the dental sac consists of several layers of long slender fibroblasts arranged parallel to the sheath. Examination of his photomicrograph shows that his connotation of dental sac is synonymous with the term investing layer used in this account, for looser connective tissue can be seen clearly on its outer aspect. Fine bundles of collagen fibres are scattered between the fibroblasts, and near the periodontal surface of the epithelial sheath. As the root sheath disintegrates collagen fibres are found between the separated epithelial cells, and between these cells and the dentine surface. These fibres are not arranged in bundles, and form an irregular meshwork on the root surface. Following the migration of the epithelial cells away from the dentine surface fibroblasts are found adjacent to the root surface, and these now became identifiable as cementoblasts. The fibrils near the tooth surface gradually became more numerous, and deposition of crystallites occurs between the fibrils to form the first layer of cementum. Significantly, this first formed cementum does not contribute to the support of the tooth as Sharpey's fibres are not found within it. Thus, from Selvig's observations it must be taken that, in the mouse at least, the connective tissue intervening between the root sheath and the root surface, and also the first formed cementum, are derived from the investing layer. Furthermore, if the hypothesis presented in this chapter is correct, this means that the first formed cementum is of ectomesenchymal derivation.

A number of authors have noticed that first-formed cementum has distinctive characteristics. Paynter and Pudy (1958) have reported the appearance of an intensely metachromatic layer against the dentine surface of the developing rat tooth concurrent with fragmentation of the root sheath. They concluded that the first-formed cementum did not originate from the dental follicle and that it was fibre-free. Although, in the light of Selvig's studies their interpretations seem erroneous, their findings support further the idea that first-formed cementum is distinctive. In a further publication, Selvig (1964) has reported formation of cementum on rodent molar roots. Here also the first-formed cementum was found to differ from that which is formed later, as it does not contain Sharpey's fibres and its matrix consists of irregularly arranged collagen fibres. Selvig concluded that precementum is formed only in the earliest stages of root formation, and that later cementum formation is a process of gradual mineralization of the periodontal ligament. Selvig's study of human cementum (1965) provides information that is significantly different from that obtained from rodent material, and which therefore does not support the hypothesis being proposed. In man the innermost layer of cementum differs from the remainder. This difference is claimed by Selvig to be due to the incorporated Sharpey's fibres being partially unmineralized. Selvig's findings may be open to criticism for a number of reasons. He examined erupted teeth only where (see later), orientation of the ligament fibres had been established. In addition, indication is not given from which part of the root the specimens were taken and, furthermore, no mention is made of intermediate cementum or the hyaline layer of dentine. This last point is of especial importance, as Selvig's electron-micrograph which illustrates the innermost layer of cementum also shows tissue which he has identified as dentine. In this photomicrograph the tissue called dentine consists of an organic matrix which is randomly orientated.

There is no visible structural element which allows unequivocal identification of this matrix as dentine. The possibility therefore exists that this matrix could be intermediate cementum. This problem requires further investigation.

(*c*) *The investing layer from the apex to the future cemento-enamel junction.* To trace the fate of the investing layer as further root growth continues,

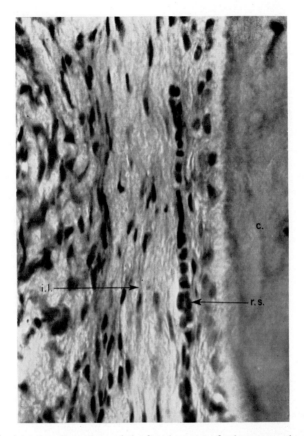

Fig. 8. The investing tissues around the forming root of a human tooth germ close to the open apex. The fragmented root sheath (r.s.) lies close to the forming cementum (c) surface. A longitudinal band of fibres (the investing layer) can be distinguished on the outer surface of the root sheath (i.l.). (H. & E.)

histological sections of unerupted human teeth which exhibit the initial stages of cementum formation, and of surgically-extracted-unerupted teeth to which some of the investing tissue still adheres, have been examined.

If, in sections of the surgically extracted teeth, the investing layer is followed occlusally, several interesting histological features can be observed. In the apical region, the tissues are arranged as already described, with the epithelial debris lying a little way from the surface of the root dentine: the fibrous investing layer lies against the outer surface of the epithelial debris (Fig. 8). External to the investing layer is connective tissue of much looser appearance. More occlusually, there is an increased separation of the cell rests and

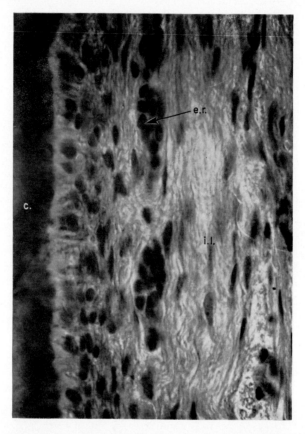

FIG. 9. The investing tissues around the forming root of a human tooth midway between the apex and the cemento-enamel junction. The longitudinal band of fibres is still present though it, and the epithelial cell rests, have migrated away from the cementum surface. c = cementum, e.r. = epithelial cell rest, i.l. = investing layer. (H. & E.)

fibrous investing layer from the root surface, with a corresponding increase in the amount of intervening connective tissue (Fig. 9). Apart from the longitudinally arranged layer of collagen fibres, which appears to increase in density as it is traced occlusually, there is no discernible orientation of the cells or fibres in the remaining connective tissue on either side of it. More occlusually still, in the region of the cemento-enamel junction, there is further drift from the root surface of the longitudinally arranged layer of collagen fibres and epithelial cell rests. At this point a change occurs in the orientation of the fibres in the collagen band; the fibres sweep around the bulbosity of the occlusal surface, and continue as a thick layer of collagen fibres over the crown of the unerupted tooth (Fig. 10). Here also there is evidence of

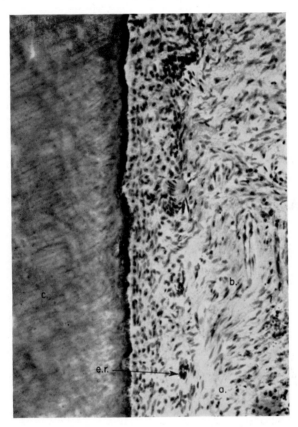

FIG. 10. The investing tissues around the forming root of a human tooth close to the cemento-enamel junction. The longitudinal band of fibres (a) becomes lost as it merges with the obliquely orientated fibres (b). c = cementum, e.r. = epithelial cell rest. (H. & E.)

orientation of the connective tissue on either side of the layer; the cells and fibres are aligned obliquely to the long axis of the tooth. This change is discussed when formation of the periodontal ligament is described. It is thus possible to trace the investing layer from the apex of the tooth as an intact structure, which runs parallel to the root surface throughout its length as far as the cemento-enamel junction, where it continues over the crown of the tooth.

If sections from similar specimens are impregnated with silver, the longitudinally arranged layer of fibres is clearly delineated from the randomly arranged fibres on either side (Fig. 11). This picture also illustrates the so-called *intermediate zone* of the dental follicle. The evidence presented in this account suggests that the investing layer surrounding the tooth germ before root formation persists throughout root formation as the pulp delineating membrane around the apex of the forming roots, and also as a longitudinally-aligned layer of older collagen fibres running parallel to the root surface. This evidence also strongly suggests that the first-formed human cementum is an ectomesenchymal derivative, as the cementoblasts

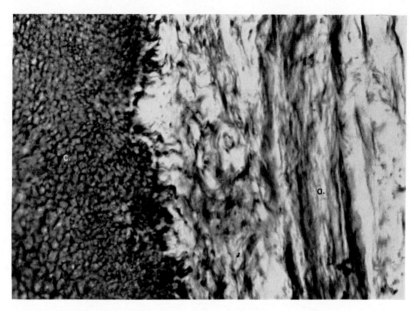

FIG. 11. Similar section as depicted in Fig. 10 impregnated with silver to depict the longitudinally orientated fibres (a). c = cementum. (Gordon & Sweets.)

apparently differentiate from the connective tissue between the investing layer and the dentine surface. It is now necessary to consider the fate of the investing layer where it surrounds the dental organ forming the crown of the tooth.

D. The Investing Layer Around the Developing Crown of the Tooth

It will be remembered that the investing layer surrounding the developing tooth prior to root formation is clearly delineated. The changes in this layer which occur to accommodate the growing roots have been described. Around the crown of the tooth the investing layer gradually increases in thickness at the expense of the loose connective tissue between it and the alveolar bone, until it eventually appears as illustrated in Fig. 12. The fine, young collagen fibres have matured into much thicker bundles. Although it cannot be stated unequivocally that this thick collagenous layer has arisen directly from the investing layer found in the earlier stages of tooth development, its anatomical relationships strongly support such a deduction. Clearly, this portion of the investing layer cannot be involved in the formation of the periodontium, but for the sake of completeness its fate during further development and eruption of the tooth is outlined.

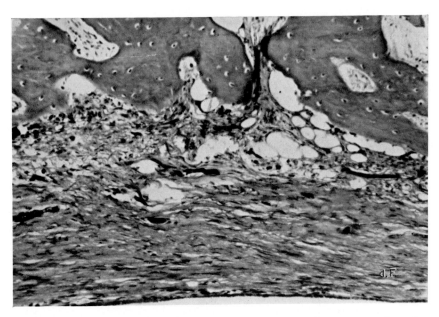

FIG. 12. The dental follicle (d.f.) surrounding the crown of an unerupted monkey premolar tooth. (H. & E.)

Figure 13 is a montage photograph of the distal surface of a monkey permanent tooth enclosed in an osseous environment beneath its deciduous predecessor. When the investing layer of the permanent tooth is followed occlusally from the region of the cemento-enamel junction, it is seen to thin out, gradually disappear, to be replaced by loose reticular connective tissue. This transition occurs first in the layer of collagen fibres adjoining the dental epithelium. Examination of the transitional zone shows that the bundles of collagen fibres have a frayed and fragmentary appearance which suggests that dissolution of the fibres is taking place. There is no definite information on how dissolution of these collagen fibres is achieved. (For a general discussion of this topic see Chapter 6.) The presence of a collagenase in connective tissue overlying erupted teeth has been postulated, but its presence here has never been demonstrated unequivocally. Over the occlusal surface of the tooth that has been illustrated, all the connective tissue is of the loose

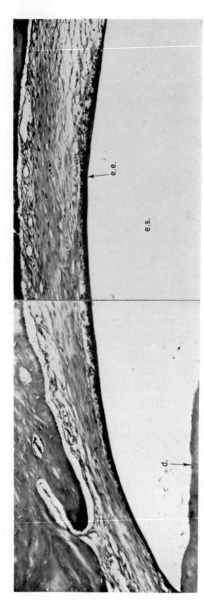

Fig. 13. Montage photomicrograph showing the dissolution of the follicular tissue surrounding the crown of an unerupted monkey tooth. e.s. = enamel space, d. = dentine, e.e. = enamel epithelium. (H. & E.)

reticular type. The author has noted that in this situation, over the occlusal surface of an erupting tooth, there is frequently gross dissolution of connective tissue with hyaline, eosinophilic masses, and sometimes free red blood corpuscles present. Recently two workers (Hodson, 1966 and Listgarten, 1966) have reported respectively that the enamel cuticle is possibly derived from the breakdown products of haemoglobin, and that free red blood cells occur on the connective tissue surface of the reduced dental epithelium. These two findings make possible the speculation that dissolution of the investing layer is non-specific and that, whatever the mechanism, erosion of capillaries also occurs.

The dissolution of the thick collagenous investing layer can also be demonstrated over the human erupting third molar tooth with no deciduous predecessor, suggesting that this is a normal occurrence. The role of the dental epithelium in the process of dissolution of the investing layer still requires elucidation. It has been suggested that the reduced dental epithelium is responsible for the connective tissue dissolution. It is well established that reduced dental epithelium proliferates into the dissolute connective tissue (Weinmann, Svoboda and Woods, 1945; McHugh, 1961; Ten Cate, 1963), and the first mentioned authors claim that this epithelial proliferation is responsible for the connective tissue breakdown. On the other hand, epithelial proliferation in the presence of connective tissue change occurs elsewhere; for example, in skin-wounds and in the inflamed periodontal ligament, where the epithelial cell rests proliferate. This suggests that epithelium, in the presence of connective tissue breakdown, has an inherent tendency to proliferate.

Thus, in tracing the ontogeny and fate of the investing layer, it has been demonstrated, mainly by histological observation, that this layer is derived from the same cellular elements as the dental papilla. It is probably ecto-mesenchymal in origin, it forms the pulp delineating membrane at the apex of the forming root, and it constitutes the so-called intermediate zone along the sides of the forming root. Furthermore, there is evidence that cementum is possibly a derivative of this layer and that this investing layer is lost from over the crown as the tooth erupts.

E. TRANSPLANTATION STUDIES

Transplantation studies of tooth germs also provide evidence in support of the thesis that the investing layer is of a distinctive character. Hoffman (1960) successfully transplanted developing molar teeth from newborn hamsters into a subcutaneous site in adult animals. The transplanted teeth were at the stage of development immediately before the beginning of amelogenesis and showed no evidence of root formation. Hoffman was careful to point out that the tooth germs were removed from their follicles before transplantation and that "only a few mesenchymal cells were seen outside the enamel organ". After transplantation to an alien site, development continued with the formation of roots, periodontal ligament and "alveolar" bone. Hoffman argued that the ability of the dental tissues proper (dental organ and dental papilla) to differentiate alveolar bone and periodontal ligament from "foreign" connective tissue indicated an organizing influence on the part of the dental tissues. He therefore regarded formation of periodontal tissue as the "efforts of a morphogenetic field to complete itself". Thus Hoffman's findings would seem to be at variance with the suggestion that the investing layer is specifically dental in nature. However, he quite properly states that

"additional evidence should be obtained to establish conclusively that no transplanted cells were the precursors to the periodontal tissues formed. Without doubt, a certain few cells adhered to the outer enamel epithelium and were transplanted. It seems improbable that these cells could have been responsible for the extensive formation of periodontium routinely seen around transplanted teeth after 28 days in the host subcutaneous tissues."

It is possible that in removing the tooth germs from their "dental sacs" Hoffman obtained the same results as removal of human tooth germs, and that the "certain few mesenchymal cells" represent the ectomesenchymal cells of the investing layer. Although it is quite possible that the alveolar bone is derived from alien connective tissue, it is by no means as certain that this is so for the entire periodontal ligament and cementum.

It is significant that Main (1966), in his culture studies of mouse tooth germs, found that when these were cultured on gelatin sponges for thirty-seven days they lost their characteristic morphology and appeared as a layer of undifferentiated epithelium on the sponge surface, with mesenchymal cells scattered throughout the interstices. When such late cultures were transplanted subcutaneously into isologous newborn recipients they developed into teeth of almost perfect shape and structure. On section such teeth were found to consist of normal dental tissues with perfectly formed dentine, predentine, odontoblasts, pulp cells and, significantly, cementum. Main points out that the tissues transplanted were undifferentiated epithelium and mesenchyme and that the mesenchyme must, in fact, have been ectomesenchyme. His photomicrograph of the base of the tooth germ developed from a transplanted culture features a prominent investing layer. This work suggests strongly the ectomesenchymal derivation of the investing layer and the cementum, and that both must be regarded as true dental tissues.

Embryological, histological, histochemical and experimental studies point to the distinctiveness of the tissue immediately encapsulating the developing tooth. The suitability of terming this tissue the inner layer of the follicle must therefore be questioned. On the contrary, the term dental follicle should be reserved for this layer as, along with the dental organ and dental papilla, it would seem to belong to the true dental tissues. Thus, the use of the word *dental* can be justified. Follicle is defined as a cocoon, and this too is an apt descriptive term for the investing layer. As it is proposed to limit the term *dental follicle* to the investing layer a term must be found for the mesodermal mesenchyme which is also involved in the formation of the periodontium. Relatively early in development alveolar bone is differentiated from this mesenchyme in relation to the developing tooth. From the evidence of Hoffman's transplanation studies this bone develops in response to the presence of the tooth germ. Where this inductive influence resides is not certain. The epithelial component of the tooth may possess this capability because of the known similar osteogenic inducing properties of other types of epithelium, especially bladder epithelium. The alveolar bone does not differentiate in contact with the tooth germ. A zone of loose mesenchyme is always retained between it and the investing layer and it is this mesenchyme which is normally designated as dental follicle. It is proposed that the term *perifollicular mesenchyme* be used instead. Tonge (1963) has described how, with growth of the alveolus, the peripheral perilaminar mesenchyme forms what is essentially the limiting layer of periosteum of the alveolus, with a vascular osteogenic zone between it and the forming bone. Thus, surrounding the early dental organ and dental papilla is the dental follicle of ectomesenchymal origin and the perifollicular mesenchyme of mesodermal origin, the periphery of which is condensed to form the periosteum of the alveolar bone. The nature and disposition of the investing tissues around the forming tooth at the stage where the crown is almost completely formed, and root formation far progressed, have already been described. Around the crown is the thick collagenous follicular layer, outside of which is successively a zone of loose mesenchyme, a periosteal zone, and finally the bone of the crypt. Around the root the follicular layer occupies an intermediate position, with loose mesenchyme followed by periosteum and then bone, on its outer aspect. On its inner aspect is cementum-forming-loose mesenchyme. It is from these tissues around the root that the functional periodontium is derived. The precise histological changes, and their timing, which bring about formation of the periodontal ligament, is in dispute.

III. The Formation of the Periodontal Ligament

A. COLLAGEN FIBRE FORMATION

The sequence of events resulting in establishment of the definitive periodontal ligament from the tissues surrounding the forming tooth germ is by no means clearly understood. There is no reason to suppose that the formation of the ligament fibres differs from fibre formation in other connective tissues as described in Chapter 6. Thomas (1965) has shown, in experiments involving the reconstitution of collagen from solutions of periodontium, that the ligament's collagen content is similar to skin connective tissue. The same author's radioactive tracer studies, in addition to those of Stallard (1966), indicate that metabolic events occurring in the periodontium, so far as the formation and maturation of collagen are concerned, are consistent with the findings of Harkness *et al.* (1954).

This concept of a viscous phase of the periodontium is probably important in the determination of the orientation of the fibre bundles. Weiss (1956) has provided evidence that fibroblast arrangement depends on the development of stress in the environment and, as pointed out in Chapter 4, root growth can provide an oblique stress sufficient to explain the oblique arrangement of fibres found in the developing periodontium of the pre-functional tooth. This latter statement, however, needs some qualification as the timing of this change is disputed. The oblique orientation of periodontal ligament fibres has been attributed to the axial load borne by the functional tooth (O'Brian, Bhaskar and Brodie, 1958) and to the resistance of the overlying tissues as the tooth erupts (Orban, 1957, Eccles, 1961). Thomas (1965) demonstrated in both human and rodent developing teeth an oblique orientation of periodontal ligament fibres concomitant with the onset of tooth eruption, and Tonge (1963) also showed this same occurrence in the developing cat's tooth. Furstman and Bernick (1965) claim that fibre orientation occurs at about the time of tooth eruption, but equate orientation with the formation of cementum on the root surface. There is general agreement that the appearance of fibres orientated in an oblique direction first occurs in the region of the cemento-enamel junction, probably at the onset of tooth eruption, and progresses apically (Tonge, 1963; Eccles, 1961). This has also been found in the material presented in this chapter (page 69). However, in this instance the first appearance of oblique fibres was not demonstrated until substantial root formation had occurred and it is difficult, therefore, to equate their appearance with the onset of tooth eruption. The causative factors bringing about the oblique orientation of the principal fibres of the periodontal ligament are therefore still not clear.

Although there is information on the formation of oblique fibres in the periodontal ligament, there is very little information on the development of the other fibre groups in this structure. It is not difficult to explain this lack of information with respect to primate development as there is an inherent difficulty in obtaining closely timed material for the study of successive stages of tooth eruption. An attempt has been made by Furstman and Bernick (1965) using the marmoset. They showed that

"before eruption all demonstrable fibres, *except those of the free gingival group*, are orientated in a superior oblique direction. With eruption of the tooth, the fibres join until they can be traced directly from the cementum to their ultimate attachment in the alveolar bone. With the continued eruption of the tooth, the oblique fibres at the alveolar crest region become more horizontal in orientation and some of these fibres become the transeptal and horizontal groups. The transeptal fibres do not become fully organized until both opposing teeth are in clinical occlusion. At this stage, fibres from one tooth pass towards the middle of the interproximal space to anastamose with the fibres arising from the cementum of the adjacent tooth. Once the teeth are in functional occlusion, these fibres become thicker and the interlacing fibres give the appearance of passing from tooth to tooth. Complete organization of the periodontal membrane fibre groups ordinarily is not achieved until the tooth reaches clinical occlusion with its antagonist."

This account has been quoted fully to emphasize the paucity of information available and to raise some queries. The first sentence referring to the free gingival fibres is difficult to comprehend. It is difficult to see how these fibres can exist before the tooth penetrates the oral epidermis. A close examination of the figures is also confusing. The first figure claims to illustrate the lack of organization in the ligament of an unerupted incisor yet the figure shows a tooth which has penetrated the oral mucosa. Even stranger is that an unerupted premolar is figured to show the organization of the oblique fibres of the periodontal ligament yet the following figure shows an erupting lower molar with no organization of the periodontal ligament. It appears therefore, that this description of periodontal ligament development is confusing and, until confirmatory work is available, the findings of Furstman and Bernick should perhaps be accepted with some reservation. The development of the fibre groups of the periodontal ligament is therefore a subject which requires further study.

B. OXYTALAN FIBRE FORMATION

Oxytalan fibres were first described by Fullmer and Lille (1958) and their properties and composition are dealt with in Chapter 6. As this chapter concerns the development of the periodontium only the development of oxytalan fibres is discussed here. The largest and most numerous oxytalan fibres are found in the transeptal region. Smaller fibres are present in the middle and apical thirds of the ligament. In deciduous teeth large oxytalan fibres are found lying free and orientated apico-occlusally.

Fullmer (1959) has investigated the development of oxytalan fibres in the human periodontal ligament. Oxytalan fibres are first found in relation to the forming periodontium adjacent and peripheral to the external dental epithelium. The time when these fibres appear is uncertain but a relationship to the developmental age of the tooth has been suggested. No oxytalan fibres could be demonstrated in the jaws of 6-month foetuses but they were demonstrable around the teeth of infants. It would seem that the location of oxytalan fibres corresponds to the thick collagenous layer surrounding the crown of the forming tooth. Fullmer states that with further development of the tooth "they (the oxytalan fibres) develop and proliferate lateral to Hertwig's epithelial root sheath as it progresses apically". Where Hertwig's epithelial root sheath had fragmented oxytalan fibres were observed embedded within the newly formed cementum.

It has also been pointed out by Fullmer that as the vascular system becomes established in the periodontium, oxytalan fibres extend from the adventitia to become attached to the teeth. Finally, in the functional periodontium, an increase in size of oxytalan fibres was noted. It is evident that knowledge concerning development of these fibres in the periodontal ligament is still fairly scanty and also that, although a relationship between oxytalan fibres and areas of stress has been postulated, their function is still enigmatic.

C. THE INTERMEDIATE PLEXUS

There is general agreement that the fibre bundles of the periodontal ligament develop in relation to alveolar bone and cementum (Fischer, 1909; Sicher, 1923; Orban, 1927; Eccles, 1959 and 1964). Ultimately these fibre bundles meet in the middle of the forming ligament, and it is in part this union of separate fibre bundles which has generated the concept of an intermediate plexus. The concept of fibre bundles interdigitating in an intermediate plexus is useful to explain the changes which must occur in the periodontal ligament to accommodate rapid vertical eruption, mesial drift and occlusal attrition. However, its presence is disputed. In the author's opinion confusion arises because of the presence of an intermediate zone in the unorganized ligament which, if it persisted, would occupy the position of the intermediate plexus in the organized ligament.

1. The Intermediate Zone in the Unorganized Periodontal Ligament

Orban (1927) has observed that, in the periodontal ligament of human teeth before eruption, three zones are present. This concept has persisted in the literature. Thus, Provenza (1964) describes how, in the prefunctional stage of development, three zones can be recognized in the tissue surrounding the tooth: a peripheral periosteal zone which lies contiguous to the developing alveolar bone; an inner pericemental zone adjacent to the developing cementum; and, between the two, an intermediate zone characterized by collagen fibres in a more advanced stage of development. The literature, however, contains little comment on the establishment of these three zones. In tracing the ontogeny of the tissues surrounding the tooth it has been suggested that the intermediate zone of more mature collagen fibres is derived from the investing layer. On the other hand Tonge (1963) considers that this intermediate zone is formed from the layer of tissue related to forming alveolar bone. This layer is pushed away from the bone surface by the appearance of engorged blood vessels between it and the bone. Whatever the correct explanation, there is little doubt that fibres form on either side of this longitudinally arranged layer of collagen fibres (Tonge, 1963; Eccles, 1959, 1964) and the problem requiring an answer is whether this persists in the form of an intermediate plexus as the definitive ligament is organized.

2. The Intermediate Plexus in the Organized Periodontal Ligament

Orban (1962) states that

"the presence of an intermediate plexus is common to the periodontium of all mammalian teeth because they move occlusally by continuous eruption during their functional period and drift mesially or distally. Their movements necessitate a continued adaptive readjustment of the suspensory ligament. How conspicuous or inconspicuous this plexus is depends on the rate of eruptive movement."

This rather dogmatic assertion must be questioned, however, as so many workers have failed to demonstrate an intermediate plexus (reviewed by Zwarych and Quigley, 1965, and see Chapters 1 and 6). At this time it is debatable whether it is worth emphasizing the controversial nature of the plexus as recent studies using radioisotopes have shown (Stallard, 1966) that there is a differential rate of fibre formation in the periodontal ligament. In experimental studies the sequence of collagen formation in various portions of the monkey periodontium were observed following the injection of H^3-proline. All the connective tissue elements were labelled after one hour, the fibrillar portions after four hours. Evidence to support the belief that labelling occurred within collagen was provided by digesting sections with bacterial collagenase. (See Chapter 6, p. 325, for discussion of this technique.) Significantly, the pattern of labelling showed collagen formation taking place throughout the entire ligament and not confined to an intermediate zone or plexus. This indicates that new unit fibrils are incorporated into pre-existing collagen fibres as well as aggregating to form new fibres, and provides an explanation for the mechanism of readjustment occurring within the ligament during tooth movement, without having to postulate an intermediate plexus. If, as these studies indicate, the intermediate plexus is non-existent, the persistence of the intermediate zone need not be postulated. Nevertheless, further information on the fate of the intermediate zone would be desirable.

IV. The Development of Cementum

This subject has already been discussed briefly (p. 66) and is also dealt with in Chapter 6, and therefore requires no further elaboration in this chapter.

V. Alveolar Bone Formation

Similarly osteogenesis is dealt with elsewhere (Chapter 6) and is not discussed.

VI. The Development of the Blood Supply to the Periodontium

The demonstration of the periodontal vascular bed is usually accomplished by means of perfusion methods, and it must be stressed that such methods demonstrate the total vascular bed, not the functional vascular bed. The anatomy of vascular supply of the periodontium is fairly well understood and there is little disagreement regarding the distribution of the principal vessels (see also, Chapter 8, Section II). The main supply of the ligament is via the dental artery. This artery initially has an intrabony course and, in this situation, gives off an interalveolar artery and two interalveolar branches. Entering the periodontium apically two longitudinal periodontal arteries are given off and the artery then enters the pulp via the apical foramen. The interalveolar arteries give off branches as they ascend to the alveolar crest. These perforate the alveolar plate to supply the periodontal ligament. In addition, the blood supply of the gingiva contributes to the ligament via anastomosis in the marginal periodontium. The longitudinal arteries run parallel to the long axis of the tooth close to the alveolar socket wall. The perforating arteries entering the ligament have been shown by Birn (1966) to increase in number from tooth to tooth towards the posterior teeth and, in single rooted teeth, to be greatest in number in the gingival third of the ligament and least in the middle third. In multi-rooted teeth, there is a greater number of perforating arteries in the gingival third, but in the apical and middle thirds of the socket the numbers correspond. It is possibly significant that whereas Birn reports fewer perforating arteries in the anterior teeth, Kindlova (1965) found that vessels from the mucous membrane were greater anteriorly and supplied a major portion of the ligament. Both the longitudinal arteries and the perforating arteries give off branches which run towards the tooth and form capillaries arranged in a flat network of rather large irregular mesh. In the region of the horizontal fibres of the ligament this capillary plexus forms a narrow band from which arise coiled single capillaries which return to the same plexus. Also in this region anastomoses between ligament vessels and gingival vessels occurs. In the gingiva two differing micro-circulations have been described. Beneath the gingiva, facing the oral cavity, there is a loose capillary plexus from which capillary loops arch up towards the epithelium between the rete pegs. Beneath the crevicular and attachment epithelium, however, a different situation exists. Kindlova (1965) describes, in the monkey, tenuously looped capillaries with clearly coiled arterial parts encircling a thick venous limb, and has related this configuration with the maintenance of the junction between soft and hard tissues. On the other hand Egelberg (1966), using a different technique, was unable to demonstrate this configuration in the gingival connective tissue of man. Instead, he found that beneath the crevicular margin there is a rich capillary plexus arranged in a layer with no capillary loops. A loop arrangement was found only in the presence of gingival inflammation.

Kindlova has suggested that, on the basis of blood supply, the periodontium can be divided into three zones

    a. the periodontal ligament,

    b. the gingiva facing the oral cavity,

    c. the gingiva facing the tooth.

Whatever the minutiae of capillary configuration, it must be emphasized that anastomoses between all three networks have been demonstrated and that this possibly allows for a considerable collateral circulation in the supporting tissues of the tooth.

A venous network, or rete, exists in the apical region of the ligament. Its presence has been linked with the provision of a steady eruptive force (Bien, 1966) (Chapter 4).

Whilst much is known of the vascular architecture of the functioning supporting tissues, little is known of its development. There are ample references in the literature to the profuse vascularity of the tissues surrounding the early forming tooth, but no study has been made of vascular development at the time the supporting tissues are formed.

Gaunt (1959), in a careful study of the vascular supply to the dental lamina of the cat during early development, showed that capillary concentrations occurred within the mesenchyme of the jaw which heralded the sites of future tooth formation. With the onset of tooth formation, it was shown that the blood supply associated with the dental lamina and its surrounding mesenchyme consisted entirely of a capillary plexus running over the surface of the perilaminar mesenchyme. A greater density of capillaries was noted on the buccal aspect of this mesenchyme. At the bell stage of tooth development a functional division of the vascular system was noted. This followed the development of an artery supplying solely the papilla, the capillary plexus persisting to supply the tooth sac, lamina and external dental epithelium. Although it might have been expected that the proliferating dental lamina would have a copious blood supply, Gaunt's findings indicate that this is not so, and Stein (1909) has made similar observations in the calf and ox. It may be that the high glycogen content (Ten Cate, 1967) of the proliferating lamina cells compensates for this lack of blood supply. Gaunt has suggested that, during the earliest stage of tooth development, the invasive blood vessels are restrained by the perilaminar mesenchyme (forming the investing layer), thus forcing the development of a capillary plexus on its outer surface.

In the developing human tooth a rich capillary plexus is found in relationship with the investing layer. Vascular osteogenic tissue is also found in association with forming alveolar bone. In the loose connective tissue between the two no marked concentration of blood vessels has been found (Tonge, 1963).

The high capillary density found in relationship to alveolar bone is most likely associated with osteogenesis. The high capillary density in relation to the dental organ can tentatively be linked with its formative function. However, occasional references in the literature (Gaunt, 1959; Thomas, 1965) point to a greater capillary density on the buccal aspect of the dental organ, and this uneven distribution blurs the exact significance of this capillary bed.

Information is lacking on the development of the vascular architecture of the supporting tissues between the stage outlined above and the vascular bed of the mature periodontium. Further information on this question would be of value in testing the postulated relationship between the vascular bed and the mechanism of tooth eruption (Chapter 4). If the apical venous rete are related to the mechanism of tooth eruption it is important to know when these rete are established in relation to the onset of eruptive movement.

VII. The Nerve Supply of the Periodontium

It is surprising how little is known concerning the innervation of the periodontium, when its important functional role is considered (see Chapter 8). In 1936 Lewinsky and Stewart wrote that little was known on this subject, and described nerve bundles in the human periodontal ligament running from the apical region of the tooth towards the gum. These nerve bundles were reinforced by fasciculi which entered the ligament through foraminae in the alveolar process. Fibres were described leaving the main bundles, branching dichotomously, and finally breaking up into fine arborizations. Many fibres were found to end in small rounded bodies. No fibres were traced entering the cementum but nerve loops were described close to the cementum surface. In the same year Bradlaw (1936) described terminal coils in the monkey periodontal ligament. Lewinsky and Stewart (1937) have described slightly different features in the innervation of the cat periodontal ligament. Nerve fibres entering the ligament from the alveolar bone divided into two components, one component running apically, the other gingivally. Furthermore, two types of nerve fibre were described; thick fibres confined to the peripheral part of the ligament with special end organs at their termination, and finer nerve fibres passing deeper into the ligament.

Bernick (1952) has described the innervation of primary teeth in the monkey. His findings were generally similar with regard to the course and distribution of nerves in the ligament. However, Bernick has also reported the termination of nerve fibres within the cementum. His explanation for this finding was that the continuous deposition of cementum embeds nerve fibres of the periodontal ligament. Bernick was unable to demonstrate specialized nerve endings in the periodontal ligament.

The same author (Bernick, 1959) has attempted to demonstrate the development of periodontal innervation in the molar tooth of the rat. He found that the overall distribution of nerves in the ligament is similar to that found in man and that no sensory innervation is established until the ligament becomes functionally organized at the time of tooth eruption. Fearnhead (1959), although primarily interested in the innervation of dentine, studied the innervation of early developing human teeth. He showed that at the "bud to cap" stage of development "pioneering" nerve fibres are present within the jaws and that these fibres lie close to the tooth germ. However, in spite of their proximity to the base of the dental papilla the axes of the nerve fibres are orientated tangentially to the tooth germ and do not enter the dental papilla. The bending of the fibres suggested that they had either deviated in their course to avoid the growing tooth germ or that the tooth germ had pushed its way between groups of fibres already present. It is of special interest that Fearnhead found a particularly rich innervation of the follicle close to the outer dental epithelium. It is difficult not to comment on the similarity between pioneering capillaries and nerves. Both fail to penetrate the papilla in the early stages of development and both ramify profusely in the follicular tissue. The rich follicular innervation was so marked that the need for a full scale study of human material was called for by Fearnhead. Such a study has not yet materialized and, as with the development of the vascular supply, a hiatus exists in our knowledge between early developmental stages and the mature ligament with respect to innervation.

VIII. The Development of the Epithelial Attachment

It has been claimed that the onset of periodontal disease can occur at the time of, or shortly after, tooth eruption (Cohen, 1959) when the epithelial attachment is being formed. If this is so there is a clear necessity for an understanding of the genesis of the attachment.

McHugh (1961) stimulated renewed interest in the development of the attachment with a careful histological description of the development of the monkey gingival epithelium. Later histochemical studies (Ten Cate, 1963) and radiobiological studies (Engler, Ramfjord and Hiniker, 1965) have clarified and extended the results of McHugh's purely morphological studies. The following account is based mainly on the above three references.

Before the tooth erupts its enamel surface is covered by reduced dental epithelium consisting of two layers, an inner layer of columnar ameloblasts and an outer layer of polygonal cells most likely derived from the stratum intermedium. Connective tissue separates the dental epithelium and the overlying oral epithelium. This connective tissue is removed as the tooth erupts and the problems associated with its removal have been briefly discussed (p. 315) and are discussed more fully by Melcher (1967). There is no dispute that, as the dissolution of this connective tissue occurs, the cells of the outer layer of the reduced dental epithelium proliferate as do the basal cells of the overlying oral epithelium. Tritiated thymidine labelling has established this unequivocally. However, the factors which initiate this epithelial proliferation are still not clear. Interesting and worthwhile speculations can be made on this subject. Grupe, Jr., Ten Cate and Zander (1967) have reported the proliferation of epithelial cell rests in a closed culture system and have suggested that local anaerobic conditions may provide the initiating factor for epithelial proliferation. Certainly disturbance in the supporting connective tissue, initiated for example by wounding, radiation or infection, seems to result in epithelial proliferation. There is a disturbance of connective tissue over the erupting tooth and it can be argued, using circumstantial evidence, that the conditions in connective tissue are anaerobic as the result of strangulation of the vascular bed. Definitive measurements would be welcomed here. If such were the case, the proliferation of both dental and oral epithelium is a fortuitous, but essential response, for this epithelial proliferation permits the erupting tooth to pierce the integument without exposing the connective tissue. Whatever the factors initiating this epithelial response, the net result is that the proliferated epithelial cells form a knot over the erupting tooth, and it is from this knot of epithelial cells that the epithelium of the attachment is ultimately derived. It will be appreciated that the situation so far described applies only over the occlusal surface of the erupting tooth. Indeed, it is only over the occlusal surface that connective tissue need be removed physically. Around the sides of the crown there is no need for removal of connective tissue. Instead an adequate seal between epithelium and tooth needs to be established. The writer was responsible (1963) for suggesting that dental epithelium behaved differently in these differing locations. This suggestion was based on the study of erupting bicuspid and molar teeth. In this situation the dental epithelium at the cemento-enamel junction was found to present a similar histological appearance to that found on the occlusal surface of the tooth. As the dental epithelium was traced coronally both cell layers were found to undergo degenerative change with no proliferative activity on the part of the cells of the outer layer. Following this degenerative change, and further coronally, viable basal epithelial cells were found on the connective tissue surface of the reduced dental epithelium. These basal epithelial cells appeared to be proliferating apically. This is a situation obviously different from that described over the occlusal surface of the erupting tooth. The same description was given by Engler et al. (1965) where, in 42 sections containing over 18,000 cells, only one labelled cell was observed in the dental epithelium applied to the sides of the crown. Labelling was however, readily demonstrated in the basal epithelial cells on the connective tissue surface of the dental epithelium. Occasional labelled dental epithelial cells were found in the junctional zone. However, this report is also, so far as can be judged from the photomicrographs, based on the study of partially erupted bicuspid and molar teeth. It is difficult to reconcile these findings with those reported for the erupting incisor tooth. McHugh (1961) has described the histology here in detail, and has shown that as the dental epithelium overlying the incisal edge approaches the overlying oral epithelium, the outer layer of cells proliferate as they do when situated over the occlusal surface of bicuspid or molar teeth. This change is described as spreading gradually down to involve enamel (dental) epithelium covering the rest of the crown. A situation slightly different from that apparently occurring over a bicuspid or molar tooth.

It is also worth noting that, if the figures illustrating Engler *et al.* (1965) paper are studied, those showing the situation over the erupting cusp tip correspond to the figures of McHugh (1961). They show proliferative activity of dental epithelium in contact with the non-occlusal surface of the crown, although this situation is not apparent when dental epithelium of the erupting tooth is traced coronally from the cemento-enamel junction.

An explanation for these differences is suggested here, but it is emphasized that further substantive studies are required. The apparent proliferative response of dental epithelium to connective tissue breakdown has already been discussed. If the morphology of the erupting tooth is considered it is apparent that there must be disruption or distortion of the surrounding connective tissue until the greatest diameter of the tooth has reached the oral epithelium. Examination of published material shows that where proliferation of dental epithelium is described this is always on the occlusal side of the plane of maximum circumference. Whereas where degeneration of both layers is described, this is always in a situation apical to the maximum circumference where there is no distortion of the connective tissue.

Although it is of interest to establish the exact origin of the cells migrating down the connective tissue surface of the dental epithelium [they must originate from the plug of cells formed from the proliferated basal oral epithelial cells and outer layer cells] this is really only an academic point. Far more important is the fact that these cells have the characteristics of basal epithelial cells. It is from these cells that the "final" viable epithelial attachment is formed.

Of course, as the tooth is in its phase of active eruption, the attachment includes reduced dental epithelium. It is the replacement of the latter by the proliferating basal cells that establishes the final attachment. The time for this replacement to occur is not yet exactly established. In the monkey (McHugh, 1963) this exchange lasts more than three years for the permanent tooth whereas with deciduous teeth the time period is about four to five months (Engler *et al.*, 1965).

Cohen (1959) has described the interproximal col area as covered by reduced dental epithelium for some time after tooth eruption, the dental epithelium being derived from the juxtaposition of the dental epithelia of both teeth. This epithelium was regarded as "ill-fitted to act as a protective integument for the col" and that in "health this is normally replaced by

4

stratified squamous epithelium". It was suggested that "before this oral epithelium has contrived to replace the reduced enamel epithelium, the col may have suffered irreparable damage and an intra bony pocket may have become established". McHugh (1963) has also suggested that the functional zone between the downgrowing basal cells and dental epithelium is the area of greatest susceptibility because of the inflammatory response *always* present in the connective tissue of this region. Both these statements are contentious and require additional substantiation. Elaboration of this theme does not properly concern us here in a discussion of the development of the attachment but there is one possibility which may be pertinent.

It is usually suggested that the inflammatory response commonly found in the supporting connective tissue is the result of a defective epithelial insulation. This may well be an incorrect assumption. The proliferative activity of the outer layer cells of dental epithelium already discussed shows that it is erroneous to consider dental epithelium as effete. Furthermore, it has also been suggested that this epithelial proliferation occurs possibly in response to a defective supporting connective tissue. It could be argued that the compression and breakdown of connective tissue above the erupting tooth leads to a non-bacterial induced inflammatory response at the periphery of this compression zone. It is over this peripheral area of connective tissue that the epithelial attachment is subsequently formed. This connective tissue response could be responsible for not only the epithelial proliferation necessary for the genesis of the attachment but could also hinder the formation of a sound attachment. This, in turn, could permit the persistence of the disturbed supporting connective tissue by the ingress of "foreign" material through a defective epithelial covering.

It is appreciated that this suggestion is highly contentious and that much additional work is needed. However, the dependency of epithelium and supporting stroma is so well established that, if the development of the epithelial attachment is being considered, it cannot be divorced from the supporting connective tissue, and the hypothesis offered here serves to emphasize this relationship.

IX. Age Changes in the Periodontium

Studies on age changes in the periodontium are, on the whole, fairly inconclusive. As the supporting tissues of the tooth, except for the epithelial attachment, consist of connective tissue, it can be anticipated that age changes in the cellular, fibrillar and ground substance components of the periodontium will be similar to changes described in connective tissues elsewhere in the body. Thus general trends that may be sought within the ageing periodontium could include a decrease in the ratio of ground substance to collagen, a decrease in the amount of soluble collagen (Banfield, 1952), decrease in collagen turnover (Neuberger and Slack, 1963), decrease in water content and increased resistance to proteolytic enzymes (Keech, 1954). In the rat molar tooth periodontium Jensen and Toto (1958) have demonstrated a steadily decreasing number of DNA-synthesizing connective tissue cells with age. Toto and Borg (1968) studying the effect of age changes on the premitotic index in the periodontium of mice were able to show that the number of synthesizing cells was significantly greater in the younger animal and that there was also a greater number of cells capable of regeneration. Also, it was shown that the cells of the periodontal ligament of old mice do not renew as rapidly as they do in young mice.

If, however, we consider the periodontium as the specialized supporting tissue of the tooth, changes occur with age which are distinctive to this structure. Most attention has been paid to the apical progression of the epithelial attachment, as for this progressive shift to occur there must also be loss of periodontal ligament and alveolar bone. This triad of events can, and does, lead to the loss of the tooth.

Controversy centres on this apical shift of the epithelial attachment and there are two questions which provide the focus for argument. First, is this shift a natural physiological phenomenon or does it only occur in the presence of inflammatory change? Second, do the epithelial cells of the attachment bring about the coincident loss of connective tissue or is there proliferation secondary to the loss of connective tissue?

It is this author's contention that the apical shift of the attachment is a secondary phenomenon occurring in response to primary factors, principally inflammatory change, in the supporting connective tissue. As Miles (1961) has stated "even if it is accepted that gingival recession is related to age, it does not necessarily follow that recession is the result of a physiological ageing process, that is a process 'built in' to the organism". Miles was of the opinion that gingival recession was the result of "repeated accounts with hard or tough foodstuffs". This is an important point for it serves to emphasize that inflammatory change need not necessarily be bacterial in origin. Indeed Baer and Fitzgerald (1964) have shown the occurrence of periodontal disease in gnotobiotic animals, is usually associated with hair or food impaction. It is true that these workers also found epithelial migration some distance away from areas of impaction but examination of the photomicrograph illustrating this also seems to show some connective tissue disturbance.

Cementum deposition continues within the periodontium throughout life. Zander and Hürzeler (1958) were able to show a straight line relationship between age and cementum thickness although, the rate of cementum deposition was not the same for every area of the tooth. It was less near the cemento-enamel junction and more in the apical area.

The epithelial cell rests within the periodontal ligament decrease with age (Reeve, 1960). The significance of this cannot be clarified until a function, if any, can be found for these structures.

So far as the writer is aware, no studies of the effects of age on periodontal circulation and innervation have been undertaken.

References

Baer, P. N. and Fitzgerald, R. J. (1964). *J. dent. Res.* **45**, 406.
Banfield, W. G. (1952). *Anat. Rec.* **114**, 157–171.
Bernick, S. (1952). *Anat. Rec.* **113**, 215–234.
Bernick, S. (1959). *Anat. Rec.* **133**, 91–104.
Bien, S. M. (1966). *Trans. N.Y. Acad. Sci.* **28**, 496–506.
Birn, H. (1966). *J. periodont. Res.* **1**, 51–68.
Bradlaw, R. (1936). *Proc. R. Soc. Med.* **29**, 507–518.
Cohen, B. (1959). *Br. dent. J.* **107**, 31–39.
Dalcq, A. M. (1953). *C. r. Séanc. Soc. Biol., Paris* **147**, 2038–2040.
Diab, M. A. and Stallard, R. E. (1965). *Periodontics* **3**, 10–14.
Eccles, J. D. (1959). *Dent. Practner* **10**, 31–35.
Eccles, J. D. (1961). *Dent. Practner* **11**, 153–157.
Eccles, J. D. (1964). *Archs. oral. Biol.* **9**, 127–133.
Egelberg, J. (1966). *J. Periodont. Res.* **1**, 163–179.
Engler, W. O., Ramfjord, S. P. and Hiniker, J. J. (1965). *J. Periodont.* **36**, 44–57.
Fearnhead, R. W. (1959). M.D.S. Thesis. Univ. of London.
Fearnhead, R. W. (1961). *J. dent. Res.* **40**, 1278.
Fischer, G. (1909). *In* "Ban und Entwicklung der Mundhohle des Menschen". Klinkhardt. Leipzig.
Fullmer, H. M. (1959). *J. dent. Res.* **38**, 510–518.
Fullmer, H. M. and Lille, R. D. (1958). *J. Histochem Cytochem.* **6**, 425–430.
Furstman, L. and Bernick, S. (1965). *Am. J. Orthod.* **51**, 482–489.
Gaunt, W. A. (1959). *Acta. Anat.* **37**, 232–252.
Gaunt, W. A. and Miles, A. E. W. (1967). In "Structural and Chemical Organization of Teeth" (A. E. W. Miles, ed.), Vol. 1, pp. 151–197. Academic Press, New York, U.S.A.
Grupe, H. E. Jr., Ten Cate, A. R. and Zander, H. A. (1967). *Archs. oral Biol.* **12**, 1321–1329.
Harkness, R. D., Marko, A. M., Muir, H. M. and Neuberger, A. (1954). *Biochem J.* **56**, 558–569.
Hodson, J. J. (1966). *Int. dent. J.* **16**, 350–384.
Hoffman, R. L. (1960). *J. dent. Res.* **39**, 781–798.
Jensen, J. L. and Toto, P. D. (1968). *J. dent. Res.* **47**, 149–153.
Keech, M. K. (1954). *Yale J. biol. Med.* **23**, 295–306.
Kindlová, M. (1965). *Archs. oral. Biol.* **10**, 869–874.
Lewinsky, W. and Stewart, D. (1936). *J. Anat. (Lond.)* **71**, 98–102.
Lewinsky, W. and Stewart, D. (1937). *J. Anat. (Lond.)* **71**, 232–235.
Listgarten, M. A. (1966). *Archs. oral. Biol.* **11**, 999–1016.
Main, J. H. P. (1965). *Archs. oral. Biol.* **10**, 343–351.
Main, J. H. P. (1966). *Science* **152**, 778–780.
McHugh, W. D. (1961). *Dent. Pract.* **11**, 314–324.
McHugh, W. D. (1963). *Periodontics* **1**, 239–244.
Melcher, A. H. (1967). *In* "The Mechanisms of Tooth Support" (D. J. Anderson, J. E. Eastoe, A. H. Melcher and D. C. Picton, eds), pp. 94–97. Wright, Bristol, England.
Milaire, J. (1959). *Archs. Biol. Liège* **70**. 587–730.

Miles, A. E. W. (1961). *In* "Structural Aspects of ageing" (G. H. Bourne, ed.). Pitman Medical, London, England.

Neuberger, A. and Slack, H. G. B. (1963). *J. biol. Med.* **23**, 295–306.

O'Brian, C., Bhaskar, S. H. and Brodie, A. G. (1958). *J. dent. Res.* **37**, 467–484.

Orban, B. J. (1927). *In* "Die Fortschritte der Zahnheilkunde" (J. Mische, ed.), **3**, 749.

Orban, B. J. (1928). *J. Am. dent. Assoc.* **15**, 1004–1016.

Orban, B. J. (1957). "Oral Histology and Embryology." The C. V. Mosby Company, St. Louis, U.S.A.

Orban, B. J. (1962). "Orban's Oral Histology and Embryology" (H. Sicher, ed.) C. V. Mosby Company, St. Louis, U.S.A.

Paynter, K. J. and Pudy, G. (1958). *Anat. Rec.* **131** (2): 233–251.

Pourtois, M. (1961). *Arch. Biol. Liège* **72**, 17–95.

Provenza, D. V. (1964). "Oral Histology, Inheritance and Development." Pitman Medical, London, England.

Reeve, M. (1960). *J. dent. Res.* **39**, 746.

Robb-Smith, A. H. T. (1957). *In* "Connective Tissue." A Symposium (R. E. Tunbridge, ed.), pp. 177–183. Blackwell, Oxford, England.

Schour, I. and Massler, M. (1940). *J. Am. dent. Assoc.* **27**, 1178.

Scott, J. H. (1953). *Dent. Practner* **3**, 345–350.

Scott, J. H. and Symons, N. B. B. (1964). "Introduction to Dental Anatomy." E. & S. Livingstone Ltd., Edinburgh and London.

Sellman, S. (1946). *Odont. Tidskr.* **54**, 1–128.

Selvig, K. A. (1963). *Acta. odont. scand.* **21**, 175–186.

Selvig, K. A. (1964). *Acta. odont. scand.* **22**, 105–120.

Selvig, K. A. (1965). *Acta. odont. scand.* **23**, 423–441.

Sicher, H. (1923). *Z. Stomat.* **21**, 580.

Sicher, H. (1942a). *J. dent. Res.* **21**, 201–210.

Sicher, H. (1942b). *J. dent. Res.* **21**, 295–402.

Stallard, R. E. (1966). Paper presented to the 54th Annual Session. F.D.I. 1966.

Stein, J. B. (1909). *Items of Interest* **31**, 1 and 81.

Ten Cate, A. R. (1957). Ph.D. Thesis. Univ. of London.

Ten Cate, A. R. (1963). *Archs. oral. Biol.* **8**, 755–763.

Ten Cate, A. R. (1965). *Archs. oral Biol.* **10**, 207–213.

Ten Cate, A. R. (1967). *In* "The Mechanisms of Tooth Support" (J. D. Anderson, J. E. Eastoe, A. H. Melcher and D. C. A. Picton, eds.), pp. 80–83. Wright, Bristol, England.

Thomas, N. R. (1965). Ph.D. Thesis. Bristol University.

Tonge, C. H. (1963). Trans. European Orth. Soc. 1–9.

Toto, P. D. and Borg, M. (1968). *J. dent. Res.* **47**, 70–73.

Weinmann, J. P., Svoboda, J. F. and Woods, R. W. (1945). *J. Am. dent. Assoc.* **32**, 397–418.

Weiss, P. (1956). Symposium on wound healing and tissue repair. (W. B. Patterson, ed.), pp. 1–7. University of Chicago Press, N.Y., U.S.A.

Zander, H. A. and Hürzeler, B. (1958). *J. dent. Res.* **37**, 1035–1044.

Zwarych, P. D. and Quigley, M. B. (1965). *J. dent. Res.* **44**, 383–391.

4 | The Mechanism of Tooth Eruption

*A. R. TEN CATE

*Unit of Anatomy in Relation to Dentistry, Anatomy Department,
Guy's Hospital Medical School, London, England*

I. Introduction

Much has been written on the mechanism of tooth eruption, and this serves to underline the complexity of the subject. The justification for another contribution to the literature might be questioned, especially as an excellent review on tooth eruption has only recently been published (Ness, 1964). However, work undertaken in this field since 1964 has produced interesting and provocative results which require critical and independent evaluation. Thus, this chapter will deal only with those theories of tooth eruption pertinent to work since 1964.

The generally accepted definition of eruption is the process of migration of the tooth from its intra-osseous location to its functional position within

---

* Present address: Faculty of Dentistry, University of Toronto, Toronto, Canada

the oral cavity (Massler and Schour, 1941). This definition embraces movements of the tooth in all planes. However, for the purposes of this discussion, only movement in an occlusal direction will be considered. It cannot be denied that the crux of the problem of tooth eruption resides in identifying the factors producing movement of the tooth in this direction. Thomas (1965) has confirmed that, during the early developmental stages, migratory movements of the tooth occur until it becomes confined in a bony crypt. One of the components of these movements is in an occlusal direction. From this time, until the onset of root formation, the tooth germ and its follicle was shown to expand equally in all directions, and this was accompanied by uniform and circumferential resorption of the bone lining the crypt. With the onset of root formation this pattern of growth was found to change. Shortly after commencement of root formation, movement of the tooth in an occlusal direction can be detected, and it is the forces responsible for this movement which are discussed.

All the tissues involved in formation of the dental alveolar complex have, at some time or another, been implicated with tooth eruption, usually on the basis of histological study. However, histological changes demonstrable as the tooth erupts are just as likely to result from, and not in, tooth movement. The most striking histological changes that occur as the tooth undergoes rapid occlusal movement are those associated with formation of the root.

II. The Root

Proliferation of Hertwig's epithelial root sheath from the cervical loop of the dental organ is usually taken to herald the onset of root formation. It is this epithelial structure that is responsible for inducing the differentiation of the odontoblasts from the undifferentiated mesenchymal cells of the dental papilla. These newly differentiated odontoblasts form root dentine. It is evident that proliferation of papillary mesenchyme must coincide with, if not precede, root sheath proliferation. Downgrowth of Hertwig's root sheath (Brodie, 1934), dentine apposition with a concomitant reduction in pulp volume, and pulpal proliferation (Pierce, 1887), have each been considered to provide the eruptive force. From the histological standpoint it is easy to understand why each of the above occurrences, all associated with formation of the root, have been linked with tooth eruption; each could reasonably be suspected of effecting movement in an occlusal direction. Jenkins (1966) has written that, while there is considerable evidence that root growth is not essential for eruption, it is difficult to prove that under normal conditions root growth plays no part in the process. This may be a result of the complexity of root formation involving, as it does, the growth of several unlike tissues. Nevertheless, if epithelial proliferation, pulpal proliferation and dentine formation are each considered separately, and also together, none can be shown assuredly to provide the eruptive force.

A. Growth of Hertwig's Root Sheath

Experimental removal of Hertwig's root sheath (Herzberg and Schour, 1941) fails to prevent tooth eruption. This finding alone would seem to mitigate against root sheath proliferation as an eruptive force. Ness (1964), however, has argued cogently that epithelial proliferation of this nature could provide an axial force. A parallel is drawn with the growing hair, where it is accepted that growth of epithelial cells generates a force which reacts against the dermis. Ness argues that the anatomical configuration of the cervical loop permits epithelial cells to react against themselves, pushing new cells away to form either ameloblasts or cells of the external dental epithelium. Although fully aware that epithelial proliferation could not be the sole source of an eruptive force, because of the results of extirpation experiments, he makes the point that epithelial proliferation can provide an axial force. It must be admitted that this is no more than ingenious speculation. Even if growth of the root sheath provides an eruptive force, this force cannot be sustained as the root sheath fragments rapidly once its organizing function is completed, thereby losing its connection with the dental organ.

B. Dentine Formation and Pulp Constriction

The critical experiment involving removal of Hertwig's root sheath also mitigates against dentine formation providing the force for tooth eruption. Furthermore, hypophysectomy, which results in increased dentine deposition (Baume, Becks and Evans, 1954), retards eruption.

C. Pulpal Proliferation

Ness (1964) believes that growth of pulpal connective tissue can in no way provide an independent force. Ness's view has been supported by the findings of Main and Adams (1966), who investigated the effect of antimitotic drugs on the rate of eruption of the rat incisor. When demecolcine was used to prolong the metaphase of dividing cells, no slowing in the rate of eruption could be detected. In contrast to the temporary effect of demecolcine, triethylene melamine halts growth. Its introduction into the experimental animal causes a complete loss of cellularity in the proliferative zone below the enamel organ and Hertwig's root sheath. Yet, even after such severe cellular damage, eruption still proceeds, though at a reduced rate. The finding of spaces, totally lacking in cells, in the bases of the pulps led Main and Adams to the conclusion that tooth movement could not be the result of pressures produced by cellular proliferation. An interesting observation made in this study was that there was "a loss of cell density, but not of cellular continuity, in the periodontal membrane" after exposure to tri-ethylene melamine. This particular observation is significant in the context

4*

of recent work, discussed below, pointing to the periodontal ligament as the tissue providing the force of eruption.

D. ROOT GROWTH

Finally, if root growth is considered as a single entity incorporating growth of the root sheath, dentine formation, and pulpal proliferation, the classical observations that some teeth erupt along a path longer than the total length of the root (Baume, 1872) and that rootless teeth erupt, give further cause to abandon the concept of root growth as the prime force of tooth eruption.

III. Bone Growth

The bone of the jaws undergoes extensive remodelling during growth, and much of this takes place while the teeth are erupting. It has been suggested that remodelling of bone causes tooth movement in two ways. First, bone deposition in the fundus of the socket may push the tooth from the socket, and second, growth of alveolar bone may pull the tooth from its socket via attached periodontal fibres.

Some of the reported observations concerning bone deposition at the base of the socket are slightly at variance, but these are not significant relative to tooth movement. Manson (1967) used tetracycline labelling to study bone deposition around the tooth in cats and rats in groups from birth to maturity. He found that there is a slow deposition of bone on the lower border of the jaw associated with resorptive activity at the bottom of the molar crypts while these teeth have roots with open apices. This finding implies that neither root growth nor bone growth is directly involved in tooth movement. Only after closure of the root apices does bone deposition occur on the socket floor. These findings have been equated loosely with the findings of Carlson (1944) who showed, by means of serial cephalometric radiographs of children, that there is a definite downward movement of the root as root growth began. However, during the period of rapid eruption of the tooth, all parts of the tooth show an increased distance from the lower border of the jaw and, when the tooth reaches its occlusal position, the root end again moves nearer to the lower border of the mandible. The equation by Manson is therefore not really justified. Nevertheless, neither study implicates bone growth as the prime mover of the tooth. Thomas (1965) has also studied bony remodelling in this region in man and rats using radiographic and histological methods. In the radiographic study, the inferior dental canal instead of the lower border of the mandible, was utilized as a fixed marker as this was shown to be a more stable reference point. The findings of both Manson and Carlson were confirmed in that resorption of fundic bone was demonstrated with the onset of root formation. Bone resorption was, however, only transient for, as the tooth entered its rapid phase of eruption (slightly after the onset of root formation), bone deposition was found to occur on the socket floor. Thomas has also demonstrated that the tooth erupts a distance equivalent to the amount of bone deposited on the socket floor, plus the amount of root formed during this rapid phase of eruption. Although this relationship would seem to implicate both bone growth and root growth as prime factors in tooth eruption, it does not mean that either provides the force of eruption. Indeed, the fact that as eruption begins there is bony resorption at the base of the socket indicates that neither root growth nor bone deposition provides the force of eruption.

The formation of alveolar crestal bone has also been considered to move teeth by pulling them from their sockets by means of the attached periodontal ligament fibres. For any credence to be given to this suggestion it must be shown that the ligament fibres are attached to both tooth and bone at the time of tooth eruption and this has not been demonstrated satisfactorily.

IV. Intervening Connective Tissue

If, as seems likely, root growth and bone growth cannot be directly implicated as prime movers of the tooth, the only remaining tissue which can be responsible is the intervening connective tissue. As a result of their findings, Main and Adams (1966) were forced to conclude that

"although the explanation of the process whereby the tooth moves through the surrounding tissues remains to be found, it has been suggested recently by Kostlan *et al.* (1960) that the mechanism of this process probably lies in the periodontal ligament. Experimental evidence in support of this hypothesis is lacking but it is felt that studies on this tissue may prove fruitful in efforts to solve the problem of tooth eruption."

Such evidence is no longer lacking. As a result of his preliminary studies Thomas (1965), like Main and Adams, was forced to the conclusion that the connective tissue surrounding the developing tooth must play the primary role in tooth eruption, and his subsequent work explored this possibility. It is therefore necessary to demonstrate that within the elements of the forming ligament some system exists which is capable of generating a force sufficient to move the tooth. On theoretical grounds it can be argued that such systems do exist.

A. THE PHYSICAL CONSISTENCY OF THE FORMING PERIODONTAL LIGAMENT

The extracellular compartment of young connective tissue has the consistency of a viscous gel organized as a heterogeneous colloid. Although the constituents of the extracellular compartment of young connective tissue from different locations may differ slightly in composition, it is reasonable to suppose that the young connective tissue forming the periodontal ligament does not differ significantly from similar young connective tissue elsewhere in the body. A similar conclusion was reached by Zerlotti (1964) in his study of pulp tissue of forming teeth. Assuming that the forming periodontal ligament has a viscous consistency, it has been argued by Thomas that with downgrowth of Hertwig's epithelial root sheath, root and pulpal tissue, flow must be introduced within the periapical gel. As there is an initial resorption of bone at the base of the socket associated with the onset of root growth, it can be deduced that flow lines developing within the gel as a result of root growth, will run obliquely upwards and outwards away from the downgrowing root. An analogous situation used by Thomas to explain this system was that of drawing a matchstick through treacle. In this instance flow lines develop in the region of the head end of the match and pass backwards and obliquely outwards in a direction opposite to that of the moving match. The flow lines develop because of friction (viscosity) between the molecules of treacle. Also the treacle develops storage energy due to the decrease in entropy of its constituent molecules. This means that when the force pushing the match through the treacle is withdrawn, the release of this storage energy causes the match to recoil. Thomas has suggested that it is possible that a similar sequence of events takes place in the periapical gel. It must be remembered that the consistency of periapical gel does not remain constant as does the treacle. Large macromolecules, the forerunners of collagen fibres, are being added to the periapical gel continuously by the fibroblasts of the forming ligament. The effect of this increasing number of macromolecules, and increased cross-linkage between the macromolecules already assembled as fibrils, within the periapical gel will be to increase its viscosity. Thus, as root growth continues in a linear fashion, and as the viscosity rises to a critical level, the tension generated will also reach a critical level and possibly bring about tooth movement as a recoil phenomenon. In theory, therefore, there is no need to postulate any connection between the elements of the forming ligament and the tooth, or for that matter bone.

This postulate seems, at first, very plausible for it would explain why initially bone resorption occurs at the base of the socket under pressure from the growing root, and is later followed by bone deposition as this pressure is removed and possibly replaced by tension. It could also explain the characteristic oblique alignment of the fibroblasts in the forming periodontal ligament. Weiss (1956) has shown that fibroblasts are aligned along lines of stress in the extracellular environment; the hypothetical flow lines developing in the apical region of the forming root coincide with the alignment of the fibroblasts in the periodontal ligament. However, before this postulate can be accepted, experimental evidence must be provided to substantiate it further, and one or two apparently contradictory facts must also be re-examined. Experimental evidence is presented later in this account, for the concept of flow in the periapical gel is intimately linked with another possible generator of force within the forming ligament, fibrillogenesis, which is best discussed first.

Before doing so it must be pointed out that, theoretically, once the recoil force has developed and the tooth starts its movement in an occlusal direction, the force will be expended. Thus, if tooth movement is to be maintained, energy must be restored to the system by further root growth and repetition of the whole cycle of events. It might be anticipated, therefore, that tooth movement would be phasic and that alternating bone resorption and deposition would be found at the base of the socket. There is some evidence that the latter may occur, as histological examination of this region demonstrates simultaneous bone resorption and deposition taking place. At any one time resorption may predominate, or vice versa, at a level not demonstrable in gross studies. Even so, the results of extirpation experiments, already quoted, present the biggest single drawback to this thesis for, with the lack of root formation, the development of flow lines within the periapical gel is precluded.

B. Fibrillogenesis in the Forming Ligament

Chapter 6 deals with collagen formation in detail. All that need be said here is that the fibroblasts synthesize and presumably secrete collagen macromolecules, which are in the form of three polypeptide chains hydrogen bonded together in a triple helix, known as tropocollagen. The tropocollagen macromolecules are secreted into the extracellular compartment where at first they are in solution. Polymerization of these macromolecules into fibrous form occurs in the extracellular compartment. Thomas (1965) has suggested that several opportunities exist during this process of polymerization for the development of a force sufficient to cause tooth eruption.

It may be assumed that, when the tropocollagen macromolecules are secreted into the extracellular compartment, they exist in a relatively disordered state due to their free mobility. These macromolecules are involved in Brownian movement. As a result, they approach each other and become aligned in a state of order (a decrease in entropy), especially as the concentration of macromolecules increases with continuing synthesis. The lines of stress allegedly present in the periapical gel also have the effect of ordering the macromolecules of tropocollagen. Thomas has argued that this decrease in disorder of the tropocollagen macromolecules will produce a force along the axis of the orientating fibres to prevent the macromolecules from returning to their disordered state. Although the mechanism whereby the intricate ordering of the tropocollagen macromolecules may be disputed, there is certainly a decrease in entropy demanding in turn a restrictive force.

Whatever the mechanism bringing about the aggregation of tropocollagen, the system of aggregated macromolecules eventually becomes stabilized by the formation of covalent cross-links, not only intramolecularly between the chains in a single helix, but also intermolecularly between those in adjacent helices. During this phase of stabilization it has been demonstrated that there is a decrease of over 10% of the molecular length of the tropocollagen unit (Olsen, 1963). To this contraction can also be added a shrinkage factor due to dehydration as lateral aggregation of the adjacent helices takes place (Tomlin and Worthington, 1956). Thus, during collagen fibril formation tension may develop due to a decrease in entropy during electrostatic attraction of disordered tropocollagen macromolecules and alignment along lines of stress; to linear polymerization producing a decrease in length of macro-molecules, and to shrinkage due to dehydration. It can be postulated that tension arising from these sources will, once the fibres of the periodontal ligament have gained attachment to both alveolar bone and cement, be dissipated in the form of tooth movement. In other words traction of the tooth from its socket.

1. Testing the Hypotheses

It is evident from the discussion so far that all the forces theoretically capable of being generated in the forming periodontal ligament depend in part upon the formation of cross-linkages between the tropocollagen macro-molecules. Thus, the development of the recoil force in the periapical gel depends not only upon the number of macromolecules but also on their degree of polymerization. The tensile force resulting from decreased entropy as linear aggregation of macromolecules occurs along lines of stress in the gel depends, for its transmission between the fixed bone surface and the mobile tooth, upon the development of cross-linkages in the forming fibres. Finally, the contraction of collagen during its polymerization also depends on cross-linkages.

Lathyritic agents exert their effect by preventing the formation of both inter- and intra-molecular cross-linkages. Thomas (1965) has utilized this property of lathyritic agents to provide evidence in favour of his postulates. Rats were used as experimental animals and the administration of lathyrogen was found to retard the eruption rate severely when compared with pair-fed control animals. On histological examination it was found that the normal oblique orientation of the cells and the fibroblasts in the periodontium was absent. Instead the fibroblasts were arranged "in the form of horizontal palisades around lakes of mainly amorphous areas". The small amount of collagen demonstrable in these amorphous areas was arranged in a highly disordered fashion. Although the normal architecture of the periodontal ligament was grossly disturbed, root formation did not seem to be affected by the lathyritic agent. Continued growth of the roots and pulpal tissue during the experimental period resulted in the growing root impinging on the fundic bone, causing its resorption with synchronous buckling of the root. Hertwig's root sheath was found to have proliferated across the open base of the tooth. The predentine and the pulpal tissue, and significantly, the blood vascular elements, appeared normal. An accumulation of bone along the external surface of the alveolar crest was found, and continuing deposition of bone along the alveolar walls produced ankylosis as a late feature. In addition, exostoses at muscle insertions and joints indicated that, under the given experimental conditions, bone formation occurred where there was an adequate stimulus.

Thus the experimental prevention of inter- and intra-molecular cross-linkages during collagen formation in the periodontal ligament gives results consistent with the postulates put forward by Thomas. A question which needs to be answered is why, in this particular experimental situation, the lathyritic agent apparently affects only collagen formed in the periodontal ligament and not the collagen formed in newly deposited dentine and alveolar bone. It is possible that dentine and bone collagen differs from the collagen of the forming ligament. Dentine collagen is known to be much more stable than any soft tissue collagens; it contains little or no extractable components and, unlike soft tissue collagens, does not swell significantly in acid solutions (Eastoe, 1967). Less is known about the stability of bone collagen, but it may be intermediate between that of dentine and skin. Significantly, a recent development has been the recognition of unusual types of cross-linkages between the polypeptide chains of the collagen in bone, dentine and cementum. The studies of Armstrong and Horsley (1967) have demonstrated a bright blue fluorescence associated with the organic matrices of calcified tissue which, it is believed, represents a distinct molecular species firmly bonded to collagen and possibly constituting cross-linkage sites within the molecule. Eastoe (1967) has suggested that the dentine collagen has an additional set of cross-links involving phosphorylserine and carbohydrate. It would certainly seem that there are differences between hard and soft tissue collagens, and that these differences probably reside at the level of the cross-linkages. However (Golub et al., 1967) have shown that lathyritic agents can affect the cross-linkages of bone collagen and, moreover, Barrington and Meyer (1966) have reported lathyritic changes in alveolar bone and cementum. The latter study, however, revealed that the periodontal ligament was the first to show evidence of lathyritic damage. It may be that the degree of lathyritic damage is the significant factor, and that the soft tissue collagens have a lower threshold to the lathyritic agent than the hard tissue collagens.

On the basis of Thomas's postulates, for eruption to be maintained, it is necessary for the forming periodontal ligament to have a rapid turnover of collagen. Radiobiological studies of the periodontium in rats, rabbits and monkeys (Thomas, 1965; Stallard, 1966) indicate that collagen synthesis is continuous in the periodontal ligament of an erupting tooth. The isolation of collagen components from the periodontal ligament (Thomas and Poole, 1965) also reveals the presence of collagen sub-units in varying degrees of polymerization. These findings imply that collagen fibres in the forming ligament are continually broken down and reformed. The mechanism of collagen breakdown is controversial. Thomas has proposed that in the ligament during tooth eruption

> "the stress across the periodontium results in the oblique orientation of the periodontal fibroblasts. The collagen deposited across the periodontium becomes cemented to the surface of the root on one side and the bone surface on the other. As the tooth erupts so the periodontal space increases and the collagen sub-units must 'snap' apart since the resultant of the contraction of the obliquely orientated collagen is perpendicular to the fibre axis. While a hydrogen bond can offer considerable resistance to a force acting along its axis, separation by as little as $1°$ A in a direction at right angles to the bond axis will cause its complete breakdown (Rice, 1959)."

This argument is not entirely valid, for as soon as the tooth moves, tension in the ligament must be dissipated. If the tension is such as to fracture cross-linkages, it is difficult to visualize how it can bring about simultaneous tooth movement.

It is more likely that the periodontal ligament behaves as other soft connective tissues undergoing remodelling (see Chapter 6) but this too is a highly debatable subject. Lapiere (1967) has written

> "the correlation between the amount of collagenese activity produced in tissue culture and the advancement of the resorbing process is the only direct evidence available to indicate the possible relevance of such demonstrable collagenolytic activity to collagen breakdown *in vivo*."

However, hydrolases and cathepsins are known to increase in amount during tissue resorption and, as such enzymes are involved in the removal of different tissue proteins, they may be involved, after the limited activity of a specific collagenase, in the complete lysis of the collagen molecule to dialysable peptides and free amino acids. Even though there is this inability to demonstrate specific collagenase activity in remodelling connective tissue, collagen synthesis seems to occur even when the connective tissue is in the steady state. Lapiere (1967) has concluded that when

> "the tissues are in a steady state it seems that a large amount of the newly synthesized collagen is degraded before its incorporation into the most ordered fibrous structures. Remodelling induces an increased incorporation of the newly synthesized collagen into the most stable fibres and a simultaneous increment of the amount of neutral salt extractable collagen which seems to be derived from pre-existing structures. This process can be interpreted as a replacement procedure

using the newly formed collagen molecules as a highly efficient means for building new structures while the pre-existent framework is progressively removed."

Thus, there could be sufficient collagen synthetic activity to account for the generation of a continuous eruptive force.

Therefore, although there are still several pertinent queries concerning Thomas's proposed mechanism of eruption, there is sufficient experimental evidence to warrant serious consideration of the hypothesis that collagen metabolism provides the force required to move the tooth, at least until more positive evidence becomes available to support the alternative theories of tooth eruption.

C. THE CELLS

Recently, Ness (1967) has expressed the idea that the fibroblasts of the periodontal ligament are the agents of force producing eruptive movement. His arguments are teleological and tenuous, and could support Thomas's hypothesis equally well. Thus, Ness argues that if the periodontium is a passive agent, a Newtonian equation can be applied to its quasi-viscous flow:

$$\text{Velocity of eruption} = \frac{\text{Eruptive force} \times \text{thickness of periodontium}}{\text{Area (volume) of periodontium} \times \text{viscosity}}$$

As the unimpeded eruption rate of the mouse and elephant incisor is quoted as roughly the same and, as the thickness and viscosity coefficient are not disparate, because the area (volume) factor differs by about 10,000 times so must the eruptive force. On this basis, a pushing force such as growth of odontogenic cell layers increasing proportionately with tooth circumference, must be inadequate. On the other hand, if the force resides in the periodontium, its proportionate increase in volume would give an increased force sufficient to move the elephant incisor. The tusk of the Narwhal, *Monodon monoceros*, rotates in its socket as it is extruded. Ness argues that it is difficult to equate a pushing force, such as pulpal hydrostatic pressure, with such a rotatory movement. Instead, Ness proposes fibroblasts pulling the tooth, with the fibroblasts sitting on spirally arranged fibre planes. Both Ness's arguments, however, are just as applicable to collagen metabolism in the ligament as they are to fibroblast contraction. The only evidence Ness could find to support the contention that the fibroblasts are capable of pulling is the unpublished work of James and his colleagues at University College, London. From work on wound contraction and on chick bone explants connected by a sheet of fibroblasts in culture, a tensile force of 3×10^4 dynes/cm^2 has been calculated, with each fibroblast exerting a force of $1 \cdot 6 \times 10^{-2}$ dynes. Again these figures could be derived from a tensile force generated by collagen synthesis in the repairing wound and in the culture. Thus, the evidence for fibroblast contraction is rather nebulous and can, in any event, be equally applied to the concept of collagen contraction.

D. The Blood Vascular/Hydrostatic Component

Within the forming ligament there is the developing vascular bed. The concept of blood pressure and tissue fluid pressure as the motivating force of tooth eruption was perhaps the most favoured until a few years ago. The evidence has been reviewed by Ness (1964) and Jenkins (1966). However, recent work raises serious objections to this concept. Thus, Main and Adams (1966) were able to show that after the introduction of hypotensive drugs, which surprisingly produced a 20% increase in capillary blood pressure (measured in the capillaries of the ear), there was no effect on the eruption rate. This finding, together with those of Thomas (1965), who showed that in the lathyritic animals there was a reduced eruption rate, although the vascular elements appeared normal, and those of Main and Adams (1966) with respect to the complete loss of cellularity (and vascularity?) in the bases of the pulps, after treatment with triethylene melamine, all cast doubt on the role of vascularity as a force of eruption.

V. Conclusion

It is thus fair to say that since the last critical review of the mechanisms of tooth eruption, which emphasized the unsatisfactory state of knowledge on this subject, most work has led to the conclusion that the connective tissue surrounding the tooth is the significant tissue with respect to tooth movement. Nevertheless, it is unwise to ignore the role played by other tissues of the attachment apparatus, for the ligament cannot function as a mover of the tooth unless there is root growth and fibre attachment to both bone and cementum. It is perhaps because of this intimate relationship between the supporting tissues of the tooth that the identification of the forces required for tooth eruption has proved so difficult.

References

Armstrong, W. G. and Horsley, J. (1967). Abstract of paper presented to the Bone and Tooth Society.

Barrington, E. P. and Meyer, J. (1966). *J. Periodont.* **37,** 453–467.

Baume, L. J., Becks, H. and Evans, H. M. (1954). *J. dent. Res.* **33,** 80–103.

Baume, R. (1872). *Mont. Rev. dent. Surg.* **495,** 552–570.

Brodie, A. G. (1934). *J. Am. dent. Assoc.* **21,** 1830–1838.

Carlson, H. (1944). *Am. J. Orthodont. and Oral Surg.* (Orthodontic Section) **30,** 575–588.

Eastoe, J. E. (1967). *In* "The Mechanisms of Tooth Support" (D. J. Anderson, J. E. Eastoe, A. H. Melcher and D. C. A. Picton, eds.), pp. 14–19. J. Wright and Sons Ltd., Bristol, England.

Golub, L., Stern, B., Glimcher, M. and Goldhaber, P. (1967). International Association for Dental Research, 45th General Meeting. Printed Abstract No. 559.

Herzberg, F. and Schour, I. (1941). *J. dent. Res.* **20,** 264–276.

Jenkins, G. N. (1966). "The Physiology of the Mouth" (Ch. VI). Blackwell, Oxford, England.

Kostlan, J., Thorova, J. and Skach, M. (1960). *Čas. Lék. čes.* **60**, 401–410.

Lapiere, C. M. (1967). *In* "The Mechanisms of Tooth Support" (D. J. Anderson, J. E. Eastoe, A. H. Melcher and D. C. A. Picton eds.), pp. 20–24. J. Wright and Sons Ltd., Bristol, England.

Main, J. H. P. and Adams, D. (1966). *Archs. oral. Biol.* **11**, 163–178.

Manson, J. D. (1967). *In* "The Mechanisms of Tooth Support" (D. J. Anderson, J. E. Eastoe, A. H. Melcher and D. C. A. Picton, eds.), pp. 98–101. J. Wright and Sons Ltd., Bristol, England.

Massler, M. and Schour, I. (1941). *Am. J. Orthod.* **27**, 552–576.

Ness, A. R. (1964). *In* "Advances in Oral Biology" (P. H. Staple, ed.), Vol. 1, pp. 33–70. Academic Press, New York, U.S.A.

Ness, A. R. (1967). *In* "The Mechanisms of Tooth Support" (D. J. Anderson, J. E. Eastoe, A. H. Melcher and D. C. A. Picton, eds.), pp. 84–88. J. Wright and Sons Ltd., Bristol, England.

Olsen, B. R. (1963). *Z. f. Zellforschung.* **59**, 199–213.

Pierce, C. (1887). *In* "The American System of Dentistry". Lea Bros. and Co., Philadelphia, U.S.A.

Rice, S. A. (1959). *Rev. mod. Phys.* **31**, 69–84.

Stallard, R. E. (1966). Paper presented at the 54th Annual Session of the F.D.I.

Thomas, N. R. (1965). Ph.D. Thesis. University of Bristol, England.

Thomas, N. R. and Poole, D. F. G. (1965). Unpublished results quoted *In* "The Mechanisms of Tooth Support" (D. J. Anderson, J. E. Eastoe, A. H. Melcher and D. C. A. Picton, eds.), p. 10. J. Wright and Sons Ltd., Bristol, England.

Tomlin, S. G. and Worthington, C. R. (1956). *Proc. R. Soc. A.* **235**, 189–201.

Weiss, P. (1956). *In* "Symposium on Wound Healing and Tissue Repair" (W. B. Patterson, ed.), pp. 1–7. University of Chicago Press, Chicago, U.S.A.

Zerlotti, E. (1964). *Archs. oral Biol.* **9**, 149–162.

5 | Gingival Epithelium

C. J. SMITH

Department of Dental Science, Royal College of Surgeons of England, London, England

I. Introduction

The epithelial components of the fully-developed periodontium comprise gingival epithelium, which is the subject of this chapter, and the epithelial rests of Malassez described previously in Chapter 3. During development, combinations of dental and oral epithelium contribute to the gingival epithelium; these have also been considered in Chapter 3.

Descriptions of normal adult gingival epithelium are frequently confused by differences of opinion arising from two major sources. The first of these is inconsistent use of anatomical nomenclature, and the other depends upon the almost invariable presence of inflammatory cells in associated connective tissue. Arbitrary subdivision of gingival epithelium, according to functional theories or morphological characteristics, has been responsible for a proliferation of overlapping anatomical terms. Inflammation of gingival tissues is so common that it is often difficult to obtain normal tissue for study purposes; this has led to the adoption of various individual criteria in defining "normal" gingiva. Moreover, it is certain that some of the diverse opinions relating to gingival epithelium stem directly from failure to exclude the influence of inflammation. The structure and metabolism of gingival epithelium are also modified by ageing, and hormonal and nutritional factors. These are discussed in Chapters 3, 9, and 10, respectively, though relevant aspects of their effects will be included here. Where information on certain topics is not available from studies on human material, research into these problems carried out on experimental animals will be discussed. In addition, data of biological significance will be drawn from studies of epithelia in sites other than the gingiva. It is recognized that extrapolation of these observations to human gingival epithelium should be undertaken with caution.

II. General

The original Greek derivation of the word "epithelium", from *epi-* (upon) and *thele* (nipple), was soon extended to apply to the tissue covering all external and internal surfaces of the body. While much epithelium is derived from embryonic ectoderm, including gingival epithelium, some epithelia have their origin in mesoderm or endoderm. The present classification of a tissue as epithelium does not, therefore, depend upon its embryological origin; rather is it determined by position, structure, and function. Characteristically epithelium is found covering a body surface, the individual cells being closely related to form a continuous avascular sheet possessing the minimum of intercellular material. This is supported by connective tissue from which the epithelial cells obtain their metabolic requirements and through which the products of metabolism are dispersed. Consequently, there is a constant interaction between the two tissues in which the intervening "basement membrane" (see Section IVA) plays an important, though somewhat obscure, part.

Epithelium performs the functions most suited to a surface tissue— secretion, absorption, and protection. The structure of various epithelia is adapted to these ends. Secretory and absorptive functions are performed to a large extent by specialized epithelial derivatives, possessing characteristic histological features, none of which are present in gingival epithelium. The property of epithelium required in the gingival region is that of protection, and, in common with other epithelia adapted for protective purposes, the gingival epithelium achieves this effect by being multilayered, capable of continuous renewal, and covered by a surface layer of keratin. The multi-layered nature and flattened appearance of the superficial cells constitute the features of stratified squamous epithelium.

It is appropriate before describing gingival epithelium in more detail, to discuss the surface characteristics of the gingiva.

III. Surface Characteristics of the Gingiva

The surface of the gingiva appears as a strip of pink mucosa immediately adjacent to the teeth (Fig. 1). The coronal margin of the gingiva is scalloped and forms a papilla on the vestibular (buccal/labial) and oral (palatal/lingual) aspects of each interdental space. On all except the palatal surface, where pink gingival mucosa merges almost imperceptibly into pink palatal mucosa, the gingival mucosa is further delineated by the gently undulating mucogingival line separating it from the dark red alveolar mucosa. This strip of gingival mucosa can be further divided according to various surface features into the attached gingiva, the free or marginal gingiva, and the interdental papillae.

Attached gingiva extends from the mucogingival line towards the teeth where its limit is formed by the free gingival groove, a shallow and narrow depression parallel to the gingival margin and 0·5–1·5 mm from it (Sicher, 1966). Often, however, the free gingival groove is not clearly marked and the transition from attached to marginal gingiva is indistinct; indeed Fehr and Muhlemann (1955), using a surface replicating technique, failed to locate this groove in non-inflamed gingiva. Ainamo and Löe (1966) could find this groove only in one-third of a collection of normal gingival specimens, its position corresponding to that of the bottom of the gingival crevice. Neither the level of the gingival margin nor mild inflammatory changes were found to influence the presence of the groove. Firm attachment of this portion of the gingival mucosa to underlying alveolar bone, and to a lesser extent to cementum, imposes the gently undulating surface of bone upon the gingival mucosa (slight depressions corresponding to inter-radicular areas and slight elevations covering tooth roots). Faint vertical striations may be seen on the surface of attached gingiva in the depressions. In addition, small, slight, indentations occur irregularly over the surface of attached gingiva; these are referred to as stippling and may be confined to, or be more prominent in, the inter-radicular areas (Rosenberg and Massler, 1967). Occasional specimens exhibit a slightly nodular surface (Rosenberg and Massler, 1967). A further feature of the gingival surface is the presence of pigmentation. The gingiva is the most frequently pigmented of all oral tissues (Dummett, 1960), pigmentation being directly proportional to that of the skin in most cases. Some very dark Negroes, however, show no clinical evidence of oral pigmentation (Dummett, 1946). The degree and extent of individual pigmentation is variable, occurring most prominently in the attached gingiva beneath interdental papillae.

As explained, the transition from attached to marginal gingiva at the free gingival groove is often obscure, so that the mucosal extent of the marginal gingiva is inconstant. Unlike attached gingiva, the marginal gingiva is slightly mobile and not stippled. Approaching the surface of the tooth the marginal gingiva becomes paler, and is often semi-translucent at the extreme margin. This is due to the lack of underlying connective tissue in this region.

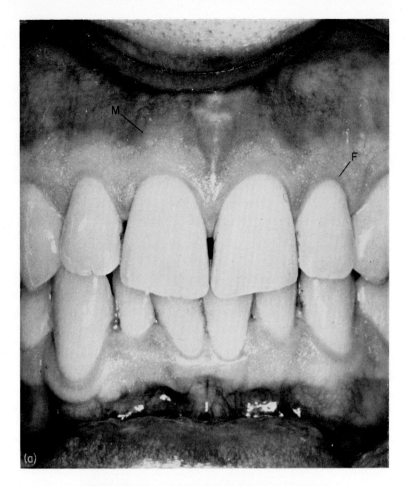

(a)

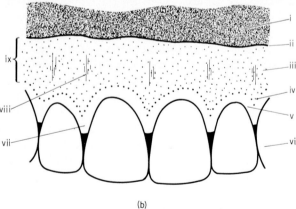

(b)

Fɪɢ. 1. (a); Some of the surface features of normal human gingiva. Both the mucogingival line (M) and the free gingival groove (F) are indistinct in parts. No vertical striae can be seen. (b); Various subdivisions of the gingiva; i. alveolar mucosa, ii. mucogingival line, iii. attached gingiva, iv. free gingival groove, v. marginal gingiva, vi. teeth, vii. interdental papilla, viii. vertical striae, ix. stippled area. (×2·5.)

Interdental gingival papillae are found on vestibular and oral aspects of interdental spaces where teeth are in close contact; if teeth are separated by sufficient space the gingival margin still has a scalloped appearance but is not sufficiently pronounced interdentally to form true papillae. The interdental papillae are often defined as that part of the gingiva occupying the space above an imaginary line drawn between the gingival margin at the centre of one tooth and the centre of the next; it thus has a triangular shape with two slightly concave sides and includes some marginal gingiva. At one time

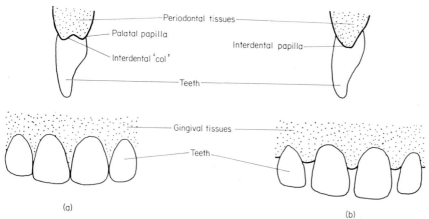

(a)   (b)

FIG. 2. (a); Diagrams to show the concave surface of interdental gingival tissue, forming a *col* between labial and palatal papillae (top diagram), when adjacent teeth are closely apposed (bottom diagram), (b); Diagrams to show the convex surface of interdental gingival tissue, forming a single interdental papilla (top diagram), when adjacent teeth are separated (bottom diagram).

it was thought that the two papillae (vestibular and oral) related to adjacent teeth rose to an even greater eminence in the interproximal region, but this is now known to be a misconception. Rather does the opposite occur in that the surface of the tissue joining the two papillae is concave and has been compared to that of a col between two mountain peaks (Cohen, 1959). Such a *col* occurs, however, only where adjacent teeth are in apposition; when teeth are spaced the interdental gingiva assumes a slightly convex form and true papillae are not present in the embrasure (Fig. 2).

The entire surface of the gingival mucosa is not visible on clinical examination but the remaining parts, crevicular epithelium and attached epithelial cuff, are microscopically discernible. A general description of the microscopic features of the gingival epithelium now follows.

IV. Components of Gingival Epithelium

A vertical section in the vestibulo-oral plane through a tooth and its supporting structures displays representative samples of all parts of the

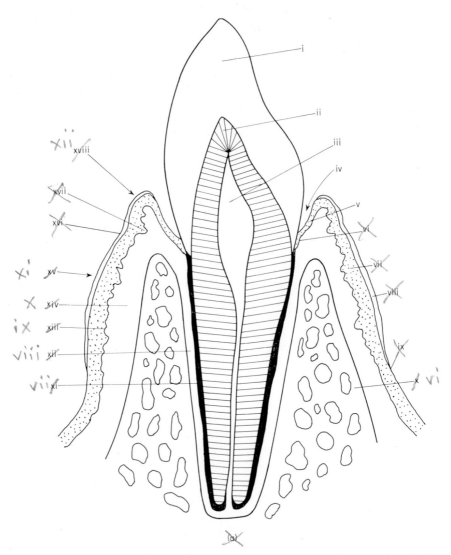

Fɪɢ. 3. (a); Diagram of a vertical section through a tooth and its supporting structures in the vestibulo-oral plane; i. enamel, ii. dentine, iii. pulp chamber, iv. gingival crevice, v. crevicular gingival epithelium, vi. attached epithelial cuff, vii. masticatory gingival epithelium, viii. keratin, ix. mucogingival line, x. alveolar bone, xi. cementum, xii. periodontal membrane, xiii. basement membrane, xiv. connective tissue, xv. attached gingiva, xvi. free gingival groove, xvii. heavy epithelial ridge, xviii. marginal gingiva.

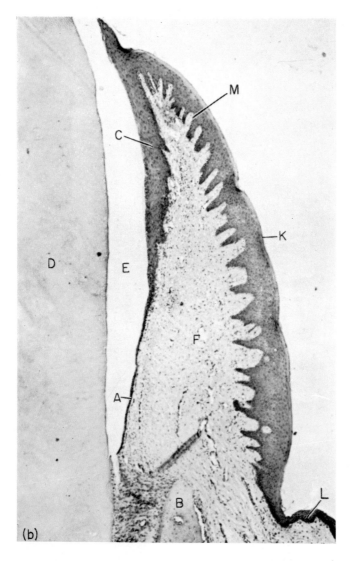

Fig. 3. (b); A histological section through the vertical plane (vestibulo-oral) of a decalcified tooth and its supporting structures showing the different elements of the gingival epithelium: masticatory gingival epithelium (M), crevicular gingival epithelium (C), and the attached epithelial cuff (A). The enamel space (E), dentine (D), alveolar bone (B), keratin (K), alveolar mucosa (L) and fibrous connective tissue (F) are also shown. Monkey (*M. irus*). Haematoxylin and eosin. (× 70.)

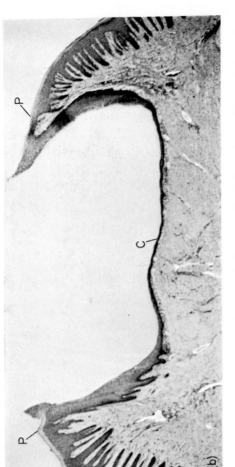

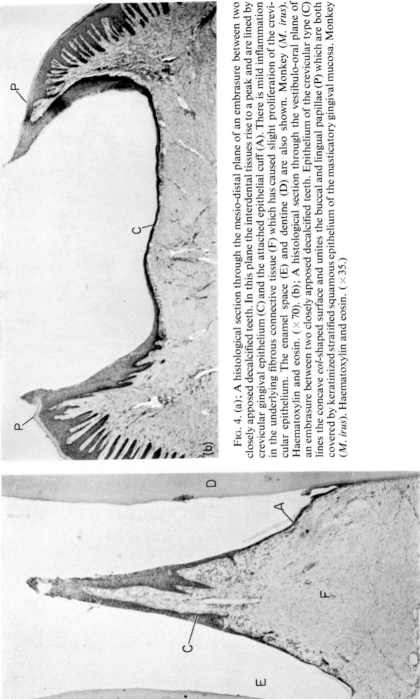

Fig. 4. (a); A histological section through the mesio-distal plane of an embrasure between two closely apposed decalcified teeth. In this plane the interdental tissues rise to a peak and are lined by crevicular gingival epithelium (C) and the attached epithelial cuff (A). There is mild inflammation in the underlying fibrous connective tissue (F) which has caused slight proliferation of the crevicular epithelium. The enamel space (E) and dentine (D) are also shown. Monkey (*M. irus*). Haematoxylin and eosin. (×70). (b); A histological section through the vestibulo-oral plane of an embrasure between two closely apposed decalcified teeth. Epithelium of the crevicular type (C) lines the concave *col*-shaped surface and unites the buccal and lingual papillae (P) which are both covered by keratinized stratified squamous epithelium of the masticatory gingival mucosa. Monkey (*M. irus*). Haematoxylin and eosin. (×35.)

gingival epithelium (Fig. 3). Oral and vestibular gingival epithelia cover the visible surfaces, extending from the mucogingival line to the gingival margin; these include attached, marginal (free), and crestal gingival epithelium, and will be described under the heading of *masticatory gingival epithelium*. At the gingival margin the characteristics of the epithelium undergo some changes as it forms the lining of the gingival crevice, a shallow channel that surrounds each tooth. Where this *crevicular gingival epithelium* terminates apically by attachment to the tooth surface, whether to enamel, dentine, cementum, or any combination of these tissues, it is called the *attached epithelial cuff* (or epithelial attachment). The crevicular epithelium and attached epithelial cuff completely encircle each tooth and are also seen therefore, unlike oral and vestibular gingival epithelium, in mesio-distal sections of a tooth and its supporting structures. In this plane the col appears as a peak-shaped process lined on each side by the crevicular gingival epithelium associated with adjacent teeth (Fig. 4a). On the other hand, a vestibulo-oral section through the col displays two papillae covered on their outer surfaces by masticatory gingival epithelium and united across the interproximal region by epithelium of the crevicular type (Fig. 4b). Only where the space between two teeth is wide enough are oral and vestibular epithelium continuous through the interdental region.

Three main components of gingival epithelium therefore can be delineated —masticatory gingival epithelium, crevicular gingival epithelium, and the attached epithelial cuff. These will be described in detail in separate sections.

A. Masticatory Gingival Epithelium

The masticatory gingival epithelium (Fig. 5) is of stratified squamous type and is supported by a dense fibrous corium. These two tissues are separated by a thin "basement membrane" which is irregularly and deeply undulated due to the presence of elevated papillae on the surface of the connective tissue. Invaginations between the papillae are occupied by downgrowths of epithelium, the rete ridges. At the mucogingival line this corrugated junction is sharply divided from the more gently undulating junction of the alveolar mucosa (Fig. 3; and Fig. 36, Chapter 6). Other microscopic differences can also be found in the tissues on either side of the mucogingival line; keratinization is observed in masticatory gingival epithelium but not in alveolar mucosa epithelium, and elastic fibres are present in connective tissue of the alveolar mucosa but not in that beneath masticatory gingival epithelium (see Chapter 6). These structural variations are admirably suited to the different functions of these tissues; extensive corrugations between epithelium and connective tissue of gingival mucosa provide protection against shearing stresses, keratinized surfaces of masticatory gingival epithelium provide protection against abrasive forces, and elastic fibres endow alveolar mucosa with its necessary flexibility. From the mucogingival line to the gingival margin most of the gingival mucosa is bound firmly to underlying alveolar bone, and some to cementum; this has led to that part being referred to as

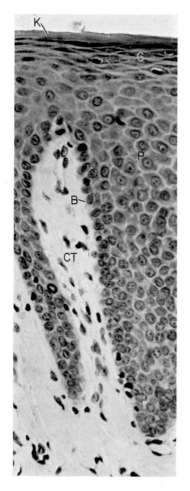

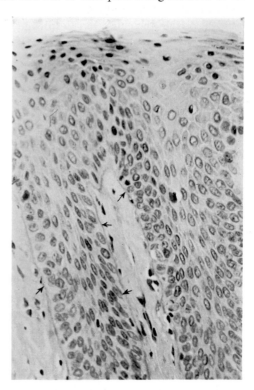

FIG. 6. A histological section of human masticatory gingival epithelium stained by the periodic acid–Schiff technique. The "basement membrane" (arrowed) forms a continuous dark line separating epithelium from connective tissue. Counterstained with haematoxylin. (×375.)

FIG. 5. A histological section of human masticatory gingival epithelium. The regular basal layer (B) supports a prickle-cell layer (P) of variable thickness, a granular cell layer (G) containing keratohyalin granules, and an amorphous superficial layer of keratin (K). The intercellular spaces between basal cells are not as marked as those between prickle-cells; occasional intercellular bridges can be seen between the latter. Connective tissue papillae (CT) are found between the epithelial rete ridges. Haematoxylin and eosin. (×100.)

"attached" gingiva. The more coronal region, not bound to alveolar bone or cementum, is called "marginal", "free", or at its apex, "crestal" gingiva. Demarcation between attached and marginal gingiva, as described previously in consideration of the surface characteristics of the gingiva, is occasionally marked by the free gingival groove. Some authorities (Orban, 1948) believe this to be associated with a marked epithelial ridge, both groove and ridge arising by virtue of functional impacts continually received by the marginal gingiva so that it hinges against the immobile attached gingiva. An alternative explanation for the presence of a free gingival groove, but implying a similar hinging mechanism, has been propounded by Ainamo and Löe (1966). They found this structure to be at the same level as the base of the gingival crevice and to be dependent upon the arrangement of supra-alveolar fibres running from cementum to marginal and attached gingiva. Though attempts have been made in many experimental studies to divide masticatory gingiva into marginal and attached components, the inconstant presence of the free gingival groove has led to the decision not to describe these parts separately in this review.

Attempts have been made to find a histological explanation for the presence of stipples on the surface of masticatory gingival epithelium. Orban (1948) believed that the epithelium surrounding a stipple was elevated from beneath by particularly high connective tissue papillae. Efforts to confirm this by histological techniques have not been successful (Rosenberg and Massler, 1967), but no alternative explanation for the presence of stipples can be offered.

Due to the relatively smooth surface of masticatory gingival epithelium and the deeply invaginated epithelial-connective tissue junction, the thickness of the epithelium varies widely; Gargiulo et al. (1961a) have estimated the average depth to be 12–13 cells. The deepest layer of these cells, the basal layer, comprises a single row of cuboidal cells resting on the "basement membrane" and following its serpentine shape. Above the basal layer is the prickle-cell layer, a multiple layer of cells clearly characterized by peripheral "prickles" (intercellular bridges) that seem to unite the cells across thin intercellular spaces. As cells of the prickle-cell layer pass peripherally their original polyhedral form becomes flattened, with long axes parallel to the epithelial surface, and their nuclei become denser and smaller. It is this prickle-cell layer that shows most variation in thickness, for its deepest cells follow the irregular line of the basal cells while its superficial cells are parallel to the smooth mucosal surface. Some parts, overlying prominent papillae, effect a rapid transition from polyhedral to flattened cells, while in regions of deep epithelial rete ridges as much as a three-fold increase in depth of the cell layers may be encountered. As the same degree of cell differentiation occurs in both cases, a more sophisticated control mechanism is implied than would depend upon progressive removal of cells from a source of nutrition. Indeed the conventional methods for studying this region may have promoted too static a view; it is not known, for example, if the deep epithelial rete ridges and prominent connective tissue papillae are maintained in a fixed position or whether they vary with normal tissue turnover and reorganization.

Superficial, flattened cells of the prickle-cell layer merge into the granular layer; this is distinguished by the appearance of keratohyalin granules, which are basophilic (staining deep blue with haematoxylin) but are not always present in masticatory gingival epithelium. By this stage cell nuclei are pyknotic. Most superficial of all is the keratinized layer which can consist of a uniform, longitudinally-striated, hyaline, eosinophilic substance (orthokeratin), may also contain some pyknotic nuclei (parakeratin), or may comprise a mixture of both these types. In common with other parts of the oral epithelium, but unlike some heavily keratinized areas of skin, there is no glassy stratum lucidum between granular and keratinized layers. Flakes of keratin are shed from the surface in the normal process of wear and tear; these are replaced by differentiation from deeper layers and the continuation of this process provides the necessity for a mechanism of cell renewal. If keratin and parakeratin are absent from the surface of masticatory gingival epithelium the most superficial layer is formed by a layer of flattened, nucleated cells corresponding to those at the top of the prickle-cell layer.

Cellular constituents of masticatory gingival epithelium that are ultimately transformed into keratin can be referred to as keratinocytes. Other cell types, however, can occasionally be found among keratinocytes; these are melanocytes, responsible for producing pigment, and high-level clear cells, or Langerhans cells, apparently related to melanocytes.

The various components of masticatory gingival epithelium are now considered in more detail.

1. *"Basement Membrane"*

Some aspects of the terminology and function of " basement membrane" have been considered previously in Chapter 2. Briefly, the term "basement membrane" refers, at the level of the optical microscope, to the material which occupies the junctional zone between epithelium and connective tissue and is stained strongly by the periodic acid-Schiff method (Fig. 6). At higher magnification, with the electron microscope, this "basement membrane" is seen to possess two distinct parts. The deeper of these is a compact network of reticulin and this is covered by a double-layered structure comprising an electron-dense proximal component (lamina densa or basement lamina) and a distal electron-lucent component (lamina lucida). Accumulated evidence, derived mainly from electron microscopic, immunohistochemical, and radioautographic studies (reviewed in Chapter 2), leads to the conclusion that the lamina densa is derived mainly, if not entirely, from the epithelial cells. Mercer (1961) has put forward the view that the "basement membrane" is formed by precipitation between two proteins, one of epithelial cell origin and the other from connective tissue. Moreover, he suggests that such a precipitate could exert a selective influence upon the transfer of molecules from connective tissue to epithelium and in this way control the behaviour of epithelium.

It is not clear whether all components revealed by the electron microscope are part of the paS-positive "basement membrane" of the optical microscope, though some have argued that the undulating nature of the lamina densa

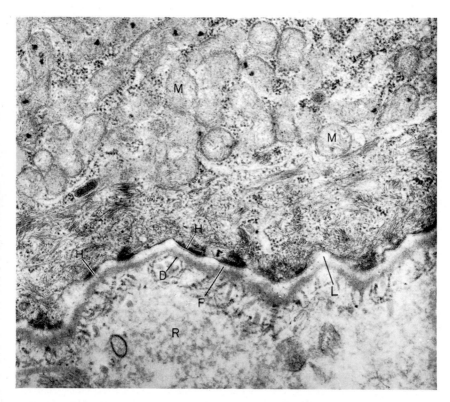

FIG. 7. Electron micrograph of the "basement membrane" region of human masticatory gingival epithelium. This shows the lamina densa (D), lamina lucida (L), reticulin (R), and hemidesmosomes (H). In some regions fine fibrils appear to cross the lamina lucida; these are marked "F". Mitochondria (M) are present in the cytoplasm of the basal epithelial cell. (×21,000.)

would enable it to be seen in the relatively thick sections used for optical microscopy (Gersh and Catchpole, 1960). As the subepithelial reticulin network is described in Chapter 6, only the lamina lucida, lamina densa, and associated structures comprising the electron microscopic "basement membrane", are considered further. Their appearance in masticatory gingival epithelium (Fig. 7) varies only slightly from that in other parts of the oral epithelium and skin (Stern, 1965).

The lamina densa seems to be of variable width, 330 Å (Melcher, 1965) to

5

400–600 Å (Listgarten, 1964) and, while apparently amorphous upon cursory examination, detailed surveys have disclosed a fine fibrillar pattern at right-angles to the connective tissue-epithelial junction. Also, occasional thread-like structures, extensions from the subepithelial reticulin, appear to pass through it and thence into the lamina lucida (Melcher, 1965). These thread-like structures, 200–400 Å in thickness, show a definite but non-periodic transverse banding and are composed of numerous, fine, closely-packed filaments which become separated into a looser spray upon approaching the lamina densa (Susi *et al.*, 1967). Some of these filaments (60 Å wide) then appear to pass across both lamina densa and lamina lucida to become in-serted into the plasma membrane of a basal epithelial cell, usually in the region of a hemidesmosome, or sometimes to simulate continuity with intra-cytoplasmic fibres of the basal cell (Melcher, 1965; Stern, 1965; and Susi *et al.*, 1967). Although Melcher (1965) originally considered the possibility that such filaments may have been an artefact, subsequent work confirming their presence in oral and gingival epithelium, and the fact that they also exist in uterine cervix (Younes *et al.*, 1965), indicates that they should be con-sidered as definite entities (see also Chapter 2). Occasional loops of material resembling lamina densa and apparently leaving its connective tissue aspect to penetrate the subepithelial reticulin are probably artefacts due to plane of section (Melcher, 1965).

The width of the lamina lucida is 400–450 Å (Listgarten, 1964; Melcher, 1965) and it has been described as containing, in addition to the fine fibrils mentioned above, fine granular (Melcher, 1965), or homogeneous (Stern, 1965), material. Indeed, it has been suggested (Pease, 1960) that the relatively constant width of the lamina lucida is maintained by the presence of such a substance. Hemidesmosomes interrupt the lamina lucida at periodic but irregular intervals (500–2000 Å apart) (Listgarten, 1964). Between the hemi-desmosomes small vesicles and invaginations can be found associated with the plasma membranes of basal cells (Schroeder and Theilade, 1966); these contain material only slightly less electron-dense than the lamina densa. It is not clear whether these vesicles are responsible for ingestion of substances by the basal cells, or for secretory activities possibly associated with main-taining the lamina densa. Microvilli, which may be cut in cross section, extend from the proximal plasma membranes of the basal cells into the lamina lucida (Stern, 1965).

2. Basal Cell Layer

A row of low columnar, cuboidal, or occasionally fusiform, cells rests on the "basement membrane" with long axes perpendicular to that structure; this comprises the basal cell layer. In tissue sections stained with haematoxylin and eosin these cells possess a homogeneous pink cytoplasm and a dense purple, round or oval, plump nucleus which occupies a large part of the cell.

Occasionally the continuity of the basal layer is interrupted by a basal cell in the process of division, by a melanocyte, or by a white blood cell migrating between epithelial cells. In the optical microscope, junctions between individual basal cells and between those cells and the "basement membrane" appear close and regular.

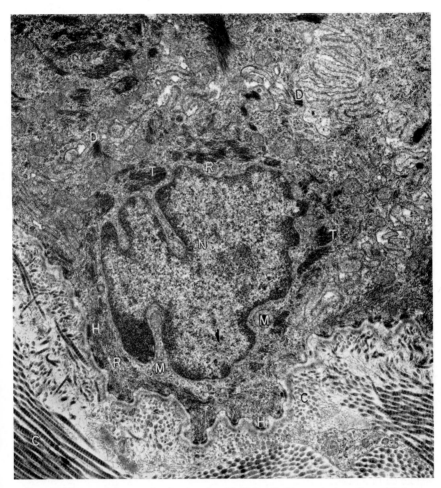

FIG. 8. Electron micrograph of a basal epithelial cell. The central nucleus (N) is surrounded by cytoplasm in which tonofilaments are collected together to form tonofibrils (T); mitochondria (M) and free ribosomes (R) can also be seen. Desmosomes (D) form junctions with adjacent cells and hemidesmosomes are present (H) at intervals along the proximal plasma membrane. Bundles of collagen fibres (C) can be seen in the underlying connective tissue. Hamster cheek pouch mucosa. (×12,000.)

The electron microscopic appearance of a typical basal cell in stratified squamous epithelium is shown in Fig. 8. The fine structure of basal cells in masticatory gingival epithelium has been described by Listgarten (1964), Stern (1965), and Schroeder and Theilade (1966); all were alike and independent of the keratinized or non-keratinized nature of the surface. Many free ribosomes occupy the cytoplasm, in spaces between loose interwoven bundles of tonofilaments. These tonofilaments (about 50 Å in diameter) are gathered into bundles, tonofibrils, which pursue a tortuous course between their two terminal insertions into the attachment plaques of desmosomes or hemidesmosomes, both in the same cell. Tonofilaments are inserted into the attachment plaques perpendicular to the cell surface. Mitochondria, which are often numerous, are found in the perinuclear and proximal regions of the cytoplasm; histochemical techniques for oxidative enzymes associated with mitochondria confirm this intracellular distribution (Nuki, 1967). Oxidative enzymes taking part in the aerobic Krebs cycle exhibit high histochemical activity in basal cells (Shahrik et al., 1964; Gerson et al., 1966; Löe, 1967 and Nuki, 1967), while those taking part in the anaerobic pentose shunt, such as glucose-6-phosphate dehydrogenase, show low activity in basal cells (Nuki, 1967). A Golgi complex, lipid droplets, glycogen granules, various types of vesicles with single or double membranes, and pigment granules, may contribute to the contents of the cytoplasm of the basal cells. Rough-surfaced endoplasmic reticulum, however, is only occasionally observed.

Radioautography of skin basal cells, following the injection of radio-actively-labelled cytidine and amino-acids into newborn rats, has shown that these cells are capable of synthesizing RNA and proteins (Bernstein, 1964; Fukuyama and Epstein, 1966). Some amino-acids seem to be localized more particularly to the basal layer than other layers of the epithelium, notably phenylalanine, leucine, valine, lycine and methionine. The large number of ribonucleoprotein granules present in basal cell cytoplasm is also indicative of protein synthesis but, as these granules are not arranged on an endoplasmic reticulum, it appears that the synthesized proteins are retained by the cells for their own use. The purposes to which such cellular proteins are directed probably include the synthesis of tonofilaments and as an adjunct to mitosis (Rowden and Budd, 1967). Basal cell nuclei contain one or more nucleoli and are bounded by a double layer of dense material constituting the nuclear membrane; this may be infolded and is occasionally perforated by nuclear pores.

The cell membrane (plasma membrane) which encloses the cytoplasm consists of an electron-lucent central lamina bounded on either side by two dense layers, the whole being 75–100 Å in thickness. Where the plasma membranes of two adjacent cells approach each other desmosomes or other junctional complexes may be found; similarly, at intervals along the proximal surfaces of basal cells the plasma membrane contributes to the formation of hemidesmosomes. These specialized structures are described in more detail later in this chapter. Between the junctional structures plasma membranes of adjacent cells are separated by the intercellular space. In these regions the surfaces of the membranes may be coated with fine granular or fibrillar material, and small projections and invaginations of the membranes may form interdigitations with neighbouring cells. However, the closest non-junctional appositions of adjacent cell surfaces are approximately 150 Å apart, except for the surfaces of basal cells near to the lamina densa where no junctional structures are formed and closer approximations of adjacent plasma membranes may occur (Schroeder and Theilade, 1966). The inter-cellular space is continuous with the lamina lucida and tends, as in other tightly bound epithelia, to be more prominent in masticatory gingival epi-thelium than in distensible epithelia. On the proximal surface of basal cells the plasma membrane may be smooth or raised into fine microvilli or pedicles. In the case of the latter these form interdigitations with connective tissue, but regardless of the smooth or ragged course followed by the plasma membrane it is pursued faithfully, at a constant distance, by the lamina densa.

There are, therefore, three levels of interdigitation between epithelium and connective tissue contributing to their ability to resist forces that may sep-arate them; interlocking connective tissue papillae and epithelial rete ridges, undulations caused by dissimilar levels of the proximal surfaces of adjacent basal cells, and fine microvilli extending into connective tissue from the proximal surface of each individual basal cell.

The masticatory gingival epithelium protects the underlying tissues by constant exfoliation of cells from its surface in response to normal wear and tear, and by restoring surface integrity in case of injury. Both of these pro-cesses are effected by new cells being formed in the basal layer by mitotic division. These new cells then gradually pass out to the exposed epithelial surface or migrate to cover the surface defect. Cell renewal for normal maintenance of masticatory gingival epithelium is now considered; its adapta-tion for healing is discussed in Chapter 12.

3. Cell Renewal

As the purpose of cell renewal is to replace the continual loss of other cells from the surface, it is important for the rate of renewal to approximate to the rate of loss so that atrophy or hyperplasia do not ensue. A state of dynamic equilibrium must therefore be maintained in the epithelium. Various tech-niques can be employed to demonstrate cell division in renewing cell popula-tions. Of these, administration of a radioactive precursor of DNA (tritiated thymidine) followed by radioautography (Messier and Leblond, 1960) (Fig. 9a), or administration of colchicine to arrest mitoses in metaphase (Bertalanffy, 1960) (Fig. 9b), are commonly employed in animal studies; for human tissues the laborious counting of cells in various stages of mitosis (Fig. 9c) and their expression as a percentage of the total pool of epithelial cells, the mitotic index, has been the most common method practised. By use of such techniques the proliferative pool of cells in the masticatory gingival epithelium has been found to comprise the basal layer and the inner layers of the prickle-cell layer. Meyer *et al.* (1956) observed that only 23% of mitotic figures were in the basal layer of normal human masticatory gingival epithelium, whereas Krajewski *et al.* (1964) found 35% in the basal layer and

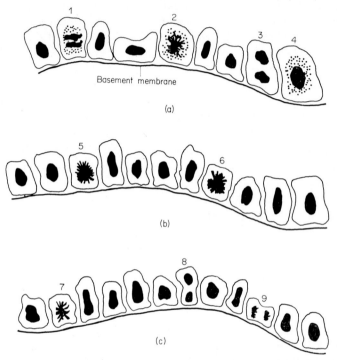

Fig. 9. (a); Diagram to illustrate labelling of basal epithelial cells by radioactive precursor of DNA. Fine dots over cells indicate the presence of radioactivity. Depending upon the time that has elapsed since injection of the isotope various patterns of labelling are obtained. In this example cells in metaphase and prophase (1, 2) are labelled whereas the cell in early telophase is not (3). This last cell would have completed DNA synthesis before administration of the isotope. On the other hand, the labelled cell in interphase (4) had incorporated some radioactive DNA precursor but had not started to divide. (b); Diagram to illustrate arrest of cells in mitosis (5, 6) by administration of colchicine. All cells entering mitosis are arrested at the same point. Counting of such cells can therefore give an assessment of the mitotic rate. (c); Diagram to illustrate some of the mitotic figures (7, 8, 9) that may be seen in basal cells. These can be counted and used to estimate the mitotic index.

Gargiulo *et al.* (1961a) 50% in the basal layer; the remaining mitotic figures were in the innermost layers of the prickle-cell layer. Such variable results may be attributable to the difficulties involved in deciding, on a visual basis, which cells are in mitosis; to the fact that inflammation may have been more prevalent in one study than another, thus elevating the mitotic index (Marwah *et al.*, 1960; and Soni *et al.*, 1965); or to other factors that will be discussed later in this section. It can be shown also, from experiments on rat oral epithelium (Sharav and Massler, 1967), that active DNA synthesis occurs in the cells of the innermost layer of prickle cells to a greater extent than in the basal layer. Masticatory gingival epithelium, therefore, seems similar to the palmar and plantar epithelium in which all cells resembling basal cells were found to be capable of synthesizing DNA (Leblond et al., 1964), regardless of the fact that they may be situated in the inner prickle-cell layers. This is in contrast to the situation that exists in some sites, as in the oesophageal epithelium of mice, where synthesis of DNA and most cell division is confined to the basal layer (Greulich, 1964; Leblond et al., 1964; and Frankfurt, 1967). Thus, although the basal layer of the masticatory gingival epithelium can be defined as that layer of epithelial cells adjacent to the connective tissue-epithelial junction, it is not correct to consider this layer as the only repository of epithelial cells capable of division. The terms *basal layer* and *stratum germinativum* should not therefore be used interchangeably in descriptions of masticatory gingival epithelium.

Gargiulo et al. (1961a) and Krajewski et al. (1964) have divided the mitotic figures in masticatory gingival epithelium into those parallel or those perpendicular to the "basement membrane". The percentages of mitoses found in either position, knowledge of which has limited value at present, can be compared with results of similar investigations on human skin (Pinkus and Hunter, 1966). Such percentages are misleading, however, for they must be interpreted with the understanding that, by virtue of the plane of section and its extreme thinness, results obtained by counting mitotic figures in different planes are biased in favour of those perpendicular to the "basement membrane". All perpendicular mitotic figures in a row of cells will be seen easily, at the expense of those parallel to the "basement membrane", some of which will not be obvious (Fig. 10).

Where analyses have been made of the various stages of the mitotic cycle represented among dividing cells of the masticatory gingival epithelium extremely erratic results have been obtained. Soni et al. (1965) found 64–69% in prophase, 27–28% in metaphase, 3–5% in anaphase, and 1–3% in telophase; Gargiulo et al. (1961a) reported corresponding figures of 27·5%, 22%, 18%, and 32·5%, and Krajewski et al. (1964) 40%, 29%, 16%, and 16% respectively. The main difficulty in any study related to distinguishing the stages of mitosis, and probably a major source of discrepancies in different studies, is that it is difficult to describe, and therefore to standardize, at which point one stage becomes the next.

No reliable information for the duration of mitosis, or its phases, seems to be available for human masticatory gingival epithelium, but synthesis of DNA takes about eight hours in marmoset masticatory gingival epithelium (Skougaard, 1965a) and in this respect resembles the time taken by other cell populations and cells from other species. The time taken for complete renewal (turnover time) of marmoset masticatory gingival epithelium, has also been studied by Skougaard (1965b); in addition, he has reviewed previous work on mitotic rates and calculated turnover times for various parts of the gingival epithelium in other experimental animals and man. A striking lack of correlation between various studies shows that no clear guidance can be

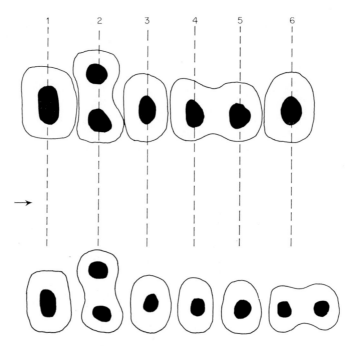

FIG. 10. Diagram of basal cell layer (top row) to show how a disproportionate assessment of perpendicular/parallel mitotic figures may be made. The bottom row of cells represents the same cells rotated through 90 degrees, as if a section was cut through each at right angles to the plane of section for the top row. Whereas the mitotic figure (2) appears perpendicular in both planes, the cell in early telophase (4, 5) appears similar to a cell in interphase if cut at right angles. This is also shown for cell 6. Therefore, although the apparent ratio of perpendicular/ parallel mitotic figures in the top row is 1:1, the true ratio is 1:2. This illustration is an example only and is not meant to convey the likely extent of the error.

given with regard to turnover time for gingival epithelium in any particular animal, though inflammation seems to induce more rapid turnover of epithelial cells.

Among the factors which influence mitotic activity in masticatory gingival epithelium are: age—the mitotic index showing a 50% increase in older subjects (Meyer et al., 1956; and Gargiulo et al., 1961a); sex—there being a slightly higher mitotic index in males than females (Soni et al., 1965); and endocrine status—oestrogen stimulating mitotic activity (Beagrie, 1966). In addition, mitotic activity is known to vary from site to site in the gingiva, and to be different from time to time during the day and night (Beagrie, 1963; Trott and Gorenstein, 1963; Hansen, 1966a; Hansen, 1966b; Irons and Schaffer, 1966; and Hansen, 1967a). This alteration in activity from time to time during the day is referred to as the diurnal variation and imposes the necessity for standardizing the time at which studies of cell turnover are made. The fact that no diurnal variation can be found in skin cultured *in vitro* has led Mercer (1961) to suggest that control of mitosis is influenced by extracellular factors.

The mechanism by which mitotic rate is controlled to meet the demands of changing circumstances has been the subject of much speculation. Bullough (1962) and Bullough and Rytömaa (1965) have proposed the presence of *chalones*, tissue specific substances normally present in cells and capable of diffusing over short distances, that act as mitotic inhibitors. When tissue is lost, by wounding or by excessive loss of cells from the surface of epithelium, then chalones are also lost. The inhibitory effect is thereby reduced and mitotic activity increases in the surrounding tissue. Bullough further maintains that the normal activity of chalones is controlled by the local concentration of adrenaline, which forms an unstable compound with chalone to act as the effective principle; when adrenaline output is low then mitotic activity increases because chalone-adrenaline complex concentration decreases. Mitotic rate returns to normal when a normal chalone-adrenaline complex concentration is re-established. This is believed to account for diurnal variations in mitotic activity, following the alterations that occur in adrenaline secretion. Recently, Hansen (1967b) has shown that mitotic activity in masticatory gingival epithelium of rats is increased by adrenalectomy and decreased by injection of adrenaline; moreover, the diurnal mitotic rhythm was eliminated by adrenalectomy. Hansen (1967c) has shown also that injection of an epidermal chalone preparation depresses the mitotic activity in masticatory gingival epithelium of rats, but has no such effect when injected into animals from which adrenals have been removed. Such observations are in general agreement with the suggested control of mitotic activity expounded by Bullough and his co-workers. Further support for this hypothesis has been given by Finegold (1965) on the basis of results from skin grafting experiments.

Whatever mechanism controls the mitotic rate, it is clear that if the proliferative pool is not to become rapidly overpopulated, there must be provision for cells to leave the basal layer, differentiate, and become exfoliated. Indeed, this is part of their function and the main purpose for constant renewal of the epithelium from the proliferative pool.

4. Differentiation

The prerequisite of differentiation is that cells should leave the basal layer and inner prickle-cell layers where cell division occurs. In a steady state

5*

renewing epithelium, for such is masticatory gingival epithelium, there are three possible ways of achieving such a result (Greulich, 1964):

(*a*) Each division of a basal cell could result in one differentiated cell ready to continue differentiation and one basal cell ready to continue the process of cell division (Fig. 11a). Such an arrangement would imply the inheritance of dissimilar genetic information by each daughter cell, a phenomenon for which no evidence seems to exist; it is not, therefore, a popular theory.

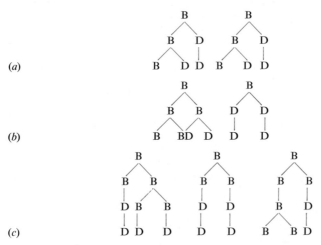

FIG. 11. Diagrams to show the possible ways in which basal cells (B) may give rise to further basal cells and differentiating cells (D): (*a*); Each division of a basal cell could give rise to one differentiating cell and one basal cell. (*b*); Some basal cells could divide to produce two new basal cells while others divide to produce two differentiating cells. (*c*); All basal cells could be capable of dividing to produce two new basal cells each; later, some of these would (in a separate process) undergo differentiation while others would remain for further division.

(*b*) Some basal cells could divide to produce two differentiating cells and a comparable number could divide to produce two new basal cells capable of further division (Fig. 11b). There is evidence, however, mainly from sites where the proliferative pool is confined to the basal layer (Greulich, 1964; Frankfurt, 1967; and Galand *et al.*, 1967), that after cell division both daughter cells are confined to the basal layer for a maturation phase before migration into the prickle-cell layer. A system whereby some daughter cells pass immediately into the prickle-cell layer for differentiation does not exist in these tissues.

(*c*) Basal cells could divide to form other basal cells, some of which, in a process separate from that of mitosis, could later enter upon the process of differentiation and migrate to the prickle-cell layer (Fig. 11c). The evidence quoted against scheme (*b*) above provides some of the evidence which supports this proposition.

Differentiation and migration of cells from the basal layer occurs in a random fashion, the length of time elapsing between the formation of new basal cells and their differentiation being indeterminate and probably varying considerably for individual cells. Greulich (1964) believes that the change of position from basal layer to a more superficial position is enough to produce cytologic differentiation and loss of the proliferative capacity of the cell. One of the factors responsible for deciding which cells leave the basal layer may be associated with overcrowding. As more basal cells divide the basal layer becomes crowded and, as the newly formed cells invariably remain in the basal layer for a while, some cells must move into the prickle-cell layer. Such cells can occasionally be seen in the process of being forced from the basal layer, and are recognizable by their constricted racket-shaped nucleus (Leblond et al., 1964). The presence of mitotic figures arranged perpendicularly to the connective tissue junction of masticatory gingival epithelium does not affect the argument in (c) above. This relates to cells leaving the complete proliferative pool, of which the innermost prickle cells are a part, not only those leaving the basal layer.

Upon leaving the proliferative pool epithelial cells commence differentiation; but there are many possibilities open to them, and for a specific tissue to be formed and maintained some disciplinary influences must prevail. Once the pattern of differentiation has been imposed upon a tissue to provide it with characteristic special features then it is necessary for this pattern to be maintained throughout life. This applies no less to masticatory gingival epithelium than to any other tissue. Two mechanisms have been postulated to explain how this process is controlled (Billingham and Silvers, 1967).

(a) All basal epithelial cells are equipotential; stimuli that determine which pathway is to be followed and constantly maintained being provided by the underlying dermal tissues. Proponents of this theory cite as evidence; (i) the histological similarity between all basal cells; (ii) the capacity of basal cells from any part of a hair follicle or sweat gland to produce a complete new pilosebaceous unit or normal stratified squamous epithelium; (iii) boundaries between epithelia of different characteristics, such as the mucocutaneous junction of the lips or the mucogingival junction, remain strictly constant; and (iv) some vitamins and hormones can interrupt normal differentiation and influence the basal cells to develop a different type of epithelium. This evidence is derived from the work and deductions of Van Scott and Reinertson (1961), Billingham and Silvers (1963), McLoughlin (1963), and Billingham and Silvers (1967).

(b) Basal cells from different types of epithelium possess intrinsic genetic differences, although they look alike, which enable them to determine the course of differentiation to be followed. Experimental evidence in favour of this hypothesis is derived from observations on the characteristics of split-thickness skin grafts; distinctive skin epithelium from sole of foot, cornea, and tongue of guinea pigs retains its specialized appearance indefinitely when transplanted to sites normally covered by epithelium of a dissimilar type (Billingham and Medawar, 1950). Similar experiments, transposing keratinized masticatory gingival epithelium and non-keratinized alveolar mucosa in monkeys, have shown that these tissues retain the characteristics of the donor site (Cohen et al., 1962). Both these studies entailed some transfer of associated dermis with the epithelium of the graft, which may have been sufficient to enable retention of its donor characteristics. An extension of these experiments on skin has shown, however, that if dermis is removed by trypsin digestion before transplantation, then in some sites the type of dermis determined the type of epithelium that developed, whereas in others the epithelium remained true to its original characteristics (Billingham and Silvers, 1967). It is of interest, with respect to the apparent histological similarity of all basal cells, that in human embryological oral epithelium at certain stages of development a clear distinction can be seen between basal cells in areas that will ultimately be keratinized and those in areas that do not undergo keratinization (Coslet and Cohen, 1967). This is indicative of a genetic predetermination in the differentiation of epithelium.

It would seem probable, therefore, that there is an interplay of factors between the basal epithelial layer and the underlying dermis that determines the specific pathway of epithelial cell development, similar to that existing between ectoderm and mesoderm in embryonic life (McLoughlin, 1963; and see Chapter 2). Whatever these factors may be, and however they act, the basal cells of masticatory gingival epithelium differentiate into a typical stratified squamous epithelium. Before the prickle-cell layer is discussed, consideration will be given to the specific junctional structures found in this type of epithelium, desmosomes, hemidesmosomes, maculae or zonulae occludentes, and zonulae adherentes.

5. Junctional Complexes

(a) Desmosomes. When the intercellular bridges between epithelial cells are examined with the aid of an electron microscope then a characteristic structure, the desmosome, becomes visible at the points where two adjacent cells are closely apposed (Fig. 12). The desmosomes consist of two dense attachment plaques, one associated with the plasma membrane of each adjacent cell, and the structure found between them. The attachment plaques each consist of a moderately dense aggregation of granular or fibrillar material (about 150 Å thick) on to the cytoplasmic side of the innermost layer of the plasma membrane. Closely packed tonofilaments extend from attachment plaques into the adjacent cytoplasm; these often run at right angles to the plasma membrane but occasionally may be seen parallel to the plasma membrane. In some instances the attachment plaque merges with the denser innermost layer of the plasma membrane, otherwise these two structures are separated by a narrow band of electron-lucent material. Between the two attachment plaques, which form the outer limits of the desmosome, is a space of about 350 Å occupied by alternate layers of light and dark material running the whole length of the desmosome. The region right in the centre, a

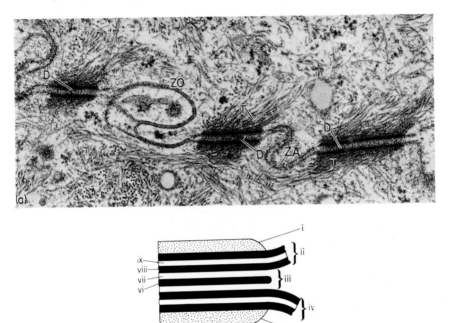

(b)

FIG. 12. (a); Electron micrograph of three desmosomes (D) between two epithelial cells. A zonula occludens (ZO) and a probable zonula adherens (ZA) are also shown. Tonofilaments (T) are concentrated in the regions of the attachment plaques. Hamster cheek pouch epithelium. (×55,000.) (b) ; A diagram to show the various components of a desmosome: i. attachment plaque, ii. unit membrane, iii. intercellular layers, iv. unit membrane, v. attachment plaque, vi. median stratum, vii. distal light zone, viii. lateral dense line, ix. proximal light zone.

dense layer 40 Å in width and called the intercellular contact layer, intermediate line, or the median stratum, is truly intercellular. This line is formed at sites where the very fine, granular, extracellular coating material of one plasma membrane contacts that of the other; these coatings are usually electron-lucent but become electron-dense where they meet (Ham, 1965). On either side of this central layer is a distal light layer (or distal light zone), about 65 Å thick and representing the extracellular coating granules not in contact with those of the adjacent cell and therefore retaining their electron-lucent appearance. The distal light layer separates the intercellular contact layers from another dense layer of 40 Å thickness, the lateral dense line (or intermediate layer). This layer has the right dimensions to be the outer layer of the plasma membrane, and is sometimes seen to be continuous with this structure. Finally, the lateral dense line is separated from attachment plaque by the proximal light layer, 50 Å in width, which appears to be continuous with the central light zone of the trilaminar plasma membrane. The dimensions of desmosome components that have been quoted above are derived from the work of Listgarten (1964) on healthy human masticatory gingival epithelium. Stern (1965) has also contributed to the information available on this topic and, in addition, has drawn attention to the fact that such measurements are necessarily inexact due to the limitations of technique which are able to show only a gradual transition from one layer to another.

These desmosomes make a contribution to adhesion between epithelial cells. This is indicated by the occurrence of intercellular bridges. The intercellular bridges are visible by optical microscopy only because the cytoplasm of the cell in the regions between them shrinks in the fixative unimpeded by adhesion to its neighbour. At one time it was thought that tonofilaments effected cellular adhesion by passing from one cell to another through the sites of desmosomes. However, electron microscopy reveals no cellular continuity and also shows that the plasma membranes of adjacent cells do not fuse. It is believed that the tonofilament-desmosome complex, as well as contributing to cell adhesion, also may serve to distribute stresses through the epithelium (Stern, 1965). Although desmosomes seem to contribute to cell adhesion it is evident, from the continual passage of lymphocytes and leucocytes between epithelial cells (often seen on routine sections), that desmosomal structures suffer repetitive breakdown and repair. The white blood cells are too large to pass between the desmosomes. This process may be identical to the passage of similar cells through the endothelium of blood vessels. The mechanism of desmosome rupture and repair, however, is ill-understood.

This account of desmosome structure applies to their appearance in the basal and prickle-cell layers. As the epithelium differentiates further the desmosomes undergo certain changes which will be described in the appropriate sections.

(b) *Hemidesmosomes.* These structures, not visible in the optical microscope, are found only in association with the basal cells and lamina densa and may assist adhesion between epithelium and connective tissue. Electron microscopy reveals (Fig. 13) an attachment plaque at intervals on the proximal surfaces of basal epithelial cells, similar to that of the desmosome but thicker, between 190 Å and 220 Å (Stern, 1965). Since this cell surface faces the lamina densa and not another plasma membrane there is no partner for the attachment plaque. Where the attachment plaque of a hemidesmosome abuts onto the inner dense layer of the plasma membrane this is denser than the outer layer. Some 60 Å beyond the outer dense layer is a structure called the peripheral density, a prominent electron-dense line (35-60 Å in thickness) corresponding to the intercellular contact layer of the desmosome.

(c) *Other junctional complexes.* Schroeder and Theilade (1966) have described a further type of cell junction in human masticatory gingival

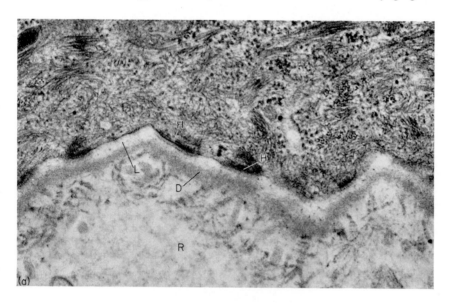

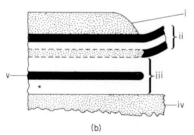

FIG. 13. (a); Electron micrograph of hemidesmosomes (H) at the proximal surface of a basal epithelial cell. The lamina lucida (L), lamina densa (D) and subepithelial reticulin (R) are also shown. Human masticatory gingival mucosa. (×33,000.) (b); A diagram to show the various components of a hemidesmosome: i. attachment plaque, ii. unit membrane, iii. lamina lucida iv. top of lamina densa, v. peripheral density.

epithelium but were undecided whether the appearance represented zonulae occludentes, maculae occludentes, or both. These structures are tight junctions formed between epithelial cells, commonly at the free margins of intestinal epithelium. In a zonula occludens (Fig. 14) the two outer layers of opposed plasma membranes fuse together and form a continuous structure in which three dense layers enclose two light layers. The distance between the inner membrane leaflets of the two cells is 100–150 Å (Thilander and Bloom, 1968). In a macula occludens, on the other hand, the fusion of adjoining cell membranes is limited to small areas or point contacts (Farquhar and

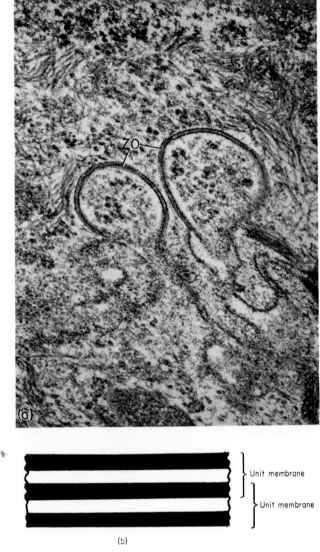

FIG .14. (a); Electron micrograph of two zonulae occludentes (ZO) between two epithelial cells. Hamster cheek pouch epithelium. (×68,000): (b); A diagram to show the structure of a zonula occludens. Three electron-dense layers enclose two electron-lucent layers after fusion of adjacent cell unit membranes.

Palade, 1965). These authors believe that zonulae occludentes, because they provide a continuous seal, divide the epithelium into sub-compartments and thus retard the passage of water, ions, and small water-soluble molecules through intercellular spaces. In addition, both zonulae and maculae occludentes are believed to facilitate ion exchange through sites of membrane contact, and to represent intercellular attachment devices.

Thilander and Bloom (1968) have reported the presence of zonulae adherentes (intermediate junctions) in human oral epithelium, including that of the gingiva. These structures are formed where adjacent cell membranes become almost exactly parallel over a distance of about 0.2μ and have an intercellular space, approximately 200 Å in width, which is occupied by a homogeneous, apparently amorphous material of low density (Fig. 12a). In the original description of intermediate junctions (Farquhar and Palade, 1963) bands of dense material were described in the subjacent cytoplasmic matrix; as these could not be found in oral epithelium Thilander and Bloom concluded that their observations had been made on a modified form of zonula adherens. Although the function of intermediate junctions is not clear it is possible that they form temporary intercellular attachment zones. It is of interest that the principal mode of attachment of clear cells to adjoining epithelial cells appears to be by this type of junction (Thilander and Bloom, 1968). These structures have all been found associated with basal cells and in other layers of the epithelium from masticatory gingival mucosa (Schroeder and Theilade, 1966; Thilander and Bloom, 1968).

6. Intercellular Spaces

Routine histological stains and light microscopy show the spaces between epithelial cells to be vacant except for interruptions by epithelial bridges; electron microscopy occasionally reveals vague amorphous fibrillae occupying these spaces, and various histochemical techniques have indicated the presence of definite chemical substances. From such techniques it is evident that the spaces between cells of masticatory gingival epithelium are occupied by proteins, carbohydrates, and mucopolysaccharides of the neutral, acidic sulphated, and acidic non-sulphated types, possibly including chondroitin sulphate B (Thonard and Scherp, 1962; Cimasoni et al., 1963; Cimasoni and Held, 1964; Toto and Sicher, 1964; Toto and Grandel, 1966a; and Cohen, 1968). Some increase in intensity of staining for mucopolysaccharides has been described as occurring towards the surface (Toto and Grandel, 1966a) and has been interpreted as an indication that these substances play a role in keratinization. However, Cohen (1968) found that the intercellular substance stained more intensely in basal and lower prickle-cell layers than in the upper layers of masticatory gingival epithelium, and this was independent of the keratinized or non-keratinized nature of the surface layer. The staining properties of intercellular substance seem to be similar to those of the light microscopic "basement membrane" and indicate that they comprise similar chemical substances.

A combination of electron microscopic and cytochemical methods (Rambourg and Leblond, 1967) has enabled a coating of glycoproteins and acidic residues to be seen outside the plasma membranes of individual epithelial cells and between the lamina densa and basal epithelial cells. This coating is continuous with the middle plate, intercellular contact layer, of the desmosomes and is believed to play a part in holding cells together and controlling reactions that occur between cells and their environment.

7. The Prickle-cell Layer (Stratum Spinosum)

When keratinocytes migrate from the basal layer to enter the deepest layer of the stratum spinosum they can still contribute to the proliferative pool and so occasional mitotic figures are seen. The most immediate effect of transition to a prickle cell is that the erstwhile basal cell exhibits more prominent spines at the cell periphery and, in addition, an increase in cytoplasmic tonofibrils, an increase in cytoplasmic-nuclear ratio, and a decrease in cytoplasmic granules (Listgarten, 1964). The prominent peripheral spines of these cells consist of cytoplasm packed with tonofibrils which terminate in the attachment plaques of desmosomes. These spines are thrown into striking relief by wide intercellular spaces which are mainly due to shrinkage artefact (Schroeder and Theilade, 1966); their greater prominence compared to the basal layer may be caused by the increased amount of cytoplasm available for shrinkage in prickle cells. The desmosomes between adjacent cells are tenaciously adherent and do not separate, so causing the cytoplasm to be drawn into fine spines wherever they are situated. The desmosomes are more frequent in the stratum spinosum than in the basal layer, and often maculae or zonulae occludentes can be found halfway between two desmosomes (Schroeder and Theilade, 1966). Histochemical observations on the site of oxidative enzymes in human masticatory gingival epithelium have shown reaction product to be associated with desmosomes; however, as no special relationship between mitochondria and desmosomes has been found it is possible that such a localization is due to an artefact (Nuki, 1967).

Though cytoplasmic granules are fewer than in basal cells, the cells of the stratum spinosum are still capable of synthesizing protein. The deepest layers show similar synthetic activity to basal cells but, in the skin of newborn rats, arginine, histidine, methionine, and serine show a slightly greater affinity for the prickle-cell layer than cells of other layers (Fukuyama and Epstein, 1966). RNA synthesis also occurs in the stratum spinosum (Bernstein, 1964).

Occasional cytoplasmic particles of glycogen have been described in the stratum spinosum cells of healthy human masticatory gingival epithelium examined by electron microscopy (Schroeder and Theilade, 1966). As the stratum spinosum forms the bulk of the epithelium it is appropriate here to discuss the presence of glycogen in masticatory gingival epithelium as detected by histochemical techniques. Such demonstration of glycogen, and of the phosphorylase enzyme associated with glycogen formation, in masticatory gingival epithelium has proved to be widely variable and dependent upon species, presence of inflammation, and degree of keratinization (Weinmann et al., 1959; Klingsberg and Butcher, 1961; Klingsberg et al., 1961; Quintarelli and Cheraskin, 1961; Cabrini and Carranza, 1966; Löe, 1967; and Weinmann and Meyer, 1959). While vagaries of technique may have been responsible for some of the equivocal results obtained, it would seem likely that the most important factor is the presence of inflammation and perhaps also the effect this has upon keratinization. Certainly where glycogen is absent keratinization is more likely to be fully developed (Weinmann and Meyer, 1959). In considering the question of the presence of glycogen in masticatory gingival epithelium it is as well to take into account the observations of Freinkel (1964) on skin epithelium. This normally contains little or no glycogen, but glycogen will accumulate in epithelial cells in response to mechanical or radiation trauma and in abnormal states of keratinization. The difficulty experienced not only in defining, but also in obtaining, normal masticatory gingival epithelium would seem to account for many of the conflicting reports in the literature. In fact, careful selection of gingiva by the use of rigid criteria for the exclusion of any inflammatory states has failed to show the presence of glycogen in any part of the human gingival epithelium (Löe, 1967).

As the cells of the stratum spinosum pass peripherally and become more superficial a variety of changes can be observed, the most obvious being a change in shape from polyhedral to squamous (scale-like). Also there are variations in the oxidative enzyme pattern, Krebs cycle enzymes exhibiting a gradual decrease in intensity while glucose-6-phosphate dehydrogenase activity shows an increase (Gerson et al., 1966; Löe, 1967; Nuki, 1967). This has been interpreted as representing a shift from aerobic to anaerobic glycolytic activity in superficial cells as they enter upon the processes of desquamation (Löe, 1967) or keratinization (Gerson, 1967). Concomitant with this altered gradient there is also a change in the intracytoplasmic distribution of histochemical reaction products for oxidative enzymes compared with that seen in basal cells. In addition to their presence at desmosomal sites, as has already been described, these are deposited only in the perinuclear regions of cells in the stratum spinosum and subsequent layers (Nuki, 1967).

Toto and Grandel (1966b) have shown that a weak reaction for sulphated mucopolysaccharides, apparently associated with keratinization, commences in the stratum spinosum. This increases in intensity through the granular layer.

In skin (Snell, 1967), and mouse oral epithelium in organ culture (Kallman and Wessels, 1967), definite cross-banding of tonofibril bundles has been demonstrated. As the cells become flattened and elongated, tonofibril bundles become orientated parallel to the epithelial surface. Another change which takes place as the cells of the stratum spinosum become more superficial concerns the plasma membrane; this begins a process of thickening which continues through the granular layer, and is associated with keratinization. Changes in the plasma membrane seem to be associated with the presence of small cytoplasmic structures most commonly called membrane coating granules or Odland bodies. These granules are sometimes reported to be visible in superficial cells of the stratum spinosum. However, as they always seem to be present in the granular layer, consideration of their properties and changes in plasma membrane structure are confined to that section. Similarly, alterations that have been described as occurring in desmosomes as part of the process of keratinization will be discussed in the section on the granular layer.

8. The Granular Layer (Stratum Granulosum)

The flattened cells of the granular layer are notable for the fact that they contain keratohyalin granules, which give the layer its name. Such granules are not, however, invariably present in keratinized epithelia (Mercer, 1961), including masticatory gingival epithelium (Cohen, 1967a), and this has been taken to indicate that they are not essential for keratinization. Support for this view is claimed from the facts that: (i) keratohyalin granules are more numerous in sites of slow keratinization, or where mitotic rate is reduced (Meyer et al., 1956), and (ii) these granules, in contradistinction to keratin, contain no disulphide or sulphydryl groups (Matoltsy and Matoltsy, 1962). It has been argued that instead of being precursors of keratin, the keratohyalin granules represent epithelial debris or areas of partially lysed cellular constituents (Jarrett et al., 1966). Further, the metal ions present in keratohyalin granules, which incidentally account for their deep staining with haematoxylin, may indicate an excretion pathway for these possibly toxic substances (Pizzolato and Lillie, 1967). On the other hand, calcium and magnesium present in keratohyalin granules may act as enzyme activators essential for normal epithelial function (Jarrett et al., 1966). Calcium has been demonstrated in the granules of masticatory gingival epithelium by Cohen (1967b). The opinion that keratohyalin granules represent areas of cell lysis or debris is not supported by the observations that these granules do not appear to be associated with digestive enzymes but in fact appear to be metabolically active. Squier and Waterhouse (1967a) found no coincidental localization of these granules and acid phosphatase in an electron cytochemical study of the oral epithelium in rats, yet it would be reasonable to expect areas of debris or lysis to be associated with deposits representing sites of acid phosphatase activity. Also, following administration of various radioactively labelled amino acids to mice, glycine, histidine, arginine and serine appear to be localized to keratohyalin granules of oesophageal epithelium (Bernstein, 1964; Fukuyama and Epstein, 1966; Rowden and Budd, 1967). Cox and Reaven (1967) and Fukuyama and Epstein (1967) have confirmed the localization of labelled histidine to keratohyalin granules by an electron microscopic technique, the latter authors demonstrating initial localization to tonofibrils with final passage of labelled material into the keratin layer. Of the other amino acids, labelled tyrosine was only inconsistently localized to keratohyalin granules and labelled proline was found between the granules. The overall pattern of selective localization of amino acids in the granular layer is at variance with that in other layers of the epithelium. It has been interpreted as implying that the keratohyalin granules are indeed active in the process of keratinization (Fukuyama and Epstein, 1966). Mechanisms that have been suggested for this process are: (a) the addition of "sulphur-rich" elements (Bernstein, 1964); (b) contribution to the matrix of the final keratin pattern (Rowden and Budd, 1967); or (c) contribution to changes in the intercellular substance following export of synthesized proteins from the granular cell (Rowden and Budd, 1967). The latter possibility presages the role of membrane coating granules, which are considered shortly, but at this juncture it is necessary to point out that observations made on radioautographs obtained after injection of radioactive amino acids should be interpreted with caution. Such factors as the variable transport of amino acids across cell membranes and the possibility of breakdown and re-incorporation into another molecule should always be considered. It seems likely, however, that those amino acids incorporated into the granular layer as early as five minutes after administration enter the cells by diffusion from the intercellular spaces (Rowden and Budd, 1967) and not by being carried up within differentiating basal layer cells. Interpretation of electron microscopic radioautographs with regard to accurate localization of label in cells containing many tonofibrils and keratohyalin granules is fraught with difficulties. The presence of RNP particles in the stratum granulosum is a further factor indicative of protein synthesis in that layer, but not necessarily in the keratohyalin granules.

Although active RNA synthesis has been judged as occurring in the stratum granulosum, by radioautography following incorporation of radioactively labelled cytidine (Bernstein, 1964), the granules have been reported as being free from both RNA and DNA (Jarrett et al., 1959). Other histochemical techniques have demonstrated that glycogen and paS-positive carbohydrates are absent from keratohyalin granules and that they are susceptible to digestion by elastase and lipase but resistant to hyaluronidase and trypsin (Matoltsy and Matoltsy, 1962; and Cohen, 1967c). Glycogen particles were occasionally found in the cytoplasm of cells of the stratum granulosum in human masticatory gingival epithelium (Schroeder and Theilade, 1966).

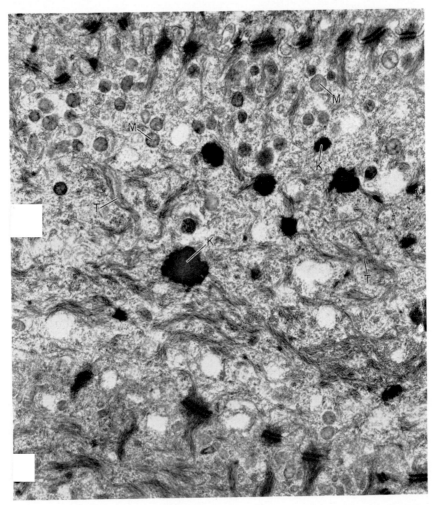

FIG. 15. Electron micrograph of an epithelial cell in the granular layer to show the variable size of keratohyalin granules (K). There is only a random association of these granules with tonofibrils (T). Membrane coating granules (M) are present almost exclusively in the distal part of the cell cytoplasm. Human masticatory gingival epithelium. (×20,000.)

According to Zelickson (1963), keratohyalin granules of skin epithelium increase in size and number as the cells approach the keratin layer, exhibit a filamentous internal structure, and are found in close association with tono-filaments. In masticatory gingival epithelium, however, Listgarten (1964) has found that the keratohyalin granules, though initially identical in size, eventually vary greatly. Also, they possess a definite granular structure, are not associated with tonofibrils, but consistently are surrounded by a clear zone of cytoplasm (Fig. 15). The tonofibrils of the stratum granulosum cells are concentrated at the periphery, especially along the border adjacent to keratin (Listgarten, 1964). Snell (1967) has also observed a close association between keratohyalin granules and tonofibrils in human skin. However, as other types of skin, such as that from guinea pig, revealed no such association he concluded that a close relationship between these two structures was not essential for keratinization.

In cells of the stratum granulosum nuclei are pyknotic and mitochondria have a degenerate appearance. Squier and Waterhouse (1967a) have shown, in rat oral epithelium, a close relationship between deposits representing sites of acid phosphatase activity and the mitochondria, indicating that acid phosphatase may play a part in the removal of these organelles prior to keratinization. Rowden (1967) has found only occasional lysosomes in the granular layers of mouse oesophageal and skin epithelium, unlike the greater number in deeper layers; on the other hand, non-lysosomal acid phosphatase was present to a greater extent in the stratum granulosum than in other layers. This observation conforms to the pattern suggested by many other histochemical studies for acid phosphatase, and also for esterases (Cohen, 1967d).

Changes in the plasma membranes of keratinocytes occur while nucleus and cytoplasm are still intact; this means that they are often first observed in the superficial cells of the stratum spinosum. Initially a moderately dense band of material, 100–150 Å thick, is seen at the periphery of the cytoplasm against the inner surface of the plasma membrane. Increase in density occurs until it becomes indistinguishable from the inner layer of the plasma membrane, causing this to appear thickened while the middle and outer layers remain unchanged (Farbman, 1966). Listgarten (1964) did not describe changes in the plasma membranes of cells in human masticatory gingival epithelium until they were part of the stratum granulosum, where thicker, denser, and straighter membranes were observed. Acid phosphatase activity has been demonstrated adjacent to the plasma membranes of cells in the stratum granulosum of rat oral epithelium and could possibly be associated with changes in these membranes or in the desmosomes (Squier and Waterhouse, 1967a). Although most observers have related changes in plasma membranes with the process of keratinization, similar thickening of the membranes has been reported in non-keratinized buccal mucosa (Hashimoto et al., 1966).

In one of the first electron microscopic studies of human skin, Selby (1957) described small uniform particles, believed then to be small keratohyalin granules, in the superficial cells of the stratum spinosum. Later, Odland (1960) presented his view that these particles are attenuated mitochondria.

They are first located in the layer immediately beneath the stratum granulosum, possess definite internal structure, and co-exist with keratohyalin
granules in the granular layer. Similar bodies have been described in superficial cells of the stratum spinosum in mouse oesophageal epithelium (Rowden,
1966), and in rat oral epithelium (Farbman, 1964), where they are associated

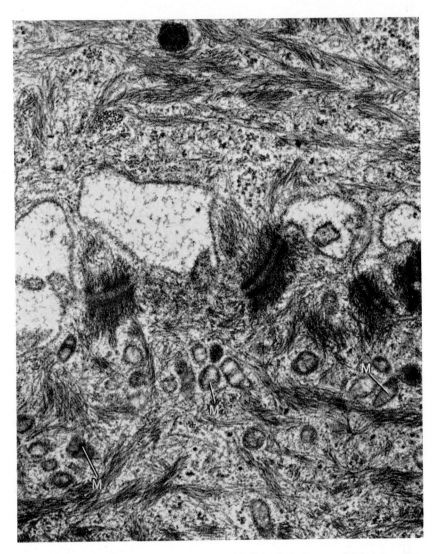

FIG. 16. Electron micrograph of part of two epithelial cells in the superficial region of the
prickle-cell layer. Membrane coating granules (M) are conspicuous in the distal cytoplasm.
Some of these can be seen to possess a definite internal lamellated structure. Human masticatory gingival epithelium. (×45,000.)

with the inner surface of the plasma membrane on the side of the cell furthest from the basal lamina. As the particles contain material structurally similar to that which, for the first time, is also present in the intercellular spaces of the same region, it has been suggested that the function of the particles is to discharge this substance into the intercellular spaces. This would perhaps be responsible for changes observed in the plasma membranes (Rowden and Budd, 1967). It is on account of this supposed function that these particles are called *membrane coating granules* (Fig. 16); in addition they are referred to as *Odland bodies* and *intracellular dense bodies*. Farbman (1964) has pointed out that these granules do not resemble attenuated mitochondria because the internal lamellae are too thin and there is not always a definite limiting membrane. The internal structure may be indicative of synthetic activity (Rowden, 1966) or protein transport (Rowden and Budd, 1967). Matoltsy and Parakkal (1965) claim to have shown that these granules initially appear in association with the Golgi apparatus and do not migrate to the cell periphery until the cell enters the granular layer.

It is highly probable that the structures described as "small dense granules", first appearing at the distal borders of superficial cells in the stratum spinosum of normal human masticatory gingival epithelium (Schroeder and Theilade, 1966), represent membrane coating granules, particularly in view of their behaviour in superficial cells of the stratum granulosum. Here granules diminish in number, and dilatations, occupied by empty microvesicles of approximately the same size as the granules and by dense material of similar consistency to that contained by the granules, are present in the intercellular spaces. Listgarten (1964) had observed these structures only occasionally, as rounded vesicles of 500–1500 Å diameter, in cells of the stratum granulosum of human masticatory gingival epithelium. Frithiof and Wersäll (1965), on the other hand, found membrane coating granules in all specimens of ortho- and para-keratotic human oral epithelium, including gingiva, of similar size, position and appearance to those described in other keratinized epithelia. The highly ordered internal lamellated structure of parallel dense layers was separated from the cytoplasm by a diffuse membrane. In the upper stratum granulosum the granules were frequently seen in intercellular spaces, with a corresponding decrease in cytoplasmic granules, and the striated material often increased considerably near the keratin layer. Interestingly Frithiof and Wersäll (1965) did not find membrane coating granules in any normal non-keratinizing oral epithelium.

The membrane coating granules produce a coating on the outer surface of the plasma membrane, which may lead to the deposition of the peripheral cytoplasmic band on the inner surface. Such processes may seal off the cells from the normal environment, or affect permeability and plasticity, in such a way that a chain of events is set in motion that will eventually lead to production of a keratinized cell (Farbman, 1966; and Rowden, 1966). It appears that at a molecular level, keratin formation begins at the cell periphery (Jarrett et al., 1966).

Changes in the desmosomes begin to appear, according to Listgarten (1964), in the superficial cells of the stratum spinosum in masticatory gingival epithelium and are continued, more markedly, in the stratum granulosum. These changes involve frequent loss of the intercellular contact layer, better definition of the proximal light layers, a thicker and straighter inner dense lamina which becomes continuous with the attachment plaque, and an apparent loss of continuity in the outer dense lamella of the plasma membrane. On the other hand, Schroeder and Theilade (1966) and Thilander and Bloom (1968) have not observed, in similar tissue, changes in the desmosomes, tight junctions and intermediate junctions until the border between the granular layer and keratin is reached. Here well-defined attachment plaques are present on the stratum granulosum side, whereas in the keratin attachment plaques are continuous with the broader and denser inner layer of the proximal plasma membrane. It has been suggested by Thilander and Bloom (1968) that the discrepancies between these two views of desmosomal changes may be due to differences in degree of keratinization in the tissues examined, or to appearances produced by oblique sectioning. Long stretches of zonulae occludentes occur between the granular and keratin layers; also, a zonula occludens often seems to form the most superficial junction between two stratum granulosum cells (Schroeder and Theilade, 1966). Intercellular spaces are considerably diminished in the stratum granulosum whereas tight and intermediate junctions are very common (Thilander and Bloom, 1968).

Cells pass from the granular layer into the keratin layer independently and randomly rather than as a single sheet of cells (Rowden and Budd, 1967).

9. The Keratin Layer (Stratum Corneum)

The final stage in the differentiation of cells in the masticatory gingival epithelium is the process of keratinization. This results in formation of a layer of fully cornified, almost featureless cells, the stratum corneum or keratin layer, which is sharply demarcated from the underlying stratum granulosum. Though often thought of as resulting from degeneration, dessication, poor nutrition or other deleterious factors, keratin is purposefully formed for a definite function (Mercer, 1961). In fact, as well illustrated in the gingiva, adverse factors have the effect of causing a reduction in keratinization while conditions of optimal health are favourable to its continued production.

Although there seems to be little doubt, on the basis of exfoliated cell smears stained by Papanicolaou's method, that the masticatory gingival epithelium can be one of the most heavily keratinized regions of the oral mucosa (Miller et al., 1951; and Montgomery, 1951), there are conflicting reports on the prevalence of keratinized, parakeratotic, and non-keratinized surfaces (Meyer *et al.*, 1956; Trott, 1957; Gargiulo *et al.*, 1961b; Schroeder and Theilade, 1966; and Sicher, 1966). In these reports it would appear that more rigorous selection of "normal" material has led to observations of more complete keratinization. This is borne out by the work of Weinmann *et al.* (1959), showing that the degree of keratinization of human masticatory gingival epithelium is inversely proportional to the severity of inflammation in the underlying connective tissue. Moreover, Weinmann and Meyer (1959) have described the condition of incomplete parakeratosis, a layer of keratin surmounted by a layer of parakeratin, in human masticatory gingival epithelium. When no inflammation was present nearly all surfaces exhibited full keratinization, incomplete, or complete parakeratosis; conversely, fully keratinized surfaces were infrequent even when inflammation was only mild. It seems possible, therefore, that the association of non-keratinized masticatory gingival epithelium with an increase in mitotic index of 50% (Soni *et al.*, 1965) represents a common cause for both of these factors, namely the presence of inflammation in underlying tissue. However, there may be an association between mitotic activity and keratinization, for both are affected by age and endocrine status. The thickness of keratin and the mitotic index are increased with age (Gargiulo *et al.*, 1961a); and the keratinization pattern of the oral mucosa is known to vary during the menstrual cycle (Main and Ritchie, 1967). Pathological and physiological factors affecting keratinization probably account for most of the reported discrepancies in the nature of the gingival surface.

It would appear that masticatory gingival epithelium naturally produces keratin, but that this process is easily inhibited. A further pointer to the validity of this view is the effect of toothbrushing or other physical stimulation in enhancing keratinization of masticatory gingival epithelium (Merzel *et al.*, 1963; and Cantor and Stahl, 1965). This is more likely to be due to stimulation of pre-existing keratinizing characteristics, by the encouragement of gingival health, than to transformation of a non-keratinizing epithelium into the keratinized type. In this respect it is of interest that non-keratinized alveolar mucosa transplanted to the site of normally keratinized gingival mucosa in a monkey retained its non-keratinized characteristics after daily toothbrushing (Ten Cate, personal communication). Brushing does not, therefore, cause keratinization but can only encourage it to occur if there is already a tissue predisposition. The fact that such a predisposition exists, and that it is at least in part genetically determined, has been implied by the observations of Coslet and Cohen (1967) that human embryological oral epithelium has a basal layer exhibiting different characteristics in sites to become keratinized compared to those remaining non-keratinized.

The keratinized cells of human masticatory gingival epithelium are shrunken, flattened, and composed primarily of packed tonofilaments embedded in a less dense matrix (Listgarten, 1964). Some authorities, working mainly on skin, believe that the tonofilaments are bound together in an inter-fibrillar matrix in the stratum granulosum (Brody, 1959; Brody, 1964; and Odland, 1964). Others are of the opinion that there is no clear evidence for tonofilaments being true precursors of keratin, as some non-epithelial cells also possess tonofilaments but never produce keratin (Jarrett et al., 1966); their alternative view is that the appearance resembling tonofilaments is a fixation, precipitation, or polymerization artefact.

Cytoplasmic organelles are rare, and difficult to recognize, in the stratum corneum; the process of keratinization seems to be carried out in conjunction with cell lysis. Synthesis of the fibrous protein, keratin, occurs at the same cellular level as hydrolytic enzymes become apparent in greatest quantity (Cabrini and Carranza, 1958; Ten Cate, 1963; Eisen et al., 1964; Riley, 1964; Jarrett et al., 1966; Cohen, 1967d; Itoiz et al., 1967; and Squier and Waterhouse, 1967a). The presence of these enzymes has been interpreted as an indication that non-keratinized cell contents are being rapidly removed, thus leaving only the keratinized periphery of the cell to contribute to the keratin layer. Such a process indicates some degree of control. However, other investigators, taking the view that keratinization is a degradative process, believe that the activity of acid hydrolases is due to an acid pH in the upper layers of the epithelium providing the right milieu, and that it is brought about by distance from supply of necessary metabolites (Dicken and Decker, 1966).

In electron microscopic studies of human masticatory gingival epi-thelium (Listgarten, 1964; and Schroeder and Theilade, 1966), nuclei and occasional cytoplasmic organelles were found in cells of parakeratotic stratum corneum, and occasional empty, round spaces of various diameter, in keratinized cells. Although the outer layer of the plasma membrane in keratinized cells is thin, the inner layer is denser and broader than usual; also, the desmosomes and maculae or zonulae occludentes remain intact right up to the surface, indicating that exfoliation is abrupt rather than gradual (Schroeder and Theilade, 1966). Conversely, Listgarten noted a continual disintegration of desmosomes, with gradual loss of adhesiveness, until the most superficial cornified cells became separated by rupture of the desmosomes. In skin it would appear that changes in desmosomes occur throughout the stratum corneum, not abruptly at the surface (Snell, 1966). Thin-walled cells without desmosomal attachments probably represent melanocytes or Langerhans cells. The electron microscopic appearance of a keratinized stratified squamous epithelial surface is shown in Fig. 17.

The final event in the life of a keratinocyte is its detachment from the sur-face. In skin this appears to take the form of variably sized flakes containing many cells rather than as individual cells (Goldschmidt and Kligman, 1967). To judge from the individual cornified cells that are usually collected from

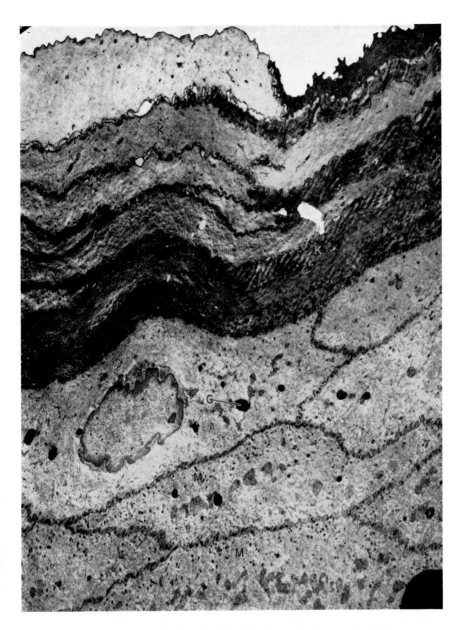

FIG. 17. Electron micrograph of keratin (K). A few keratohyalin granules (G) are present in the underlying granular layer and membrane coating granules (M) are again seen to be concentrated in the distal part of the cytoplasm. Hamster cheek pouch epithelium. (× 4,000.)

the surface of oral epithelium in exfoliative cytology studies, it seems likely that such cells are shed individually rather than in larger flakes (Fig. 18).

The physical, chemical, and biological properties of keratin that enable it to fulfil its protective function have been extensively reviewed by Mercer (1961), Kligman (1964), and Malkinson (1964). It is apparent that the chemical composition of keratin varies from animal to animal, site to site, and time to time, being less constant than many other tissues of the body.

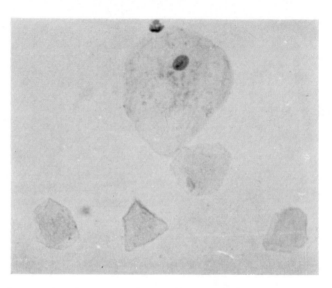

FIG. 18. Four anucleated squames, keratinized cells, in a smear from the surface of human masticatory gingival epithelium. The larger, nucleated cell at the top of the plate is probably a cell from the prickle-cell layer. Papanicolaou's stain. (×410.)

Keratin comprises a fibrous protein that contains eighteen amino acids arranged as polypeptide chains. Parallel polypeptide chains are united by disulphide bonds, one part of which is in each chain. The bonds are formed by the diamino acid cystine and arise by the oxidation of sulphydryl groups in two molecules of the amino acid cysteine, one in each of two adjacent polypeptide chains. Conversion of sulphydryl (SH) groups to disulphide (—S—S—) bonds most probably occurs in the granular layer, with magnesium and calcium acting as catalysts (Jarrett et al., 1966). However, some workers are of the opinion that such a conversion could not occur above the basal layer (Van Scott and Flesch, 1954). Histochemical studies of sulphydryl groups and disulphide bonds in masticatory gingival epithelium have not given consistent results but generally seem to show an increase of either disulphide bonds, or sulphydryl groups, or both, concomitant with keratinization (Turesky et al., 1957; Cancellaro et al., 1961; and Cohen, 1967e). Although keratin relies largely upon the disulphide bond for its physical strength this bond is extremely vulnerable to disruption by reduction and oxidation (Mercer, 1961).

The cell membranes of the stratum corneum are also protein but have an amino acid composition different from that of keratin (Matoltsy and Matoltsy, 1966), particularly in having a higher proline and cystine content. Fortunately the cell membranes enclosing keratin, although physically weaker, are much more resistant to the chemical processes attacking keratin, and will not dissolve in strong reducing or oxidizing agents (Mercer, 1961). Proteolytic enzymes, however, will digest cell membranes, except where these are incorporated into a solid intact tissue like keratin. An efficient, well-integrated system of protection is therefore provided by the simple expedient of enclosing a substance of physical strength, but certain chemical frailty, within membranes that are resistant to the reagents most likely to damage their contents.

10. Pigmentation

This section is concerned with the microscopic features of pigmentation and the associated cells, melanocytes and Langerhans cells; the distribution of pigment visible upon clinical examination of the gingiva has been described in the section dealing with surface characteristics. The pigment concerned is melanin, which ranges in colour from light brown to almost black, and is found in the form of fine granules, mostly in the basal cells. In human masticatory gingival epithelium melanin is distributed evenly throughout the basal cell cytoplasm (Squier and Waterhouse, 1967b), differing from the situation in skin where the pigment forms a cap over the superficial aspect of the nucleus. The function of melanin seems to be concerned with protection of basal cell nuclei and underlying connective tissue from the harmful effects of ultraviolet light (Seiji and Itakura, 1966). While this would account for its presence in skin, particularly "on the sunny side of the nucleus", it hardly explains pigmentation of some parts of the gingiva, particularly on the lingual or palatal aspects and in the molar regions, where little protection from such stimuli is required. As keratinocytes pass peripherally the melanin granules disappear in much the same way as other organelles, and it is rare for melanin granules to be seen in exfoliated cells (Cohen, 1967f; and Squier and Waterhouse, 1967b). Although many basal keratinocytes may contain pigment granules they are not responsible for manufacture of the granules, this function being performed by a specialized cell, the melanocyte.

(a) *Melanocytes.* In embryonic life certain cells of the neural crest epithelium, melanoblasts, migrate to the epidermal-dermal junction where they insinuate into the basal epithelial layer and differentiate into melanocytes. A melanocyte has characteristic long cytoplasmic processes that extend between or under keratinocytes to terminate on any epithelial cell surface. These processes used to be called *dendrites* and the melanocytes *dendritic cells*, but such terminology is now falling into disuse. Transfer of melanin granules from their site of manufacture in melanocytes to other epithelial cells is effected through the melanocyte processes. A graphic illustration of this procedure has been provided by Cruickshank and Harcourt (1964) in

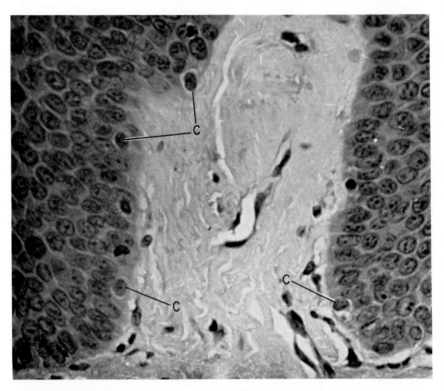

FIG. 19. Basal region of human masticatory gingival epithelium exhibiting some "clear cells" (C) which are probably melanocytes. Haematoxylin and eosin. (×660.)

time-lapse cinematographic studies on cell suspensions. Within the limits of the experimental conditions they found that a melanocyte could donate melanin pigment to more than one cell at a time and an epithelial cell could receive pigment from more than one melanocyte at a time. The recipient cell rather than the donor seems to be the active partner in the process. In relation to this it appears that intensity of pigmentation in any site is not so much dependent upon the number of melanocytes present as upon the capacity of melanocytes to transfer melanin to keratinocytes, the capacity of those cells to receive melanin, and the functional activity of melanocytes (Szabo, 1967).

The presence of pigment granules in keratinocytes as well as melanocytes often causes difficulty in distinguishing between these two types of cells in sections stained by routine methods, for these only reveal the presence of melanin if there are heavy deposits (Squier and Waterhouse, 1967b). It may be possible, however, to recognize a melanocyte from its "clear cell" appearance (Fig. 19), a characteristic that depends upon the greater contraction of cytoplasm upon fixation in melanocytes than in keratinocytes. Absence of desmosomes, hemidesmosomes, and tight junctions from the plasma membrane of melanocytes allows this shrinkage to occur; apparently the intermediate junctions around these cells (Thilander and Bloom, 1968) do not prevent their contraction. Melanocyte processes are therefore not seen in routine histological preparations but may be visible, extending through many layers of prickle cells, in cold-microtome sections not subjected to chemical fixation (Squier and Waterhouse, 1967b). Attempts to recognize melanocytes in this way may be confounded by their similarity in these respects to Langerhans cells. It is possible, however, by the use of a special histochemical technique, to distinguish active melanocytes from all other epithelial cells. This technique, the DOPA-reaction, relies for its effect upon the presence of tyrosinase, the enzyme or enzyme complex responsible for the last stage of the melanin-producing pathway in functioning melanocytes. Histologically-recognizable pigment is produced by tyrosinase still present in active melanocytes in tissue sections if dihydroxyphenylalanine (DOPA) is provided.

Melanin and melanocytes are largely concentrated in the basal layer of human masticatory gingival epithelium where the melanocytes account for about one in every fifteen cells (Barker, 1967; and Squier and Waterhouse, 1967b). Electron microscopic examination of melanocytes in this site reveals that they contain dense, slightly angular, melanin granules in a cytoplasm that is less dense than adjacent keratinocytes due to the absence of tonofilaments. Characteristically, there are no desmosomes at the cell periphery (Squier and Waterhouse, 1967b). An electron micrograph of a melanocyte is shown in Fig. 20. The presence of centrioles and occasional mitotic figures (Mitchell, 1963) indicates that melanocytes are able to divide, thereby replacing those lost superficially. Some workers have speculated upon a role for melanocytes in keratinization (Riley, 1964). Various possible mechanisms to explain the mode of development of melanin granules and synthesis of melanin have been discussed by Moyer (1963), Seiji et al. (1963), Zelickson et al. (1965), and Fitzpatrick et al. (1967).

(b) Langerhans cells. The presence of dendritic cells in a supra-basal position in human skin epithelium was first described by Langerhans (1868). By light microscopy these cells resemble melanocytes, consisting of contracted cytoplasm around a rod-shaped or elongated nucleus, and occupying a clear space enclosed by keratinocytes. They are, however, more superficial then melanocytes and hence have acquired an alternative name of *high-level clear-cells*. The explanation for this clear zone surrounding them is, as for

6

melanocytes, lack of desmosomes and consequent contraction of cytoplasm upon fixation (Breathnach, 1965). Unfixed cold-microtome sections, however, reveal the dendritic nature of these cells, again betraying a similarity to melanocytes, but they do not stain with the DOPA-reaction because tyro-

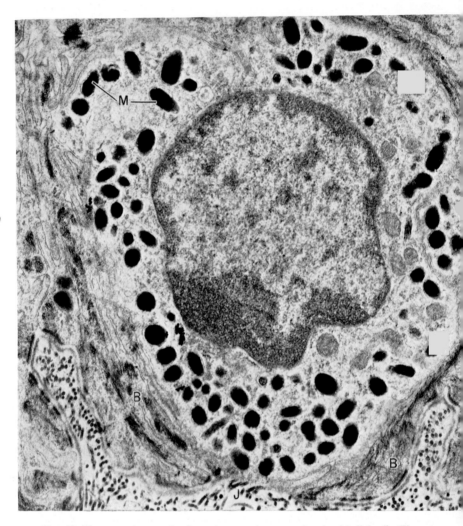

FIG. 20. Electron micrograph of a melanocyte in among basal epithelial cells. The cytoplasm contains numerous melanin granules (M) but no tonofilaments. No desmosomes are visible at the periphery of this cell. The melanocyte is cradled by two projections from adjacent basal cells (B) so that the junction between melanocyte and connective tissue is reduced to a small area. This area (J) has no lamina lucida, lamina densa, or hemidesmosomes, in contrast to the adjacent basal epithelial cells. This cradling effect of melanocytes can also be seen in Fig. 19 and is therefore unlikely to be due to plane of section artefact. Guinea pig ear skin. (×17,000.)

sinase is not present. However, another staining technique which relies upon the presence of gold chloride in the staining medium can be used (Waterhouse and Squier, 1967). This stains Langerhans cells but apparently not melanocytes. Such a technique applied to human masticatory gingival epithelium shows that Langerhans cells occur mainly in the superficial prickle-cell layers and only rarely among basal cells (Waterhouse and Squier, 1967).

Identification of Langerhans cells is most reliable in the electron microscope, their unique character having been revealed initially in skin epithelium

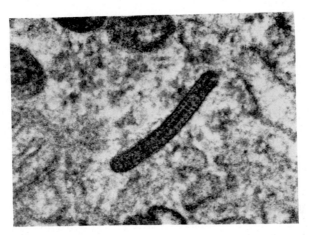

FIG. 21. An electron micrograph of a Langerhans cell granule. Guinea pig ear skin. (×120,000.)

(Breathnach, 1964 and 1965) and more recently in masticatory gingival epithelium (Waterhouse and Squier, 1967). The nucleus of the cell is indented, there is a well-developed Golgi region and centriole, tonofilaments and desmosomes are absent, and the cytoplasm contains distinctive granules. These granules have been reconstructed as a three-dimensional model by Sagebiel and Reed (1968), though as usually seen in two dimensions by electron microscopy they are mostly rod-shaped, about 4000 Å × 400 Å (Fig. 21). They sometimes have inflated vesicles at one end indicating an overall shape like a tennis racket. These granules occasionally are continuous with the plasma membrane (Breathnach, 1964; Zelickson, 1965; Waterhouse and Squier, 1967; and Wolff, 1967). Such an appearance may be interpreted in two ways; either the granules fuse with the plasma membrane or they are derived from it. However, Zelickson (1966) has claimed to show that these granules are produced by the smooth-walled vesicles of the Golgi apparatus. Similar granules have been reported as occurring rarely in epithelial cells that are obviously not Langerhans cells, presumably having entered these cells by a process of injection by Langerhans cells (Waterhouse and Squier, 1967) but

Zelickson (1965) does not believe that the granules can be secreted into other cells. A second type of granule also appears to be present in Langerhans cells of skin epithelium (Zelickson, 1966), distinct and separate from the characteristic granule previously described. This has a triple-layered membrane enclosing a matrix of homogeneous material or small vesicles, appears round or oval depending upon plane of section, and is formed by budding from the outer cisternae of the Golgi complex.

Other organelles, resembling melanin granules (but not pre-melanosomes) and lysosomes, have been described in Langerhans cells of skin epithelium (Zelickson, 1965) and masticatory gingival epithelium (Waterhouse and Squier, 1967). Cytoplasmic lipid droplets and a convoluted plasma membrane produce a vacuolated appearance in superficial Langerhans cells of skin epithelium (Zelickson, 1965). As these cells pass to the surface some changes take place, but they do not become keratinized and are not found in recognizable form in the stratum corneum (Breathnach, 1964). Identification of nucleoside polyphosphatase and adenosine triphosphatase activity in Langerhans cells, including those in masticatory gingival epithelium (Cohen, 1967f), has been taken as an indication that these cells are motile (Riley, 1966).

Riley (1967) has observed that the population of Langerhans cells varies in different parts of the skin, fewer being present where keratinization is heaviest. He has suggested that this may indicate some effect by these cells upon the removal of keratinocyte cytoplasm and organelles during the final stages of keratinization. A reduction in number of Langerhans cells is presumed to cause a reduction of lysis in keratinocytes, and consequently to allow more time for keratinization to take place, thus allowing a thicker layer of keratin to be produced. On the other hand, variations in number of Langerhans cells may simply reflect the fact that, in various parts of the epithelium, their stem cells have mitotic rates different from those of the keratinocyte stem cells (Riley, 1967). A further possible explanation of the function of Langerhans cells is that they act as epithelial macrophages. This view is supported by evidence that typical granules are found in some connective tissue macrophages under certain pathological conditions (Tarnowksi and Hashimoto, 1967; and de Man, 1968), and takes into account the presence of lysosomes in Langerhans cells.

(c) *The relationship between melanocytes and Langerhans cells.* The suggestion that Langerhans cells represent effete melanocytes (Billingham and Medawar, 1953) is supported by morphological similarities between melanocytes and Langerhans cells, predominance of melanocytes in basal layers and Langerhans cells in superficial layers, the mutual presence or absence of both types of cell in most sites, and their presence in similar quantities. It is now clear, however, from ultrastructural appearance, ability to synthesize protein in production of typical granules, high level of adenosine triphosphatase activity, and possession of mitotic capacity (Giacometti and Montagna, 1967), that Langerhans cells can no longer be considered effete, though the problem of their origin remains to be settled. The presence of melanin granules in a Langerhans cell need not imply that they were synthesized when that

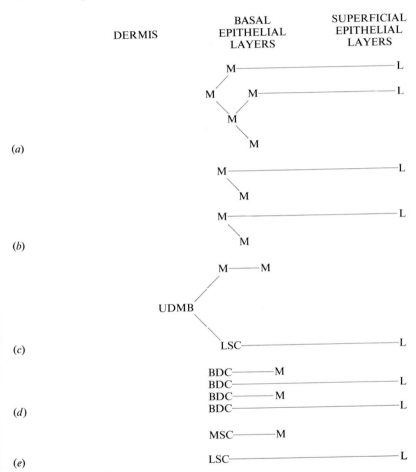

FIG. 22. Diagram to show some of the schemes suggested for the relationship between melanocytes (M) and Langerhans cells (L). (a); Basal melanocytes may divide to produce other melanocytes which either become Langerhans cells as they pass peripherally or divide to produce two more melanocytes. (b); Basal melanocytes may divide to produce one melanocyte and one Langerhans cell. (c); Undifferentiated melanoblasts (UDMB) may differentiate into either basal melanocytes or Langerhans stem cells (LSC) from which further melanocytes or Langerhans cells develop separately. (d); A uniform population of basal dendritic cells (BDC) may develop into either melanocytes or Langerhans cells. This scheme is similar to that shown in (b) but does not imply that Langerhans cells develop from mature melanocytes. (e); Langerhans cells and melanocytes may be two separate and distinct cell lines developing from unrelated Langerhans stem cells (LSC) and melanocyte stem cells (MSC).

cell was a melanocyte; it is quite possible that other melanocytes could have injected melanin granules into the Langerhans cell in the same way as into any other epithelial cell (Breathnach and Wyllie, 1965).

Although Langerhans cells are not effete melanocytes it still seems probable that both types of cell are in some way related to each other. It is unlikely, however, that a basal melanocyte would divide to produce one Langerhans cell unable to synthesize melanin and one melanocyte, as this would require transmission of a different set of genetic instructions to each daughter cell. A more acceptable possibility is that superficial Langerhans cells may be derived from a stem cell other than the melanocytes, but that both Langerhans stem cells and melanocytes arise from undifferentiated melanoblasts (Zelickson, 1966). There is some evidence in favour of this view: (i) in some situations Langerhans cells are present without melanocytes also being found (Zelickson, 1966); (ii) in such sites the number of Langerhans cells can be increased by irradiation, yet without pigment production (Riley, 1967); and (iii) selective histochemical methods for Langerhans cells and melanocytes reveal that there are more dendritic cells in the basal layers than there are melanocytes (Riley, 1967). Interpretation of this latter observation should be undertaken with caution as the non-melanogenic basal dendritic cells may represent pre-melanocytes in which tyrosinase activity has not been induced, or basal Langerhans cells in which tyrosinase activity has ceased. Finally, there remain the possibilities that basal dendritic cells may differentiate into either superficial Langerhans cells or acquire the ability to synthesize melanin and become melanocytes (Waterhouse and Squier, 1967), or that Langerhans cells and melanocytes represent two distinct and independent cell lines (Wolff and Winkelmann, 1967). The possible relationships between melanocytes and Langerhans cells are represented diagrammatically in Fig. 22.

B. CREVICULAR GINGIVAL EPITHELIUM

Extending from the gingival margin to the most coronal point of the attached epithelial cuff is a thin layer of stratified squamous epithelial cells, 5–15 cells in depth (Löe, 1967), the crevicular gingival epithelium (Fig. 23). This forms the soft tissue lining of the shallow gingival crevice encircling each tooth. The crevicular gingival epithelium gradually becomes thinner as it extends from the gingival margin towards the attached epithelial cuff. It is supported by dense fibrous connective tissue, though it is too coronal to be related to alveolar bone. Distinctions are soon apparent when crevicular and masticatory gingival epithelia are compared. The crevicular type, as well as being thinner, is devoid of rete ridges except where the undulating character of masticatory gingival epithelium may sometimes extend over the gingival margin for a short distance. Consequent upon the lack of rete ridges, the "basement membrane" of crevicular gingival epithelium appears by optical microscopy to be smooth and regular. At ultrastructural level the composition of lamina densa, lamina lucida, and basal cells in this region are similar to those of masticatory gingival epithelium.

Above the basal cell layer, cells of the stratum spinosum are slightly smaller than their counterparts in masticatory gingival epithelium (Löe, 1967) and, though the deepest layers may be polygonal, there is a rapid transition to flattened cells which lie parallel to the tooth surface. Tonofilaments and tonofibrils are more prevalent in prickle cells than basal cells, and have no particular intracytoplasmic orientation prior to insertion into attachment plaques, except in superficial cells where they are mainly parallel to plasma membranes and tooth surface. Desmosomes are in plentiful supply in the deeper cell layers, being fairly evenly distributed around plasma membranes (Thilander, 1963), but as the cells become more superficial the spaces between them diminish and intercellular bridges become less conspicuous. There is no information on the changes undergone by desmosomes in this site prior to desquamation (Löe, 1967). Histochemical demonstration of oxidative enzyme activity has illustrated similar staining in basal and prickle cells of crevicular and masticatory gingival epithelium, except that the association of granular reaction products with desmosomal sites was hardly visible in crevicular gingival epithelium (Nuki, 1967). Various observations (Person et al., 1961; and Felton et al., 1965) of stronger oxidative enzyme activity in crevicular gingival epithelium and the attached epithelial cuff compared with masticatory gingival epithelium possibly reflect the presence of inflammation in the tissue chosen for study.

Crevicular gingival epithelium has no granular layer and is not keratinized (McHugh, 1964). This explains the comparatively weak reactions for hydrolytic enzymes in this tissue (Cabrini and Carranza, 1958; and Itoiz et al., 1967), and could possibly account for the weak oxidative enzyme reaction at desmosomal sites should these be concerned with the process of keratinization. It would appear that no glycogen is present in cells of the crevicular gingival epithelium (Klingsberg et al., 1961; and Löe, 1967).

Desquamation of cells from the surface implies the presence of dividing cells in some part of the epithelium. These are found in the basal layer and divide at a rate as great as, or greater than, dividing cells in the masticatory gingival epithelium in rats (Trott and Gorenstein, 1963; and Hansen, 1966b), in mice (Beagrie, 1963), in marmosets (Beagrie, 1966), and in monkeys (Engler et al., 1965; and McHugh and Zander, 1965). Unlike the situation in masticatory gingival epithelium Trott and Gorenstein (1963), and Irons and Schaffer (1966), could find no evidence of diurnal variation in the mitotic activity of cells in the crevicular gingival epithelium of rats; Hansen (1966b), however, found evidence of a diurnal variation in all parts of the gingival epithelium of rats. In view of the fact that crevicular gingival epithelium in various animals often seems to have greater mitotic activity than masticatory

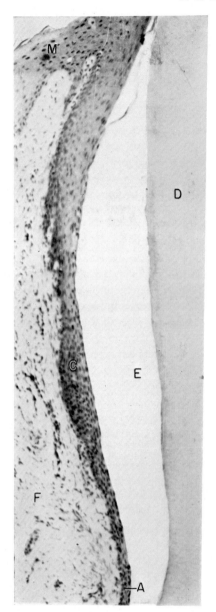

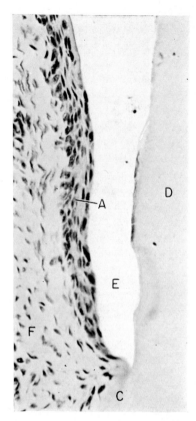

Fig. 24. A histological section of the attached epithelial cuff (A) which, in this decalcified section, is not shown in its true relationship adjacent to enamel. The enamel space (E), dentine (D), cementum (C) and fibrous connective tissue (F) are also shown. Monkey. Haematoxylin and eosin. (×585.)

Fig. 23. A histological section of crevicular gingival epithelium (C) to show its relatively smooth "basement membrane", and that it becomes thinner apically where it joins with the attached epithelial cuff (A). The enamel space (E) and gingival crevice are indistinguishable in this decalcified section. At its coronal end the crevicular gingival epithelium unites with masticatory gingival epithelium (M) in the region sometimes called the crestal gingiva. Dentine (D) and fibrous connective tissue (F) are also shown. Monkey. Haematoxylin and eosin. (×175.)

gingival epithelium it may be expected that desquamation of superficial cells from this site is also more rapid.

Melanocytes are not present in crevicular gingival epithelium (Squier and Waterhouse, 1967b), except occasionally in that part nearest to the gingival margin (Barker, 1967). Other dendritic cells, presumably Langerhans cells, have been found in more apical parts than the melanocytes, though still not further than 1 mm from the gingival margin (Barker, 1967).

C. Attached Epithelial Cuff

The term *attached epithelial cuff* was first employed by Orban *et al.* (1956). This was in a restatement of the traditional view that had been challenged by Waerhaug (1952), that a definite attachment apparatus exists between gingival epithelium and the tooth surface. As used in this Chapter, the term *attached epithelial cuff* describes the apical extension of the crevicular gingival epithelium which is not separated from the tooth surface by the gingival crevice but which is actually attached to the tooth (Fig. 24). Thus the relationships of the attached epithelial cuff are: coronally, the apical end of both the gingival crevice and the crevicular gingival epithelium; peripherally, dense fibrous connective tissue; apically, the superficial fibres of the periodontal ligament; and centrally, the tooth substance to which it is attached, which may be enamel, dentine, or cementum, or any combination of these tissues. The length of epithelial surface attached to tooth shows marked differences at various stages of passive eruption. When entirely confined to cementum it is reduced to nearly half of its length when entirely confined to enamel. On the other hand, the distance from the base of the attached epithelial cuff to the crest of alveolar bone remains remarkably constant through all stages of passive eruption (Gargiulo *et al.*, 1961b).

The general morphology of the attached epithelial cuff is similar to that of crevicular gingival epithelium in that the "basement membrane" is smooth, there is a definite basal layer, and superficial cells rapidly become flattened. Its unique features are all associated with the area of attachment of superficial cells to tooth surface. Ultra-microscopic investigation of this area shows that two cuticular structures, one believed to represent the primary enamel cuticle and the other to be derived from tissue fluid or saliva, can often be found between epithelium and tooth surface (Listgarten, 1966). Neither of these cuticular structures appear to be produced or secreted by the cells of the attached epithelial cuff so warrant no further consideration here; further information of relevance to their form and derivation may be obtained from Chapters 3 and 11, and from Löe (1967). Regardless of whether the superficial cells of the attached epithelial cuff are attached directly to either of the cuticular structures mentioned, or to any of the three possible dental tissues (enamel, dentine, or cementum), the manner in which such an attachment is

6*

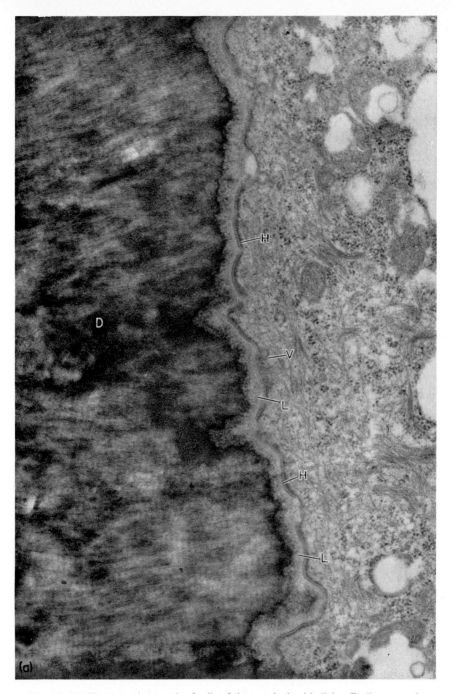

Fig. 25. (a); Electron micrograph of cells of the attached epithelial cuff adjacent to dentine (D). Reproduced by courtesy of M. A. Listgarten, *J. periodont. Res.* **2**, 46–52, 1967. Human. (×22,000.) Hemidesmosomes (H) are frequent along the interface and indistinct material thought to represent both lamina densa and lamina lucida (L) can be seen. Vesicles (V) along the cell periphery have been interpreted as contributing material to the junctional zone.

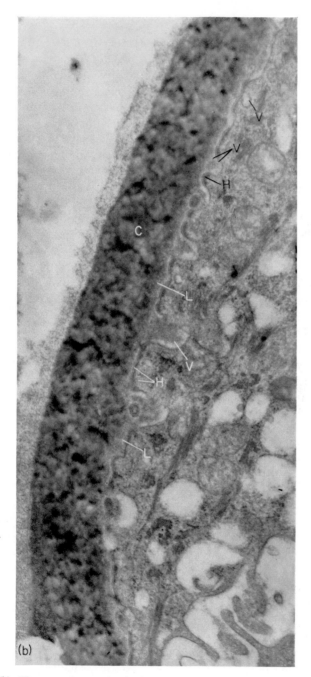

FIG. 25. (b); Electron micrograph of cells of the attached epithelial cuff adjacent to a cuticular structure (C). Reproduced by courtesy of M. A. Listgarten, *Am. J. Anat.* **119,** 147–178, 1966. Human. (×28,000.) Hemidesmosomes (H) are frequent along the interface and indistinct material thought to represent both lamina densa and lamina lucida (L) can be seen. Vesicles (V) along the cell periphery have been interpreted as contributing material to the junctional zone.

effected remains the same. A thin granular layer, 400–1200 Å in thickness, and resembling the lamina densa beneath basal epithelial cells, is always present between the superficial cells of the attached epithelial cuff and the tooth or cuticular surface. This granular structure is not divided into a lamina densa and lamina lucida but its average width is similar to the total width of lamina lucida and lamina densa (about 800 Å) in other sites. It is possible that the greater variation in thickness and uniform structure of this material may be due to decalcification procedures employed. A more likely prospect, however, would seem to be related to the observation that where the lamina densa is free from underlying unmineralized collagen, as in the lens capsule, Descemet's membrane of the cornea, or the vitelline membrane, it is thick or multilayered (McLoughlin, 1963). It is clear that the granular material associated with the attachment apparatus resembles the morphological appearance of a lamina densa (Fig. 25). Confirmatory evidence, other than that relying upon its structure, is also available. For example, distal plasma membranes of superficial cells of the attached epithelial cuff adjacent to the granular material exhibit hemidesmosomes (Fig. 25); occasional invaginations of plasma membranes adjacent to the granular material are filled with a morphologically identical substance (Fig. 25); and circular vesicles in the granular material resemble microvillous projections of basal epithelial cells described by Stern (1965) in the lamina lucida of masticatory gingival epithelium. Techniques other than electron microscopy can also be used to glean information on this subject. Radioactive proline, administered to mice and traced by radioautography, accumulates in sites of the "basement membrane", including that between the attached epithelial cuff and the tooth surface (Stallard et al., 1965). Continuous replacement of labelled material in the region of the "basement membrane" can be interpreted as an indication that the attachment between epithelium and tooth is a product of the epithelial cells. If the "basement membrane" of the attachment region was being manufactured apically and being drawn up between tooth and epithelial cuff, progressive labelling would be seen; in fact the all or none labelling that seems to occur enhances the view that "basement membrane" is a product of the epithelial cells (see also Chapter 2). Histochemical methods show that intercellular substance in the attached epithelial cuff, and the material between cuff and tooth surface, react in a similar manner to intercellular material and "basement membrane" material of masticatory gingival epithelium (Thonard and Scherp, 1962; Cimasoni et al., 1963; Toto and Sicher, 1964; and Toto and Sicher, 1965).

There is, therefore, ample evidence to indicate that the granular material present between superficial cells of the attached epithelial cuff and tooth surface is equivalent to the lamina densa of the "basement membrane" associated with other epithelia, and that this material is a product of the adjacent epithelial cells. This provokes a piquant morphological argument—

should the superficial cells of the attached epithelial cuff, having hemidesmosomes, resting on a "basement membrane", and contributing material to that "basement membrane", be considered as basal cells? There is no doubt that, although it is rare to find a lamina densa without underlying connective tissue, the mode of attachment of epithelium to calcified tissue as in this site, is unique and of biological importance. It is also clear that the nature of the attachment is in the form of a cementing substance and not a physical continuity of structure. However, during eruption, while reduced enamel epithelium still lines the gingival crevice, there is evidence that physical bonds do exist between enamel and epithelium (Cohen, 1962). These are not present for long, a rapid (Engler *et al.*, 1965), or gradual (McHugh and Zander, 1965), replacement of the reduced enamel epithelium being effected by oral squamous epithelium. Also, there is some evidence that cells of the stratum intermedium may play some part in replacement of reduced enamel epithelium, and combine with oral epithelium in forming crevicular gingival epithelium and the attached epithelial cuff (Hunt and Paynter, 1963; and Diab *et al.*, 1966). Although the nature of the attachment of epithelium to the tooth surface is that of a glue rather than a fibrous insertion, it does not follow that this state implies physical frailty.

Radioautographic studies have shown that cells of the attached epithelial cuff are capable of DNA synthesis and mitosis. In monkeys (Engler *et al.*, 1965; and McHugh and Zander, 1965) the attached epithelial cuff exhibited less labelling than any other part of the gingival epithelium; in marmosets (Beagrie, 1963; and Skougaard, 1965b) labelling was greater in the attachment region than in masticatory gingival epithelium; and in mice (Beagrie, 1963) and rats (Trott and Gorenstein, 1963), which have a completely different cellular organization in the attached epithelial cuff compared with primates, the cells of the cuff exhibit more frequent mitoses than other regions of the gingival epithelium. This illustrates the hazard of comparing the attached epithelial cuff of rodents with that of primates, but is sufficient to show that cells of this region undergo mitosis, thus implying, if overcrowding is to be avoided, that exfoliation of cells from this area must take place. In this respect it is of interest that in his study on marmosets, Beagrie (1963) described labelled cells in the superficial layers of the epithelial cuff adjacent to tooth surface, these migrating in a coronal direction as time elapsed. Skougaard (1965b) has compared turnover time in the attached epithelial cuff of marmosets with results from workers using other animals. He showed a widely variable pattern and concluded that this may be due partly to the effect of inflammation in reducing turnover time. Moreover, this could account for the frequent observations of more rapid turnover in the attached epithelial cuff than in masticatory gingival epithelium, the former site being subjected to more frequent and severe inflammatory insults.

Reconciliation of the evidence that an attachment apparatus exists and that its cells are in a constant state of division and exfoliation into the gingival crevice is not difficult. Such a dynamic attachment, in which strong adherence is maintained while movement of cells occurs, is no different from that existing between the nails and epithelial cells of the skin on fingers and toes, or between individual cells of the epithelium. The fact that there is a continual breakdown and reformation of lamina densa, hemidesmosomes, and desmosomes, obviously allows cells to alter their relationships to each other as they migrate through the attached epithelial cuff. As these processes occur in all other epithelia without loss of strong adhesion between individual cells, between epithelium and connective tissue, and between epithelial cells and keratin (which includes the finger- and toe-nails), it is safe to assume that similarly strong forces of adhesion are present in the attached epithelial cuff.

No melanocytes or Langerhans cells appear among cells of the attached epithelial cuff (Barker, 1967; and Squier and Waterhouse, 1967b), nor do any of these cells undergo keratinization, probably accounting for the weak hydrolytic enzyme activity in the region (Cabrini and Carranza, 1958; and Itoiz et al., 1967).

The passage of tissue fluid and cells, such as lymphocytes, into the gingival crevice is probably no more marked than similar transport through the intercellular spaces of other epithelia. Löe (1967) believes, with considerable justification, that fluid only passes into the gingival crevice from surrounding soft tissue in pathological conditions, and he further suggests that the absence of tissue fluid from the crevice is the best clinical indication of gingival health. There is no evidence that the cells of the attached epithelial cuff secrete substances into the gingival crevice, indeed any indication that such cells have secretory activity would have to be carefully screened to exclude the possibility that this was involved only in maintaining the granular lamina densa material effecting the attachment. (See Chapter 11.)

Acknowledgements

The electron micrographs comprising Figs. 7, 8, 12(a), 13(a), 14(a), 15, 16, and 17, were provided by Dr. D. Woods, and Figs. 20 and 21 by Mr P. Seal, both of the Electron Microscopy Unit, Imperial Cancer Research Fund, Lincoln's Inn Fields, London. Their help has been invaluable.

References

Ainamo, J. and Löe, H. (1966). *J. Periodont.* **37**, 5–13.
Barker, D. S. (1967). *Archs oral Biol.* **12**, 203–208.
Beagrie, G. S. (1963). *Dent. Practnr dent. Rec.* **14**, 18–26.
Beagrie, G. S. (1966). *Br. dent. J.* **121**, 417–420.
Bernstein, I. A. (1964). *In* "The Epidermis" (W. Montagna and W. C. Lobitz, Jr., eds.), pp. 471–483. Academic Press, New York and London.
Bertalanffy, F. D. (1960). *Acta anat.* **40**, 130–148.

Billingham, R. E. and Medawar, P. B. (1950). *J. Anat.* **84,** 50–56.
Billingham, R. E. and Medawar, P. B. (1953). *Phil. Trans. R. Soc. B.* **237,** 151–171.
Billingham, R. E. and Silvers, W. K. (1963). *New Engl. J. Med.* **268,** 477–480 and 539–545.
Billingham, R. E. and Silvers, W. K. (1967). *J. exp. Med.* **125,** 429–446.
Breathnach, A. S. (1964). *J. Anat.* **98,** 265–270.
Breathnach, A. S. (1965). *Int. Rev. Cytol.* **18,** 1–28.
Breathnach, A. S. and Wyllie, L. M. A. (1965). *J. invest. Derm.* **45,** 401–403.
Brody, I. (1959). *J. Ultrastruct. Res.* **2,** 482–511.
Brody, I. (1964). *In* "The Epidermis" (W. Montagna and W. C. Lobitz, Jr., eds.), pp. 251–273. Academic Press, New York and London.
Bullough, W. S. (1962). *Biol. Rev.* **37,** 307–342.
Bullough, W. S. and Rytömaa, T. (1965). *Nature (Lond.)* **205,** 573–578.
Cabrini, R. L. and Carranza, F. A. Jr. (1958). *J. Periodont.* **29,** 34–37.
Cabrini, R. L. and Carranza, F. A. (1966). *Int. dent. J., Lond.* **16,** 466–479.
Cancellaro, L. A., Klingsberg, J. and Butcher, E. O. (1961). *J. dent. Res.* **40,** 436–445.
Cantor, M. T. and Stahl, S. S. (1965). *Periodontics* **3,** 243–247.
Cimasoni, G. and Held, A-J. (1964). *Archs oral Biol.* **9,** 751–752.
Cimasoni, G., Fiore-Donno, G. and Held, A-J. (1963). *Helv. odont. Acta* **7,** 60–67.
Cohen, B. (1959). *Br. dent. J.* **107,** 31–39.
Cohen, B. (1962). *Br. dent. J.* **112,** 55–64.
Cohen, B., Ten Cate, A. R. and Donaldson, K. I. (1962). *Proc. Br. Soc. Study Prosth. Dent.* pp. 30–32.
Cohen, L. (1967a). *Dent. Practnr dent. Rec.* **18,** 134–138.
Cohen, L. (1967b). *Archs oral Biol.* **12,** 569–570.
Cohen, L. (1967c). *J. dent. Res.* **46,** 630.
Cohen, L. (1967d). *J. periodont. Res.* **2,** 317–322.
Cohen, L. (1967e). *Archs oral Biol.* **12,** 769–771.
Cohen, L. (1967f). *Archs oral Biol.* **12,** 1241–1244.
Cohen, L. (1968). *Archs oral Biol.* **13,** 163–169.
Coslet, J. G. and Cohen, D. W. (1967). *J. periodont. Res.* **2,** 297–316.
Cox, A. J. and Reaven, E. P. (1967). *J. invest. Derm.* **49,** 31–34.
Cruickshank, C. N. D. and Harcourt, S. A. (1964). *J. invest. Derm.* **42,** 183–184.
de Man, J. C. H. (1968). *J. Path. Bact.* **95,** 123–126.
Diab, M. A., Stallard, R. E. and Zander, H. A. (1966). *Oral Surg.* **22,** 241–251.
Dicken, C. H. and Decker, R. H. (1966). *J. invest. Derm.* **47,** 426–431.
Dummett, C. O. (1946). *J. dent. Res.* **25,** 421–432.
Dummett, C. O. (1960). *J. Periodont.* **31,** 345–385.
Eisen, A. Z., Arndt, K. A. and Clark, W. H. (1964). *J. invest. Derm.* **43,** 319–326.
Engler, W. O., Ramfjord, S. P. and Hiniker, J. J. (1965). *J. Periodont.* **36,** 44–57.
Farbman, A. I. (1964). *J. Cell Biol.* **21,** 491–495.
Farbman, A. I. (1966). *Anat. Rec.* **156,** 269–282.
Farquhar, M. G. and Palade, G. F. (1963). *J. Cell Biol.* **17,** 375–412.
Farquhar, M. G. and Palade, G. F. (1965). *J. Cell Biol.* **26,** 263–291.
Fehr, C. and Muhlemann, H. R. (1955). *Oral Surg.* **8,** 649–655.
Felton, J., Persson, P. A. and Stahl, S. S. (1965). *J. dent. Res.* **44,** 1238–1243.
Finegold, M. J. (1965). *Proc. Soc. exp. Biol. Med.* **119,** 96–100.
Fitzpatrick, T. B., Miyamoto, M. and Ishikawa, K. (1967). *Archs Derm.* **96,** 305–323.
Frankfurt, O. S. (1967). *Expl Cell Res.* **46,** 603–606.
Freinkel, R. K. (1964). *In* "The Epidermis" (W. Montagna and W. C. Lobitz, Jr., eds.), pp. 485–492. Academic Press, New York and London.

Frithiof, L. and Wersäll, J. (1965). *J. Ultrastruct Res.* **12**, 371–379.
Fukuyama, K. and Epstein, W. L. (1966). *J. invest. Derm.* **47**, 551–560.
Fukuyama, K. and Epstein, W. L. (1967). *J. invest. Derm.* **49**, 595–604.
Galand, P., Rodesch, F., Leroy, F. and Chretien, J. (1967). *Expl Cell Res.* **48**, 595–604.
Gargiulo, A. W., Wentz, F. M. and Orban, B. (1961a). *Oral Surg.* **14**, 474–492.
Gargiulo, A. W., Wentz, F. M. and Orban, B. (1961b). *J. Periodont.* **32**, 261–267.
Gersh, I. and Catchpole, H. R. (1960). *Perspect. Biol. Med.* **3**, 282–319.
Gerson, S. J. (1967). *Archs oral Biol.* **12**, 891–900.
Gerson, S. J., Meyer, J. and Mattenheimer, H. (1966). *J. invest. Derm.* **47**, 526–532.
Giacometti, L. and Montagna, W. (1967). *Science, N.Y.* **157**, 439–440.
Goldschmidt, H. and Kligman, A. M. (1967). *Archs Derm.* **95**, 583–586.
Greulich, R. C. (1964). *In* "The Epidermis" (W. Montagna and W. C. Lobitz, Jr., eds.), pp. 117–133. Academic Press, New York and London.
Ham, A. W. (1965). "Histology", 5th edn., Pitman Med. Pub. Co. Ltd., London.
Hansen, E. R. (1966a). *Odont. Tidskr.* **74**, 196–201.
Hansen, E. R. (1966b). *Odont. Tidskr.* **74**, 229–239.
Hansen, E. R. (1967a). *Odont. Tidskr.* **75**, 28–32.
Hansen, E. R. (1967b). *Odont. Tidskr.* **75**, 467–472.
Hansen, E. R. (1967c). *Odont. Tidskr.* **75**, 480–487.
Hashimoto, K., DiBella, R. J. and Shaklar, G. (1966). *J. invest. Derm.* **47**, 512–525.
Hunt, M. A. and Paynter, K. J. (1963). *Archs oral Biol.* **8**, 65–78.
Irons, W. B. and Schaffer, E. M. (1966). *Periodontics* **4**, 316–321.
Itoiz, M. E., Carranza, F. A. and Cabrini, R. L. (1967). *J. Periodont.* **38**, 130–133.
Jarrett, A., Spearman, R. I. C. and Hardy, J. A. (1959). *Br. J. Derm.* **71**, 277–295.
Jarrett, A., Spearman, R. I. C. and Riley, P. A. (1966). "Dermatology. A Functional Introduction", pp. 5–13. E.U.P., London.
Kallman, F. and Wessels, N. K. (1967). *J. Cell Biol.* **32**, 227–231.
Kligman, A. M. (1964). *In* "The Epidermis" (W. Montagna and W. C. Lobitz, Jr., eds.), pp. 387–433. Academic Press, New York and London.
Klingsberg, J. and Butcher, E. O. (1961). *J. dent. Res.* **40**, 682.
Klingsberg, J., Cancellaro, L. A. and Butcher, E. O. (1961). *J. dent. Res.* **40**, 461–469.
Krajewski, J. J., Gargiulo, A. W. and Staffelino, H. (1964). *Periodontics* **2**, 267–271.
Langerhans, P. (1868). *Virchows Arch. path. Anat. Physiol.* **44**, 325–337.
Leblond, C. P., Greulich, R. C. and Pereira, J. P. M. (1964). *In* "Advances in Biology of Skin" (W. Montagna and R. E. Billingham, eds.), Vol. 5, pp. 39–67. Pergamon Press, London.
Listgarten, M. A. (1964). *Am. J. Anat.* **114**, 49–69.
Listgarten, M. A. (1966). *Am. J. Anat.* **119**, 147–178.
Löe, H. (1967). *In* "Structural and Chemical Organization of Teeth" (A. W. Miles, ed.), Vol. 2, pp. 415–455. Academic Press, New York and London.
Main, D. M. G. and Ritchie, G. M. (1967). *Br. J. Derm.* **79**, 20–30.
Malkinson, F. D. (1964). *In* "The Epidermis" (W. Montagna and W. C. Lobitz, Jr., eds.), pp. 435–452. Academic Press, New York and London.
Marwah, A. S., Weinmann, J. P. and Meyer, J. (1960). *Archs Path.* **69**, 147–153.
Matoltsy, A. G. and Matoltsy, M. N. (1962). *J. invest. Derm.* **38**, 237–247.
Matoltsy, A. G. and Matoltsy, M. N. (1966). *J. invest. Derm.* **46**, 127–129.
Matoltsy, A. G. and Parakkal, P. F. (1965). *J. Cell Biol.* **24**, 297–307.
McHugh, W. D. (1964). *J. Periodont.* **35**, 338–348.
McHugh, W. D. and Zander, H. A. (1965). *Dent. Practnr dent. Rec.* **15**, 451–457.
McLoughlin, C. B. (1963). *Symp. Soc. exp. Biol.* **17**, 359–388.
Melcher, A. H. (1965). *Archs oral Biol.* **10**, 783–792.

Mercer, E. H. (1961). "Keratin and Keratinization." Pergamon Press, Oxford, England.

Merzel, J., Reis Viegas, A. and Munhoz, C. O. G. (1963). *J. Periodont.* **34**, 127–133.

Messier, B. and Leblond, C. P. (1960). *Am. J. Anat.* **106**, 247–285.

Meyer, J., Marwah, A. S. and Weinmann, J. P. (1956). *J. invest. Derm.* **27**, 237–247.

Miller, S. C., Soberman, A. and Stahl, S. S. (1951). *J. dent. Res.* **30**, 4–11.

Mitchell, R. E. (1963). *J. invest. Derm.* **41**, 199–212.

Montgomery, P. W. A. (1951). *J. dent. Res.* **30**, 12–18.

Moyer, F. H. (1963). *Ann. N.Y. Acad. Sci.* **100**, 584–606.

Nuki, K. (1967). *Dent. Practnr dent. Rec.* **17**, 245–250.

Odland, G. F. (1960). *J. invest. Derm.* **34**, 11–15.

Odland, G. F. (1964). *In* "The Epidermis" (W. Montagna and W. C. Lobitz, Jr., eds.), pp. 237–249. Academic Press, New York and London.

Orban, B. J. (1948). *Oral Surg.* **1**, 827–841.

Orban, B. J., Bhatia, H., Kollar, J. A. and Wentz, F. M. (1956). *J. Periodont.* **27**, 167–180.

Pease, D. C. (1960). *In* "Fourth International Conference on Electron Microscopy" (W. Bargmann, D. Peters and C. Wolpers, eds.), Vol. 2, pp. 139–155. Springer-Verlag, Berlin.

Persson, P. A. Stahl, S. S. and Scapa, S. (1961). *J. dent. Res.* **40**, 304–310.

Pinkus, H. and Hunter, R. (1966). *Archs Derm.* **94**, 351–354.

Pizzolato, P. and Lillie, R. D. (1967). *J. Histochem. Cytochem.* **15**, 104–110.

Quintarelli, G. and Cheraskin, E. (1961). *J. Periodont.* **32**, 338–342.

Rambourg, A. and Leblond, C. P. (1967). *J. Cell Biol.* **32**, 27–53.

Riley, P. A. (1964). *Nature (Lond.)* **201**, 1031.

Riley, P. A. (1966). *J. invest. Derm.* **47**, 412–420.

Riley, P. A. (1967). *J. invest. Derm.* **48**, 28–38.

Rosenberg, H. M. and Massler, M. (1967). *J. Periodont.* **38**, 473–480.

Rowden, G. (1966). *J. invest. Derm.* **47**, 359–362.

Rowden, G. (1967). *J. invest. Derm.* **49**, 181–197.

Rowden, G. and Budd, G. C. (1967). *J. invest. Derm.* **48**, 571–586.

Sagebiel, R. W. and Reed, T. H. (1968). *J. Cell Biol.* **36**, 595–602.

Schroeder, H. E. and Theilade, J. (1966). *J. periodont. Res.* **1**, 95–119.

Seiji, M. and Itakura, H. (1966). *J. invest. Derm.* **47**, 507–511.

Seiji, M., Shimao, K., Birbeck, M. S. C. and Fitzpatrick, T. B. (1963). *Ann. N.Y. Acad. Sci.* **100**, 497–533.

Selby, C. C. (1957). *J. invest. Derm.* **29**, 131–149.

Shahrik, H. A., Eichel, B. and Lisanti, V. F. (1964). *Archs oral Biol.* **9**, 1–15.

Sharav, Y. and Massler, M. (1967). *Expl Cell Res.* **47**, 132–138.

Sicher, H. (1966). "Orban's Oral Histology and Embryology", 6th edn., pp. 213–265. C. V. Mosby Co., St. Louis, U.S.A.

Skougaard, M. (1965a). *Acta odont. scand.* **23**, 615–622.

Skougaard, M. (1965b). *Acta odont. scand.* **23**, 623–643.

Snell, R. S. (1966). *J. invest. Derm.* **47**, 598–602.

Snell, R. (1967). *Z. Zellforsch. mikrosk. Anat.* **79**, 492–506.

Soni, N. N., Silberkweit, M. and Hayes, R. L. (1965). *J. Periodont.* **36**, 15–21.

Squier, C. A. and Waterhouse, J. P. (1967a). *Nature (Lond.)* **215**, 644–645.

Squier, C. A. and Waterhouse, J. P. (1967b). *Archs oral Biol.* **12**, 119–129.

Stallard, R. A., Diab, M. A. and Zander, H. A. (1965). *J. Periodont.* **36**, 130–132.

Stern, I. B. (1965). *Periodontics* **3**, 224–238.

Susi, F. R., Belt, W. D. and Kelly, J. W. (1967). *J. Cell Biol.* **34**, 686–690.

Szabo, G. (1967). *Phil. Trans. R. Soc. B.* **252**, 447–485.

166   C. J. SMITH

Tarnowski, W. M. and Hashimoto, K. (1967). *Archs Derm.* **96,** 298–304.
Ten Cate, A. R. (1963). *Archs oral Biol.* **8,** 747–753.
Thilander, H. (1963). *Acta odont. scand.* **21,** 431–451.
Thilander, H. and Bloom, G. D. (1968). *J. periodont. Res.* **3,** 96–110.
Thonard, J. C. and Scherp, H. W. (1962). *Archs oral Biol.* **7,** 125–136.
Toto, P. D. and Grandel, E. R. (1966a). *Periodontics* **4,** 127–130.
Toto, P. D. and Grandel, E. R. (1966b). *J. dent. Res.* **45,** 211.
Toto, P. D. and Sicher, H. (1964). *Periodontics* **2,** 154–156.
Toto, P. D. and Sicher, H. (1965). *J. dent. Res.* **44,** 451.
Trott, J. R. (1957). *Br. dent. J.* **103,** 421–427.
Trott, J. R. and Gorenstein, S. L. (1963). *Archs oral Biol.* **8,** 425–434.
Turesky, S., Crowley, J. and Glickman, I. (1957). *J. dent. Res.* **36,** 255–259.
Van Scott, E. J. and Flesch, P. (1954). *Archs Derm. Syph.* **70,** 141–154.
Van Scott, E. J. and Reinertson, R. P. (1961). *J. invest. Derm.* **36,** 109–117.
Waerhaug, J. (1952). *Odont. Tidskr.* **60,** Supplement 1.
Waterhouse, J. P. and Squier, C. A. (1967). *Archs oral Biol.* **12,** 341–348.
Weinmann, J. P. and Meyer, J. (1959). *J. invest. Derm.* **32,** 87–94.
Weinmann, J. P., Meyer, J., Mardfin, D. and Weiss, M. (1959). *Am. J. Anat.* **104,** 381–402.
Wolff, K. (1967). *J. Cell Biol.* **35,** 468–473.
Wolff, K. and Winkelmann, R. K. (1967). *J. invest. Derm.* **48,** 531–539.
Younes, M. S., Steele, H. D., Robertson, E. M. and Bencosme, S. A. (1965). *Am. J. Obstet. Gynec.* **92,** 163–171.
Zelickson, A. S. (1963). "Electron microscopy of skin and mucous membrane." C. C. Thomas, Springfield, Illinois.
Zelickson, A. S. (1965). *J. invest. Derm.* **44,** 201–212.
Zelickson, A. S. (1966). *J. invest. Derm.* **47,** 498–502.
Zelickson, A. S., Hirsch, H. M. and Hartmann, J. F. (1965). *J. invest. Derm.* **45,** 458–463.

6 | The Connective Tissues of the Periodontium

*A. H. MELCHER AND J. E. EASTOE

Department of Dental Science, Royal College of Surgeons of England, London, England

I. Organization of the Periodontium

The morsels of food which animals must eat to survive are cut or torn from unwieldy chunks and, in many animals, need then to be pulverized further before swallowing. The whole of the masticatory apparatus is involved in this process of aquisition and trituration of food, but direct responsibility for these tasks devolves on the enamel and dentine of the teeth. These tissues are admirably endowed with the requisite physical properties, but they can function properly only if adequately supported. In man, and in other higher animals, this support is provided by an organ comprising soft and hard connective tissues, the periodontium (Fig. 1).

* Present address: Faculty of Dentistry, University of Toronto, Toronto, Canada

A. H. MELCHER AND J. E. EASTOE

The periodontium attaches the teeth to the bone of the jaws, providing a resilient suspensory apparatus resistant to normal functional forces. It allows the teeth to adjust their position when under stress. The periodontium comprises hard connective tissues (cementum and bone) and soft connective tissues (the periodontal ligament and the lamina propria of the gingiva),

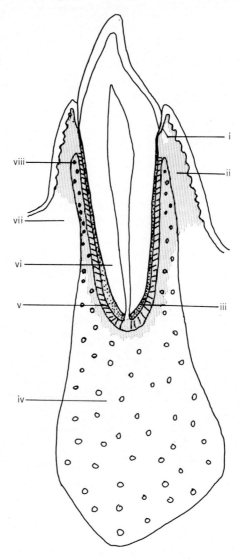

FIG. 1. A diagram of a mandibular incisor and its supporting structures. The connective tissues of the periodontium are shaded: i. Marginal gingiva; ii. Attached gingiva; iii. Cementum; iv. Mandibular bone; v. Periodontal ligament; vi. Dentine; vii. Alveolar mucosa; viii. Alveolar process.

which are covered by epithelium (Chapter 5). It should be regarded as a functional unit, although developmentally, its tissues may be derived from more than one germ layer (Chapter 3). It is attached to dentine by cementum and to the jaw-bone by the alveolar process. Continuity between these two hard tissue components is maintained by the periodontal ligament and the lamina propria. The organization and maintenance of the periodontium and its constituent tissues will be described in this chapter.

A. CEMENTUM

Cementum, one of the hard tissue components of the periodontium, is firmly attached to the radicular dentine of the tooth. The boundary between the two tissues follows a wavy course in permanent teeth, but may be scalloped in primary teeth. Peripherally, cementum is contiguous with the soft connective tissues comprising the periodontal ligament and the gingival lamina propria, providing attachment for some of their fibres. Cementum is of two types, acellular and cellular. A thin layer of acellular cementum usually covers the cervical $\frac{1}{3}$ to $\frac{1}{2}$ of the root dentine. Cellular cementum is found on the remainder of the root, and also on the surface of acellular cementum. Sometimes the two types occur in alternating layers (Chapter 12).

Cementum extends from the cervical limits of the enamel to the apex of the root. Cervically it can either meet the enamel in a butt joint, overlap it, or be overlapped by it, and all three of these relationships may occur around the periphery of a single tooth. Apically it covers the end of the root, extending into and lining the root-canal for a short distance.

Cementum is first laid down on the surface of the dentine after disorganization of Hertwig's epithelial root sheath. It is the least hard of the hard connective tissues, having some properties of bone, and is usually regarded as a modified form of bone. Although yellow in colour, it has a lighter hue and is more translucent than dentine, but is darker than enamel.

Deposition of cementum continues throughout life (Section IV), so that the thickness of the tissue varies. It is usually much thinner in the cervical part of the root (where it may measure as little as 10 μ), than in either the apical region (where its thickness may exceed 600 μ (Kronfeld, 1931)), or the interradicular area of multi-rooted teeth. Deposition of cementum does not appear to rely on function, as thick layers are found on roots of functionless teeth. (Kronfeld 1931).

B. PERIODONTAL LIGAMENT

The periodontal ligament is bounded centrally by the cementum and peripherally by the alveolar bone, while cervically it merges into the lamina propria of the gingiva. Although separation of the soft connective tissues of the periodontium into periodontal ligament and gingival lamina propria is of value in description, the two tissues should not be regarded as separate entities but as two anatomical parts of the same functional system. The periodontal ligament may be defined as the soft connective tissue extending between cementum and alveolar bone (Goldman, 1962), and consequently its cervical limit is marked by the most superficial fibres extending from the cementum to the crest of the alveolar bone.

The connective tissue extending between cementum and alveolar bone has been described by many names; for example, gomphosis, desmodont, pericementum, dental periosteum, periodontal membrane, alveolo-dental ligament and periodontal ligament. The tissue has a number of functions, including support, nutrition, formation and removal of tissue, and proprioception. None of the names adequately describe all of these functions, nevertheless, a number of them provide a useful anatomical description, so that terminology has become a matter of personal preference and usage. Wakely (1953) has defined a ligament as "a structure mainly or entirely composed of connective tissue connecting skeletal or other parts". In the light of this definition, the term *periodontal ligament* seems to us to be an appropriate name, and will be used in this book. This terminology is also discussed in Chapters 1 and 8.

The principal fibres of the periodontal ligament are embedded in cementum and in the bone lining the sockets of the teeth. The space occupied by the periodontal ligament is usually widest cervically, and wider both cervically and apically than at mid-root (Kronfeld, 1931; Coolidge, 1937). This hourglass shape appears to be associated with the location, midway along the root, of the fulcrum about which the tooth moves. Occasionally the periodontal space is tapered, and the fulcrum is then situated more apically (Kronfeld, 1931). This conforms with the view expressed by Mühlemann and Houglum (1954) that a tooth does not necessarily move around its biological rotation centre.

The width of the periodontal ligament depends on the load carried by the tooth in function, and also on age. A narrow periodontal ligament is found when dental function is decreased and in the elderly. The average width has been found to be about 0·2 mm, but may be more than 0·3 mm in teeth subject to heavy function. It may be as narrow as 0·12 mm, or less, in functionless or unerupted teeth (Kronfeld, 1931; Coolidge, 1937). (See also Tables 5–11 in Chapter 8). Tooth function also affects the quantity and calibre of the fibre bundles in the periodontal ligament; greater function leading to increased development, and disuse to atrophy.

C. The Lamina Propria of the Gingiva

The gingiva covers the external aspects of the alveolar bony process and the cervical aspect of the cementum, rising as a wedge-shaped sheet to surround the necks of the teeth. Its connective tissue, or lamina propria, is continuous with the periodontal ligament. Anatomically, the gingiva may be divided into two regions: the *attached gingiva*, which covers the alveolar bone and cementum, and which varies in width (Bowers, 1963); and the *marginal gingiva*, which covers the necks of the teeth (Fig. 1). The marginal gingiva lying between teeth is called specifically the *interdental gingival septum* (Chapter 5). In the young individual, the cementum is covered by attached gingiva only; in the older, by attached and marginal gingiva (Chapter 3).

The lamina propria of the gingiva is limited by the epithelium lining the gingival crevice, the epithelium of the attached epithelial cuff (Chapter 5), cementum, periodontal ligament, alveolar bone, the connective tissue of the alveolar mucosa, and the masticatory epithelium (Fig. 1) (Chapter 5). The lamina propria of the interdental gingival septum is limited medially and distally by the epithelium lining the gingival crevice and that forming the attached epithelial cuff, and by cementum, and apically by the alveolar bone crest and the periodontal ligament on either side of it. When adjacent teeth are in contact, the interdental lamina propria rises to a mesio-distal knife-edge, but vestibulo-orally it follows the shape of the interdental gingival septum, that is, two papillae joined by a depression (Chapter 5). When teeth are separated, the mesio-distal contour of the connective tissue is blunted or flat, depending on the degree of separation, and the vestibulo-oral contour flat or convex.

D. ALVEOLAR PROCESS

The alveolar process is an integral part of the maxilla and mandible, and not separated from the jaw bone by any obvious boundary such as a suture.

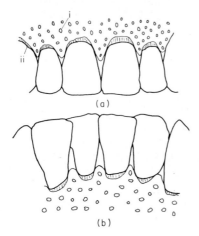

FIG. 2. The scalloped margin of the alveolar bony process at the necks of the teeth. (a) Vestibular aspect of maxillary incisors; (b) Oral aspect of mandibular incisors; i. Alveolar process; ii. Cementum.

As a result, a junction between the two cannot be identified. The alveolar process may be defined as the bone surrounding and supporting the teeth. It envelops the roots of the teeth, extending between them, and covering their interproximal, vestibular, oral and apical surfaces. It is recognized as an entity because its existence depends on the presence of erupted teeth; development of the alveolar process is associated with eruption of the teeth (Chapter 3), and loss of teeth precipitates its resorption. Furthermore, it has been shown that alveolar bone may exert some influence on developing teeth (Weinreb *et al.*, 1967).

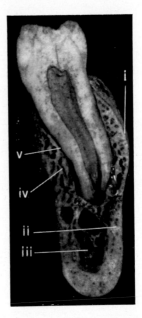

Fig. 3. A section of a mandibular molar showing the alveolar bone, outer cortical plate and spongiosa of the alveolar process, and the cortical and cancellous bone of the mandible. i. Outer cortical plate of alveolar process; ii. Cortex of jaw bone; iii. Cancellous bone; iv. Spongiosa; v. Alveolar bone (cribriform plate).

From its base, where it is continuous with the bone of the jaws, the alveolar process rises to surround the roots of the teeth. On the vestibular and oral surfaces it terminates slightly apical to the amelo-cemental junction in a thin scalloped edge (Fig. 2), with the high points of the contour situated between the teeth. The scalloped contour is much more marked vestibularly than orally. The vestibular and oral plates of the process are joined by inter-dental bone septa. The crests of the interdental septa are convex vestibulo-orally, and this is much more marked anteriorly than posteriorly. Between the anterior teeth the crests taper to a thin mesio-distal edge of bone. This dimension increases posteriorly and, between the molar teeth, the septal crests are in the form of elongated plateaus, the mesio-distal inclination of which may vary with the inclination of the adjacent teeth (Ritchey and Orban, 1953).

Except at its base, the outer layer of the alveolar process comprises compact bone. That on the vestibular and oral surfaces, and on the crests of the inter-dental septa, is termed the *outer cortical plate*. That lining the sockets of the teeth and crests of the inter-radicular septa of multi-rooted teeth, which may

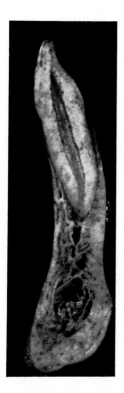
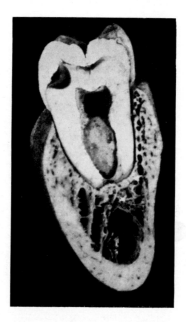

FIG. 4. Sections of Mandibular central incisor and mandibular first molar showing the variation in thickness of the alveolar process.

be very thin, is termed the *alveolar bone* or *cribriform plate*. The outer cortical plate of the alveolar process is continuous with that of the jaw-bone, and with the alveolar bone at the rims of the sockets of the teeth. In some situations, the outer cortical plate and alveolar bone are fused. When they are separated, the space between them is filled by cancellous bone which is continuous with that of the jaw (Fig. 3).

Functionally, the alveolar process is divided into the alveolar bone, to which the fibres of the periodontal ligament are attached, and the supporting bone which comprises the outer cortical plate and the spongiosa (cancellous bone). The spongiosa is perforated by the interdental and inter-radicular vessels and nerves. Further in their course, these vessels and nerves perforate the alveolar bone and the outer cortical plate of the crests of the interdental septa to supply the soft connective tissues of the periodontium. The term cribriform plate arises from the numerous perforations in the alveolar bone which transmit these structures.

The thickness of the alveolar process investing the teeth varies considerably (Fig. 4). For example, the vestibular alveolar process of both maxillary and mandibular anterior teeth tends to be very thin and, particularly in the latter case, may be perforated; whereas more posteriorly, and particularly in the mandible, it may be very thick. The width of the outer cortical plate, and the quantity of spongiosa present between it and the alveolar bone, is also variable. Frequently, where the alveolar process is thin, there is no spongiosa, and the outer cortical plate and the alveolar bone are fused. In other situations, where the alveolar process is thicker, the spongiosa may be replaced largely or entirely by a greatly enlarged cortical plate. The thickness of the alveolar bone also varies.

The spongiosa consists of a honeycomb of bone trabeculae, between which lies red haemopoietic marrow in young subjects and yellow marrow in older ones. The trabeculae buttress the outer cortical plate and the alveolar bone, and their disposition and state of development are dependent upon the forces which are exerted on the alveolar process (Fig. 28, Chapter 8). The width of the compact bony plates is probably governed in the same way.

II. Organization of the Connective Tissues of the Periodontium

A. General Structure of Connective Tissues

Connective tissue comprises cells and extracellular substance. The latter, which is produced by the cells, confers upon the connective tissue its physical properties, and is composed of fibres and ground substance.

1. The Cells of Connective Tissues

Connective tissue cells may conveniently be grouped into two categories: those having a main function concerned with synthesis and removal of extracellular substance, and those which perform other functions. Only some of these cells need be discussed here.

(a) Synthetic cells
   Fibroblasts
   Osteoblasts
   Cementoblasts

(b) Other cells
   Osteoclasts
   Macrophages or histiocytes
   Mast cells

(a) *Synthetic cells.* These cells, as will be discussed more fully below, are concerned with formation and maintenance of the soft and hard connective tissues. To fulfil this responsibility, they require apparatus for synthesizing and secreting structural proteins, carbohydrates and possibly lipids, and their involvement in these tasks could consequently be expected to be reflected in their architecture. Expressed differently, the structure of cells should be seen as an expression of their function. For this reason, the organelles responsible for synthesis of the components of the extracellular substance will be considered before discussing the detailed morphology of the synthetic cells. Synthesis of protein which, in varying forms, is probably the largest constituent of the extracellular substance is particularly important. Comprehensive discussions of this topic have been provided by Arnstein (1965), Smellie (1965), Watson (1965), and Crick (1967).

i. Organelles concerned in synthesis of extracellular substance

The cell's store of genetic information is resident in the genes, which are made of desoxyribonucleic acid (DNA). The DNA, which is located in the nucleus, occurs as double stranded molecules comprising repeating units, each of which consists of desoxyribose, phosphate and nitrogenous base. The bases found in DNA are adenine, guanine, cytosine an l thymine. The DNA is not itself directly involved in protein synthesis but, thi ugh the agency of ribonucleic acid (RNA), it ultimately dictates the nature of the protein to be formed. RNA is synthesized in the nucleus on a temp ate provided by specific areas of DNA. This reaction is effected by a special enzyme, polynucleotide polymerase, and the process is called transcription. Duplication of DNA prior to cell division is known as replication. RNA is single stranded, and differs further from DNA in that it contains ribose instead of desoxyribose, and uracil instead of thymine. The RNA of the cell is found almost entirely in two compartments, in the nucleolus and in the cytoplasm (Siekevitz, 1959).

RNA is transported to the cytoplasm of the cell. Here it performs two functions, both of which are concerned directly with the synthesis of protein. The essential step in protein synthesis is linking amino acids one to the other in appropriate order, forming chains which, at first, are called polypeptides and later, as their length increases, proteins. Linking of amino acids (formation of peptide bonds) involves in principle the reaction of the α-amino group of one amino acid and the carboxyl group of another with the elimination of a water molecule. One fraction of the RNA, the soluble RNA (sRNA) (also called transfer RNA (tRNA)) is concerned with conveying the appropriate amino acid to the place where it will be incorporated into the protein. The other RNA fraction, the messenger RNA (mRNA), holds information obtained from DNA which dictates the order in which the amino acids are to be incorporated into the protein. As the amino acid sequence largely determines the properties of the protein, the information conveyed by the RNA dictates the protein to be made. This could be, for example, a particular enzyme, or a structural protein.

The molecular weight of sRNA is about 25,000. It comprises approximately 80 polynucleotide residues, and all but the terminal bases are arranged in varying order. Each amino acid interacts with a specific sRNA, or at most a small number of sRNA's. The amino acid is first "activated" by reaction of its carboxyl group with a molecule of adenosine triphosphate (ATP) to form an amino-acyl adenylate, the reaction being catalyzed by an enzyme specific for each amino acid. The enzyme, which remains tightly bound to the transient amino-acyl adenylate, then transfers it to the terminal ribose of an appropriate molecule of sRNA, to give an amino-acyl-sRNA. The enzymes belonging to the group involved in these two reactions are amino-acyl-sRNA synthetases. The base sequence of the sRNA confers structural specificity between the appropriate sRNA and the particular amino-acyl-sRNA synthetase.

The actual site of protein synthesis, that is the situation where peptide bonds are formed between the amino acids, is on ribonucleoprotein (RNP) particles or ribosomes. These are almost spherical, complex structures, comprising about equal proportions of protein and RNA, but no detectable phospholipid (Siekevitz, 1959). They consist of two parts, one about twice the size of the other, having diameters between 200×170 Å and 240×180 Å, and are attached to strands of mRNA. The 'plan' of the order in which amino acid are to be incorporated into nascent protein is contained in a message coded by the arrangement of the bases in the mRNA. Each amino acid is described in a sequence of three bases; the base triplets being known as codons. The bases in the sRNA are also arranged in specific triplets called anticodons. The bases of the anticodons interact with the bases of the codons, base pairs being formed only between "matching" bases. This mechanism ensures correct positioning of the particular amino-acyl-sRNA on the strand of mRNA, and subsequent incorporation of the contained amino acid at the appropriate site in the protein chain.

Proteins are formed on aggregates of ribosomes (polysomes) attached to a single strand of mRNA, and these may be large, particularly when involved in the synthesis of high-molecular weight proteins such as myosin (Breuer et al., 1964) and collagen (Kretsinger et al., 1964; Gould et al., 1965; Fernández-Madrid, 1967). Although Manner and Gould (1965) claim that synthesis of a protein can sometimes take place on a single ribosome, the functional unit in protein synthesis is thought to consist of an aggregate of several ribosomes (a polysome) (Arnstein, 1965; Manner et al., 1967).

Synthesis of a protein is initiated by a ribosome attaching itself to the beginning of a strand of mRNA. The first amino-acyl-sRNA containing the required amino acid then attaches itself to the ribosome, with the amino end of the amino acid free and the carboxyl end involved in the structure of the amino-acyl-sRNA (Figs 5 and 6). Thus, synthesis of a polypeptide starts at the amino end. The ribosome moves along the strand of mRNA, and an amino-acyl-sRNA containing the amino acid required next in sequence takes its place on the ribosome (Figs 5 and 6), the selection each time relying

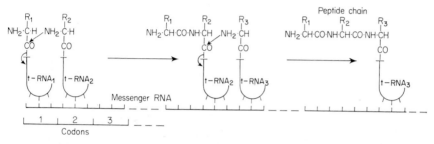

Fig. 5. Peptide bond formation from amino-acyl-tRNA. (Reproduced with permission from Arnstein, *Brit. Med. Bul.* **21**, 217–222, 1965.)

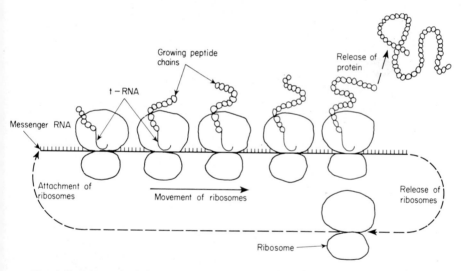

Fig. 6. Protein synthesis by polyribosomes. (Reproduced with permission from Arnstein, *Brit. Med. Bul.* **21**, 217–222, 1965.)

on the matching of the codon of the mRNA and the anticodon of the sRNA (Fig. 5). A peptide synthetase, which appears to be attached firmly to the ribosome (Arlinghaus *et al.*, 1964) then catalyzes formation of a peptide bond between the carboxyl group of the first amino-acyl-sRNA and the α-amino group of the incoming amino-acyl-sRNA (Fig. 5). This reaction requires the release of the sRNA from the first amino-acyl-sRNA and its return into solution. The ribosome then moves further along the strand of mRNA, and with the inclusion of each new amino-acyl-sRNA a new peptide bond is formed between the carboxyl group of what is now a peptidyl-sRNA and the α-amino group of the new member. In this way, the peptide chain is gradually

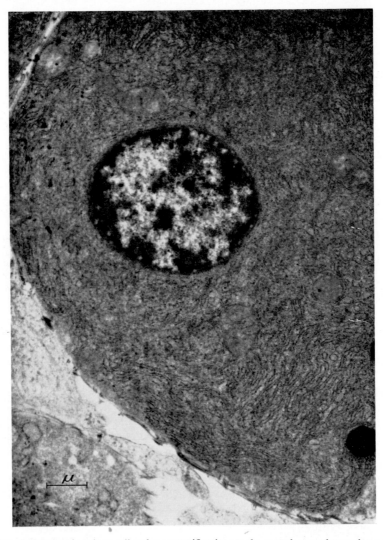

Fig. 7. Pancreatic acinar cell at low magnification to show nucleus and cytoplasm containing GER. Compare with Fig. 8. (Courtesy, Professor Gilbert Causey.)

lengthened until the end of the strand of mRNA is reached, when the poly-peptide chain and the ribosome are believed to be released simultaneously (Fig. 6). Finally, the last molecule of sRNA is cleaved from the polypeptide chain to expose the terminal carboxyl group of the latter, and the empty ribosomes are apparently available for reattachment to mRNA.

It is of interest that some cellular proteins can be synthesized outside this system. There is evidence that the nucleus and the mitochondria of some cell types can synthesize their own protein (Siekevitz, 1959, Campbell, 1960 and

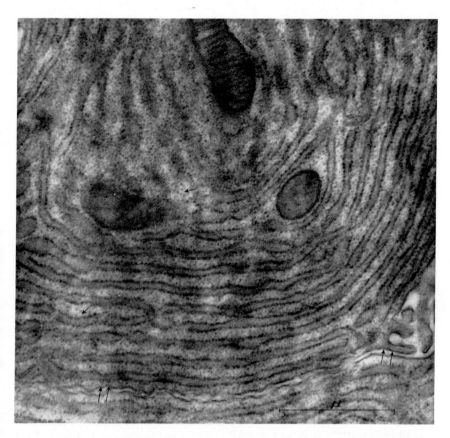

FIG. 8. Higher magnification than in Fig. 7 of cytoplasm of a pancreatic acinar cell. The GER is evident, and some loose ribosomes are present (single arrow). Part of the plasma membrane of the cell can be seen in the lower part of the electronmicrograph (double arrows). (Courtesy, Professor Gilbert Causey.)

Tapley et al., 1967). Nevertheless, as has been shown particularly by Caspersson et al. (1963), interference with DNA-dependent synthesis of RNA will inhibit synthesis of cellular proteins.

Electron microscopy has revealed that ribosomes occur in two situations, either lying free in the cytoplasm or associated with cytoplasmic membranes (Figs 7 and 8). The membranes studded with ribosomes constitute the granular endoplasmic reticulum (GER), and are present in the cell in varying amounts. The "microsomal fraction", isolated by fragmentation of cells and differential centrifugation, is derived from the GER (Palade and Siekevitz, 1956a,b; Siekevitz, 1959). The membranes of the endoplasmic reticulum (ER), which are $\sim$100 Å thick, enclose areas which vary in diameter up to $\sim$ 1000 Å (Ito, 1962), and the whole system constitutes the ergastoplasm. The attachment of polysomes to the GER, at least in liver, is believed by Benedetti et al. (1966) to be effected by a single ribosome. Palade (1958a) has pointed out that the granules of the ER tend to be arranged in regularly spaced rows, and that parallel double rows are seen particularly in fibroblasts.

It has been suggested that protein for export is synthesized by ribosomes attached to the membranes of the ER, whereas ribosomes lying free in the cytoplasm are concerned in synthesizing protein for use in the cell (Siekevitz, 1959). However, more recently, Palade is reported to have expressed the view that protein synthesized on membrane-bound ribosomes may be destined for use either extracellularly or intracellularly (Palade and Porter, 1967). It is apparent that cells actively producing protein will be well endowed with ribosomes; if the protein is to be secreted they will also be particularly rich in GER.

Protein synthesized by ribosomes of the GER is apparently transferred across the membranes into the cisternae of the GER (Siekevitz, 1959) which form a labyrinth of channels in the cytoplasm (Palade, 1956; Freeman, 1964). Here the proteins may condense out of solution, and are sometimes seen as "dense bodies" or granules (Palade, 1956). Some, but apparently not all proteins (see below), are then transported through the cisternae to the elements of the Golgi complex (Siekevitz, 1959) with which they communicate (Fawcett, 1961).

A cell possessing the potential to synthesize protein may exhibit little GER while developing or resting, but requires an extensive GER when in full production. It is possible that new GER is synthesized by existing GER. Dallner et al. (1966) have shown that new ER in rat hepatocytes is synthesized in the GER, and is subsequently transferred to the smooth part of the system. While the protein required for these membranes is probably synthesized by the ribosomes on the GER, it is not known where the lipid with which it becomes associated is produced. However, interaction between the two to form membrane appears to take place in the GER. There does not appear to be much information on how ribosomes subsequently become attached to the ER. According to Palade it is possible that other cellular membranes, such as those of the Golgi complex and plasmalemma, are also synthesized in the GER (Palade and Porter, 1967).

Agranular endoplasmic reticulum (AER), at least in liver cells, is continuous with the GER (Jones and Fawcett, 1966), and Yamada maintains that its identification depends on recognizing this continuity (Palade and Porter, 1967). It is most abundant in cells of sebaceous glands and steroid producing organs, in retinal pigment cells and gastric parietal cells. This membrane system may be considered to be the centre of the specialized processes carried out by the cell. In liver cells it hypertrophies when called upon to metabolize certain drugs, and it may also be associated with glycolysis (Jones and Fawcett, 1966). The Golgi complex possibly represents a specialized form of the AER (Freeman, 1964).

Protein in pancreatic acinar cells is "parcelled" in the Golgi complex for secretion, forming zymogen granules (Fawcett, 1962). The Golgi has also been found to participate in the secretion of protein by connective tissue cells (Revel and Hay, 1963; Ross and Benditt, 1965), as will be discussed in more detail below. In cells which secrete protein-polysaccharide complexes it is probably also the site where carbohydrate is synthesized, where the carbohydrate and protein moieties are linked, and, if appropriate, where the carbohydrate moieties are sulphated (Petersen and Leblond, 1964).

It is apparent from the foregoing that the different connective tissue cells actively synthesizing intercellular substance of bone, cementum or soft connective tissue, must have some morphological features in common. The GER and Golgi complex, and also the mitochondria, which are concerned in cell respiration and regeneration of ATP (Lehninger, 1964) might all be expected to be prominent in electronmicrographs. But, of these, a well developed GER is regarded as the predominant morphological feature of cells synthesizing protein for export (Karrer, 1960). Characteristics of active protein production can also be recognized in the light microscope. The most striking of these is an increase in cytoplasmic basophilia (Weiss, 1953), and this is usually demonstrated by strong affinity for haematoxylin. Strong basophilia is indicative of a high concentration of ribosomes, either attached or free. Basophilia does not reflect the state of development of the ER (Porter, 1954; Palade, 1958b; Fawcett, 1961), and is characteristic not only of cells synthesizing protein for secretion but also of those synthesizing protein for internal use, as for example rapidly dividing cells. The cisternae of the ER and the Golgi complex of living cells can be identified by using phase contrast microscopy (Rose and Pomerat, 1960). The Golgi "vacuole" and mitochondria of fixed cells can be demonstrated by appropriate staining techniques (Lillie, 1954).

ii. Fibroblasts, osteoblasts and cementoblasts

Useful observations on the morphology of fibroblasts have been made on living cells (Stearns, 1940a,b), squashes of cellular connective tissue (Moore and Schoenberg, 1960), and teased preparations (Ham and Leeson, 1965). These observations have shown that the cells are pleomorphic (Fig. 9);

7

fusiform or tripolar with long fine cytoplasmic processes, or stellate with numerous short processes. Active cells are rich in cytoplasm and exhibit a low nuclear to cytoplasmic ratio. The nucleus, which is oval and vesicular, is often folded, and contains one or more prominent nucleoli. Active osteoblasts are also plump cells (Fig. 10) and are rich in cytoplasm which is continued into processes. These processes are largely restricted to the aspect of

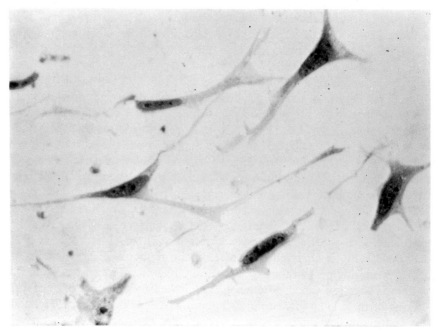

Fig. 9. Fibroblasts from embryonic mouse gingiva grown *in vitro*. Haematoxylin and eosin. (×430.)

the cell adjacent to bone, the matrix of which they penetrate (Dudley and Spiro, 1961; Cooper *et al.*, 1966) (Fig. 11). The round or oval, vesicular nucleus which is eccentrically placed, not necessarily in the part of the cell most distant from the bone surface, usually exhibits at least one prominent nucleolus. The nucleus of both fibroblasts and osteoblasts is surrounded by a double-membraned nuclear envelope which is perforated by nuclear pores. Cementoblasts are identified by their proximity to the surface of cementum, but are similar in character to osteoblasts (Linghorne, 1954). They have distinct vesicular nuclei with one or more nucleoli. Cells actively depositing acellular cementum do not exhibit prominent cytoplasmic processes. However, cells depositing cellular cementum exhibit abundant basophilic cytoplasm and cytoplasmic processes, and their nuclei tend to be folded and irregularly shaped.

As might be expected from observations on other protein-secreting cells, the most striking electronmicroscopic feature of active fibroblasts (Chapman, 1962; Fernando and Movat, 1963a,b; Goldberg and Green, 1964) (Fig. 12), osteoblasts (Sheldon and Robinson, 1957; Dudley and Spiro, 1961; Cooper et al., 1966) (Fig. 11), and cementoblasts (Selvig, 1963; Stern, 1964) is the extensively developed and abundant GER. Essentially similar descriptions of

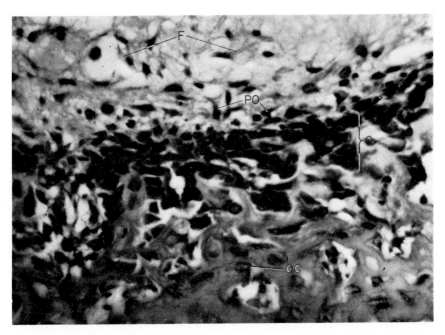

FIG. 10. Young soft and hard connective tissues in a healing wound. Fibroblasts (F), osteoblasts (O), osteocytes (OC), and cells which appear to be pre-osteoblasts (PO), are illustrated. Haematoxylin and eosin. (×375.)

the ergastoplasm of fibroblasts, osteoblasts and cementoblasts have been given by numerous workers. Indeed, the ergastoplasm of osteoblasts has been said to resemble that in fibroblasts, odontoblasts and pancreatic acinar cells (Sheldon and Robinson, 1957; Decker, 1966), and although there is very little detailed information available about the fine structure of cemento-blasts, its ergastoplasm has been compared with that of fibroblasts (Selvig, 1963).

The GER comprises membranes ~75 Å thick enclosing spaces which, in fibroblasts, may vary in width from ~400 Å to ~2,000 Å (Peach et al., 1961) or more. The membranes of the GER are continuous with the cytoplasmic layer of the nuclear envelope (Dudley and Spiro, 1961; Chapman, 1962; Stern, 1964), and the lumen of the GER is continuous with the lumen of the nuclear envelope. The membranes of the GER may approach the plasma membrane closely, and sometimes are in contact with it (Ross and Benditt, 1964 and 1965) (see below). The GER and the cytoplasmic surface of the nuclear membrane are covered with ribosomes 100–150 Å in diameter. In

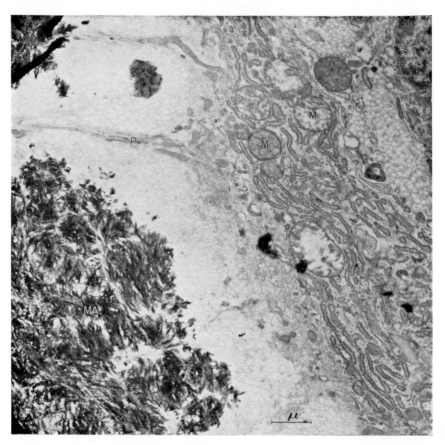

FIG. 11. Part of an active osteoblast in the developing Haversian canal of a puppy. There is abundant GER and many mitochondria (M). The osteoblast process (P) extends through the unmineralized matrix and into a canaliculus in the mineralized matrix (MA) of the bone. (Reproduced with permission from R. G. Cooper, J. W. Milgram and R. A. Robinson, *J. Bone Jt Surg.* **48A,** 1239–1271, 1966.)

fibroblasts, these are arranged in parallel chains, each having a characteristic contour (Palade, 1958a; Cameron, 1961; Goldberg and Green, 1964; Ross and Benditt, 1964; Stern, 1964) (Fig. 12). Loose ribosomes are also present, and these may be grouped in clusters or rosettes (Sheldon and Robinson, 1957; Goldberg and Green, 1964; Ross and Benditt, 1964; Cooper *et al.,* 1966).

The GER may be distributed varyingly; either as narrow elongated profiles in relatively ordered parallel array and showing comparatively little communication, or as grossly distended profiles forming a continuous series of interconnected channels and occupying a considerable part of the cytoplasmic volume, or in a transitional pattern (Karrer, 1960; Chapman, 1961; Ross and

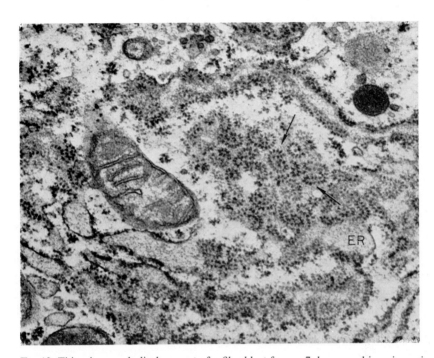

FIG 12. This micrograph displays part of a fibroblast from a 7-day wound in guinea pig skin. The region of the cell depicted shows part of a mitochondrion, as well as several profiles of rough endoplasmic reticulum (ER). Where the cisternae are sectioned normally, a single layer of ribosomes may be seen attached to the membranes. However, there are many regions (arrows) where the ergastoplasmic membranes have been grazed tangentially, presenting an *en face* view of the orientation of the ribosomes attached to the membranes. Here the membrane appears as an increased area of density around the ribosomes. The ribosomes are arranged in characteristic curved and spiral patterns, some of which are in double rows. In some regions (arrows) a fine thread appears to connect these ribosomes. (×46,000.) (Reproduced with permission from R. Ross and E. P. Benditt, *J. Cell Biol.* **22**, 365–390, 1964.)

Benditt, 1961; Stern, 1964; Cooper *et al.*, 1966). The second arrangement appears to be characteristic of cells actively secreting protein (Peach *et al.*, 1961; Ross and Benditt, 1961). The cisternae of the GER are usually filled with material which is more electron dense than the remaining cytoplasm; this material may be granular or filamentous (Chapman, 1961; Stern, 1964; Cooper *et al.*, 1966). The protein secreting role of osteoblasts is also reflected by the high level of H^3 uridine that they transfer from nucleus to cytoplasm (Owen, 1967).

Continually moving granules can be seen in the cytoplasm of living fibroblasts and osteoblasts (Stearns, 1940a; Fitton Jackson, 1955). Periodic acid-Schiff (paS) positive granules can be demonstrated in histological preparations of these cells (Gersh and Catchpole, 1949; Heller-Steinberg, 1951), and cementoblasts (Paynter and Pudy, 1958). Fitton Jackson (1955) believes that the continually moving granules are similar to those that react with paS, and that they both correspond to granules which can be identified in the electron microscope. This view has been disputed by Sheldon (1959), Cameron (1961) and Chapman (1962) who think that the granules correspond with the dilated cisternae of the GER. Fitton Jackson (1964) has refuted this explanation on the grounds that the granules are freely movable in the cell. However, Ito (1962) has stated that observations on the ER of living cells using phase contrast microscopy strongly suggest that the form of the ER is constantly changing. This observation implies therefore, that mobility of the granules does not necessarily exclude the possibility that they and the paS positive granules are the light microscopic image of the dilated cisternae of the ER.

Agranular endoplasmic reticulum is not generally abundant in these cells, but has been identified particularly where it connects the GER and Golgi complex (Dudley and Spiro, 1961; Ross and Benditt, 1964). The latter authors have also pointed out that membranes of the GER in close proximity to the plasma membrane are devoid of ribosomes. In contrast to these observations, however, Goldberg and Green (1964) have seen many examples of AER in continuity with GER in cultured fibroblasts. The cisternae of the AER were found to contain material of similar electron density to that in the GER.

The Golgi complex is a smooth-membraned system comprising elongated sacs, small round vesicles and large vacuolated vesicles. The elongated sacs are each about 1 μ long and are sometimes stacked closely together. The large vacuolated vesicles are found in differentiated cells (Fitton Jackson, 1964). The elements of the Golgi complex form an extensive complicated system which has a typical juxta-nuclear location in active fibroblasts and osteoblasts, but parts of the complex may extend between the cisternae of the GER into the peripheral cytoplasm (Fernando and Movat 1963a,b; Goldberg and Green, 1964; Decker, 1966). There appears to be scant information on the distribution of the Golgi complex in cementoblasts.

When observed by light microscopy, a pale-staining area in the vicinity of the nucleus, the so-called juxta-nuclear vacuole, corresponds with the location of the Golgi complex. The site of the Golgi complex can be recognized under phase contrast (Rose, 1961), and may be seen to comprise a series of fine canals (Hancox and Boothroyd, 1964).

Mitochondria are numerous in active connective tissue cells (Fitton Jackson, 1964; Han et al., 1965; Cooper et al., 1966). They tend to be oval in shape, but may be elongated or branched, exhibit short well developed cristae and a pale intercristal space, and appear to be scattered randomly in the ergastoplasm (Kajikawa et al., 1959; Cameron, 1961; Peach et al., 1961; Ross and Benditt, 1961; Fitton Jackson, 1964; Decker, 1966). Continuity between the membranes of the mitochondria and GER has not been recognized (Dudley and Spiro, 1961).

Vesicles of different types are present in the cytoplasm of active cells, and lysosome-like bodies have been reported in osteoblasts (Cooper et al., 1966). Membrane-bound osmiophilic bodies, probably lipid in nature, occur in the cytoplasm of fibroblasts. Movat and Fernando (1962) regard these structures as characteristic of fibroblasts.

The presence of numerous bundles of fine intracytoplasmic filaments ($\sim$20–$\sim$80 Å in diameter) are an exclusive feature of fibroblasts (Chapman, 1961; Ross and Benditt, 1961; Goldberg and Green, 1964). These tend to be concentrated peripherally, may be orientated parallel to the cell boundary, and are present in the cell processes. Cameron (1961) and Hancox and Boothroyd (1965) have described the presence of intracytoplasmic filaments in osteoblasts, but say that they do not appear to be a prominent feature of the peripheral cytoplasm of these cells. There appears to be no information on the presence of these filaments in cementoblasts. Intracytoplasmic filaments have not been seen to exhibit the periodicity of collagen fibrils but, because of their small diameter, this does not exclude the possibility of their being collagen (Ross and Benditt, 1961). However, Goldberg and Green (1964) have presented chemical evidence suggesting that the intracytoplasmic filaments of fibroblasts are not collagen, and believe that they may be concerned in cell motility. Hancox and Boothroyd suggest that they may serve as a cytoskeleton for osteoblasts.

The plasma membrane of active fibroblasts is indistinct (Peach et al., 1961; Goldberg and Green, 1964), but this is not emphasized as a feature of active osteoblasts, and there is little information about the plasma membrane of cementoblasts. Stearns (1940a,b), in observations on fibrogenesis in vivo, noted that it was difficult to see the entire boundary of the fibroblast.

iii. Pre-fibroblasts, pre-osteoblasts and pre-cementoblasts

The precursor cells of active fibroblasts (Goldberg and Green, 1964; Han et al., 1965) and active osteoblasts (Cooper et al., 1966) appear to be morphologically similar, and will be discussed in Section IVA. Little seems to be known about the cells which precede cementoblasts; Selvig (1963) associates them with fibroblasts and Linghorne (1954) with osteoblasts. The precursor cells (Fig. 10), which do not actively produce extracellular substance, are polygonal and of irregular outline and have a well defined plasma membrane. Their cytoplasm, which appears pale in sections stained with haematoxylin and eosin, is characterized in electronmicrographs by small amounts of GER having mainly tubular or vesicular profiles containing material of low density. The cells may exhibit numerous loose ribosomes, many of which are arranged in clusters or rosettes, but have a poorly developed Golgi complex. The mitochondria are small and spherical. Cells destined to become fibroblasts contain intracytoplasmic filaments ~50 Å in diameter, which are often concentrated in bundles beneath the plasma membrane (Goldberg and Green, 1964). Although pre-osteoblasts also contain intracellular filaments (Cooper *et al.*, 1966) there does not appear to be any evidence that they show a characteristic peripheral distribution.

The cells which line and cover resting bone are fusiform with tapering pale cytoplasm and oval nuclei and, according to Ham and Leeson (1965), are pluripotential. Those that line Haversian canals (Cooper *et al.*, 1966) have a high ratio of nucleus to cytoplasm, the plasma membrane being sometimes separated from the nuclear membrane by only a thin tract of cytoplasm which contains little GER. Cytoplasmic processes from these cells extend through canaliculi into the adjacent bone.

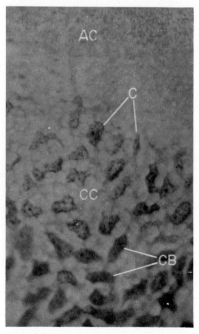

FIG. 13. An oblique section of developing cementum showing acellular cementum (AC) cellular cementum (CC), cementoblasts (CB) and cementocytes (C). Haematoxylin and (eosin. × 500.)

iv. Fibrocytes, osteocytes and cementocytes

Many of the cells that have completed their task of secreting extracellular substance remain surrounded by the tissue that they have synthesized; the fibroblasts as fibrocytes, the osteoblasts as osteocytes (Fig. 10) and, sometimes (see below) the cementoblasts as cementocytes (Fig. 13). The fibrocytes (Kajikawa *et al.*, 1959; Porter, 1964; Stenger, 1965), which lie between the

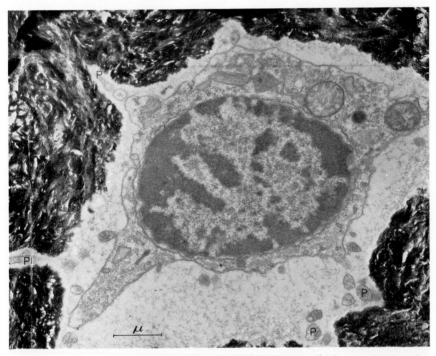

FIG. 14. An osteocyte in its lacuna. There is a relatively large nuclear/cytoplasmic ratio. The cytoplasm contains some mitochondria and free ribosomes. There are a number of cell processes (P) cut in cross section or obliquely, and a portion of one (P1) is lying in a canaliculus. (Reproduced with permission from R. R. Cooper, J. W. Milgram and R. A. Robinson, *J. Bone Jt Surg.* **48A**, 1239–1271, 1966.)

bundles of collagen fibres in soft connective tissues, show elongated, slender cytoplasm with long thin processes which entwine bundles of collagen fibres and contact one another (Van Winkle, 1967). Fibrocytes in loose connective tissue are generally plumper than those in densely fibrous connective tissue (Movat and Fernando, 1962). The GER and Golgi elements are sparse, the mitochondria small, and there are comparatively few loose ribosomes. These features suggest that the cell is not very active.

The morphology of the osteocyte (Fig. 14), which is enclosed in a lacuna by the extracellular substance of bone, probably varies with the age of the cell (Dudley and Spiro, 1961). Osteocytes have a smaller ratio of cytoplasm to nucleus than osteoblasts (Cooper *et al.*, 1966), and this ratio decreases as the cell ages (Wassermann and Yaeger, 1965). The cells are surrounded by a distinct plasma membrane (Wassermann and Yaeger, 1965). Cytoplasmic

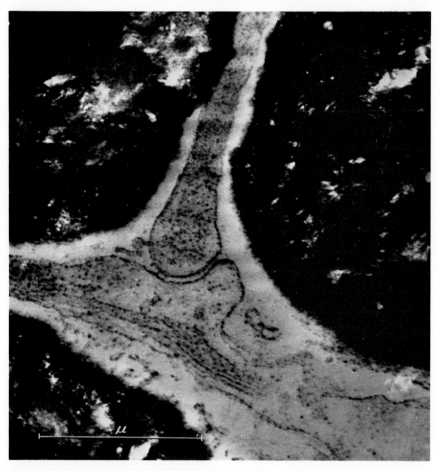

FIG. 15. Junction of osteocyte processes at the edge of a lacuna. (Reproduced with permission from R. R. Cooper, J. W. Milgram, and R. A. Robinson, *J. Bone Jt Surg.* **48A,** 1239–1271, 1966.)

processes extend into the canaliculi of the surrounding extracellular substance, forming junctions with processes from other osteocytes (Fig. 15) and bone cells at the surface.

The state of development of the intracytoplasmic membrane system and the organelles of osteocytes appears to vary between that exhibited by actively synthesizing cells and that seen in resting cells. Periodic acid-Schiff positive granules have been seen within their cytoplasm (Lipp, 1954). The finding of characteristics suggesting activity similar to that exhibited by osteoblasts is not surprising. As will be discussed in Section **IV**, osteocytes are believed by some investigators to be capable of considerable activity. Although smooth-walled vesicles and granules resembling ribosomes have been identified in the cytoplasm of the cell processes, Cooper *et al.* (1966) have not seen ER in this situation. In this connection, it is of interest that Herold and Kaye (1966) have recently reported the presence of GER, loose ribosomes and mitochondria in odontoblastic processes of human dentine.

The osteocyte is separated from the mineralized matrix by material which Wassermann and Yaeger (1965) think resembles the organic matrix of bone, and which they call the capsule. They find that the capsule has a mean width of 0.7μ. Similar material separates the processes of the osteocytes from the mineralized bone matrix. According to Cooper *et al.* (1966) however, extra-cellular fluid fills this space in life and, *post mortem*, its contents are structure-less.

v. Attachment between connective tissue cells

Approximation of the plasma membranes of adjacent fibroblasts (Devis and James, 1964; Ross and Greenlee, 1966), adjacent osteoblasts (Dudley and Spiro, 1961) and adjacent osteocytes (Cooper *et al.*, 1966) may be seen before and after deposition of extracellular substance. This involves close proximity of parallel segments of plasma membranes of contiguous cells. The apposed membranes may be unembellished, or comprise or be punctuated by specialized structures such as attach adjacent epithelial cells (Farquhar and Palade, 1963) (see also Chapter 5). Structures resembling zonula adherens have been found between fibroblasts (Ross and Greenlee, 1966) and between osteoblasts (Dudley and Spiro, 1961); Devis and James (1964) have described structures resembling zonula occludens between fibroblasts cultured *in vitro* under vitamin C deficient conditions. Macula adherens (desmosomes) do appear to effect contact between connective tissue cells. We have seen zonula adherens and plaque-like structures between adjacent fibroblasts in developing mouse gingiva (Figs 16 and 17). Specialized structures have not been identified in contacts between the intercannalicular processes of osteocytes (Cooper *et al.*, 1966).

(b) Other cells

i. Osteoclasts (and cementoclasts)

Osteoclasts are found in areas where bone is being resorbed. Until recently proof that osteoclasts actively participate in the process was lacking, but modern evidence clearly points to their having a direct role in the removal of

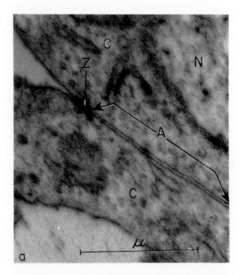

Fig. 16a

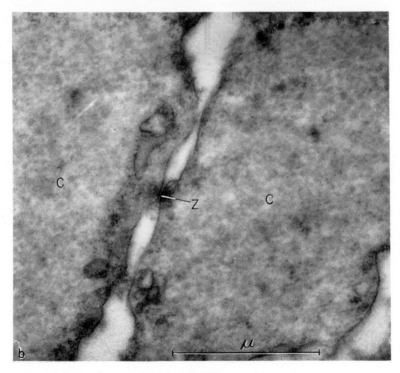

Fig. 16b

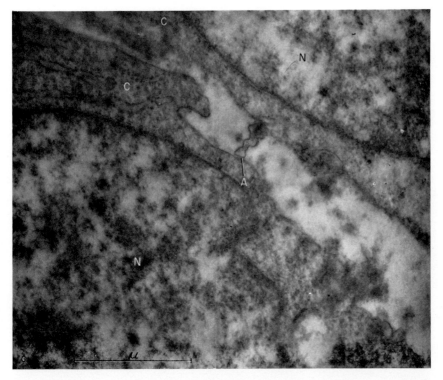

FIG. 16c

FIG. 16a,b,c. Contacts between fibroblast-like cell surfaces in developing mouse gingiva. Close approximation between cell surfaces without evident specialization (A): specialized areas resembling zonula adherens (Z). Cell cytoplasm (C) and cell nucleus (N).

bone (Kirby-Smith, 1933; Goldhaber, 1960; Hancox and Boothroyd, 1961; Hancox, 1965). However, as Hancox points out, their mere presence does not signify that bone is being removed at that moment. The cells are found in association with bone surfaces, lying either in Howship's lacunae (Fig. 18) or on flat surfaces, or enveloping the ends of spicules. Alternatively they may be found at short distances from bone surfaces, or surrounded by soft connective tissue in areas where bone apparently has been resorbed completely (Fig. 19).

Osteoclasts show considerable variation in size and shape, from small mononuclear cells to very large multinuclear cells. According to Hancox (1956), the latter are the largest of mammalian cells. They may attain dimensions of $\sim 105\,\mu \times \sim 85\,\mu$ with a volume calculated at $\sim 200,000\,\mu^3$, and may contain 100 or more nuclei. Large cells may be divided into two or more lobes connected by thin cytoplasmic bridges, each lobe containing its own quota of nuclei (Hancox, 1965). Much of our knowledge of osteoclasts has

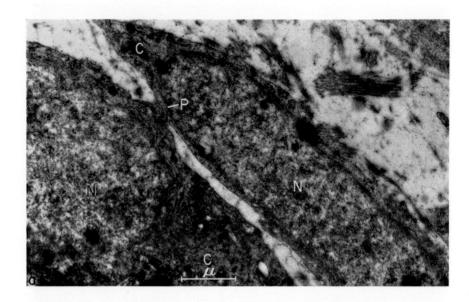

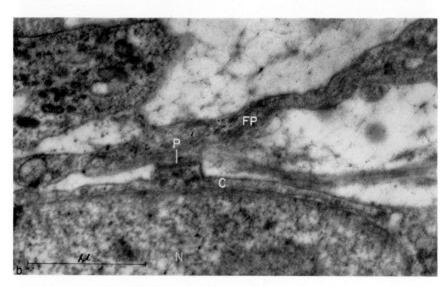

FIG. 17a and b. Contacts between fibroblast-like cell surfaces in developing gingiva. Specialized areas resembling plaques (P). Cell cytoplasm (C), cell nucleus (N), process of fibroblast (FP).

been obtained from observations made, especially by Goldhaber and Hancox, on material growing *in vitro*; the observed variation in shape of the cells when seen in histological section reflects their active motility *in vitro* (see Hancox, 1965) and *in vivo* (Kirby-Smith, 1933).

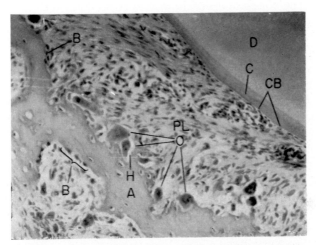

FIG. 18. Periodontium, showing dentine (D), cementum (C), resting cementoblasts (CB), periodontal ligament (PL), and alveolar bone (A) undergoing resorption. Osteoclasts (O), some in Howship's lacunae (H), and osteoblasts (B), are evident. Haematoxylin and eosin. (× 100.)

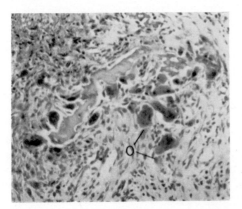

FIG. 19. Osteoclasts associated with a spicule of bone. Some of the cells (O) lie in an area from which bone appears to have been removed completely. Haematoxylin and eosin. (× 100.)

The cytoplasm may be slightly haematoxyphilic in young cells, but becomes increasingly eosinophilic with age. It tends to have a foamy appearance and to exhibit numerous vesicles, the contents of which may be PAS positive (Heller-Steinberg, 1951; Kroon, 1954) or metachromatic (Young, 1963a).

Effete cells are riddled with vacuoles (Fig. 20). The part of the cell which lies adjacent to bone often has a striated appearance when viewed in the light microscope, the so-called ruffled or brush border. The reason for this appearance, though still debated (Ham and Leeson, 1965), is generally accepted to be due to the unique contours of the plasma membrane which can be resolved by electron microscopy (Scott and Pease, 1956; Cameron and Robinson, 1958; Gonzales and Karnovsky, 1961; Hancox and Boothroyd, 1961). It can be seen at high magnifications that adjacent to bone, but in no other part of the periphery of the cell, the plasmalemma is thrown up into a complicated system of folds and deep penetrating clefts. Some of the clefts have been seen to communicate with intracytoplasmic vesicles, and Hancox (1956) has drawn attention to the orderly series of vacuoles which may be seen in the light microscope to lie just beneath the ruffled border. However, the plasmalemma applied to bone is not always arranged in this way as in some sections it may follow closely the contour of the bone edge, only occasionally being thrown up to form a blunt channel (Hancox and Boothroyd, 1963). The rest of the plasma membrane is relatively regular in outline (Cooper et al., 1966), but may be raised in microvilli (Gonzales and Karnovsky, 1961).

Osteoclasts contain numerous mitochondria scattered throughout the cytoplasm (Scott and Pease, 1956), having closely packed cristae with characteristic dense granules $\sim$550 Å in diameter (Cooper et al., 1966), and abundant ribosomes lying free and arranged in rosettes (Dudley and Spiro, 1961). The profusion of mitochondria is indicative of high metabolic activity, and is reflected in the cells' strong reactivity with histochemical techniques demonstrating oxidative enzymes (Burstone, 1960; Goldhaber and Barrnett, 1960; Walker, 1961; Irving and Handelman, 1963). The cytoplasm contains many vesicles. However, there is a paucity of GER; the small amount present is located in areas remote from the ruffled border. The Golgi lamellae occur in small aggregates. The cells contain many lysosome-like bodies of varying size and structure (Fell, 1964; Scott, 1967). The latter author believes that these are derived from the Golgi apparatus and that their contents may either be secreted by way of the vesicles associated with the brush border, or else utilized in intracellular digestive mechanisms. The presence in the cells of hydrolytic enzymes usually associated with lysosomes has been demonstrated chemically (Fell, 1964a,b; Susi et al., 1966) and histochemically (Lipp, 1959; Burstone, 1960; Hancox and Boothroyd, 1963; Irving and Handelman, 1963).

According to Hancox (1956) the nuclei are of varying appearance and may reflect the age of the cell. Nuclei which are round or oval, vesicular, and which contain one or two nucleoli, are probably found in young cells. The nuclei in ageing cells may be shrunken, crenated or box-like, and in cells at the end of their life-span, possibly pyknotic. Mathews et al. (1967) maintain that osteoclasts contain pairs of centrioles corresponding in number to the nuclei. They have found that these are localized to a single centrosphere, and in this respect differ from the scattered distribution of these organelles in foreign body giant cells.

Direct participation of osteoclasts in removal of bone has been ascertained from study of living cells *in vivo*, and particularly *in vitro*, and from morphological studies of dead cells. Goldhaber (1960; 1961; 1965; 1966) has observed

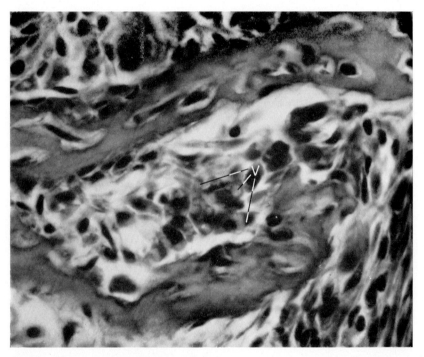

FIG. 20. Effete osteoclasts showing extensive vacuolation (V). One week organ culture of mandible from mouse embryo 18 days *in utero*. Haematoxylin and eosin. (× 300.)

that, *in vitro*, osteoclasts applied to bone exhibit an unusual "back and forth" sliding motion, and that their cytoplasm "bubbles and boils". Intracellular vacuoles tend to stream inwards from the periphery of the cell adjacent to bone, and small vacuoles fuse to form giant vacuoles. He believes that there is evidence that these giant vacuoles are present in osteoclasts *in vivo*. Bone adjacent to cells exhibiting this behaviour is seen to "melt away". The giant vacuoles eventually contract, an occurrence possibly accompanying the terminal phase in the life-cycle of osteoclasts (Fig. 20). Osteoclast death has been observed following rapid resorption. Crystals of inorganic material, believed to have been derived from resorbed bone, have been identified in osteoclasts (Arnold and Jee, 1957). They have been seen between the channels and folds of the ruffled border, in intracytoplasmic vesicles, and in mitochondria (Scott and Pease, 1956; Cameron and Robinson, 1958; Gonzales and Karnovsky, 1961; Hancox and Boothroyd, 1961; Lehninger, 1964; Anderson and Parker, 1966; Cooper *et al.*, 1966). Similar material has been identified in macrophages found in the vicinity of osteoclasts (Mclean and Bloom, 1941; Arnold and Jee, 1957; Anderson and Parker, 1966).

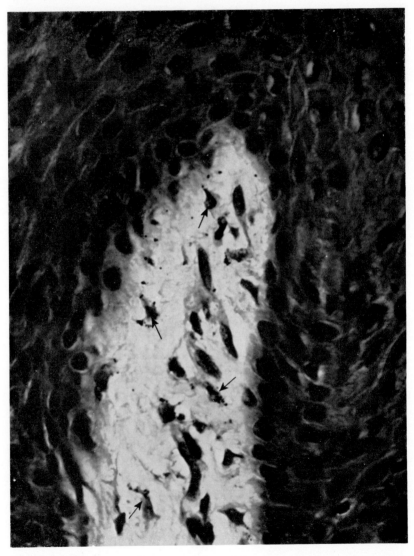

Fig. 21. Tattoed monkey gingiva. Carbon particles in the cytoplasm of macrophages. Haematoxylin and eosin. (×530.)

The giant cells associated with resorption of cementum do not appear to have been described in detail, although Provenza (1964) says that these cells exhibit the same cytological features as osteoclasts. In this connection, it is of interest that Takuma (1962) has found chondroclasts to have the same cytological organization as osteoclasts. It is significant that, although soft connective tissue is resorbed (as will be described in Section **IV**) multinucleated giant cells do not appear to be associated with this process.

ii. Macrophages or histiocytes

The terms macrophage and histiocyte are used interchangeably for a cell whose function is to ingest alien material or the debris of cells and their products. Macrophages may be resident in connective tissue, or they may be of haematogenous origin, but cells from the two sources are indistinguishable morphologically. The cells are large, thereby differing from so-called "microphages" which emigrate from the blood into the connective tissue when required. They are often difficult to differentiate from fibroblasts at light microscopic magnifications. However, they can be distinguished readily in preparations of tissues which have been exposed to foreign material during life. They ingest this material and can then be identified by its presence in their cytoplasm (Fig. 21).

Macrophages are ovoid, but may be elongated or angular when crowded by other tissue components. Cytologically, Ham and Leeson (1965) distinguish them from fibroblasts by their smaller, more intensely stained and indented nucleus, which tends to be located towards one end of the cell with its convex surface facing the nearest cell margin. At the higher magnifications of the electron microscope, the plasma membrane is seen to be thrown up into short projections, folds and clefts. Characteristics which distinguish them from fibroblasts (Ross and Benditt, 1961) are: their rich content of vacuoles that contain ingested matter and which may be lysosomes; the occasional presence of myelin figures within these vacuoles; the presence in the cell of irregularly shaped, very dense amorphous masses of varying size; a relative paucity of GER; and the absence of marginal intracytoplasmic filaments (Fig. 22).

iii. Mast Cells

Ehrlich (1877) is credited with the first description of mast cells. In the ninety-year period since his discovery a large number of publications concerning mast cells have appeared (for reviews see Selye, 1965; Goffman, 1966). Although these have elucidated the morphology and distribution of the cells, and, more recently, their chemical components, this mass of work has not shed much light on their function. More than thirty theories concerning their purpose have been reviewed by Selye (1965), and new hypotheses

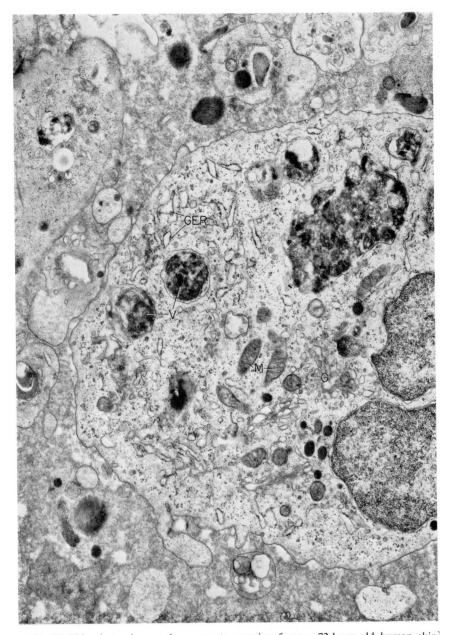

FIG. 22. This photomicrograph represents a region from a 72-hour old human skin
wound, in which part of a large macrophage can be seen. Profiles of cisternae of rough
endoplasmic reticulum (GER), containing small numbers of attached ribosomes, are
apparent. Mitochondria (M) and large cytoplasmic vacuoles (V) are present that contain
dense material, some of which have an appearance similar to the granules seen in intact
neutrophilic leukocytes. Numerous free cytoplasmic ribosomes and a portion of the Golgi
complex (G) are also apparent. ($\times 4,600$.) (Reproduced with permission from R. Ross.
J. Dent. Res **45**, 449–462, 1966.)

continue to be put forward (Chayen *et al.*, 1966; Selye, 1966). Indeed, at the conclusion of a long and comprehensive review, Smith (1963) was constrained to say that although it seems certain that tissue mast cells release some of their constituents under a variety of experimental conditions, it has not been established definitely that they play a role in the everyday life of the organism. An annotation on mast cells (*Lancet*, 1967) concluded with the assertion that there is still no obvious prospect of a unifying concept of mast-cell function.

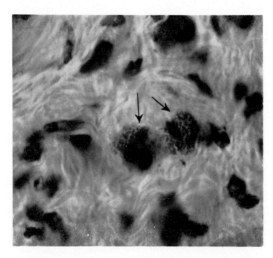

FIG. 23. Mast cells. Harris's haematoxylin and eosin. (×530.)

Mast cells occur in a variety of connective tissues in man, other mammals, amphibia and fishes (Smith, 1963), and there are marked species differences in their composition, distribution, and staining (Fullmer, 1965; 1967). They have an oval or polymorphous form, and are characterized by the presence of numerous large intracytoplasmic granules which stain with basic dyes and sometimes with haematoxylin (Fig. 23). The ultra-structural features of mast cells have been reviewed by Smith (1963). The mature cell is surrounded by a plasma membrane having numerous villous processes, which Fawcett (1955) regards, at least in rats, as being more fragile than that of other cell types. The cytoplasm is largely obscured by the characteristic granules which vary between 0·25 μ and 1·3 μ in diameter (Fernando and Movat, 1963b; Weinstock and Albright, 1967). The latter authors have found that there may be variation in the morphology and internal structure of the granules in cells in adult human gingiva. Combs (1966) has described the differences between the cytoplasm in young and mature cells. The granules appear to develop in saccules of the Golgi apparatus of young cells, and in mature cells are membrane-bound. In young cells, where granules are being formed, GER and elements of the Golgi apparatus are abundant, and continuity has been established between the cisternae of the GER and the Golgi saccules in which granules are being formed. In the mature cell, according to Combs, there is virtual absence of GER and a diminutive Golgi. However, Weinstock and Albright have found a well developed Golgi complex, a paucity of GER, but numerous free ribosomes in the cytoplasm of mast cells in gingiva from human adults. They have also described the presence of typical mitochondria in these cells.

The nucelus appears to be of unexceptional morphology. Fernando and Movat (1963b) report that nucleoli are present only in immature cells, and Weinstock and Albright observed them occasionally in cells obtained from adults.

Mast cells contain heparin (Jorpes et al., 1937), which Julén et al. (1950), Sylven (1951) and Hedbom and Snellman (1955) thought was contained in the cytoplasm but not in the granules. However, it is now clear that this conclusion is mistaken (Smith, 1963), and Lagunoff et al. (1964) have found that the granules of rat mast cells contain 30% heparin (dry weight). It is this content of sulphated acid mucopolysaccharide that accounts for the metachromasia, which Benditt (1958) says is resident entirely in the granules, and their staining with alcian blue. However, Riley (1953) has found that elongated, probably developing, mast cells in the adventitia of blood vessels are orthochromatic. Fawcett (1955) has expressed the view that young mast cells are not metachromatic but are paS positive, and Hall (1966) has ascribed this variation in histochemical reaction to the degree of sulphation of the contained heparin. Ultrastructurally, Gustafson and Pihl (1967a,b) have localized "staining" by a method believed to demonstrate sulphated acid mucopolysaccharides to the granules of rat mast cells.

Schiller and Dorfman (1959) and Parekh and Glick (1962) have found that heparin is the only sulphated acid mucopolysaccharide occurring in mast cells. Sulphur has been shown to be incorporated into mast cells (Jorpes et al., 1953; Curran and Kennedy, 1955), and more rapidly into the cells of young rats than into those of old rats (Guidotti, 1957), but Glücksmann et al. (1956) have denied that the cells contribute to the sulphur-containing compounds of the connective tissue.

Mast cells are rich in histamine (Riley and West, 1953; Benditt et al., 1955), and Lagunoff et al., (1961) have described a histochemical method for its demonstration. Histamine has been isolated from the granules of rat mast cells, and found to account for about 10% of their dry weight (Lagunoff et al., 1964). Histidine decarboxylase, an enzyme concerned in the synthesis of histamine, has been found to be associated with mast cells (Schayer, 1956). Serotonin (5-hydroxytryptamine), which was first isolated from mast cells by Benditt et al. (1955), is also stored in the granules (Smith, 1963), and ascorbic acid has recently been identified in rat mast cells (Glick and Hosoda, 1965).

Several uncharacterized proteolytic enzymes (Ende *et al.*, 1964), a trypsin-like enzyme (Glenner and Cohen, 1960; Glenner *et al.*, 1962), and a chymotrypsin-like enzyme (Benditt and Arase, 1959) have been identified in mast cells. The chymotrypsin-like enzyme has been demonstrated histochemically (Lagunoff *et al.*, 1962); Hall (1966) has suggested that this is the most specific method for identifying mast cells histologically. The chymotrypsin-like enzyme has also been localized to the granules (Budd *et al.*, 1967). Daržyn-kiewicz and Barnard (1967) have estimated that enzymes resembling chymotrypsin make up 85% of all the proteases, and these account for at least 10% of the total dry mass of the rat mast cell. They have found that the enzyme is active in the cell, suggesting the absence of a zymogen precursor, and that 5-hydroxytryptamine appears to inhibit protease activity in the intact mast cell. Leucine amino-peptidase and non-specific esterase, the latter of which is clearly localized to the granules, have been identified histochemically (Keller 1962), as have other enzymes (Fullmer, 1967).

Many different cells have been suggested as the precursors of mast cells (Smith, 1963; Fullmer, 1967; Ginsburg and Lagunoff, 1967). Mature mast cells are long-lived and stable (Miller and Cole, 1968). However, they appear to be able to divide mitotically. Evidence to support this belief has been obtained following experimental depletion of mast cells (Hunt and Hunt, 1957), from observations on cells underlying experimentally-produced epitheliomas (Asboe-Hansen and Levi, 1962; Sawicki, 1967b), in growing mice (Blenkinsop, 1967), and in lymph nodes stimulated by antigen (Miller and Cole, 1968). One of the great difficulties besetting observations of this type is the problem of distinguishing between mast cells and cells that have ingested mast cell granules.

Although the function of mast cells is unknown, their products can be released by degranulation following disruption of the cells, by degranulation from an intact cell, or by merocrine secretion of histamine or 5-hydroxytryptamine (Smith, 1963). Shed granules are taken up and digested by many cell types (Smith and Lewis, 1958), but particularly by fibroblasts (Higginbotham *et al.*, 1956) and this may give them the appearance of mast cells.

2. Extracellular Substance of Connective Tissues

The extracellular substance of connective tissue comprises fibres and ground substance and in mineralized connective tissues, mineral salts. The morphological characteristics of fibres and ground substance will be described in this section, while their chemical properties will be discussed in Section **III**.

(*a*). *The fibres of connective tissues.* There are two major groups of fibres in connective tissues, collagen fibres and elastic fibres. Collagen fibres, which are present in virtually all connective tissues, are the most numerous and important. Elastic fibres are restricted to tissues exhibiting elasticity.

i. Collagen fibres

Collagen fibres are composed largely, but not entirely, of the unique protein, collagen. The collagen macromolecules are assembled to form fibrils which, when examined in the electron microscope, show a characteristic band pattern which repeats every ∼640 Å. This periodicity, which provides

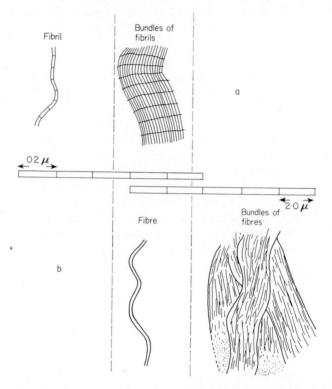

FIG. 24. Diagrammatic comparison between the appearance of collagen fibres in the (a) electron and (b) light microscopes. Collagen fibr*ils* ∼100 Å or more in diameter, are gathered into bundles. When the bundles of fibr*ils* reach a diameter of 0·2 *μ* they can be resolved as collagen fibr*es* in the light microscope. These, in their turn, are gathered into bundles of collagen fibr*es*.

the only hall-mark by which collagen fibrils can be recognized at high magnification, becomes evident in positively-stained material when the fibrils attain a thickness of ∼100 Å (Ross and Benditt, 1961). As a result, the nature of both thinner unbanded fibrils, and fibrils cut in cross section, cannot be determined with certainty. The diameter of the fibrils increases with age, the final thickness varying with the tissue. For example, in developing avian tendon the fibrils attain a diameter of 750 Å (Fitton Jackson, 1957a,b), but in healing guinea-pig skin they reach 1300 Å (Ross and Benditt, 1961). The

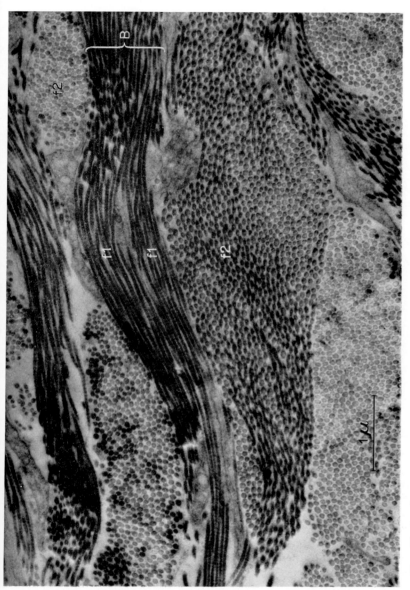

Fig. 25. An electronmicrograph of collagen fibres in monkey gingival connective tissue. The fibrils which are cut longitudinally show the periodicity that is characteristic of collagen fibrils, and the bands of adjacent fibrils are frequently found to be in register. The fibrils cut transversely can be presumed to be collagen on account of their situation. The fibrils are gathered together to form fibres. Some of the fibres (f1) forming bundles (B) converge and diverge slightly, while others (f2) run in a direction very different from these.

collagen fibrils are gathered together in bundles, with the bands of adjacent fibrils often in register (Figs 24 and 25). These bundles of fibrils may also reach varying thicknesses in different tissues, but are only recognizable in the light microscope when they attain a diameter of 0·2–0·3 μ (Fig. 24). They are then called fibres. All collagen structures resolvable in the light microscope are conveniently called fibres, the term fibril being reserved for the banded structure resolvable only in the electron microscope. The fibres, in their turn, are gathered together in bundles (Figs 25 and 26). In the light microscope,

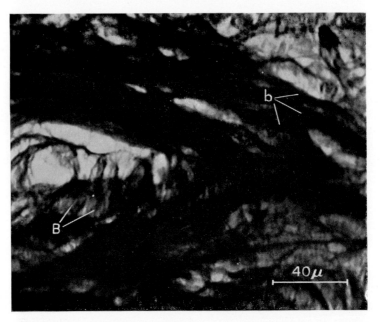

Fig. 26. Collagen fibres in gingival connective tissue. Large bundles of collagen fibres (b). Small bundles (B) approximately the same thickness as that marked B in Fig. 25. Van Gieson's picro-fuchsin. ($\times$ 500.)

many of the fibres making up these bundles often appear to be more or less parallel. However, the thinner sections and the higher magnifications of electron microscopy show that the fibres do not follow a straight course but tend to converge and diverge. Adjacent bundles of fibres which, in the light microscope, can be seen to run in different directions, comprise fibres whose fibrils are orientated very differently from one another.

At light microscope magnifications, collagen fibres cannot be identified positively as there is no known histochemical technique for demonstrating collagen. Collagen does not contain any chemical group absent from surrounding substances by which it can be identified selectively. It does contain significant amounts of the comparatively rare amino acid, hydroxyproline.

The chemical tests for collagen utilize this content of hydroxyproline. As yet, it has not been possible to adapt these methods to histochemistry because they require hydrolysis of the collagen macromolecule, and this is incompatible with its morphological localization. Collagen fibres are therefore recognized by their morphology. The bundles are frequently wavy, although they may sometimes run a straight course, and are rarely seen to branch. A number of histological stains show them to advantage but it is not known whether these stains react with chemical groups of the collagen molecule, or with chemical groups of intimately associated ground substance, or with both. The chemical groups of the substrates involved in staining by a number of the common methods have been reviewed by Fullmer (1965; 1966; 1967). Perhaps the most widely and easily used method utilizes van Gieson's picro-fuchsin mixture, the acid fuchsin component of which appears to react with hydroxyl groups. Amphoteric dyes, such as aniline blue and light green, are also useful and are widely employed in the methods described by Masson and Mallory. These dyes are used in conjunction with a mordant, phospho-tungstic acid or phosphomolybdic acid, which is believed to react with amine groups, and perhaps guanidino groups. Another dye of this type is haematoxylin, as used in the phosphotungstic acid-haematoxylin method. Haematoxylin, when used in the traditional technique, also stains collagen fibres lightly but is displaced when followed by eosin (Melcher, 1966a). Salthouse (1965 and 1966) has found recently that a saturated solution of Luxol fast blue G in methanol can be used to demonstrate collagen fibres.

Silver impregnation is another method for demonstrating fibres of connective tissue. The methods of Gordon and Sweets (1936) and Gömöri (1937) are well known and particularly useful. Provided that the "toning" step is omitted, mature collagen fibres are coloured golden-brown. The identity of the chemical groups involved in the reaction is obscure. When viewed in polarized light, collagen fibres show form and intrinsic birefringence which is positive with respect to the fibre-axis. They also show dichroism and anomalous colours when stained with certain acid and basic dyes (Brewer, 1957).

Collagen could conceivably also be identified in both the light and electron microscopes by techniques utilizing suitably labelled antibody. For light microscopy the antibody is attached to a fluorescent material, and for electron microscopy to an electron-dense substance. But this technique is dogged by two great difficulties; preparation of pure collagen for use as antigen, and preparation of pure antibody (O'Dell, 1965). Impurities result in additional labelling of substances other than collagen. It used to be believed that collagen is non-antigenic, but a number of workers have now produced antibodies to collagen (Watson et al., 1954; Rothbard and Watson, 1962 and 1965; Mancini et al., 1965a,b; O'Dell, 1965), and to a group of polar peptides obtained from the collagen macromolecule (Seifter, 1965).

Schmitt *et al.* (1964) and Rubin *et al.* (1965) have found that the antigenicity of collagen macromolecules resides in terminal extrahelical peptides. The rewards that might accrue from successful development of this technique are manifold, but will be obtained only after a number of technical difficulties have been overcome, and by the use of rigorous controls.

In light microscope sections of connective tissue that have been impregnated with silver, two other types of fibres belonging to the collagen family are demonstrated (Fig. 27). These fibres, which are argyrophilic (i.e. coloured

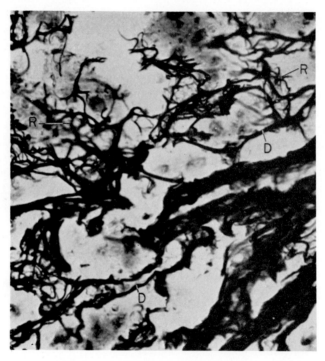

Fig. 27. Reticulin (R) and argyrophilic developing collagen fibres (D) in the liver of an aged rat. Gordon and Sweets silver impregnation. (× 530.)

black instead of golden brown), have been the subject of great controversy (Melcher, 1966b) and will be discussed fully in Section **IV**. The first of these, the argyrophilic developing collagen fibres, have the morphology of mature collagen fibres, and occur in developing connective tissue. The second type, reticulin, is characteristically branched, forming networks (Robb-Smith, 1957 and 1958), and is most readily seen in the stroma of parenchymatous organs and at the junction of epithelium and connective tissue. A staining method for differentiating between "precollagen" and mature collagen has been described by Herovici (1963), but this technique does not differentiate between developing collagen fibres and reticulin (Melcher, 1966a). Reticulin is poorly stained by the van Gieson method, but staining is improved by increasing the picric acid content.

ii. Elastic fibres

Elastic fibres contain a protein, elastin, the chemistry of which will be discussed in Section **III**. Ultrastructural studies have been carried out on elastin isolated after vigorous chemical treatment (Partridge, 1962; Ayer,

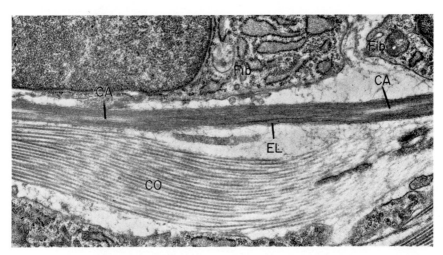

FIG. 28. This micrograph shows a longitudinal section of a digital flexor tendon of a newborn rat in which a long elastic fibre (EL) appears to consist primarily of densely stained 100 Å fibrils with occasional lighter areas (CA) that represent the non-staining central areas. A somewhat beaded appearance can be seen in the fibrils of the elastic fibre, similar to that seen in ligamentum nuchae. Collagen fibrils (CO) with their characteristic banding can be seen. The elastic fibre follows a straighter course than the collagen and lies in proximity to two fibroblasts. Fixed in OsO_4. Stained with uranyl acetate and lead. ($\times$ 6,500.) (Reproduced with permission from T. K. Greenlee, Jr., R. Ross and J. L. Hartman, *J. Cell Biol.* **30**, 59–71, 1966.)

1964; Cox and O'Dell, 1966), but this description will be confined to elastic fibres studied in histological sections. Three papers (Greenlee *et al.*, 1966; Fahrenbach *et al.*, 1966; Taylor and Yeager, 1966), which appeared almost simultaneously, have elucidated the ultrastructure of developing and mature elastic fibres. Very young elastic fibres have been found to be composed of groups of apparently hollow filaments. The filaments are 100–140 Å thick and the apparently hollow central core is ∼40 Å in diameter. As the fibre matures, it acquires a granular central area, which Fahrenbach *et al.* consider to be elastin and which could be derived from crosslinking of the material comprising the hollow fibrils. The fibres, according to these workers, are between 700–1000 Å in diameter and are gathered in bundles which, in developing bovine ligamentum nuchae, are at first ~0·4 μ in diameter and may reach 9·9 μ in diameter. The central material increases in diameter as the fibres thicken, but is always surrounded by a mantle of hollow filaments. During this process of enlargement, according to Greenlee *et al.*, the central material of adjacent fibres may coalesce. They point out that mature elastic fibres therefore contain two morphological components, a large central area

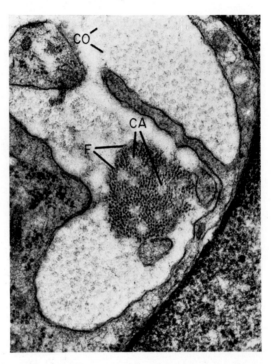

Fig. 29. Cross-section of an elastic fibre from a tendon of a new-born rat. Double-staining (uranyl acetate and lead) appears to be additive in that the fibrils (F) of the elastic fibre are more intensely stained than the central areas (CA) of the elastic fibres or the collagen (CO). (×41,000.) (Reproduced with permission from T. K. Greenlee, Jr., R. Ross and J. L. Hartman, *J. Cell Biol.* **30**, 59–71, 1966.)

of material surrounded by a thin layer of hollow fibrils which, in longitudinal sections, shows no cross-banding but may, in some regions, be regularly beaded.

Greenlee *et al.* have found that the fibrils and the material in the centre of the fibre have different "staining" properties. The fibrils have little or no affinity for phosphotungstic acid, in contrast to the central material, which takes it up strongly. On the other hand, lead salts and uranyl acetate do not demonstrate the central material, but show the peripheral fibrils well (Figs 28 and 29).

Unstained elastic fibres are slightly yellow in colour, and at the magnifications of the light microscope are seen to branch. A number of so-called elastic stains, orcein, resorcin fuchsin, aldehyde fuchsin, orcinol-new fuchsin and Verhoeff's iron haematoxylin, stain them selectively (Fig. 30) but by no means specifically. The precise mechanism by which the stains react with elastic fibres is obscure. This topic has recently been discussed fully by Ayer (1964) and Fullmer (1965) and will not be repeated here. Gillman *et al.*

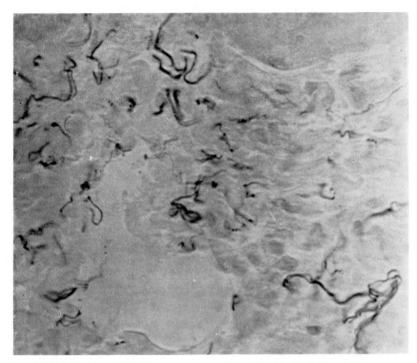

Fig. 30. Elastic fibres. The fibres are frequently found to be curled probably as a result of their contracting when the specimen is excised. Orcein. (× 530.)

(1955a,b) have stressed the need to identify elastic fibres on the basis of their morphology as well as by their staining reaction. This is because collagen fibres which have been altered in pathological conditions (Gillman *et al.*, 1955a,b; Newton, 1964), and experimentally (Burton *et al.*, 1955; Fullmer and Lillie, 1956 and 1957), will also take up elastic stains (Section **IIIA**). Furthermore, there is some evidence that aldehyde fuchsin and resorcin fuchsin can stain sulphated acid mucopolysaccharides (Melcher, 1967c).

iii. Oxytalan fibres

These fibres, first described by Fullmer and Lillie (1958) and Fullmer (1959a, and 1960), and recently reviewed by Fullmer (1965 and 1967), were given their name on account of their resistance to destruction by formic acid. They have been found in human periodontium, in tendons, ligaments, the adventitia of blood vessels, the epineurium and perineurium, and surrounding appendages of skin. They are stained by some elastic stains (resorcin fuchsin, aldehyde fuchsin and orcein), but only after they have been oxidized by peracetic or performic acid. They are also stained by some basic stains after oxidation with oxone (Rannie, 1963). They are digested by elastase, and their stainable component by β-glucuronidase, but again, only after oxidation.

Based on observations using the electron microscope, they are believed to consist of fibrils 150–160 Å thick gathered together in bundles (Carmichael and Fullmer, 1966). Fullmer (1967) has drawn attention to their resemblance to previously published electronmicrographs of elastic fibres, and Greenlee et al. (1966) have pointed out the similarity between one of their electron-micrographs of an immature elastic fibre and Carmichael and Fullmer's picture of an oxytalan fibre.

In some animal species oxytalan fibres have been found in tissues which, in other species contain elastic fibres. Developing elastic fibres can be stained by the oxytalan methods (i.e. after oxidation) at an earlier stage in their development than their aquisition of a direct affinity for traditional elastic stains. These findings, and the ultrastructural appearance of the fibres, have led Fullmer to suggest that oxytalan fibres are related to elastic fibres, possibly representing incompletely developed or modified elastic fibres. Despite Selvig's (1966) suggestion that they might represent degenerated collagen fibres, the evidence seems to support strongly the view that they are immature elastic fibres. Persistence of immature elastic fibres in mature connective tissue has a possible analogue in reticulin which, as will be discussed in Section **IV**, may be an immature precursor of collagen fibres persisting in mature connective tissues.

iv. Cellulose-protein fibres

These fibres were identified in mammalian dermis by Hall et al. (1958 and 1960), and have been discussed by Hall (1961). The fibres, which are aniso-tropic, appear to occur in pathologically involved connective tissue and to comprise degraded collagen fibres to which are attached deposits of cellulose.

(b). The ground substance of connective tissues. Ground substance completely envelops the other connective tissue constituents; the cells and the fibres. All metabolites and other substances moving to or from cells must pass through the ground substance, as must motile cells and the moving processes of cells. Thus, the environment of connective tissue cells is largely governed by the nature of the ground substance. Ground substance is a part of both mineralized and soft connective tissues. In the former it is intimately associated with crystals of mineral salts, and the resulting fabric probably greatly restricts the changes that can take place in the ground substance and its effect on the properties of the mineralized connective tissue.

The ground substance was formerly described as *amorphous*, but there is increasing evidence to show that it is highly organized at the macromolecular level (e.g. Smith *et al.*, 1967). It is composed of proteins, carbohydrates which are both acidic and neutral, and probably lipids, and these are usually combined in macromolecular complexes. Some of the polysaccharides are sulphated, and these have a high capacity for binding water and cations (Muir, 1961). Although Fitton Jackson (1964) has described the appearance in the electron microscope of protein-polysaccharide complexes obtained from cartilage, there are as yet no standard morphological criteria for identifying the components of ground substance at light or electron microscopic magnifications. Their microscopic identification therefore depends on histochemical techniques. The chemical composition of the ground substance and the mineral crystals, will be discussed in Section **IIIB**.

The structural components of the ground substance are closely associated with the interstitial fluid with which they are permeated. Indeed, variation in the relative concentrations of the two will produce marked changes in the consistency of the connective tissue. Other components of the extracellular compartment include plasma proteins, electrolytes, hormones, vitamins, enzymes, and substances for anabolism and products of catabolism. Thus, the texture, permeability, metabolism and reactions of all connective tissues are influenced greatly by the metabolism of the organism as a whole.

(c). *The inorganic phase of bone.* One of the earliest papers concerning the morphology of the crystallites of bone was that of Robinson (1952) who described them as tablet-shaped, and measuring ~500 Å long, ~250 Å wide and ~100 Å thick. Cameron (1963) has recently reviewed the literature on this topic and has pointed out that many subsequent investigators have described them as needle or rod-shaped. However, the weight of evidence appears to support Robinson's original concept, their shape in electron-micrographs possibly being determined by the profile they present to the electron-beam. Different estimations of their dimensions have been given, these varying between 150 and 1500 Å in length and 15 and 75 Å in thickness. Cameron suggests that the wide range that has been reported may result from differences in the age and source of materials examined. It is of interest that Johansen and Parks (1960) have found the crystallities of human alveolar bone to be plate-like structures with a maximum length of 1,000 Å and a thickness of 25–40 Å.

It is generally agreed that the long (or C) axis of the crystallites lies parallel to the axis of the collagen fibrils. The crystallites are intimately associated with collagen fibrils, actually lying within them or on them (Glimcher, 1960; Cooper *et al.*, 1966). The crystallites in fully mineralized tissue obscure the band-pattern of the collagen fibrils. However, the intimate association between the two has been demonstrated elegantly by Quigley and Hjørting-Hansen (1962), who have shown that the inorganic framework of bone exhibits the electronmicroscopic periodicity of the collagen fibrils after the latter have been removed by chemical means.

3. The Effects of Structure on the Physical Characteristics of Connective Tissues

Connective tissue is almost ubiquitous in the human body, but it occurs in many different guises. This is well illustrated by comparing the gelatinous consistency of Wharton's jelly in the umbilical cord with the harsh, fibrous texture of the Achilles tendon; the delicate, sticky, connective tissue of the superficial fascia with the tough, resilient, lamina propria of the attached gingiva; and all of these with the hard, resistant, mineralized connective tissues, bone, dentine and cementum. These tremendous variations within a single family of tissues are achieved by alterations in the numbers of cells present per unit volume and the nature of the extracellular substance.

Tendon, which has great tensile strength, is relatively acellular and possesses a high content of collagen (Fitton Jackson, 1964). The collagen fibres generally run in the direction of pull. Hyaline cartilage, on the other hand, can resist compression. It has a comparative paucity of collagen fibres (about 40%), but a relatively high concentration of ground substance (about 50%) of firm consistency (Fitton Jackson, 1964), much of which consists of chondroitin sulphates. In some situations the cartilage is, in addition, required to be particularly elastic, as in the external ear and the epiglottis. In these situations numerous elastic fibres are present in the extracellular substance. When cartilage requires especially great tensile strength, as for example at tendon insertions, there is a marked increase in its content of collagen fibres. Areolar connective tissue, such as constitutes the superficial fascia, requires relatively little mechanical strength, and here there are few collagen fibres amidst much ground substance of tacky consistency. The great strength and resistance of bone is provided by a dense network of collagen fibres braced with mineral crystals. The orientation of the bundles of collagen fibres is influenced by the direction of the forces acting on the bone. A further example of the versatility of connective tissue is provided by that present in the cornea. This connective tissue must be transparent. It is avascular and relatively acellular. The collagen fibrils are thin and of uniform diameter, and are arranged in highly ordered fashion (Jakus, 1961), and the ground substance is of characteristic composition (Anseth, 1965). It is significant that alterations in the size and distribution of the collagen fibrils, or in the composition of the ground substance, lead to opacity (Anseth, 1965).

Thus, although all connective tissue is organized from cells and intercellular substance, it is able to perform a wide variety of functions through great variation in the content, distribution and architecture of these constituents. The collagen fibres in different connective tissues are present in varying concentrations and, where necessary, are orientated in a manner which enables the tissue to resist prevalent forces acting upon it. Variations in concentration and make-up of the ground substance greatly influence the texture of the connective tissue, and the type and proportions of mucosubstances vary not only from connective tissue to connective tissue, but also with age in a given connective tissue (Lloyd, 1965; Kent, 1967).

4. Organization of the Components of Bone

Bone is a highly specialized connective tissue. Its unique organization and properties stem from the rigid nature of its extracellular substance. A canalicular system which transmits the processes of the osteocytes, and which connects adjacent osteocyte lacunae with each other and with the soft connective tissue surrounding blood vessels, allows the movement of metabolites to and from bone cells incarcerated in the mineralized extracellular substance. This arrangement conceivably sets a limit on the distance separating an osteocyte from its source of nutrition, as metabolites have to pass between blood vessels and cells by diffusing through canaliculae. Consequently, the cellular components of bone are organized around the blood vessels.

The bone deposited initially in the developing embryo, or in repair of a bone wound, is termed woven bone (Fig. 31a). It is laid down as a network of fine trabeculae. The system of connecting channels between the trabeculae is occupied by vascular connective tissue. The osteocytes of woven bone tend to be numerous, large and round, and are disposed irregularly. The collagen fibres show no preferred orientation and, when seen in the light microscope, appear to be large and of varying diameter (Pritchard, 1956; Smith, 1960). A characteristic feature of these trabeculae is their penetration by extrinsic collagen fibres which have been incorporated from the surrounding connective tissue; that is, by Sharpey's fibres. The collagen fibrils of woven bone have a diameter up to ~ 600 Å (Cameron, 1963). Woven bone is stained strongly with haematoxylin, and is highly coloured by the paS reaction (Young, 1963a).

More mature bone occurs in the form of lamellae or sheets (Fig. 31b). These are first laid down on the surface of trabeculae of woven bone. When deposited on free surfaces, they constitute circumferential lamellae; when deposited on internal surfaces they colonize the soft connective tissue occupying the channels between the woven bone trabeculae. The trabeculae being laid down in the latter situation slowly encroach on blood vessels, around which they are laid concentrically, eventually enclosing them in a central canal, the Haversian canal. The Haversian canal, and its contents, and the surrounding bone lamellae constitute a primary osteone (or primary Haversian system). Secondary osteones are laid down only following prior removal of bone during remodelling. An area of bone is resorbed and replaced by soft connective tissue. The new intrabony channel thus formed is then colonized by new bone lamellae which form a new (secondary) osteone.

Circumferential lamellae may be periosteal or endosteal. Lamellar bone is also found in random situations between osteones. These are interstitial

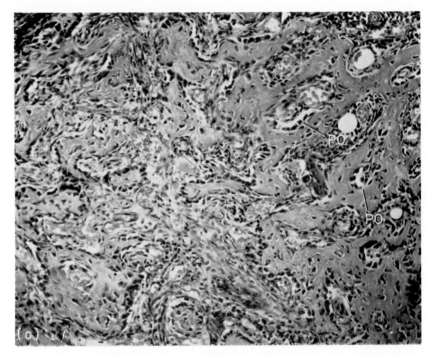

FIG. 31a. Trabeculae of woven bone deposited in repair of a bone wound. Primary osteones are present (PO). Haematoxylin and eosin. (×110.)

lamellae, and represent fragments of osteones or circumferential lamellae that have been spared the ravages of resorption occurring as part of remodelling processes.

Primary and secondary osteones can be differentiated readily (Smith, 1960; Amprino, 1963). Primary osteones are usually surrounded by primary spongiosa (woven bone) and, unlike secondary osteones which develop subsequent to a period of resorption, their periphery is not demarcated by a reversal line which stains with haematoxylin. Furthermore, particularly at their periphery, the lamellae of primary osteones contain Sharpey's fibres, many of which are continuous with those of the primary spongiosa.

Because bone is organized entirely around its blood supply, osteones branch, bifurcate and anastomose, and vary in length, diameter and shape.

Furthermore, interstitial lamellae are practically always structurally continuous with intact osteones (Cohen and Harris, 1958). The vessels of the Haversian canals in long bones are derived mainly from the nutrient vessel via the medullary sinusoids and, secondarily, from the periosteal vessels (Cohen and Harris, 1958; Trueta, 1964). Circulation of blood through these

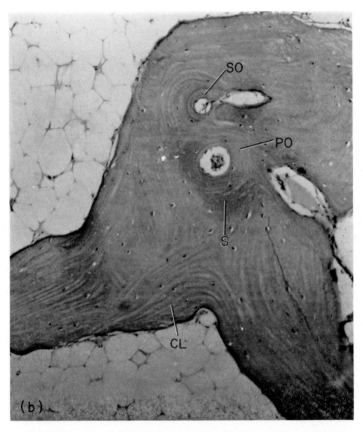

Fig. 31b. Trabeculum and yellow marrow from alveolar process of young adult. The trabeculum contains primary osteones (PO), secondary osteones (SO), woven bone (S) and circumferential lamellae (CL). Haematoxylin and eosin. (× 80.)

vessels, which do not have valves, appears to be dependent largely on the effect of intermittent contraction of the overlying muscles and, to a lesser extent weight-bearing, on the pressure in the marrow (Trueta, 1963; McPherson, 1967). The vessels in the Haversian canals are surrounded by concentric layers of bone. Anastomosing with these are other vessels lying in the Volkman's canals which cut across the lamellae of osteones. It is important to realize that the vessels in the Volkman's canals, while supplying those in the Haversian canals, do not really occupy a special position for, through the processes of remodelling, they may be derived from, or may themselves come to occupy, Haversian canals. Vessels are also found in association with circumferential lamellae, but these are not arranged in any special system and merely pass between adjacent lamellae (Cohen and Harris, 1958; Smith, 1960).

The lamellae of osteones in dogs average $\sim 3\mu$ in width, and adjacent lamellae have their collagen fibrils orientated in different directions. No amorphous zone separates individual lamellae, and the collagen fibrils of adjacent lamellae intermingle near the boundary (Cooper et al., 1966). The collagen fibrils appear to be of greater diameter than those of young bone, up to 1500 Å (Cameron, 1963), but the fibres have been reported as thinner from light microscope observations (Pritchard, 1956). Ascenzi (1964) has found that there is less interfibrillar cementing substance than in young lamellae. All lamellae may be permeated by osteocytes (Cooper et al., 1966) which, in contrast to those of woven bone, are fusiform with their longest diameter parallel to the axis of the lamella (Dudley and Spiro, 1961). Mjör (1962 and 1963) believes that the matrix bordering osteocyte lacunae and canaliculi is hypermineralized. However, Cooper et al. (1966) have found that the matrix adjacent to canaliculi appears to be fully mineralized, in contrast to the unmineralized matrix bordering some lacunae. Wassermann and Yaeger (1965) have noticed that the mineral crystals in the matrix bordering the lacunae are arranged in a less orderly fashion than those elsewhere in the matrix. The observations of the last two groups of workers appears to be in keeping with the observed activity of some osteocytes (Section **IVC**), and it is possible that mineralization of this area of the matrix varies.

At the hub of the osteone is the Haversian canal, the diameter of which varies with development of the osteone. Cooper et al. have examined the contents of Haversian Canals in the electron microscope, and have found them to contain one or two vessels. When two vessels were present, one was often seen to be large and thin-walled and the other smaller and thick-walled. Smooth muscle was not identified in their walls. These investigators found unmyelinated nerves in the canals of adult dogs but, strangely, could not identify neural elements in this situation in puppies. The presence of lymphatics does not appear to have been demonstrated. Osteoblasts, osteoclasts, undifferentiated (or osteoprogenitor) cells and, in the mature osteone, flattened attenuated cells, are also present.

Woven bone and lamellar bone are found in both cancellous and compact types of bone. The trabeculae of mature, cancellous bone are much coarser than are those of immature bone, and surround large marrow spaces (Fig. 31). Mature cancellous and compact bone are made up of secondary osteones and circumferential lamellae; but both may contain primary woven bone and primary osteones until remodelling processes eliminate and replace these by secondary osteones.

The external surfaces of bones are covered by periosteum. Periosteum comprises an inner or cambium layer of active or resting osteogenic connective tissue, and an outer fibrous layer of varying thickness which transmits vessels and nerves. The cambium layer, when active, comprises a layer of plump osteoblasts applied to the bone surface (Pritchard, 1952) and, peripheral to these, differentiating spindle-shaped osteogenic cells, supported by loosely arranged collagen fibres orientated more or less perpendicular to the bone surface. When resting, the osteoblasts on the bone surface become flattened and the osteogenic cells constitute a single layer of fusiform cells similar in appearance to fibroblasts. The fibrous layer is made up of a dense sheet of collagen fibres arranged parallel to the bone surface, between which lie fibrocytes. The periosteum is loosely attached to the underlying bone except where it is concerned in the attachment of muscles. Internal surfaces of bone are covered by a layer of active or resting osteogenic cells, the endosteum.

5. Functions of Connective Tissue

The functions of connective tissue are many and varied, and for convenience may be grouped in four categories:

(a) Supportive
(b) Locomotor
(c) Protective
(d) Nutritive

(a) *Supportive*. The form of the human body is dictated by the bones of the skeleton, themselves connective tissue, and these are held together by soft connective tissue ligaments and tendons. The contours of the body depend on the form of the bones, and the muscles and soft connective tissues which cover them. Bone, cartilage and fibrous connective tissue play an essential part in bearing the weight of the body and in resisting deformity by external forces applied to it. Organs and structures are held in place by ligaments, for example, the liver and the teeth. Soft tissue organs and structures, such as liver, kidney, blood vessels, nerves and muscles, are further supported by capsules or frameworks of connective tissue. Thin layers of connective tissue also provide support for specialized cells, as in liver and in endocrine and salivary glands.

(b) *Locomotor*. Locomotion in human beings is dependent in great measure on connective tissues. Mastication might be regarded as being a part of this activity. Locomotion is achieved by co-ordinated movement of the bones of the skeleton. This is brought about by transmission of forces from muscles through tendons to bones. Excess movement of bones is restricted by ligaments. A connective tissue, synovial fluid, supplies the lubrication which facilitates movement of bones at joints.

(c) *Protective.* Connective tissues protect the organism from damage by external forces. Vital organs are protected by skeletal structures, and also by the corium of the skin and mucous membranes. The ground substance of the connective tissues of the skin and mucous membranes hinders invasion by noxious organisms which have penetrated the overlying epithelium. Soft connective tissues contain macrophages which phagocytose extraneous material. Haemopoiesis is an important protective function of connective tissue; this phenomenon ensures that a supply of cells capable of producing antibodies and ingesting foreign substances is maintained. Connective tissue cells also play a large part in the repair of damage to tissues and organs (Chapter 12). Some connective tissues store energy in the form of fat, which also insulates the body against cold.

(d) *Nutritive.* Haemopoiesis provides the erythrocytes that transport oxygen around the body. Soft connective tissues are also responsible for transmitting the various gases and other substances which pass from the blood to the cells of the body, and in the reverse direction.

As will become apparent, the connective tissues of the periodontium perform many, though not all, of these functions.

B. The Connective Tissues of the Periodontium

1. Cementum

Cementum fills a number of roles. It attaches the collagen fibres of the periodontal ligament to the dentine of the root. It also plays a part in maintaining the width of the periodontal ligament, and the length of the root available for support of the tooth (Section **IV**). It effects repair of damage to the root (Chapter 12). Cementum is thought to be a modified form of bone. Linghorne (1954) suggests that the different structure of cementum may be related to its avascularity and lack of remodelling. Cementum, like bone, is softer than dentine (Hodge and McKay, 1933; Rautiola and Craig, 1961) (see p. 224 for chemical composition), and is permeable to dye (Stones 1934) and to various elements (Wainwright, 1952; Sognnaes *et al.*, 1955).

(a) *Microscopic appearance.* Acellular cementum, in which no cells can be recognized, is often confined to a thin layer covering the cervical half of the root dentine. However, it may occasionally cover the whole root or be interleaved between layers of cellular cementum. Cellular cementum, which contains within its substance irregularly distributed cementocytes lying in lacunae, forms the bulk of the cementum. It usually covers the dentine of the apical part of the root as well as the acellular cementum. At light microscopic magnifications both types of cementum exhibit incremental lines, but those of cellular cementum are generally more widely spaced. This is probably due to the more rapid deposition of cellular cementum, which is believed to lead to cementoblasts being trapped within its substance. Both types of cementum are of granular appearance, are coloured blue by haematoxylin, and are separated from the cementoblasts lined up in the adjacent connective tissue by a layer of eosinophilic precementum (Fig. 32).

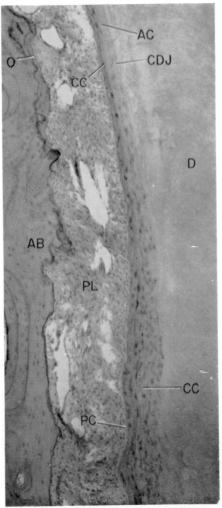

FIG. 32. An area of human periodontium. There is a thin layer of acellular cementum (AC) cervically, but not apically. It is covered by cellular cementum (CC), which is much thicker apically then cervically. The precementum (PC) is also much thicker apically than cervically. Alveolar bone (AB) is covered by a layer of cells (O) of the periodontal ligament (PL). D. dentine. CDJ. cemento-dentinal junction. (H & E.) (× 70.)

Much has been written on light microscopic investigations into the distribution and orientation of the collagen fibres in cementum, and while examination in polarized light has helped to elucidate this problem (Gustafson

8*

and Persson, 1957), recent electron microscopic reports, particularly by Stern (1964) on rat cementum and Selvig (1965) on human cementum, have greatly clarified the situation. Selvig has pointed out that no region of the intercellular matrix of cementum is free from collagen fibrils. The dense mass of collagen fibrils in cementum is orientated in two ways, which suggests that it is composed of two groups of fibrils of different origin. One group, Sharpey's fibres, runs at right angles to the cementum surface. These are fibres of the periodontal ligament which are probably laid down by periodontal fibroblasts, but incorporated into cementum during its development. The fibres of the other group run predominantly parallel to the surface of the cementum. These are the intrinsic fibres of cementum, and probably are laid down by cementoblasts. Selvig has found that much of the acellular cementum contains only Sharpey's fibres (Chapter 3). Where both groups of fibrils are present, they tend to run at right angles to one another.

Stern and Selvig have found that, irrespective of the orientation of the fibres in the periodontal ligament, they always enter the cementum at right angles to its surface (Fig. 33); turning if necessary, to do so. Stern has noticed in the rat incisor that, after penetrating some distance into the cementum, they may bend again. He suggests that these bends result from changes in the position of the tooth. This view is similar to that of Gustafson and Persson (1957) who examined the orientation of the fibres of cementum in polarized light. However, Listgarten (1966) has found that the fibrils of human cervical cementum tend to run a straight course from the surface to the cemento-dentinal junction. This finding must be considered in the light of the fact that Listgarten examined teeth from comparatively young people. Stern has not found any evidence for the presence of isolated ends of Sharpey's fibres in cementum. He believes that the absence of fibre-fragments contradicts the view that Sharpey's fibres become detached from the fibres of the periodontal ligament during tooth movement. Stern's belief is supported by observations which suggest that fibres in the part of the periodontal ligament adjacent to the cementum of the continuously erupting rodent incisor are carried in the direction of eruption (Melcher, 1967d).

Fibrils belonging to Sharpey's fibres, and fibrils apparently laid down by cementoblasts, can be seen at the surface of cementum. In man, these fibrils probably belong to the precementum, a layer varying in width up to about 5μ. The surface of the cementum is marked by small conical projections, each associated with the entry into cementum of a single collagen fibril. Occasionally a bundle of fibrils is associated with a large projection. Collagen fibrils do not cross the cemento-dentinal junction (Selvig, 1965; Listgarten, 1966), which Stern has found in the rat incisor to be marked by a slightly irregular opaque line, possibly representing the "basement membrane" of Hertwig's sheath.

Little information appears to be available about the fine structure of

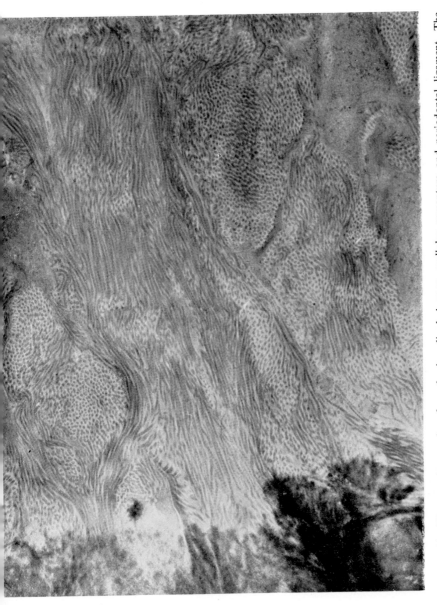

Fig. 33. Electronmicrograph of undemineralized human acellular cementum and periodontal ligament. The collagen fibrils of the ligament enter the cementum more or less at right angles to its surface. (Reproduced with permission from K. A. Selvig, *Acta Odont Scand.* **23**, 423–441, 1965.)

cementocytes and their lacunae. Frank and Nalbandian (1963) have observed that the structure of cementocytes is not unlike that of osteocytes; Amazawa (1963) has described canaliculi radiating from lacunae and connecting with one another. The last-named author believes that the walls of the lacunae are more highly mineralized than the rest of the tissue, and the presence of unmineralized collagen fibrils in the space between the cementocyte and the walls of the lacuna has been described by Albright and Flanagan (1962). On morphological grounds, Paynter and Pudy (1958) claim that cementocytes entrapped in lacunae remain alive for at least 101 days. The cells have been shown to react positively to a number of histochemical tests for enzymes, but those in the deeper part of the cementum are generally less active than those located more superficially (Fullmer, 1967).

Observations based on microradiographic studies suggest that the layer of acellular cementum nearest the dentine has a lower mineral content than the more peripheral layers, and that cellular cementum is more irregularly and less well mineralized than acellular cementum (Selvig, 1965). (See Chapter 3 for a discussion on the uniqueness of first-deposited cementum.) The basic relationship between the mineral crystals and collagen fibrils appears to be similar to that found in bone and dentine (Albright and Flanagan, 1962). Selvig (1965) has found that although the intrinsic collagen fibrils of cementum are wholly mineralized, Sharpey's fibres are mineralized only peripherally; he suggests that this might be explained by the origin of Sharpey's fibres as a possibly non-mineralizeable soft connective tissue. He has also noticed that the cementum surface is covered by a zone of very small mineral crystals, supporting the concept of continual cementum deposition throughout life. The dimensions of the hydroxyapatite crystals at the surface of acellular and cellular cementum do not appear to exceed $400 \times 200 \times 20$ Å.

Cementum does not appear to be innervated, nor to have a blood supply or lymphatic drainage. Nerves or vessels seen in cementum probably are incorporated from the adjacent periodontal ligament by rapidly proliferating cellular cementum. The cementum appears to be nourished by diffusion, probably from the adjacent periodontal ligament.

(b) *Chemical composition*. There is comparatively little information on the chemical composition of cementum, but that which is available points to a close similarity with bone. Cementum thus consists of a primarily collagenous matrix mineralized with small hydroxyapatite crystals to a slightly lower degree than dentine. Selvig and Selvig (1962) found a combined calcium plus magnesium value ranging from 25·7 to 26·6% in the cementum of healthy human teeth compared with 26·8 to 27·6% for the dentine. Corresponding values for phosphorus were 11·8 to 12·5 and 12·2 to 13·2% respectively. Glimcher *et al.* (1964) found 72% of ash in bovine coronal cementum compared with 77% in bovine dentine, both values being expressed in terms of

Amino acid composition of collagens from periodontal and other tissues

	Bovine coronal incisor cementum (Glimcher et al. (1964))	Bovine cemental gelatin (1964)	Bovine bone collagen cortical Eastoe (1955)a	Bovine bone collagen Piez and Likins (1960) cortical	Bovine bone collagen cancellous	Human bone collagen Eastoe (1955)a	Human renal reticulin Windrum et al. (1955)a
Alanine	113	115	109·7	109	101	113·5	96·5
Glycine	291	307	314	337	333	319	309
Valine	26	21	21·2	20	22	23·6	26·8
Leucine	31	27	27·9	25	26	25·5	35·8
Isoleucine	14	12	12·3	11	11	13·3	18·0
Proline	122	124	118·8	123	118	123·4	97·2
Phenylalanine	16	14	16·3	13	14	13·9	18·1
Tyrosine	5	3	2·9	4·3	4·0	4·5	3·0
Serine	38	39	37·8	34	36	35·9	42·8
Threonine	21	19	19·7	16	18	18·4	21·9
Cystine (half)	4	<0·5					
Methionine	3	3	5·1	5·0	5·3	5·3	8·6
Arginine	49	51	49·0	50	49	47·1	45·3
Histidine	—	—	5·8	4·1	4·0	5·8	5·3
Lysine	28	25	26·2	26	28	28·0	21·6
Aspartic acid	53	50	49·8	45	46	47·0	52·9
Glutamic acid	81	80	75·8	74	78	72·2	76·7
3-hydroxyproline	0·5	1					
4-hydroxyproline	91	105	100·8b	98b	102b	100·2b	107·7b
Hydroxylysine	9	11	6·4	5·7	5·0	3·5	12·2
Amide			(41·8)	(38)	(39)	(37·3)	(43·0)

(Values are expressed as numbers of amino acid residues per 1000 total residues).
a Recalculated (Eastoe and Leach, 1958).
b Total hydroxyproline.

dry weight of tissue. The weight ratio of Ca:P was 2·08 for both tissues. The powder X-ray diffraction pattern showed the principal inorganic constituent of this cementum to be an apatite. The pattern exhibited a broadening of the bands and loss of resolution of fine details of the spectrum, indicative of the small size and relatively poor crystallinity of the apatite crystals. In these respects the cementum pattern is closely similar to those of dentine and bone, but markedly different from that of enamel.

Following decalcification the organic portion of the tissue shows the characteristic wide angle reflections of collagen. Several orders of the low-angle X-ray diffraction spectrum are also shown; these correspond to the 640 Å axial period revealed as banding in the fibrils by electron microscopy. The amino acid composition of an acid hydrolysate of whole decalcified coronal cementum (Table 1) is characteristic of collagen, indicating that the organic matrix contains at least 90% of this protein. Like the collagens from bone and dentine, it is essentially insoluble in neutral buffers and acetic acid. It gives rise to a gelatin of characteristic composition, similar to the collagen but with slightly larger amounts of the most dominant amino acid constituents (Table 1). Glimcher et al. undertook this work to characterize cementum in a somewhat unexpected site. However, the data probably represents the composition of cementum generally, as the bovine coronal cementum is continuous with, and histologically similar to, the more typically situated cementum overlying the dentine of the root.

2. Periodontal Ligament

The periodontal ligament performs a number of functions. Its most apparent role is to provide continuity between the hard tissues of the teeth and the alveolar process, and hence, resilient support for the tooth during function. It would seem that the capacity of the periodontal ligament to fill this role depends largely on the integrity of its collagen fibres, ground substance and blood supply (Chapter 8). The periodontal ligament transmits blood vessels and lymphatics (Chapter 3). It probably also provides the substances which diffuse through and nourish the cementum, and removes the catabolites of the cementocytes. Nerves in the periodontal ligament appear to have a proprioceptive role in the control of masticatory movement, and a protective function through transmitting pain impulses (Chapter 7). Finally, the cells of the periodontal ligament are responsible for maintaining and remodelling the soft and hard connective tissues in the functioning periodontium (Section IV).

The periodontal ligament comprises soft connective tissue, but also contains a network of epithelial cells, the rests of Malassez (Chapter 3). In histological section, orientated bundles of collagen fibres, the principal fibres, appear to be the predominant constituent. Between these are collections of loose, less fibrous, connective tissue with which blood vessels are associated (Fig. 34). The principal fibres of the periodontal ligament which sometimes appear to extend between cementum and alveolar bone are embedded at both ends in hard tissue. The embedded parts of the fibres are termed Sharpey's

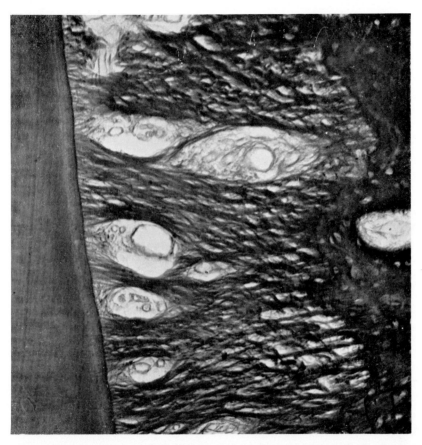

FIG. 34. Horizontal section of monkey periodontal ligament. Some wavy fibre bundles appear to extend from cementum to bone, and fibres run from bundle to bundle. The fibre bundles on the cementum side of the ligament tend to be gathered together in small tufts. The blood vessels are surrounded by loose connective tissue. Van Gieson's picro-fuchsin. (×215.)

fibres. The bundles of fibres are arranged in groups having varying orientation. Cervically, the alveolar crest fibres run from the crest of the alveolar process coronally towards the cementum. Slightly nearer the root apex, an adjacent group run horizontally; while apically to this, most of the bundles are seen to run obliquely from the alveolar bone in an apical direction. Around the apex, and around the crests of the inter-radicular bony septa of multi-rooted teeth, the bundles of fibres have a fan-like arrangement. The course of the collagen fibres from cementum to bone is not straight but tends to be wavy (Figs 34 and 35). This allows some movement of the tooth in the bony socket (Chapter 8). The fibroblasts and fibrocytes tend to be orientated parallel to the fibre bundles.

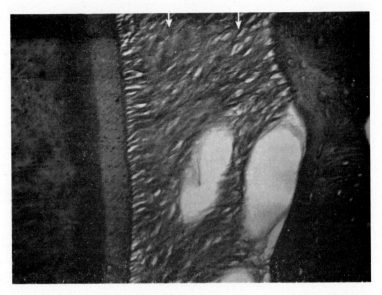

Fig. 35. Longitudinal section of monkey periodontal ligament. The tufts of fibre bundles on the cementum side are not illustrated in this plane of section, but the "intermediate plexus" is evident (↓ – ↓) Van Gieson's picro-fuchsin. (×215.)

It is impossible to assess the length of any individual collagen fibril, and the question of whether single collagen fibres span the interval between the cementum and bone has not been resolved. It has been suggested that, in the periodontal ligament of teeth of limited eruption, short bundles of collagen fibres embedded in cementum are joined to other fibres embedded in bone by an intermediate plexus of fibrous connective tissue (Sicher, 1959) (Fig. 35) (see also Chapter 3). However, the existence of this intermediate plexus has been disputed (Trott, 1962), and it is probable that its appearance is an artefact arising from the plane in which the principal fibres are sectioned (Zwarych and Quigley, 1965; Ciancio et al., 1967). Zwarych and Quigley claim to have traced some fibres from cementum to bone in sections cut parallel to the fibres. They suggest that other fibres pass from bundle to bundle, so effecting a transition from the grouping of the fibres in many small bundles on the tooth side of the ligament to their distribution in few, large bundles, on the bone side (Fig. 34). Although the appearance of a specific arrangement of fibres in an intermediate plexus is evidently artefact, there is some evidence to suggest that alterations in the principal fibres of the periodontal ligament to accommodate changes in tooth position can occur in this area of the ligament. This problem will be discussed in Section **IV**.

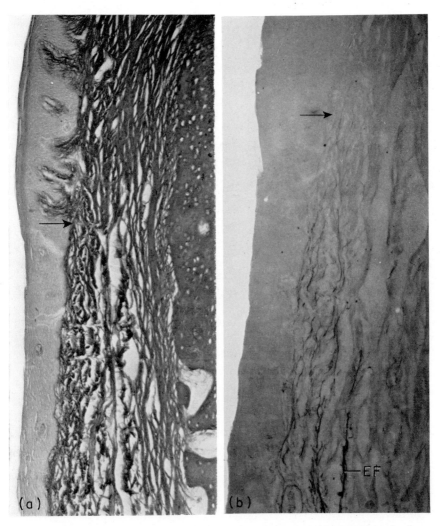

FIG. 36. Junction of attached gingiva and alveolar mucosa (→) (a) Van Gieson's picro-fuchsin. (b) Orcein. ef-elastic fibres. (a). ×75: (b). (×90.)

Elastic fibres in the human periodontal ligament are generally restricted to the walls of the blood vessels. This is not true of the periodontal ligaments of all mammals, some of which may contain elastic fibres (Fullmer, 1960). By contrast, oxytalan fibres are relatively abundant in the human periodontal ligament. They tend not to cross the periodontal space directly. Instead, they run a rather more vertical course, with only one end embedded in either cementum or bone, or form a complex network at the apex of the tooth (Fullmer, 1967). Their function is obscure.

3. The Lamina Propria of the Gingiva

(a) *Microscopic appearance.* The functions of the lamina propria of the gingiva are twofold: firstly, to provide additional support for the teeth and, secondly, to protect the underlying alveolar bone. As in the periodontal ligament, collagen fibres are the predominant constituent, and elastic fibres are rarely seen except in the walls of the blood vessels. The collagen fibres occur as a densely woven mat and the cells tend to be orientated parallel to the fibre bundles. The junction of the attached gingiva and the alveolar mucosa is marked by a transition from the dense connective tissue of the former to the loose connective tissue, and rich content of elastic fibres, of the latter (Figs 36 and 41) (see also Chapter 5). The lamina propria also contains a network of reticulin. The component of the network which lies beneath the epithelium, the subepithelial reticulin, can be seen easily in the light microscope (Fig. 37). This is in contrast to the components lying more deeply which can be identified only with difficulty (Melcher, 1964; 1965a).

The distribution of blood vessels, nerves and lymphatics have been described in Chapter 3.

Several discrete groups of fibres have been described in the vicinity of the necks of the teeth (Goldman, 1951; Arnum and Hagerman, 1953; Melcher, 1962). The lamina propria does not consist of a few bundles of clearly orientated fibres amidst a welter of randomly arranged bundles; there appear to be two systems of fibres, the members of which interweave within each system and between the systems. Functionally, these are an extension of the fibre system of the periodontal ligament. The more predominant system has a horizontal component; the other is orientated predominantly in a vertical direction (Fig. 38). It seems likely that the orientation of each fibre bundle is determined by the forces which act upon it, but as yet there is no direct experimental evidence to support this belief. It is of interest to note that when *in vitro* cultures of chick bone are subjected to tension, highly organized fibrous tissue, with cells and fibres orientated parallel to the lines of tension, is formed instead of bone (Bassett, 1962).

The fibres having a horizontal component (Fig. 38) are most conveniently described in layers, starting with the most superficial. However, it must be stressed that there is extensive intermingling between the various groups. Beneath the epithelium of the interdental gingival septum, fibres run in a vestibulo-oral direction. The most superficial bundles bend crownwards in the vestibular and oral papillae, appearing to terminate beneath the epithelium

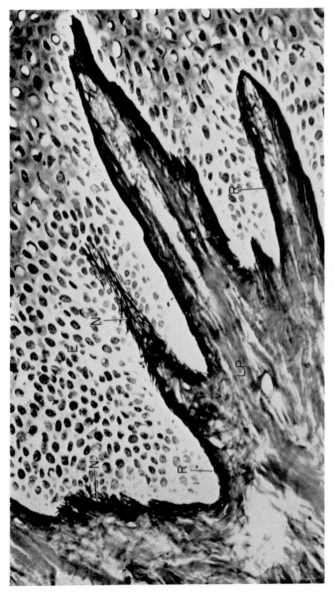

FIG. 37. Subepithelial reticulin of gingiva. When cut at right angles to the epithelium-connective tissue junction, the reticulin appears as a line (R); when cut obliquely, the constituents of the network (N) are revealed. E—epithelium LP—lamina propria. Gordon and Sweets silver impregnation. (×220.)

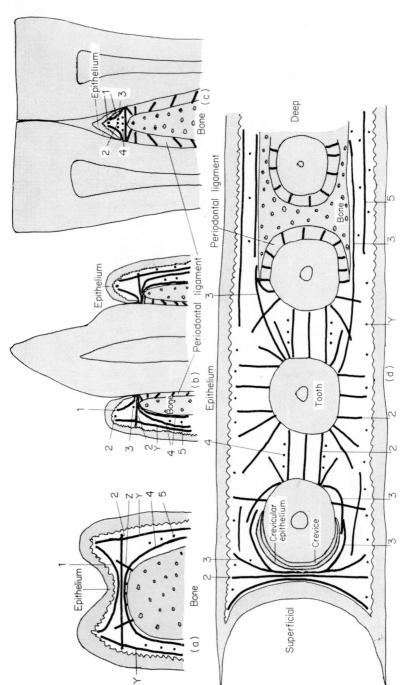

FIG. 38. Diagrammatic representation of the two fibre systems in the lamina propria of the gingiva. (a) vestibulo-oral section of an interdental gingival septum; (b) vestibulo-oral section through a tooth; (c) mesio-distal section through an interdental gingival septum; (d) horizontal section running obliquely through a length of gingival corium. The gingival corium is unshaded and the orientation of fibre bundles is indicated by thick black lines. Bundles *with a horizontal component*: 1, curving crown-wards; 2, running straight; 3, curving mesially or distally; 4, curving apically; 5, running horizontally in the attached gingiva. Bundles *without a horizontal component*: Y, running vertically in the lamina propria; Z, attached to bone and running vertically in the attached gingiva.

(Fig. 39). Although many of the bundles of fibres of the gingival connective tissue appear to end in the lamina propria beneath the epithelium, the

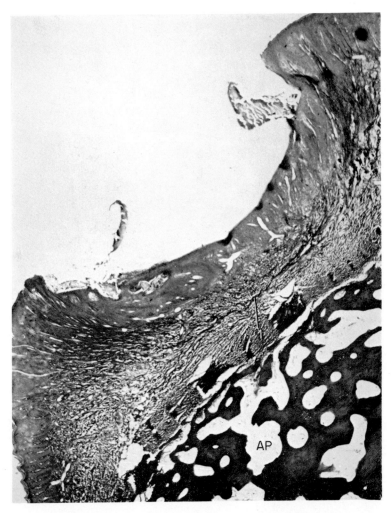

FIG. 39. A vestibulo-oral section of an interdental gingival septum, showing a band of fibres running horizontally and turning crownwards to ramify in the vestibular and oral papillae (1). AP, alveolar process. Van Gieson's picro-fuchsin. (× 15.)

precise site of their termination has not been determined. Electronmicroscopy has shown clearly that they do not end in the epithelium itself, as is sometimes stated. Slightly deep to these, bundles of fibres run in the same direction but do not bend crownwards. Some of these are straight, appearing to terminate beneath the vestibular and oral epithelium. Others bend mesially or distally to course through, and anastomose with other bundles, in the thin wedge of lamina propria in the vestibular and oral marginal gingiva (Fig. 40). These fibre bundles tend to run circumferentially around the teeth, and some may eventually terminate in alveolar bone or cementum.

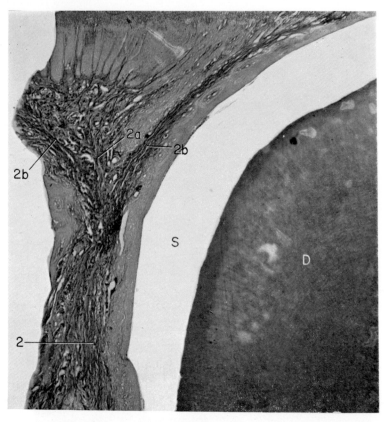

Fig. 40. Horizontal section through the vestibular part of an interdental gingival septum illustrating horizontally-disposed fibre bundles (2). Some of these run straight (2a), while others bend mesially or distally (2b). S, area formerly occupied by enamel and gingival crevice; D, dentine. Van Gieson's picro-fuchsin. (×35.)

The next stratum of fibres lies parallel to those in the interdental gingival septum. They arise from the whole circumference of the cementum immediately apical to the last of the cells of the attached epithelial cuff, passing out at right angles to the surface of the cementum. They run horizontally for a short distance, and then bend crownwards to pass parallel to the crevicular epithelium. These fibres also appear to terminate beneath the gingival epithelium. There is, immediately deep to these, a layer of fibres which does not bend crownwards. These may be divided geographically into three groups. The first pass horizontally to terminate vestibularly and orally beneath the epithelium. The second run mesially and distally (the transeptal fibres) to terminate in the cementum of the adjacent teeth. The third group of fibres, which arises from the cementum between the first two groups, passes

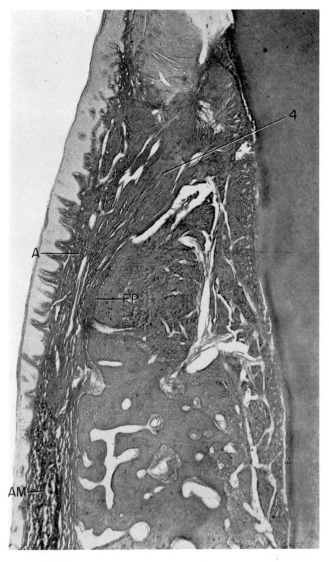

FIG. 41. Oblique section showing fibre bundles passing from the cementum, over the crest of the alveolar process, and into the attached gingiva (4). The bundles interweave with bundles of the fibrous layer of the periosteum (FP) and contribute to the body of the attached gingiva (A). AM-alveolar mucosa. Van Gieson's picro-fuchsin. (×15.)

circumferentially to anastomose with the circumferentially running bundles described above, or to ramify with bundles embedded in nearby bone, or to ramify with bundles running on the vestibular or oral surfaces of the alveolar process, possibly to be embedded at a distance.

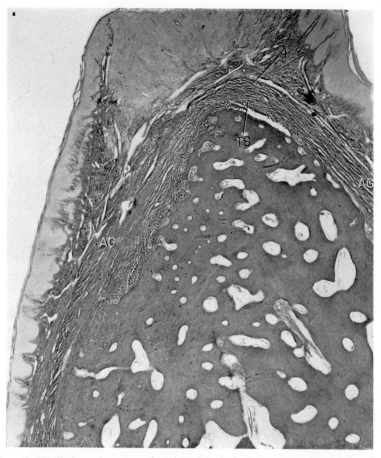

FIG. 42. Vestibulo-oral section of an interdental gingival septum showing bundles of fibres passing over the crest of the alveolar process (4) and into the attached gingiva (AG). TS, transseptal fibres cut in cross section. Van Gieson's picro-fuchsin. (× 5.)

The next layer of the horizontally arising system also runs vestibulo-orally, and is present in the vestibular and oral marginal gingiva and in the interdental gingival septum (Figs 41 and 42). These bundles, in the presence of teeth, take origin from cementum and then pass over the crest of the vestibular and oral alveolar processes. However, interdentally, they appear to lie superficial to the transseptal fibres. They then bend apically to ramify over the vestibular and oral surfaces of the alveolar process, it frequently being possible to trace the continuity of successive bundles into the alveolar mucosa. The bundles run in intimate relationship with the fibrous layer of the periosteum, or contribute to the body of the lamina propria of the attached gingiva. Associated with these, there is the last group of horizontal fibres which run parallel to the surface of the attached gingiva (Fig. 43). Numerous fibre bundles pass obliquely from one group to the other, helping to bind the

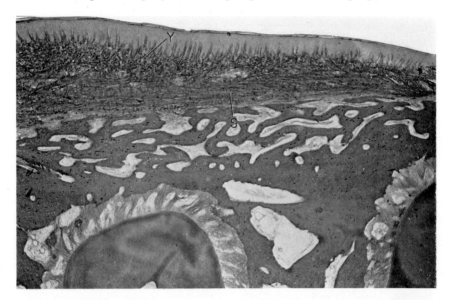

FIG. 43. Horizontal section showing fibres of the attached gingiva disposed horizontally (S), and those disposed vertically (Y) cut in cross-section. Van Gieson's picro-fuchsin. (×16.)

attached gingiva to the alveolar process, but there appear to be surprisingly few bundles which run perpendicularly to the vestibular or oral surfaces of the alveolar bone.

The other system of fibres, composed of those that run in the main vertically (Fig. 38), is very much smaller and intermingles with the first system. One group of fibres in this system originates from the interdental, vestibular and oral crests of the alveolar process, and passes coronally into the lamina propria. The other arises in the alveolar mucosa or attached gingiva, and passes coronally, the bundles frequently being traceable to the subepithelial connective tissue of the marginal gingiva, or vestibular or oral papilla.

The distribution of these fibre systems is such that the stresses of all tooth movement must be assumed to be conveyed to the marginal and attached gingiva, and to the outer cortical plate of the alveolar process. The continuity also extends to the connective tissue of the alveolar mucosa; so, similarly, activity of the muscles associated with the alveolar mucosa must be transmitted to the lamina propria of the marginal and attached gingiva, and possibly to the teeth.

Plasma cells, lymphocytes and macrophages have frequently been reported as invariably present in the connective tissue beneath the base of the crevicular epithelium. It has often been suggested that their presence should be regarded as anatomically normal. However, the associated connective tissue nearly always exhibits signs of destruction. Their presence therefore probably indicates an inflammatory reaction resulting from damage to gingiva which clinically appears healthy (Cattoni, 1951; Bernier, 1952). Several investigators have reported the presence of large numbers of mast cells in human gingiva (Hall, 1966) but, as has been discussed above, their function is unknown.

(b) Chemical composition of the soft connective tissues of the periodontium. Very few chemical investigations of the soft connective tissues in the periodontium have been undertaken. This is due to the difficulty of obtaining sufficient material and of separating by dissection, a suitably well characterized and uniform sample for chemical analysis. Connective tissue in gingiva has been examined more often than that from the region of the periodontal ligament. Most of the material examined has come from tissues resected during gingivectomy for the treatment of periodontal disease. Unfortunately, in many of these investigations, the adjacent gingival epithelium has not been separated from the connective tissue, so that the composition of the latter has to be largely inferred from observations on the combination of tissues. However, some clue to the probable distribution of chemical components in connective tissue and epithelium can be obtained from investigations of completely separated tissues from other regions of the body.

As in all connective tissues, collagen is the major constituent. Schultz-Haudt and Aas (1960) found an average value of 31·0% collagen in normal gingiva, calculated from the hydroxyproline content of tissue hydrolysates. Gingiva from humans with various kinds of periodontal disease had rather lower contents of collagen (Table 2). From and Schultz-Haudt (1963) subsequently determined by the same method the collagen content of gingiva from a range of positions in the mouth of a patient with chronic periodontitis. The results were corrected for the presence of epithelium by calculating in histological sections the percentage of the total area of the gingiva which actually consisted of connective tissue. There was a considerable local variation in the corrected value for the collagen content of the connective tissue which ranged from 36 to 61 %, the average being 48·8 % with a standard deviation of ±8·9. From the (uncorrected) earlier values (Table 2) the corrected value for the collagen content of healthy gingival connective tissue would be expected to be somewhat higher, perhaps around 60%. A comparison was made between the corrected values and visual observations of the amount of collagen present in stained histological sections (the individual specimens being classified into five groups). Correlation was not good, only 26 of the possible 80 combinations showing agreement between the two methods. Lack of correlation was possibly due to the less fibrous states of collagen, including degraded collagen, not being demonstrated by staining procedures.

TABLE 2

Collagen content of human gingiva (Schultz-Haudt and Aas (1960))

	A Acid citrate extractable collagen	I Insoluble collagen	Total of $A+I$	Total determined directly
Normal gingiva	1·7	30·8	32·5	31·0
Paradontitis marginalis chronica profunda	1·3	25·3	26·6	24·5
Paradontitis marginalis chronica profunda regressiva.	(1·3)	(29·3)	(30·6)	24·9
Paradontitis marginalis chronica profunda exudativa	(0·5)	(23·0)	(23·5)	22·4
Paradontitis marginalis chronica profunda mixta	1·6	24·5	26·1	27·0
Paradontitis marginalis chronica profunda superficialis	1·0	14·2	15·2	17·9
Hyperplastic gingivae (sodium diphenylhydantoin)	(1·3)	(30·1)	(31·4)	29·9

Values are expressed as % of dry weight of whole gingiva, including epithelium.
Values in brackets are single values, not averages.

The proportion of total collagen in gingiva which is soluble in acid citrate buffer and less vigorous solvents (Tables 2 and 3) is quite small, and in this respect gingival connective tissue resembles most other collagenous tissues. Salt-soluble collagen is generally considered to represent newly synthesized collagen which has not yet become insoluble through the 'maturation' process, which probably involves cross-linking (Section **IIIA**). It could conceivably also represent matured collagen which has subsequently been broken down again, though this idea is not supported by any increase in the values for acid citrate soluble collagen (Table 2) in periodontal disease when compared with normal gingiva. Recently, there has been some evidence to suggest that there is a particularly high rate of collagen synthesis in part of the connective tissue of the periodontal ligament (Section **IVD**), and it is therefore interesting that Michi *et al.* (1963) found an increased proportion of neutral salt soluble collagen in periodontal ligament, compared with that found in gingiva, subcutaneous tissue and Achilles tendon. The fraction of collagen extracted from periodontal ligament by 5% trichloracetic acid was associated with a higher proportion of polysaccharide material than that from the other three tissues. Possibly differences in the rate of turnover of collagen from the region of the periodontal ligament may have an important bearing on the homeostasis of the periodontium (Section IV), but unfortunately no reliable quantitative data are available.

TABLE 3

Soluble and total collagen content of human gingiva (Schultz-Haudt and Aas (1960))

		Collagen content					
Age of patient	Sex	Water soluble	Neutral-salt soluble	Acid citrate soluble	Total soluble	Insoluble	Total
47	F	—	0·04	0·23	0·27	2·57	2·84
38	M	0·04	0·05	0·20	0·29	2·90	3·19
29	F	0·04	0·06	0·14	0·24	7·00	7·24
37	M	0·02	0·07	0·12	0·21	4·30	4·51
35	M	0·05	0·05	0·10	0·20	2·86	3·06

Values are expressed as % of wet weight of whole gingiva; including epithelium.

Mucopolysaccharides and glycoproteins have also been shown to occur in human gingiva, probably in the connective tissue. Schultz-Haudt (1958) extracted diseased human gingiva using 0·5N sodium hydroxide solution, after removing fat by means of acetone, and obtained 1·1–1·5% of the dry weight as a crude polysaccharide. Various polysaccharide preparations contained 1·6–2·2% of total nitrogen, 11·6–12·7% of hexuronic acid, 10·6–12·3% of hexosamine and a glucosamine to galactosamine ratio of 1·5–1·9. These values suggest that human gingiva contains a higher proportion of acid mucopolysaccharides than skin and that, whereas chondroitin sulphate predominates in skin, hyaluronic acid is more abundant in gingiva. The average content of total acid mucopolysaccharides in the crude gingival polysaccharide was calculated as 27·3%.

Two polysaccharide-protein complexes with different electrophoretic mobilities were extracted from human gingiva by Schultz-Haudt et al. (1961). In addition to glucuronic acid and glucosamine, these contained the neutral sugars galactose, glucose, mannose and possibly ribose and fucose. One of the complexes contained hydroxyproline, suggesting that soluble collagen might be associated with it. Both complexes gave a positive periodic acid-Schiff reaction under conditions where chondroitin sulphate and hyaluronic acid do not. This reaction is also given by bone sialoprotein (Herring, 1964c) and the finding of sialic acid, amounting to approximately 1·41–1·67% of the total mucopolysaccharide fraction, in gingival tissue by Thonard and Blustein (1965) supports the idea of a sialoprotein constituent of gingiva.

The histochemical staining properties of polysaccharides that had been chemically isolated from human gingiva were studied by Schultz-Haudt et al. (1964) as a guide to the interpretation of histochemical staining reactions when used for the localization of components in tissue sections. The results, summarized by Schultz-Haudt (1965), showed that when gingival tissues were homogenized in a hammer-mill and extracted with either (i) 5% aqueous trichloracetic acid, (ii) 0·14 M sodium chloride, (iii) trypsin, or (iv) papain solutions, the extracts contained three substances which were separable by electrophoresis: (a) The slowest band, which was stained only by the periodic acid-Schiff reagent and conventional protein stains, was considered to be a glycoprotein. After acid hydrolysis of this glycoprotein, the sugars galactose, mannose and fucose could be identified by paper chromatography. The slow band separated from the trichloracetic acid extract contained hydroxyproline, and was disintegrated by bacterial protease and collagenase, whereas hyaluronidase did not affect it. (b) A faster band which stained with colloidal iron, toluidine blue (but not metachromatically), and faintly with alcian blue was identified as hyaluronic acid. (c) The fastest band of the three (absent in trichloracetic acid extracts), which also stained with colloidal iron, toluidine blue (with marked metachromasia) and strongly with alcian blue, was identified as chondroitin sulphate. Both the hyaluronic acid and chondroitin sulphate were associated with non-collagenous protein. Neither of these fractions stained with the periodic acid-Schiff reagent and, apart from hyaluronidase, they were little affected by enzymes. Hyaluronidase is known to attack hyaluronic acid, chondroitin sulphates A and C but not chondroitin sulphate B.

There is little information available about the lipid component of the extracellular constituents of the lamina propria and periodontal ligament. Material, believed to be bound lipid, has been demonstrated histologically in both of these tissues (Melcher, 1966c; 1967d).

In summary, though insufficient data is available to attempt to account for the entire weight of periodontal connective tissue in the form of an analytical "balance sheet", collagen is undoubtedly the predominating constituent. In addition there appear to be significant amounts of mucopolysaccharides, including hyaluronic acid and chondroitin sulphate, and probably glyco- and sialoproteins. The proportion of these minor components may be higher than in other comparable soft connective tissues such as skin and tendon, but the fact that many investigations have been carried out on

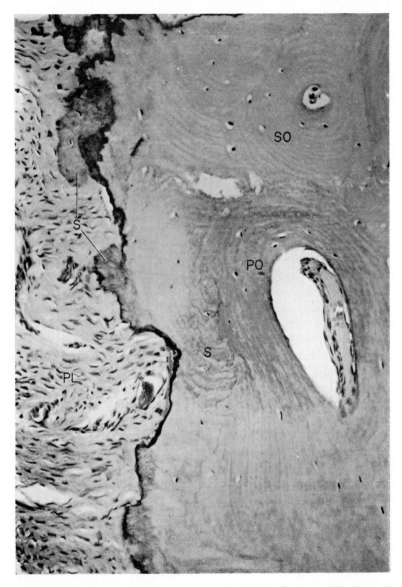

FIG. 44. Alveolar process and periodontal ligament (PL) of young adult. Woven bone (S) is present in the alveolar bone, as well as an obliquely cut primary osteone (PO) and a secondary osteone (SO). Haematoxylin and eosin. (×130.)

pathological rather than normal gingival tissue, often without removal of epithelium, sets a limit to the accuracy of these general conclusions.

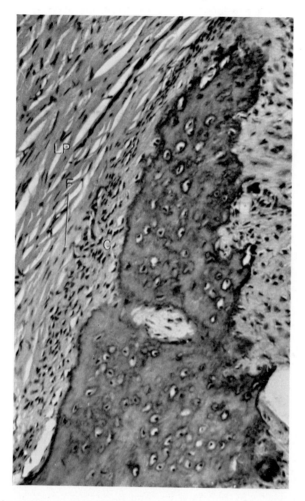

Fig. 45. Woven bone in developing alveolar crest of a young monkey. The cambium layer of the periosteum (C) is very cellular, and the fibrous layer (F) is continuous with the collagen fibres of the overlying lamina propria (LP). Haematoxylin and eosin. (×130.)

4. The Alveolar Process

(a) *Microscopic appearance.* The function of the alveolar process is supportive. In general, its bone is organized similarly to that elsewhere in the skeleton. The compact bone and cancellous trabeculae comprise woven bone and lamellar bone arranged in primary and secondary osteones, interstitial lamellae and circumferential lamellae (Figs 44, 45 and 46).

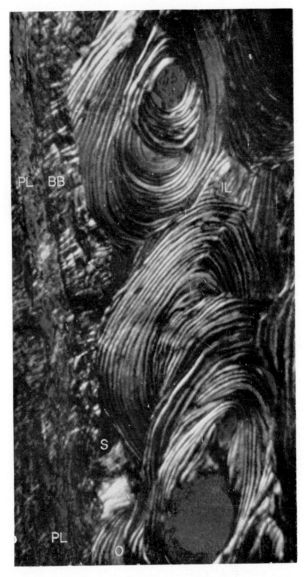

FIG. 46. Periodontium of a young adult photographed in polarized light. The fibres of the periodontal ligament (PL) are embedded in "bundle bone" (BB), in osteones (O) the lamellae of which are well illustrated, as well as in woven bone (S). IL, interstitial lamellae. (×300.)

Of particular interest is the organization of the alveolar bone, which Manson (1963) has pointed out may, in places, consist of only one trabeculum. The principle fibres of the periodontal ligament are embedded in this bone and, comparable with the situation in cementum, most of these fibres have unmineralized cores (Frank *et al.*, 1958; Selvig, 1965). These authors have also confirmed Weinmann and Sicher's (1955) finding that many of the

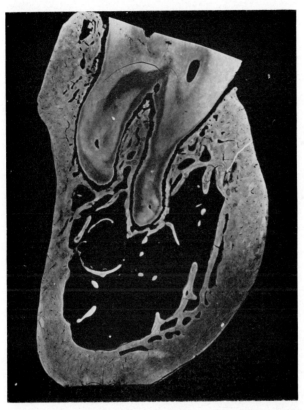

FIG. 47. Microradiograph of transverse section of mandible from a 42 year-old man. The molar tooth was functional and healthy. There is no evidence of highly mineralized "bundle bone". (Reproduced with permission from J. D. Manson, *Oral Surg. Oral Med. Oral Path.* **16**, 432–438, 1963.)

intrinsic fibres of this bone run parallel to its surface, at right angles to the Sharpey's fibres; that is, in lamellae. However, they have found in addition that there are large areas in which the intrinsic fibres are randomly arranged, and it seems possible that these are remains of primary spongiosa.

Weinmann and Sicher (1955) have called bone having this peculiar arrangement of intrinsic and Sharpey's fibres, *bundle bone*, and maintain that it contains a higher than usual amount of bone salts per unit volume. However,

9

microradiography has supported neither this claim nor the belief that the layer of bone lining the tooth socket, termed by radiologists the *lamina dura*, is more densely mineralized than the rest of the bone (Figs 47 and 48) (Manson, 1963; Ishikawa *et al.*, 1964). Furthermore, Manson has pointed out that the alveolar bone may be made of either circumferential lamellae or

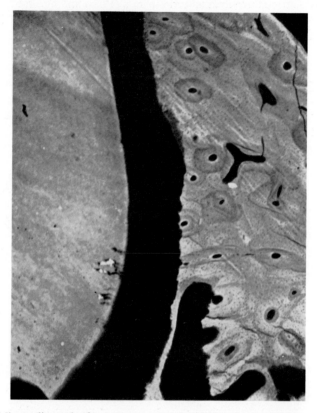

FIG. 48. Microradiograph of a transverse section of mandible containing a molar tooth from a 35-year-old woman. There is no evidence of highly mineralized "bundle bone" and osteones form part of the socket wall. (Reproduced with permission from J. D. Manson. *Oral Surg. Oral Med. Oral Path.* **16**, 432–438, 1963.)

osteones (Figs 46 and 48), and we have found that woven bone also occurs in this situation (Figs 45 and 46). It is well known that the architecture of bone is affected by stress. This has been most elegantly shown by the *in vitro* experiments of Glücksmann (1938; 1941–42), and is illustrated by Fig. 28, Chapter 8.

The external surfaces of the alveolar process are covered by mucoperiosteum; that is by periosteum, the fibrous layer of which is intimately associated with the collagen fibres of the lamina propria (Figs 45 and 49). The

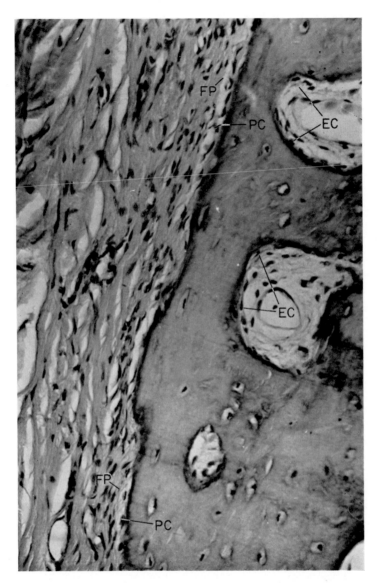

FIG. 49. Vestibular aspect of the alveolar process. Cells of the cambium layer of the periosteum (PC) and of the endosteum (EC) are illustrated. The fibrous layer of the periosteum (FP) is continuous with the collagen fibres of the lamina propria. Haematoxylin and eosin. (× 220.)

periodontal surface of the alveolar bone is covered by cells which appear to be a part of the periodontal ligament (Fig. 32), and not by any specialized structure. The internal surfaces of the bone of the alveolar process, as elsewhere, are covered by endosteal cells (Fig. 49) and the marrow cavities of mandible and maxilla contain yellow rather than red marrow (Cahn, 1940) (Fig. 31). While numerous blood vessels can be seen entering and leaving the alveolar process, no report of work such has been carried out on long bones (Trueta, 1963) describing the origin of the blood supply to its various parts, has been found.

(b) Chemical and histochemical composition of bone. Little chemical work has been undertaken on the composition of alveolar bone. Consequently, it is necessary to consider here the composition of mammalian bone tissue generally. This will provide a plausible basis for the more detailed studies concerning local variations of composition which might, in the future, be undertaken profitably. Fortunately, in the last decade, renewed interest has been taken in the chemistry of bone, and a number of reviews of the subject have appeared (Eastoe, 1956, 1961a; Glimcher, 1959; Herring, 1964a; Johns, 1967).

TABLE 4

Composition of air-dried compact bone tissue (bovine femur diaphysis)
(Eastoe and Eastoe, 1954; Leach, 1958)

	% by Weight
Inorganic matter, insoluble in hot water (probably including up to 1 % of citrate)	69·66
Inorganic matter, soluble in water	1·25
Collagen	18·64
Mucopolysaccharide-protein complex	0·24
Resistant protein material	1·02
Total lipid	0·07
Sugars other than mucopolysaccharide, etc.	0·00
Water (lost below 105°C)	8·18
Total	99·06

Most analytical investigations have been carried out on compact rather than cancellous bone because it is more easily freed from soft extraneous tissues, marrow and periosteum. The diaphysis of the bovine femur readily provides large amounts of relatively uncontaminated bone powder. Eastoe and Eastoe (1954) attempted to account for as much as possible of the entire weight of air-dried bovine bone by identifying constituents (Table 4). Their value for lipid has been corrected from the later work of Leach (1958) on the same tissue preparation. Almost the whole weight of the bone is accounted for in this analysis, although some of the items listed must be regarded as categories rather than simple chemical entities. However, it is clear that the inorganic components account for the greater part of the weight of the tissue (approx. 70%), while collagen makes up over 90% of the organic constituents and nearly 20% of the whole tissue.

Since the density of the inorganic material is approximately 3·18 (see Deakins, 1942) while that of collagen is only 1·62, the proportions of the total volume of bone tissue occupied by these two constituents will be more nearly equal—inorganic 50%, collagen 28% and water approximately 20% of the volume of air-dried bovine bone. The degree of mineralization of bone, which is a measure of its inorganic content, varies substantially with species, the particular bone, the site within the bone, and the age of the bone tissue actually being analysed. The average inorganic content of oven-dried human, ox and rabbit femur shaft bone, is 73·5, 80·0 and 84·2% by weight respectively (Eastoe, 1956, based on data of Rogers *et al.*, 1952). Compact bone from rabbit scapula, tibia and femur contains 78·6, 81·5, and 84·2% of inorganic matter respectively, while cancellous bone from the tibia and femur is rather less mineralized with 76·3 and 75·0% respectively. Soon after its deposition by osteoblasts, a given portion of bone tissue becomes rapidly mineralized, attaining within a short period some 90% of its maximum possible inorganic content. The final 10% of mineralization occurs more and more slowly; possibly because the tissue becomes less permeable, so decreasing the rate of diffusion of calcium and phosphate ions to the sites of deposition. Thus, the degree of mineralization of any piece of bone tissue will increase with the age of that *tissue*. Within a single bone, the net effect of this process will, of course, affect the average degree of mineralization. However, the continuous acquisition of inorganic matter will be interrupted by the processes of resorption and redeposition in response to cellular activity. All newly deposited bone tissue is young as regards its degree of mineralization, and will consequently tend to reduce the average mineral content of the organ of which it forms a part. Any given bone will thus contain zones of bone tissue having various ages, with different degrees of mineralization, nearly all above 90% of the final maximum limiting value. Usually, a slow upward trend in the inorganic content of a bone can be observed with the age of the individual; e.g. in the human femur from 72·6% at 7 years to 74·2% at 65. Changes in the degree of mineralization within bone tissue should be distinguished carefully from osteoporosis, a process involving resorption whereby an old bone comes to possess a smaller percentage by volume of bone tissue (i.e. larger marrow spaces) than it had when young. Both processes occur simultaneously as the individual ages, but they have opposite effects on the weight of inorganic matter in a bone.

There is a scarcity of chemical data regarding the degree of mineralization of bone in various parts of the alveolar process. The factors outlined in the previous paragraph should however, enable some estimate of relative mineralization to be made from the histology of the tissue. Thus surfaces where the processes of resorption and deposition are occurring actively will tend to contain new bone of somewhat low inorganic content, whereas areas where there is little bone-forming activity, will be more highly mineralized.

The main features of the various chemical constituents of bone are summarized briefly below:

i. Inorganic material

The inorganic constituents make up some 65 to 84% of dry, defatted bone tissue (Eastoe, 1961a). The principal ions present are calcium (25·6% of dry human bone; 35·6–36·3% of mammalian bone ash), phosphate (12·3; 15·5–16·4% as P), carbonate (0·39; 0·4–0·7%) and magnesium (0·39; 0·4–0·7%). Minor constituents include sodium, potassium and chloride, while fluoride, iron, zinc, boron and strontium are present in trace amounts. Though there are slight variations in the relative proportions of the principal ions present, the overall composition is reasonably constant and this has led to the idea of a "bone salt". Considerable attention has been paid to its crystal structure and attempts have been made to identify it with various chemical substances. Its X-ray diffraction diagram (de Jong, 1926), and to a lesser extent its chemical composition (Klement, 1929), indicate that it has a crystal lattice of the *apatite* type, analogous to the mineral fluorapatite (Mehmel 1930). It is at present widely, though not universally, agreed that the structure of the inorganic phase of bone is best represented, though only approximately, by the hydroxyapatite lattice (Neuman and Neuman, 1953; Carlström and Engström, 1956) which corresponds to the empirical formula $3Ca_3(PO_4)_2 Ca(OH)_2$. Other suggested representations for bone salt, tricalcium phosphate hydrate or α-tricalcium phosphate, $3Ca_3(PO_4)_2 . H_2(OH)_2$ (Dallemagne, 1952) and dahllite, a "carbonate apatite" (McConnell, 1965) suffer from various objections and have not been accepted widely. Hydroxyapatite is a more likely structure since this substance is an end-product of hydrolysis of most calcium phosphates and is stable above pH7·0. Nevertheless, it is only an approximate representation of the inorganic phase in bone. Termine and Posner (1967) consider that up to 40% of bone calcium phosphate is amorphous.

The extremely small size of the crystallites in bone has two consequences. Firstly, the X-ray diffraction pattern of bone mineral is diffuse compared with those of synthetic and mineral apatites and dental enamel. This prevents the resolution of fine details of the structure and reduces the accuracy of measurements of the lattice dimensions. The second consequence is that the ratio of crystal surface to volume is very high. This results in a substantial proportion of all the ions present being on the surface of the crystal with comparatively few in the interior (Neuman and Neuman, 1953). Ionic surfaces are highly reactive, and ions from such a surface can readily be exchanged for other ions of the same or another species in the surrounding milieu. In addition, foreign ions can become adsorbed to such a surface. Where a high proportion of all the ions present are on the surface, such hetero-ionic exchange or adsorption has a marked effect on the stoichiometry of the compound (i.e. the precise whole number relationship in the ratios of different elements). This is known to occur in the inorganic phase in bone where, for example, the ratio of calcium to phosphorus is lower than would be expected from the empirical chemical formula. The relatively enormous surface of bone crystallite (approximately 100 sq. m/g) means that very rapid exchange of ions can occur between bone and the circulating body fluids, having important consequences for the homeostasis of both bone and blood.

It is admittedly difficult to reconcile the high proportion of carbonate present in the inorganic phase with the apatite structure. The suggestion that there is a separate phase of calcium carbonate seems unlikely, unless this is in an amorphous form, as the amount of carbonate present would be detectable by the X-ray diffraction method if it occurred as crystalline calcite or aragonite. Attempts have been made to devise structures in which carbonate is fitted into apatite or similar lattices in place of other ions. However, the replacement of as much as the necessary 10 atomic per cent (as $CaCO_3$) of an ion having such different characteristics as carbonate would be expected to cause a marked and certainly an observable difference in the X-ray diffraction diagram. The remaining possibility, that carbonate is adsorbed on the crystallite surfaces and does not enter the crystal lattice, seems more probable and best accounts for the experimental data concerning the preferential solubility of carbonate compared to phosphate when bone is treated with acids (Carlström and Engström, 1956). It is also possible that some of the carbonate is present in the lattice and the remainder adsorbed at the crystal surface.

ii. Collagen

The composition of the collagen which is the principal organic constituent in bone, is very similar to that in other tissues (Table 1), and shows the characteristic features which distinguish collagens from other proteins (page 259). Piez and Likins (1957) have pointed out that the mineralized mesodermal tissues of the rat have substantially lower ratios of lysine to hydroxylysine, 1·9 in bone and 1·1 in dentine, than the soft tissues, skin (6·0) and tail tendon (3·9). Human and bovine bone collagens, however, do not show this peculiarity, the proportions of lysine and hydroxylysine being similar to those in the soft tissues.

Bone collagen appears to differ from collagens of the soft tissues in that soluble collagens cannot be extracted readily from it (Glimcher, 1959; Piez, 1963) although Araya et al. (1961) claimed to have obtained small quantities of soluble collagen from bone. Collagen in bone may, to some degree, resemble that in dentine (Veis and Schlueter, 1964) in being more stable than soft tissue collagens, possibly as a result of possessing an extra system of cross-linkages (Section III). Glimcher et al. (1965) have achieved solubilization of 30% of bone collagen in dilute acetic acid after a procedure involving freezing decalcified chicken bone to −70°C. The work of Mills and Bavetta (1966) suggests that the fall in soluble collagen content of newly laid down rat bone occurs simultaneously with mineralization.

iii. Water

Water, another relatively abundant constituent of bone tissue, is necessary for the diffusion of calcium and phosphate ions and the various nutrients essential for the osteocytes. Bone contains a much lower proportion of water than soft tissues. Values ranging from 5·9 to 59% have been reported (Eastoe, 1961a), but the extremes of this range probably reflect unsuitable methods of tissue preparation. The value of approximately 8% (Table 4) for ox bone is for bone which has been powdered and allowed to reach equilibrium with laboratory air. Some water would be lost from the original living bone during this equilibration, the initial water content probably being of the order of 15–20%. The overall range of values for the water content of bone *in vivo* could realistically be assumed to range from 15 to 45%. The water content of young bone (34%) diminishes as it ages (22%) and falls further after a long period (16·6%). Water is frequently determined by measuring the loss of weight following drying at 100–110°C. The small amount of firmly bound water retained at this temperature can be removed completely only by ashing at 500–550°C.

iv. Citrate

The presence of approximately 1% of citrate in bone was first demonstrated by Dickens (1940, 1941). The proportion of citrate varies with species and the particular bone (Thunberg, 1948), quoted values being man 0·89–1·87, other mammals 0·27–1·3, gull 0·6–2·67 and herring 5·25%. Citrate is also found in the mineralized dental tissues, enamel (human 0·10–0·21), dentine (human 0·8–0·9), and cementum (whale 1·08%). The proportions of citrate in the midshaft region of the human femur increases with age from 0·82% at 12 years to 1·25% at 77 years (Hartles, 1964). Citrate appears to be mainly associated with the inorganic phase of bone. It is co-precipitated with calcium phosphates under neutral or slightly alkaline conditions. All the citrate is extracted from dentine during demineralization with acid or with ethylenediaminetetra-acetate (EDTA) at pH 7·4. However, only 7–15% is removed from bone and dentine powder by boiling water.

It is uncertain whether incorporation of the citrate ion into the calcified tissues of the skeletal system is largely accidental, a necessary consequence of its properties and presence in blood, or whether it has a definite function to perform in the mechanism or control of the mineralization process. The extent of citrate accumulation in bone is certainly influenced by both vitamin D and parathyroid hormone. Vitamin D apparently stimulates osteocytes to produce citrate which, in turn, may directly mediate the increase in bone resorption known to occur following administration of vitamin D and parathyroid hormone. Interacting effects which occur in the complex problem of citrate metabolism in mineralized tissues have been discussed by Hartles (1964). Smaller amounts of lactate are present in compact bone from the human femur shaft (Leaver et al., 1963). The proportion of lactate appears to decrease with age from 0·11% at 12 years to 0·05% at 77 years.

v. Mucopolysaccharides

The limited amount of work carried out on the mucopolysaccharide fraction of bone has indicated that these substances are rather less abundant in bone than in unmineralized connective tissues. Hawk and Gies (1901) obtained by mild alkaline extraction of demineralized compact bone a complex material which they designated "osseomucoid", and which was later shown to contain both mucopolysaccharide and mucoprotein components. Hisamura (1938) separated from "osseomucoid" a substance similar in composition to chondroitin sulphate from bovine tracheal cartilage. The presence of chondroitin sulphate as the predominant mucopolysaccharide of compact bone has subsequently been confirmed by Rogers (1951) and Herring and Kent (1963). Meyer et al. (1956) identified 0·25% of chondroitin sulphate A as the sole mucopolysaccharide in ox shaft bone. From growing calf epiphysial bone, which contained about 20% of epiphysial plate, they obtained a much larger proportion (3·2%) of total mucopolysaccharides. The main constituent was again chondroitin sulphate A but chondroitin sulphate C, hyaluronic acid and a hexose-containing fraction, with properties similar to keratosulphates, were also identified in this developing region by chemical methods.

vi. Mucoproteins

A second fraction obtained from "osseomucoid" by Hisamura (1938) contained 12·6% of N, and was therefore assumed to contain a high proportion of protein. The sugar galactose was also present in addition to galactosamine, glucosamine and glucuronic acid (Masamune et al., 1951). Eastoe and Eastoe (1954) subsequently found the sugars mannose and xylose to be present, and characterized the protein moiety which accounted for 70% of "osseomucoid" by amino acid analysis (Table 5). Its composition somewhat resembled that of the mucoprotein from bovine nasal septum cartilage studied by Partridge and Davis (1958).

TABLE 5

Composition of mucoproteins from bovine compact bone and nasal septum cartilage

	Compact bone (*Eastoe and Eastoe, 1954*)	Nasal septum cartilage (*Partridge and Davis, 1958*)
Alanine	3·70	4·11
Glycine	2·65	3·46
Valine	4·50	4·54
Leucine	7·27	7·73
Isoleucine	3·65	3·50
Proline	4·24	7·86
Phenylalanine	2·86	7·42
Tyrosine	1·98	4·54
Serine	3·61	2·65
Threonine	4·13	3·27
Cystine	1·13	—
Methionine	0·84	1·22
Arginine	3·87	2·3
Histidine	2·65	1·83
Lysine	4·26	3·50
Aspartic acid	9·66	7·3
Glutamic acid	11·67	12·4
Hydroxyproline	0	0
Glucosamine	1·23	0·61
Galactosamine	7·67[a]	0·56

Values are expressed as grams of amino acid per 100 grams of material.
[a] Mainly from chondroitin sulphate, present as a contaminant.

Glegg *et al.* (1954, 1955) investigated the composition and staining properties of two types of fraction which they obtained from a variety of connective tissues, including alkaline extracts of decalcified bone. The first fraction from bone probably consisted of chondroitin sulphate and gave the metachromatic staining characteristic of acidic mucopolysaccharides. The second bone fraction which, judged from its nitrogen content, had a high proportion of protein, contained also the "neutral" sugars fucose, galactose and mannose together with glucosamine. It gave a positive periodic acid-Schiff reaction which was considered to be due to the free 1:2 glycol sites on these sugar units (Leblond *et al.*, 1957). This work is important in providing a practical histochemical basis for distinguishing the acidic muopolysaccharides from muco and glyco proteins which contain neutral sugars.

Herring and Kent (1963) isolated two mucoprotein fractions, a sialoprotein and chondroitin sulphate, from an extract of compact bovine bone made under comparatively mild conditions with EDTA solution at pH 7·9. The mucoprotein fractions contained sialic acid, galactose, glucose, mannose,

TABLE 6

Composition of bovine bone sialoprotein and orosomucoid (Herring, 1964b)

	Sialoprotein %	Orosomucoid %
Nitrogen	10·4	11·2
Hexose	10·3	13·3
Methylpentose	2·3	0·8
Glucosamine	3·9	7·2
Galactosamine	3·8	0·7
Sialic acid	17·1	11·5
Phosphate	1·8	0·2

fucose and amino sugars (Herring, 1964a), while the presence of hydroxyproline indicated contamination with soluble collagen. The sialoprotein behaved as a single component on ultracentrifugation and electrophoresis (Herring, 1964b), and differed from serum orosomucoid by staining with toluidine blue, but not light green, and in several quantitative features of its chemical composition (Table 6). Both substances contained N-acetyl neuraminic acid (sialic acid), although the larger proportion in bone sialoprotein reflects its more acidic nature. They are both stained by the periodic acid-Schiff technique. They are separable by moving boundary electrophoresis, and clearly represent distinct substances, suggesting that bone sialoprotein arises in bone itself and not from the blood. The composition of two preparations of bovine bone sialoprotein, including the amino acids present in the protein part of the molecule, is given in Table 7 (Andrews and Herring, 1965).

Carbohydrate material remaining attached to collagen which is insoluble after treatment of calf femur shaft with EDTA solution, pH 8·5, has been analysed by Dische et al. (1958). On the basis of an incomplete fractionation resulting from treatment with 80% ethanol, containing 5% potassium hydroxide followed by dialysis of the extract, they reached the conclusion that two types of heteropolysaccharide occurred in close association with collagen. One of these contained approximately equal quantities of galactose, mannose and hexosamine with a little fucose, and the other mainly galactose and glucose. The proportion of carbohydrate present in this relatively young tissue may have been higher than in more mature bone. A small amount of carbohydrate (approximately 0·4%) appears to be firmly bound as part of the collagen molecule in many vertebrate tissues (Eastoe, 1967a).

TABLE 7

Amino acid and sugar units in bovine bone sialoprotein (Andrews and Herring, 1965)

	Bovine bone sialoprotein	
	Extracted with 0·1 M—Na₂HPO₄, pH7·4	*Extracted with* EDTA, pH 7·9
Alanine	5·2	3·5
Glycine	10·1	10·7
Valine	3·9	2·6
Leucine	3·0	2·5
Isoleucine	2·9	2·2
Proline	6·7	4·3
Phenylalanine	1·9	1·0
Tyrosine	1·4	2·0
Serine	7·4	7·0
Threonine	9·2	9·7
Cysteic acid	—	1·1
Tryptophan	—	1·0
Arginine	2·1	1·0
Histidine	1·9	1·1
Lysine	2·6	2·5
Aspartic acid	17·0	15·2
Glutamic acid	19·8	20·0
Ammonia	15·3	14·5
Sialic acid	14·9	15·3
Hexose	14·6	14·4
Galactose	—	10·0
Mannose	—	3·0
Hexosamine	11·2	11·2
Glucosamine	—	5·6
Galactosamine	—	5·6
Fucose	0·6	1·0

Values are expressed as moles/23,000 g of dry sialoprotein.

vii. Resistant protein

After demineralization of both bone (Rogers *et al.*, 1952) and dentine (Stack, 1951), followed by autoclaving with excess water, which treatment gradually dissolves collagen, an insoluble residue remains. The residue from bovine compact bone (Eastoe and Eastoe, 1954) consists partly of a stringy, elastic mass and partly of an amorphous powder. The high total nitrogen content (14·6%) suggests that the residue consists mainly of protein.

viii. Lipids

Leach (1958) has demonstrated the presence of approximately 0·07% of lipids in compact bovine femur bone tissue. This consisted mainly of neutral fats and cholesterol with very small amounts of phospholipids. Large amounts of glycerides are present in the marrow spaces of bones. The lipids of hard tissues are discussed further in Section **III**.

III. Organization of Macromolecular Constituents of the Periodontium

A. FIBRES

1. Collagen

(a) *Chemical composition of collagen.* When a protein is heated at 100°–120°C. with 6N-hydrochloric acid for a period of 24–72 hours, its constituent polypeptide chains are gradually broken down by hydrolysis (Fig. 50) to the amino acids from which they were originally synthesized by the organism.

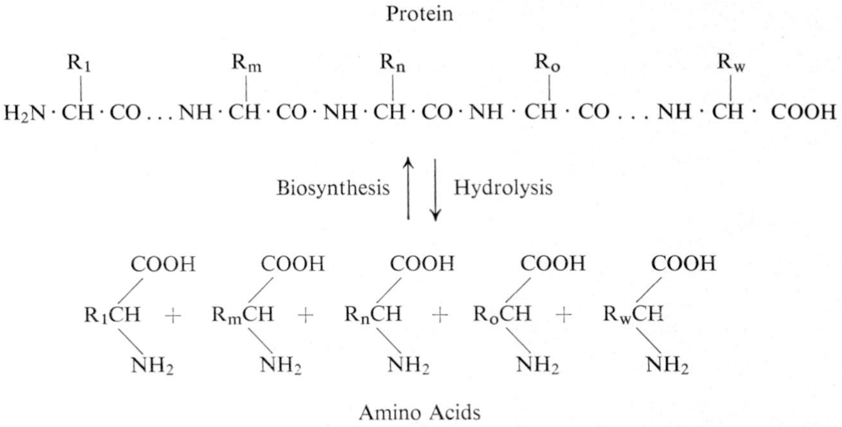

Protein

$$
\begin{array}{ccccc}
R_1 & R_m & R_n & R_o & R_w \\
| & | & | & | & | \\
\end{array}
$$

$H_2N \cdot CH \cdot CO \ldots NH \cdot CH \cdot CO \cdot NH \cdot CH \cdot CO \cdot NH \cdot CH \cdot CO \ldots NH \cdot CH \cdot COOH$

Biosynthesis ↑ ↓ Hydrolysis

$$
\begin{array}{ccccc}
COOH & COOH & COOH & COOH & COOH \\
\diagup & \diagup & \diagup & \diagup & \diagup \\
R_1CH & + \; R_mCH & + \; R_nCH & + \; R_oCH & + \; R_wCH \\
\diagdown & \diagdown & \diagdown & \diagdown & \diagdown \\
NH_2 & NH_2 & NH_2 & NH_2 & NH_2 \\
\end{array}
$$

Amino Acids

FIG. 50. Biosynthesis and hydrolysis of the polypeptide chain of a protein from and to free amino acids. Only three amino acid units in the middle of the chain are shown, together with the terminal units. A protein chain contains 100–1000 such units. Only the overall reactions are shown, the biosynthetic one involves the stepwise addition of amino acid units (Figs 5 and 6), while intermediate steps in hydrolysis result in formation and subsequent destruction of a variety of peptides.

Side reactions in which some of the amino acids themselves are slowly destroyed also occur, but their effects are small and can be allowed for. The relative numbers of the different kinds of amino acid present in the protein molecule (as amino acid residues) are thus easily ascertained by analysis of the hydrolysate. The various amino acids differ from each other only in the

TABLE 8

Structure of the amino acid side chains in collagen

Glycine	Gly	H—	Simple
Alanine	Ala	CH_3—	

$$\text{Valine} \quad \text{Val} \quad \begin{matrix} CH_3 \\ \diagdown \\ CH- \\ \diagup \\ CH_3 \end{matrix}$$

$$\text{Leucine} \quad \text{Leu} \quad \begin{matrix} CH_3 \\ \diagdown \\ CH \quad CH_5- \\ \diagup \\ CH_3 \end{matrix} \quad \text{Hydrocarbon}$$

$$\text{Isoleucine} \quad \text{Ileu} \quad \begin{matrix} CH_3 \\ \diagdown \\ CH- \\ \diagup \\ C_2H_5 \end{matrix}$$

Methionine   Met $CH_3 \cdot S \cdot CH_2 \cdot CH_2$—   Sulphur containing

$$\text{Proline} \quad \text{Pro} \quad \begin{matrix} CH_2-CH \\ | \qquad \diagdown \\ | \qquad \quad N- \\ | \qquad \diagup \\ CH_2-CH_2 \end{matrix}$$
(pyrollidine group)

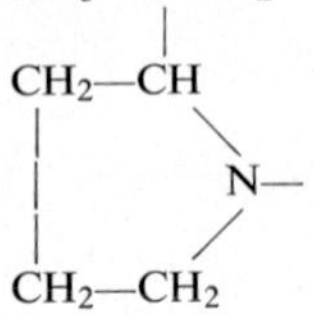

Imino

$$\text{Hydroxyproline} \quad \text{Hypro} \quad \begin{matrix} CH_2-CH \\ | \qquad \diagdown \\ | \qquad \quad N- \\ | \qquad \diagup \\ HO-CH-CH_2 \end{matrix}$$

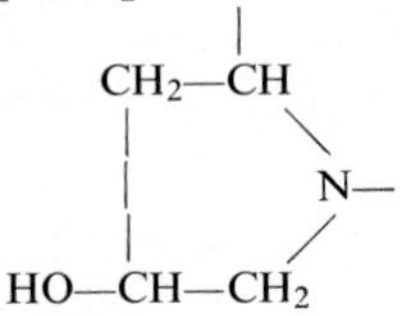

Serine   Ser $HO \cdot CH_2$—

Hydroxy

$$\text{Threonine} \quad \text{Thr} \quad \begin{matrix} HO \\ \diagdown \\ CH- \\ \diagup \\ CH_3 \end{matrix}$$

Tyrosine	Tyr	$HO \cdot C_6H_4 \cdot CH_2$—	Aromatic
Phenylalanine	Phe	$C_6H_5 \cdot CH_2$—	
Aspartic acid	Asp	$^-OOC \cdot CH_2$—	Acidic
Glutamic acid	Glu	$^-OOC \cdot CH_2 \cdot CH_2$—	

$$\text{Histidine} \quad \text{His} \quad ^+\begin{bmatrix} CH-NH_2 \\ \| \qquad \diagdown \\ \| \qquad \quad C \cdot \\ \| \qquad \diagup \\ N--CH \end{bmatrix} CH_2-$$
(imidazole group)

Lysine	Lys	$^+NH_3(CH_2)_4$—
Hydroxylysine	Hylys	$^+NH_3 \cdot CH_2 \cdot CH(OH)(CH_2)_2$—

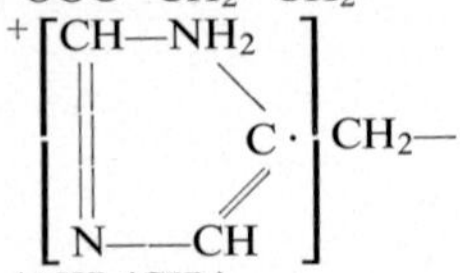

Basic

$$\text{Arginine} \quad \text{Arg} \quad ^+\begin{bmatrix} NH_3 \\ | \qquad \diagdown \\ | \qquad \quad C \cdot NH \\ | \qquad \diagup \\ NH \end{bmatrix} (CH_2)_3-$$
(guanidino group)

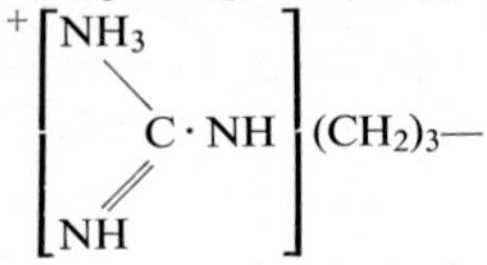

chemical structure of their side chains (R). These side chains behave as functional groups attached to the uniformly repeating structure $(-NH \cdot CH(R) \cdot CO^=)_n$ of the polypeptide backbone of the protein (Table 8).

The amino acid composition of collagens has been studied in a wide range of species and tissues. Recent summaries of results have been given by Lowther (1963), Tristram and Smith (1963) and Eastoe (1967a). A recognizable pattern is present in the composition of collagens from animals belonging to diverse phyla, although substantial variations occur within this. Vertebrate collagens form a closely knit group with smaller, well-defined variations in composition. In the mammals, collagens show only very minor variations in composition between species. Similar small differences occur between some tissues in the same species (Piez and Likins, 1957), but the significance of this is not yet known. The chemical composition of collagen is unique amongst proteins and thus has an important bearing on its structural organization. The main compositional features of mammalian collagens are typically exhibited by the proteins for which data are given in Table 1. These are summarized, as follows:

i. The most abundant unit is *glycine*, the simplest amino acid. It has no hydrocarbon side chain but a second hydrogen atom attached to the backbone carbon atom. Almost exactly one third of all the amino acid units in collagen consist of glycine (Fig. 51). Astbury (1940) suggested that glycine occupies every third position in the polypeptide chain, with two different kinds of amino acid unit between successive glycines. Recent studies of the sequence of units along the polypeptide chain have supported this idea.

ii. Collagen contains two amino acids which are not found in other animal tissue proteins. The more abundant of these is the imino acid *hydroxyproline*, which accounts for approximately one eleventh of all the amino acid units in collagen. It is derived from another imino acid, proline (which is a common constituent of most proteins), by the substitution of a hydroxyl group in the 4-position (or much more rarely the 3-position (Ogle *et al.*, 1962; Piez *et al.*, 1963) (Table 1) of its pyrrolidine ring. This ring is the distinguishing feature of imino acids. It may be visualized as being formed by joining the end of the side chain to the nitrogen atom attached to the α-carbon atom of the amino acid, so giving rise to a close ring of five atoms, four carbon and one nitrogen (Fig. 52). The second unusual amino acid in collagen is *hydroxylysine* which is much rarer, accounting for only one residue in 150. It results from addition of a hydroxyl group to the penultimate carbon atom of the common protein constituent lysine. The other sixteen amino acids found in collagen occur commonly in most proteins.

Neither hydroxyproline nor hydroxylysine can be incorporated directly into collagen during its biosynthesis. These amino acids are incorporated respectively in the form of proline (Stetten and Schoenheimer, 1944) and lysine (Piez and Likins, 1957), and are specifically hydroxylated after formation of the polypeptide chain. The recent

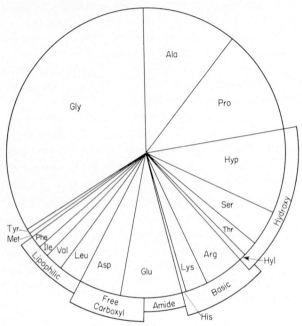

FIG. 51. Diagrammatic representation of the relative abundance of the various amino acid units in ox hide collagen. The areas of the sectors are proportional to the frequency in which the different amino acids occur. The amino acids are designated by their standard abbreviations. (From Eastoe, 1967a.)

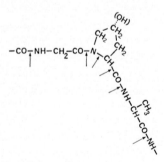

FIG. 52. Effect of the introduction of an imino acid into the protein backbone. Instead of a side chain, the imino acid has a pyrrolidine ring, formed by the side chain being bent back on itself, its δ C atom being bonded to the N attached to the α C atom. Rotation is restricted about those bonds in the backbone denoted by arrows. This imposes an overall stiffness and obligatory change in chain direction wherever proline (or hydroxyproline) occurs.

isolation of *protocollagen* containing unhydroxylated proline supports the idea that hydroxylation occurs subsequent to, rather than in conjunction with, incorporation (Kivirikko and Prockop, 1967).

Deficiency of ascorbic acid has long been known to result in defective connective tissue (Gould, 1960). For many years it has been suspected that ascorbic acid plays an essential part in the oxidation of proline to hydroxyproline after its incorporation into the protein chain. This has been proved conclusively by Hutton *et al.* (1967), who have shown that ferrous ions, α-ketogluturate and molecular oxygen are also essential. They suggest that an enzyme, *collagen proline hydroxylase*, operates as a mixed function oxidase by mediating a reaction in which one molecule of oxygen oxidizes one peptidyl proline unit to hydroxyproline together with one molecule of ascorbate to dehydroascorbate. If hydroxylation of proline to hydroxyproline is prevented by exclusion of oxygen from embryonic cartilage growing in tissue culture, the protocollagen formed in the initial stage of collagen synthesis accumulates within the fibroblasts and is not secreted into the extracellular region as collagen normally is (Juva *et al.*, 1966). Subsequent incubation in the presence of oxygen results in the hydroxylation of some of the proline in this protocollagen and the secretion of the collagen so produced. The connective tissue lesions found in scurvy thus clearly arise from the arrestment of collagen synthesis at the protocollagen stage, resulting in no newly formed collagen being available for tissue growth, remodelling, or repair. Defects in the dental tissues of the scorbutic guinea pig have been studied by Fish and Harris (1935). This topic is discussed in Chapter IX. The effects of scurvy are quite different from those of lathyrism (see page 275), another connective tissue defect in which young collagen is formed but does not mature. In lathyrism, hydroxyproline is synthesized normally but the cross-linkages which normally stabilize insoluble collagen, subsequently fail to form.

iii. The proportion of *imino acids* is higher in collagen than in most other proteins. Proline and hydroxyproline together account for two ninths of the amino acid units in collagen. Wherever one of these imino acids occurs, the presence of the pyrrolidine ring results in a loss of free rotation about four successive bonds in the polypeptide chain (Fig. 52). In consequence, the chain is both stiff and kinked at these points, with important consequences to the stability of the collagen molecule.

iv. Collagen has a relatively high proportion of amino acids with hydroxyl groups in their side chains (hydrophilic groups) and a low proportion of amino acids with hydrocarbon side chains (lipophilic groups) as illustrated in Fig. 51. It is thus on balance a hydrophilic protein (Tristram, 1949), and tends to remain in extended form when in contact with an aqueous environment, rather than rolling up on itself like a globular protein. It may be noted that the "unusual" amino acids hydroxyproline and hydroxylysine both contribute to the excess of hydrophilic groups over hydrophobic groups on collagen side chains.

v. Most of the constituent amino acids of collagen can be divided sharply into two groups: (a) those present in large amounts and (b) those present in small amounts only (Fig. 51). This is in direct contrast to other fibrous proteins such as keratin, where there is a broad spectrum of amino acids present in moderate amounts. In collagen just four amino acids—glycine, alanine, proline and hydroxyproline—together occupy two thirds of the positions in the protein chain. Thus, only one third of the positions are available for the remaining fourteen amino acids.

vi. There is a slight excess in the total of amino acids with basic groups on their side chains (arginine, lysine, hydroxylysine and histidine) compared with those with free carboxyl groups (glutamic and aspartic acids minus amide). In consequence, collagen may be regarded as a basic protein with an isoionic point in the region of pH 9·4 (see Eastoe et al., 1961).

vii. Small amounts of the hexose sugars glucose and galactose, together accounting for approximately 0·3–0·5% by weight, appear to be covalently bound to both soluble and insoluble vertebrate collagens. Cunningham et al. (1967) have shown that at least 75% of the hexose of the soluble collagen is attached to hydroxylysine by an o-glycoside linkage. The sugar-peptide combinations at these highly specific sites were shown to be of two kinds, D-glucosyl 1→6, D-galactosyl, 1→ o-hydroxylysine and D-galactosyl, 1→o-hydroxylysine.

Each of the three polypeptide chains of collagen is made up of approximately 1,000 amino acid units joined together by peptide linkages (Fig. 50) which are strong covalent chemical bonds. The total length of these chains thus exceeds 3000 Å, the width being of atomic dimensions. Recently, end-group techniques have made it possible to find the order or sequence in which the amino acid units occur along the chains. The complete sequence of collagen has not yet been determined owing to technical complexities resulting from the large size of the collagen chains. Considerable progress is currently being made on this problem (Hannig and Nordwig, 1967; Piez, 1967). Early chemical investigations of the sequence in collagen were based on the identification of the more abundant small peptides in partial hydrolysates (Schroeder et al., 1954; Kroner et al., 1955). They supported the suggestion of Astbury (1940) that glycine occupies every third position, and indicated further that the imino acids tended to be concentrated in particular regions as implied by the frequent occurrence of the sequence Gly-Pro-Hypro-Gly. The results of Grassmann et al. (1960) on the composition of some 50 larger peptides isolated from partial trypsin hydrolysates of collagen showed that all of these contained approximately 33% of glycine, whereas the proportion of imino acids varied between peptides, ranging from extreme abundance (28 out of 62 residues) to almost complete absence. Recently Kang et al. (1967) have made a promising new attack on the problem of the complete amino acid sequence of collagen by using the reagent cyanogen bromide. This reagent breaks the protein chain wherever a methionine unit occurs. Fortunately, this amino acid occurs very infrequently in collagen (Fig. 51 and Table 1) so that each chain is broken down into 8 or 9 large peptides of approximately equal size. These peptides are then separated from one another on a chromatographic column and their individual sequences determined by standard methods. Considerable progress has been made and the results have also given useful information concerning the position and nature of cross linkages between the polypeptide chains (page 273).

(b) *Structure of collagen macromolecules.* The main characteristic of the collagen macromolecule is that it contains three polypeptide chains, which are arranged in compound helices, entwined round each other like a three-stranded rope. This results in a long (3000 Å), narrow (13·5 Å), pencil-like structure, which, unlike its component chains, is stiff or only very slightly flexible.

Several early attempts were made to discover a spatial structure for the collagen molecule which would completely account for its observed X-ray diffraction pattern, but none of those suggested was satisfactory (see Bear, 1952). When it was discovered that some proteins have a helical arrangement of their chains in space (Pauling and Corey, 1951) the idea was applied to collagen for which single-helical (Huggins, 1954) and double-helical (Crick, 1954) models were proposed, neither of which fitted the experimental data in all respects.

The triple-helical structure of collagen, which is now widely accepted, was first rigorously worked out as regards all its essential features by Ramachandran and Kartha (1954 and 1955). Reference to Fig. 53 will help to give an approximate idea of how the amino acid units in the three constituent chains fit together to form the complete structure. Each of the three polypeptide chains is wound around its own (chain) axis in a simple left-handed helix of pitch approximately 9 Å with three amino acid units per turn (Fig. 53a). Three such helices may be imagined as being placed with their axes parallel to one another along the edges of an equilateral triangular prism. The axis of the molecule passes through the centre of this prism parallel to the chain axes. Each of the chains is arranged with one stack of amino acid units (representing every third residue in the chain) pointing towards the molecular axis. The closest possible proximity between the chain axes is achieved by staggering the chain helices by 3 Å in a direction parallel to the axis, so that the amino acid units pointing towards the central molecular axis are arranged in order, equally spaced along the axis. This results in a compact arrangement of the three simple helices in a system with a central molecular axis

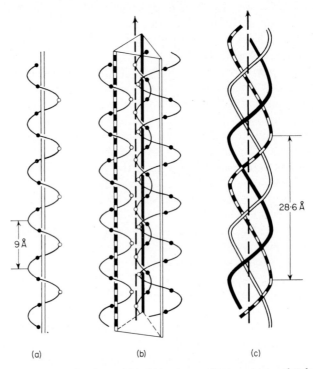

(a)   (b)   (c)

FIG. 53. Arrangement of polypeptide chains in a collagen macromolecule: (a) Single polypeptide chain arranged in a left-handed simple helix of pitch 9 Å about an axis. The circles denote amino acid units, every third unit being glycine, shown by open circles. (b) Three helices of the type shown in (a), placed with their axes along the edges of a triangular prism. The glycine units point inwards so that they are regularly spaced along the prism axis (denoted by the broken arrow). (c) The axes of the polypeptide chains in (b) given a slight twist to form right-handed simple helices of pitch 28·6 Å about the prism axis, which becomes the axis of the macromolecule. The individual polypeptide chains (not shown) form compound helices with the glycine units near the molecular axis.

(Fig. 53b). The structure of the collagen molecule is easily derived from this system by giving it a slight twist so that the chain axes form gentle right-handed helices of pitch 28·6 Å around the straight central axis of the macromolecule (Fig. 53c).

In arriving at this structure, Ramachandran and Kartha took into account not only the X-ray diffraction data but also the probability, shown by analytical and sequence studies, that every third amino acid unit along the polypeptide chain is glycine. Since glycine has no side chain, it is the only amino acid which is sufficiently small that, when situated in the special set of positions near the molecular axis, it permits sufficiently close dovetailing of the three component helices. The criterion of closeness is such that it must be possible for a set of hydrogen bonds, capable of holding the structure together, to be formed. Hydrogen bonds are individually weak, but are collectively strong enough to maintain the systematic arrangement of various biological structures, including proteins. The possibility exists of their being formed between NH and C=O groups in the backbones of different poly-peptide chains in the collagen molecule. A set of such bonds would thus stabilize the three chains as a single molecular system—the macromolecule. Studies with molecular models show that the atomic dimensions and bond lengths are such that a series of hydrogen bonds can just, but only just, be formed, provided that glycine occupies the critical positions near the molecular axis. The direction of the hydrogen bonds is at right angles to the axis. This structure can also accommodate the pyrrolidine rings of the imino acids proline and hydroxyproline which, as already mentioned, are not only bulky but impose an obligatory bend in the direction of the polypeptide chain. These will fit into either or both of the two positions in the sequence between successive glycines. Proline and hydroxyproline are unable to form stabilizing hydrogen bonds in the protein backbone because there is no hydrogen atom on the imino group, when it is involved in the peptide linkage. Despite this, Piez and Gross (1960) have shown that the thermal stability of collagens in a series from different vertebrates increases with their content of total imino acids. This is probably explained by the absence of free rotation about four adjacent bonds in the polypeptide chain at points where imino acid units occur, which helps to lock the molecular structure more firmly in place against the disordering action of thermal energy. A sufficient content of imino acids is thus an essential feature of collagen structure. No specific structural roles have yet been assigned to hydroxyproline and hydroxylysine in collagen but they may represent a means of increasing the overall hydrophilic potential, while retaining the desirable characteristics of the pyrrolidine ring and amino group in their side chains. Gustavson (1958) considers that the radially directed hydroxy group of hydroxyproline may provide intermolecular stabilization.

The broad picture of the structure of the collagen molecule outlined above has been accepted generally, although some of the details are still controversial. Thus Rich and Crick (1955 and 1961) consider that only one hydrogen bond is formed for every three amino acid units whereas Ramachandran (1967) continues to support his original view that there are two hydrogen bonds per three units except where proline or hydroxyproline occurs. His article gives a lucid and detailed exposition of collagen structure.

The concept of the collagen macromolecule is valuable in relation to the development and maintenance of connective tissues. Although the point is not completely proved, the weight of current evidence suggests that after synthesis, a particle of about the size of the molecule is secreted into the extracellular environment, where it undergoes aggregation with other such particles, resulting eventually in the formation of fibres (Fitton Jackson, 1967). The macromolecule is thus a building block for collagen; it is formed within the cell but used extracellularly (Section IV).

TABLE 9

Amino acid composition of α subunits from human, rat and cod skin collagens

	Human skin Bornstein and Piez (1964)		Rat skin Piez et al. (1963)		Cod skin Piez (1965)		
	α1	α2	α1	α2	α1	α2	α3
Alanine	115	105	112	102	119	107	101
Glycine	333	337	330	336	339	348	347
Valine	20·5	33·3	19·6	32·0	15·5	19·5	20·1
Leucine	19·5	30·1	18·1	32·4	18·8	24·4	17·5
Isoleucine	6·6	14·8	6·4	16·1	10·8	9·2	8·9
Proline	135	120	129	113	98	97	96
Phenylalanine	12·3	11·7	11·6	10·1	13·2	9·1	11·0
Tyrosine	2·1	4·6	2·1	2·4	1·8	4·7	2·6
Serine	36·8	35·1	42	43	70	73	73
Threonine	16·5	19·2	19·9	19·8	23·4	26·9	24·5
Methionine	4·9	5·2	8·0	6·1	16·7	18·3	16·8
Arginine	50	51	49	51	51	54	51
Histidine	3·0	9·7	1·9	8·5	5·2	11·5	7·0
Lysine	30·0	21·6	30·4	22·4	31·3	20·6	30·3
Aspartic acid	43	47	46	44	50	54	51
Glutamic acid	77	68	74	66	76	62	78
3-Hydroxyproline	0·8	0·9	1·0	0·0			
4-Hydroxyproline	91	82	96	86	55	52	58
Hydroxylysine	4·4	7·6	4·3	8·0	5·5	9·5	5·3
Amide	(37·9)	(45)	(42)	(43)	(43)	(46)	(54)
Tryptophan	—	—	—	—	0·5	0·2	1·0

Values are expressed as numbers of amino acid residues per 1000 total residues.

When collagenous tissues, particularly those in a young or actively developing state, are extracted with various cold electrolyte solutions, a small proportion of the total collagen of the tissue dissolves as *soluble collagen.* Thus, neutral sodium chloride solution dissolves some 1% and acid citrate buffer approximately 5% of calf skin (Bowes *et al.*, 1955). The material dissolved in neutral sodium chloride extracts has been shown to contain a high proportion of newly-formed collagen, recently synthesized in the microsomes of fibroblasts (Lowther *et al.*, 1961). It consists largely of isolated macromolecules (with the triple helical structure intact) in free solution. The manner in which light is scattered by these solutions indicates the presence of long narrow rod-like particles randomly oriented (Doty and Nishihara, 1958). When soluble collagen solutions are heated above 40°C. the hydrogen bonds which hold the polypeptide chains together in the triple helix break down and allow the chains to separate; in this manner the soluble collagen is converted to *parent gelatin*. The three chains (designated α-sub units—α1, α2 and α3) from one macromolecule are not all identical and have been separated from the "parent gelatin" by chromatography on carboxymethyl cellulose columns (Piez *et al.*, 1960). Although the composition of all the chains conforms in general to the picture of collagen composition already described, significant differences in the content of certain amino acids occur between the sub-units (Table 9). This is most marked for amino acids present in small amounts. The α2 chain of human skin collagen contains three times as much histidine and twice as much tyrosine and hydroxylysine as the α1 chains. The α2 chains appear to be more basic than the α1 chains. In mammalian tissues, two of the three α sub-units are either identical or else resemble each other so closely that they have not yet been separated. These are designated α1, α1 while the third chain is referred to as α2. In cod skin collagen all three chains differ in composition and have been separated as α1, α2 and α3 (Piez, 1965).

(*c*) *Aggregation of collagen macromolecules to form fibrils.* (See also Section **IV**). Collagen fibrils having a characteristic 640 Å periodicity (as revealed by electron microscopy and low-angle X-ray diffraction techniques) are known to form in the neighbourhood of, but probably outside, fibroblasts. The mechanism of fibrilogenesis probably involves side by side aggregation of collagen macromolecules, mainly under the influence of electrostatic forces between charged groups on the side chains of neighbouring macromolecules. The evidence for this is based upon experiments for the reconstitution *in vitro* of collagen fibres from solutions containing soluble collagen. The form in which collagen is reconstituted varies with the electrolyte concentration of the solution in which aggregation of macromolecules occurs (Schmitt, 1956). In the presence of 1% of sodium chloride, the "native-type" fibril with a 640 Å axial repeat distance is formed. By changing the conditions, fibrous long spacing and segment long spacing forms with a period of 2800 Å are produced instead (Fig. 54). The concentration and type of electrolyte added to the soluble collagen thus has an important effect on the structure of the collagen fibres formed, the native type of fibril being produced only over a restricted range of sodium chloride concentration. The critical effect of the electrolyte environment on aggregation of collagen macromolecules *in vitro* is consistent with a mechanism involving electrostatic interaction. It seems likely that a similar mechanism operates *in vivo* but in addition to the effect of small ions, the presence of negatively charged polyelectrolytes of high molecular weight, such as chondroitin sulphate, may need to be taken into account. These will affect not only the distribution of charge, but also the rate of diffusion and possibly the orientation of collagen molecules in their extracellular environment (Kent, 1967).

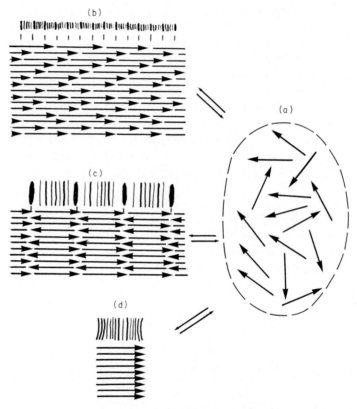

FIG. 54. Probable modes of aggregation of collagen macromolecules (a) in solution to form native type fibrils (b) with 640 Å spacing, fibrous long-spacing (c) and segment long-spacing (d) varieties, each with a period of 2800 Å. (After Schmitt and Hodge, 1960.)

True end-to-end aggregation of collagen macromolecules into *proto-fibrils* would appear to be a statistically improbable mechanism for the beginning of fibril formation, owing to the comparatively remote chance of the ends of the long macromolecules coming into sufficiently close proximity. Side-by-side aggregation has recently come to be accepted as the most probable mechanism, though there are a number of views on how this operates.

i. Hodge and Schmitt (1960) have suggested, as a result of comparing the fine structures of *native fibrillar* and *segment long spacing* collagen that each macromolecule in a fibril overlaps the next by approximately one quarter of its length, the so-called *quarter stagger* arrangement. Hodge and Petruska (1962) reached the conclusion that the length of the macromolecule (L) was approximately 4·40 D, where D is the repeat distance of the typical pattern of cross striations observed in collagen fibrils. The finding that L is not integral with D, in conjunction with

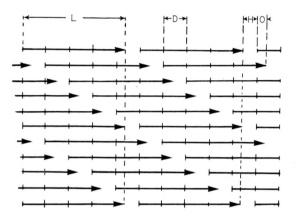

FIG. 55. Systematic aggregation of collagen macromolecules (after Hodge *et al.* 1965) D, repeat distance of fibril, 640 Å; L, length of macromolecule, 4·4D; H, hole, 0·6D; O, overlap, 0·4D.

the quarter-stagger arrangement, led to the conclusion that there is a gap or "hole" equal in length to 0·6 D between the ends of successively aligned macromolecules and that the effective overlap for bond formation is only 0·4 D (Fig. 55). A detailed analysis of the quantitative electron microscopy of the collagen fibril in terms of a model macromolecule with two α1 chains, each having five identical sub-units, and one α2 chain with seven identical sub-units is given by Hodge *et al.* (1965). Smith (1965) has pointed out that when the packing of macromolecules is considered in three dimensions, instead of only two, it becomes evident that not all of them can be accommodated in a quarter-overlapping system. In a fibril of average size, it would appear that only 67–68% of the molecular contacts can be of this nature.

ii. It has been pointed out by Grant *et al.* (1965) that such a systematic arrangement of macromolecules as that illustrated in Fig. 55 is statistically improbable. Following examination of negatively-stained preparations using the electron microscope, they suggested, instead, a more random aggregation mechanism, in which any one of five possible degrees of overlap may occur between neighbouring macromolecules (see also Cox *et al.*, 1967). Each molecule is considered to possess five *bonding zones* (*a*) alternating with four *non-bonding zones* (*b*) (Fig. 56). Aggregation consists of one or more bonding zones of parallel oriented macromolecules coming into register to give a system without systematically arranged holes.

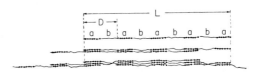

Fɪɢ. 56. Random aggregation of collagen macromolecules (after Grant *et al.* 1965). L, length of macromolecule, 2800 Å; D, repeat distance of fibril, 640 Å; a = bonding zone, approx. 265 Å; b = non-bonding zone, approx. 375 Å.

iii. Veis *et al.* (1967) have produced evidence suggesting that the α1 chains are aligned with their lengths in register whereas the α2 chains are arranged parallel but in quarter-staggered array. Instead of considering only a single plane as in the model of Hodge *et al.* (1965), they point out that there must be a regular spiralling of any given bonding positions around the macromolecules if bonding contact is to be maintained in three dimensions. On the basis of the isolation of stable δ-components (containing 12 α-chains) they propose that four macromolecules are first aggregated side by side into a tetramer in a right handed helical arrangement with the successive macromolecules displaced longitudinally by the repeat distance D along the axis and angularly by 90° around it. Tetramers then fit together, end to end, with 0.4 D overlaps of molecules and 0.6 D holes to make "limiting microfibrils of indefinite length" (Fig. 57).

It is difficult on the evidence available to decide between the relative merits of these three models. It is doubtful whether any of them fully represents the arrangement of the collagen macromolecules within the fibril, more data being needed for an unequivocal solution. Nevertheless, taken together, they account for many of the known facts of collagen fibrilogenesis, as well as emphasizing some of the difficulties which need to be resolved in this central problem of connective tissue organization.

Fɪɢ. 57. Spiral aggregation of collagen macromolecules (Veis *et al.* 1967). Models of the limiting microfibril. (*a*) The fundamental tetrad of collagen monomer units. The α 2 chains are blackened. Each monomer is displaced by D from the A end of the adjacent monomer unit; (*b*) two tetrads packed together into a continuous filament showing the positions of the 0·6D holes and the overlap between the tetrads.

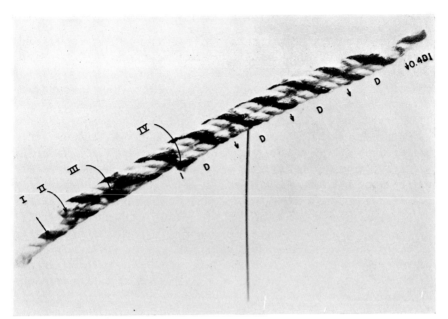

Fig. 57 (a)

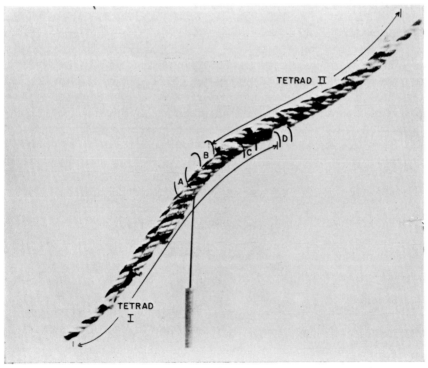

Fig. 57 (b)

[See caption opposite

(d) *The maturation of collagen and formation of cross-linkages.* The only covalent bonds (i.e. strong linkages involving the sharing of electron pairs) whose existence has been taken into account, so far, in this description of collagen structure, are those linking atoms together within the individual polypeptide chains. The triple helix of the collagen macromolecule has been considered as being held together by hydrogen bonds and the fibrillar aggregate of macromolecules mainly by electrostatic bonds between ionized groups, although the roles of these two bond types must to some extent, overlap. A structure held together only in this way would, if treated with warm neutral salt solution, completely dissolve, forming a solution of detached single chains. The collagen structure is only in this state at the moment of its formation, after which it becomes increasingly stable and insoluble, as the result of a *maturation* process. This involves the gradual formation of an increasing but, even ultimately, quite small number of covalent bonds between neighbouring protein chains. These *cross-linkages* lock the complex structure of insoluble collagen in position, so that it is stable to denaturation by electrostatic or thermal forces. Cross-linking bonds in collagen are not the disulphide linkages contained in cystine units, which are the commonest type of interchain bond found in proteins, but involve less well-known linkages, which have been investigated only recently. They join protein chains together both within the triple helix (intramolecular) and between neighbouring helices (extramolecular).

After a piece of collagenous tissue has been laid down it becomes increasingly inert and stable. This is exemplified by its decreasing solubility in neutral salt solution and dilute acids, and by the greater difficulty with which it is converted to gelatin by heating, following acid or alkaline pretreatment. This period of maturation coincides with formation of a gradually increasing number of cross-linkages. It overlaps, but perhaps should be distinguished from, very long-term ageing which may also include processes which have a deleterious effect on connective tissue integrity. The chemical nature of the cross-linkages in collagen has been under investigation for only about ten years (Harding, 1965). Such studies are experimentally difficult owing to the comparative sparsity of the linkages (of the order of two per 300,000 molecular weight), the hitherto unknown nature of their structures, and the general absence of specific and readily detectable chemical entities associated with them. The following main types of cross-link have been reported in collagen.

i. Cross-linkages derived from ε-amino group of lysine side-chains

An *amide* cross link $(-(CH_2)_4 NH \cdot CO \cdot (CH_2)-)$ in which the ε-amino group of lysine in one chain is joined to the side chain carboxyl group of glutamic or aspartic acid in another chain, was proposed by Ames (1952) to explain in terms of structure, differences in the physical properties of gelatins obtained after acid and alkaline treatment of collagen. The evidence for the chemical nature of this linkage was largely speculative.

Kang *et al.* (1967) have succeeded in determining the amino acid sequences of the pentadeca and tetradecapeptides at the N-terminal ends of the α1 and

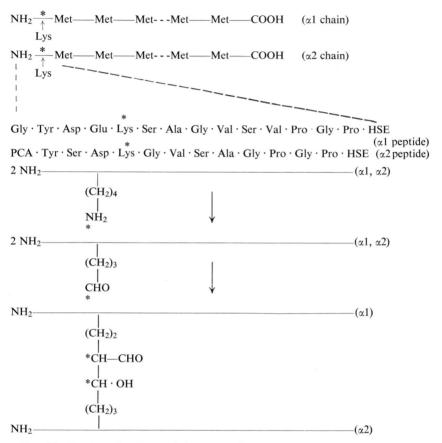

$$NH_2 \overset{*}{\underset{Lys}{\uparrow}} Met —— Met —— Met- - -Met —— Met —— COOH \quad (\alpha 1 \; chain)$$

$$NH_2 \overset{*}{\underset{Lys}{\uparrow}} Met —— Met —— Met- - -Met —— Met —— COOH \quad (\alpha 2 \; chain)$$

Gly · Tyr · Asp · Glu · Lys · Ser · Ala · Gly · Val · Ser · Val · Pro · Gly · Pro · HSE

(α1 peptide)

PCA · Tyr · Ser · Asp · Lys · Gly · Val · Ser · Ala · Gly · Pro · Gly · Pro · HSE (α2 peptide)

FIG. 58. Cleavage of collagen chains at methionine units by cyanogen bromide. The sequences of the N-terminal peptides in α 1 and α 2 chains and possible mechanism of formation of an aldehyde cross-linkage are shown (after Kang *et al.* 1967). The position of the lysine unit which eventually gives rise to a cross-linkage is denoted by an asterisk, and that of the cross-linkage by two asterisks. HSE, homoserine; PCA, pyrrolidine carboxylic acid.

α2 chains respectively of rat skin collagen, after detaching them from the remainder of the molecule by attacking the methionine units with cynanogen bromide (Fig. 58). Though these N-terminal regions of the α1 and α2 chains are not identical, they possess some sequences in common. They are atypical of the greater part of collagen in both amino acid composition and sequence, since they completely lack hydroxyproline and do not have glycine in every third position. Both the $\alpha 1$ and $\alpha 2$ chains have a lysine residue situated in the fifth position from the amino-terminal end. Evidence was obtained that this is readily oxidized in the intact chain to the corresponding aldehyde, i.e. the δ-semialdehyde of α-aminoadipic acid. Isotope studies (Piez *et al.*, 1966) have suggested that the aldehyde groups can react with one another, possibly undergoing condensation, to form an intramolecular cross-linkage near the N-terminal end of the macromolecule. A condensation of this type would leave one aldehyde group free to react (Fig. 58) giving rise to the possibility that a second cross-linkage, either intra- or intermolecular, could subsequently be formed at the same point. A study of the position of the cross link in relation to the point of cleavage of insoluble collagen by tadpole tail collagenase supports the above-mentioned conclusion that the cross link is near the N-terminal group; it is no more than three quarters of the chain's length from it (Gross and Nagai, 1965).

ii. Linkages derived from the carboxyl groups of amino acids

Blumenfeld and Gallop (1962) investigated the reactions of lithium borohydride, hydroxylamine and hydrazine on collagen and derived gelatins. From the nature of the reaction products, they reached the conclusion that both α- and β-carboxyl groups of aspartic acid participate in *ester-like* linkages of the type $R \cdot CO \cdot OR'$. The evidence indicated that such linkages occur in pairs at the carboxyl end of the collagen chains, the α-carboxyl group involved being the nominal terminal carboxyl group. Preparations of mammalian collagen invariably contain a small amount of carbohydrate even when highly purified (Eastoe, 1967a), and it is probable that at least some of this is firmly bound to the macromolecule (page 262). Hydroxyl groups of sugar units may participate in the "ester-like" linkages of collagen (Harding, 1965); the possession of several hydroxyl groups by each sugar molecule giving rise to the possibility of both intra- and intermolecular cross linking through either ester or glycosidic bonds (Hörmann, 1960).

iii. A specific linkage in dentine involving phosphate and a sugar unit

Veis and Schlueter (1963) noticed that when dentine is demineralized with ethylenediamine-tetra acetic acid, the remaining collagen retains firmly bound phosphate. They suggest that this might participate in a special type of cross-linkage, possibly involving hydroxyproline linked through a phosphoric acid and a hexose group to serine.

It is not easy to assess the relative claims of these various chemical groupings as effective cross-linkages in collagen. However, the aldehyde groups derived from specific lysine units have so many points in their favour that their relevance seems likely to become rapidly acknowledged:

The chemical evidence for their existence is definite and detailed, making it possible to establish their exact position in a molecule of known structure.

The presence of aldehyde groups in some gelatins has long been reported as an empirical observation (Landucci et al., 1958) to which biological significance may now be attributed.

The structural possibility of intra- and intermolecular cross-linking occurring at the same point may permit biological control of the order in which these processes occur.

The nature and mechanism of lathyrism is completely explained.

Lathyrism is a rare disease found in animals fed on the pea plant *Lathyrus odoratus*. It is characterized by the connective tissues having a high water content, being mechanically weak, and having brittle collagen, an unusually high proportion of which is extractable (Levene and Gross, 1959). Lathyrism can be induced artificially in animals by administering various nitriles of organic acids such as aminoacetonitrile and β-amino-propionitrile. While these have no effect on collagen which has already matured, they prevent the maturation of young collagen by interfering with the formation of both intra- and intermolecular cross linkages (Martin et al., 1963). Bornstein and Piez (1966) have found that β-amino-propionitrile inhibits the conversion of the single specific lysine unit to an aldehyde in lathyric rats and so stops, at its first stage, the reaction which normally leads to the formation of cross-linkages. The rate of formation of that stage of collagen in which lysine has been converted to aldehyde (as shown by incorporation of labelled glycine) was shown to be greatly reduced in lathyritic compared with normal rats (Piez et al., 1966). The administration of organic nitriles to animals has thus provided a valuable experimental tool for preventing the maturation of collagen, while leaving the early stages of its biosynthesis unaffected. This technique has been applied to the investigation of collagen maturation in the periodontium of rats, where it causes widening of the periodontal space and deformation of bone of the alveolar process (Marwah et al., 1963; Barrington and Meyer, 1966). Connective tissue damage is almost completely repaired within one week of discontinuing administration. Elastin is also affected in lathyrism. Lysine side chains are also involved in formation of cross links in elastin (Miller et al., 1964), but not in the same way as in collagen (page 280).

It is possible that more than one type of cross-linking occurs in collagens, and the absence of swelling of dentine collagen in acid solution (Veis and Schlueter, 1964) certainly implies a higher degree of stabilization than is found in the collagens of soft tissues. Though this could reasonably be explained by an additional set of cross-linkages mediated through phosphate and hexose, more chemical evidence is required before their existence can be established fully. The reactions of collagen with lithium borohydride, hydroxylamine and hydrazine when considered together, strongly support the existence of "ester-type" links. Whether these represent true cross-linkages, or some other perhaps equally interesting structures near the terminal carboxyl end of the molecule, is still not clear, however.

2. Reticulin

(a) *Chemical composition.* There has long been considerable controversy over the chemical nature of reticulin. This resulted firstly from reticulin being primarily a histological concept and, secondly, from the difficulty of preparing sufficient uncontaminated material for chemical analysis (Robb-Smith, 1958). Two opposing views—(i) that reticulin is chemically identical with collagen and, (ii) that it is entirely different from collagen—have been contended for half a century. The staining of reticulin by the Bielschowsky silver impregnation technique (Maresch, 1905) did not clarify this problem, as it eventually resulted in the confusion of the most typical kind of reticulin (characteristically found in basement membranes) with developing fibres of young collagen (Section IV).

Robb-Smith (1945) made an important advance by showing that both collagen and reticulin are attacked by the highly specific clostridial collagen-ases, indicating a close relationship between the composition of these entities. Reticulin was, however, shown to be strongly stained by the periodic acid-Schiff reaction, suggesting the presence of protein-bound carbohydrate. Furthermore, reticulin is metachromatic in the sulphation metachromasia reaction whereas collagen is orthochromatic (Kramer and Windrum, 1954); both these staining reactions indicate a definite difference between these two elements of connective tissue. Kramer and Little (1953) made a preparation of reticular tissue from the subcortical region of the human kidney. This site was carefully selected as it is particularly rich in basement membrane reti-culin and contains only a minimum of collagen around the blood vessels which is easily removed by dissection. This preparation, when examined with the electron microscope, showed a feltwork of interlacing fibrils of very small diameter, but having the 640 Å collagen periodicity, embedded in a homo-genous ground substance. Similar structures were seen in material from other sites known to contain reticulin.

A quantitative analysis of renal reticulin was carried out by Windrum *et al.* (1955) on a similar preparation which had also been treated with cold, very dilute, sodium hydroxide solution to remove cellular material, and boiling chloroform-methanol to extract lipids. A surprising finding was that the reticulin contained some 11% of phosphorus-free bound lipid, liberated on hydrolysis with hot, moderately concentrated acid. This was shown not to be cholesterol, and was provisionally identified as myristic acid. The reticulin contained approximately 4·2% of total carbohydrate, a value considerably greater than that for mammalian collagens, the carbohydrate content of which does not exceed 0·5% (Eastoe, 1967a). The sugar units galactose, mannose, fucose and glucosamine were identified, but uronic acid and ester sulphate were absent, suggesting the absence of chondroitin sulphate. The amino acid composition of the protein portion of reticulin (Table 1) is quantitatively similar to collagen. The analysis accounted for over 97% of the total nitrogen content of the reticulin preparation. The main constituent of renal reticulin is thus a protein having a composition almost identical with collagen, and this accounts for 85% of the weight. It is rather firmly bound to lipid and carbohydrate moieties, which rationally account for the differences in hydrothermal stability, X-ray diffraction pattern (Little and Windrum, 1954), and staining reactions observed between these two connective tissue constituents.

(b) *Structure of reticulin and its behaviour* in vitro. Very little information is available concerning the chemical and structural relationships of the protein, carbohydrate and lipid components of reticulin. From the chemical viewpoint they appear to be rather closely associated with one another.

Snellman (1965) has claimed to have isolated and determined the structure of a water soluble glycoprotein from spleen reticulin. Its molecule consists of two nonadecapeptides, very rich in asparagine and glutamine units, joined by three pairs of tetrasaccharides, each containing one unit of galactose or mannose and three of N-acetylglucosamine. He has also reported the separation on a carboxymethylcellulose column of a series of peaks from a dialysate of reticulin, dissolved in ammonium acetate solution. The ultra-violet absorption spectra of these peaks suggested that they contained equimolar quantities of guanosine triphosphate (GTP) which was bonded to peptides containing the amino acids found in collagen. In an *in vitro* experiment, a mixture of GTP peptides, and glycoprotein from reticulin was incubated with ascorbic acid and a general peptide synthetase prepared from calf liver (Snellman, 1963). The resulting reduction of free amino group concentration and release of guanosine monophosphate were considered to represent the biosynthesis of collagen, the reaction rate being greatest at pH 7·6 in the presence of magnesium ions. This experiment has important implications concerning the possibility of collagen synthesis from peptides in reticulin. It also suggests that this could occur extracellularly instead of, or in addition to, synthesis within fibroblasts, which is the site now generally favoured. However, we believe that before this new concept can be accepted, the work on the extracellular biosynthetic system should be shown to be capable of repetition, while appropriate control experiments need to be carried out.

3. Elastin and Oxytalan Fibres

The third type of connective tissue fibres, the elastic fibres consist predominantly of the protein elastin, the composition and properties of which are

10

quite different from those of collagen and reticulin. The amino acid composition of elastin (Table 10) is characterized by unusually high proportions of glycine and the amino acids with hydrocarbon side chains—alanine, valine and leucine—and an extremely low proportion of amino acids with ionizable groups on their side chains, whether basic or acidic. The content of amino

TABLE 10

Composition of elastin from chicken aorta at various ages (Miller et al. 1964)

	12-day embryo	16-day embryo	20-day embryo	3-week chick	4-week chick	1-year chicken
Alanine	172	176	180	175	177	177
Glycine	352	352	351	352	352	352
Valine	177	177	177	176	176	174
Leucine	62	59	56	58	57	58
Isoleucine	19	19	19	19	20	20
Proline	122	123	124	128	126	124
Phenylalanine	22	22	22	22	22	22
Tyrosine	11	11	12	12	12	12
Serine	5·4	4·1	3·2	5·1	5·7	4·1
Threonine	4·2	3·4	3·6	3·1	3·5	4·6
Cystine (half)	0·5	0·5	0·6	0·4	0·3	0·6
Arginine	4·9	4·2	5·6	4·5	4·1	4·5
Histidine	<0·2	<0·2	<0·2	<0·2	<0·2	<0·2
Lysine	5·7	4·6	3·9	3·6	3·5	1·6
Aspartic acid	1·9	1·9	1·8	1·9	1·9	1·8
Glutamic acid	12	12	12	12	11	12
Hydroxyproline	24	25	22	23	22	23
Desmosine (quarter)	4·3	5·7	6·7	6·8	7·1	9·3
Amide N	37·7	21·4	25·1	25·4	21·3	19·6

Values are given as numbers of amino acid units per thousand total units.

acids with side chain hydroxyl groups is also low. Hydroxyproline is present, though at a much lower level than in collagen, and it is not entirely clear whether it is an essential part of the elastin molecule or whether it represents contamination by collagen.

The predominance of hydrocarbon side chains in elastin together with the very low level of hydrophilic (ionizable and hydroxy groups) results in elastin being a lipophilic protein in contrast to collagen which is hydrophilic. The side chains of elastin will therefore tend to be attracted to one another within the fibre by van der Waal's forces rather than to the environmental water by hydrogen bonds. This partially accounts for the unusually high hydrothermal stability of elastin, which greatly exceeds that of collagen. Thus, the original method of obtaining purified elastin preparations was to autoclave tissues rich in elastin (e.g. aorta and ligamentum nuchae) with excess water for some hours. The collagen dissolved as degraded gelatin leaving the highly resistant elastin as an insoluble residue.

Another reason for the high stability of elastin is its highly cross-linked structure. Until recently the nature of this stabilization was not understood— the common type of disulphide cross-linkages being absent from elastin. Two new amino acids were found by Thomas et al. (1963) in acid hydrolysates of elastin, and these probably represent a special kind of cross-linkage in the

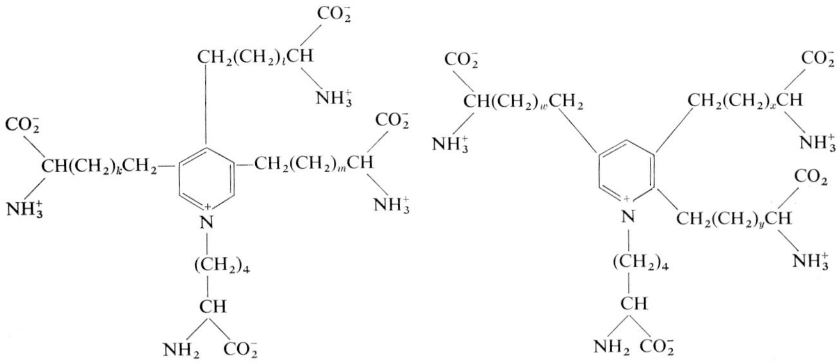

FIG. 59. Structural formulae of desmosine and isodesmosine. (Thomas et al. 1963.)

intact protein. These new substances were designated *desmosine* and *isodesmosine*; they are similar isomers both consisting of a 6-membered pyridinium ring having four side chains, each terminating in a carboxyl group and an α-amino group (Fig. 59). Their structures suggest that the ends of the side chains were originally joined in peptide linkage within the polypeptide chains of intact elastin. If this is so the desmosine structures would act as cross-links, joining four protein chains together at a single point in such a way as to give a structure with a rubber-like elasticity, assuming that there are no systematically arranged bonds between other parts of the protein chains.

Miller et al. (1964) analysed elastin from the aortas of chick embryos and chickens of various ages (Table 10). The amino acid composition was constant with age except for the content of desmosines and lysine. The lysine values gradually decreased with age while there was a corresponding increase in the desmosine content. The total of lysine and "quarter-desmosine" remained constant at 10–11 units per 1000. These investigators also cultured embryonic aortas in a medium containing radioactively labelled lysine. Although the labelled lysine was incorporated rapidly into the elastin, the desmosine took up the label more slowly. It thus appears that the cross-linkages in elastin are slowly formed by the reaction of four lysine units to form desmosines. The "maturation" process in elastin thus depends on lysine, the same amino acid unit which is initially involved in the maturation of collagen. The structure of the cross-linkages ultimately formed is, however, different, the bulky desmosine group being too large to fit into the collagen structure. This cross linking of maturing elastin is possibly reflected in the morphological changes which have been observed in tissues studied by electron microscopy (Section IIA).

Elastin is converted into a soluble form by partial hydrolysis with 0·25M oxalic acid at 100°C (Partridge et al., 1955). Addition of increasing concentrations of ammonium sulphate to the solution separates the soluble elastin into α and β fractions of molecular weight 60,000–84,000 and 5,500 respectively. The composition of these fractions is very similar to that of the insoluble parent elastin and quite unlike collagen (Partridge and Davis, 1955).

From time to time it has been suggested that collagen may be converted to elastin in old and degenerating tissues where denaturation is likely to occur. This idea has been based largely on the morphology (Burton et al., 1955) and staining of denatured collagen. Since elastin has few ionizable groups, it does not stain readily with acidic or basic dyes but takes up phenolic dyes such as orcein and resorcinfuchsin, the so-called elastin stains, which are compatible with its lipophilic side chains. Native collagen, on the other hand, stains with acid or basic dyes but does not readily take up phenolic stains. On partial denaturation some of the inter-chain hydrogen bonds of collagen are broken down, permitting the penetration of phenolic dyes which can come into proximity with small groups of lipophilic side chains. The same process may result in the denatured collagen acquiring some rubber-like elasticity. The chemical composition of collagen is hardly altered by these changes, which affect mainly the spatial arrangement of the chains. Since the amino acid composition of elastin is entirely different from that of collagen, the true interconversion of these proteins would seem to be most unlikely because of the fundamental differences between their chemical constitutions. Partridge (1958) has pointed out that whereas elastin contains more valine than any other protein, collagen can provide very little of this amino acid. Even if the whole of its valine were utilized in a hypothetical collagen-elastin conversion, the yield of elastin would be limited to approximately 14%.

Oxytalan fibres, which are considerably more numerous than elastic fibres in the human periodontium (Fullmer, 1967) have been distinguished from elastin, collagen and reticulin mainly by their histochemical staining reactions. There are indications that they represent an early stage of elastic fibre formation but their chemical constitution has not been investigated.

B. GROUND SUBSTANCE

1. Carbohydrate—Protein Compounds

(a) *Types and chemical composition.* Animal tissues contain a great variety of complex substances, usually of high molecular weight and containing both sugar and amino acid units, which are associated with the "structureless" rather than the demonstrably fibrous tissue elements. The complexity of these substances and the impossibility of obtaining them in a crystalline state has made a study of their nature difficult. While increasing knowledge has placed more and more emphasis on their biological importance, it has also led to their repeated reclassification with consequent confusion of terminology. They were originally designated as mucoproteins by Levene (1925), a term which, if broadened to mucosubstances, aptly describes their physiological properties without overemphasizing one aspect of their composition. The prefix *muco* now seems to be falling into disfavour and the general term carbohydrate-protein compounds (or complexes) has come into use. Several attempts have been made to classify these compounds using well defined criteria. Unfortunately, these have had to be successively abandoned when further research has shown them to be inapplicable, either because known substances have been shown to differ in constitution from that previously assumed, or because, new substances have been discovered which overlap several categories of the classification.

Despite these difficulties, it is possible to divide the non-lipidic mucosubstances known at the present time into two main groups (Gottschalk, 1966).

i. Polysaccharide—protein compounds

These are best known by their traditional name, mucopolysaccharides, and have also been termed glycosaminoglucuronoglycans. They are best represented by chondroitin sulphate and hyaluronic acid, the compositional features of which are included in Table 11. These substances are characterized by highly polymerized carbohydrate chains (containing from 150 to several thousand sugar units) having a regularly repeating sequence, usually with two kinds of sugar unit alternating along the whole length of the chain (... A.B.A.B.A.B....). One of these sugar units is usually a hexosamine and the other a hexuronic acid. Hexosamines are derived from simple hexose sugars by the replacement of one of the hydroxyl groups (usually that on C2, the carbon atom attached to the aldehyde group of an aldohexose) by an amino group, NH_2. In addition, the amino group may have an acetyl group attached so that the resulting structure $(-NH \cdot CO \cdot CH_3)$, is not capable of ionization and so, unlike an unsubstituted amino group, cannot acquire a charge. Hexuronic acids are derived from hexose sugars by oxidation of C6 to a carboxyl group. This group confers weakly acidic properties on polymers containing it, provided it is free to ionize. Another feature of some of these high polymers is the possession of ester sulphate groups. A molecule of sulphuric acid is attached through the oxygen atom of one of the sugar hydroxyl groups (usually to the hexosamine unit) with the result that ionization of the remaining hydrogen atom of the sulphate group confers strongly acidic properties on the polymer. Polysaccharide accounts for the greater part of

TABLE 11

Compositional features of polysaccharide-proteins (mucopolysaccharides) of connective tissues

| | Monosaccharide components | |
| | | |
Polysaccharide	Hexosamine	Uronic acid (or hexose)
Hyaluronic acid	N-acetyl-D-glucosamine (1:3 linkages, SO_4 absent)	D-glucuronic acid (1:4 linkage)
Chondroitin sulphate A (chondroitin-4-sulphate)	N-acetyl-D-galactosamine (1:3 linkage, 4-SO_4)	D-glucuronic acid (1:4 linkage)
Chondroitin sulphate B (derman sulphate)	N-acetyl-D-galactosamine (1:3 linkage, 4-SO_4)	L-iduronic acid (1:4 linkage)
Chondroitin sulphate C (chondroitin-6-sulphate)	N-acetyl-D-galactosamine (1:3 linkage, 6-SO_4)	D-glucuronic acid (1:4 linkage)
Chondroitin	N-acetyl-D-galactosamine (1:3 linkage, SO_4 absent)	D-glucuronic acid (1:4 linkage)
Heparan sulphate	N-aceytl-D-glucosamine (partially sulphated)	glucuronic acid
Keratosulphate (keratan sulphate)	N-acetyl-D-glucosamine (1:4 linkage, 6-SO_4	D-galactose (1:3 linkage)

most compounds in this group, especially when the traditional method of extraction from tissues by the use of alkali is employed for their isolation. It has been realized that this carbohydrate is nearly always associated with a smaller amount of protein. This was considered to be a loose association due to electrostatic bonds, but recent evidence suggests that in several polysaccharide-protein complexes, the polysaccharide is covalently bound through an alkali-labile o-glycosidic linkage to a serine (or threonine) group on the protein (Gottschalk, 1966). When this is so, the polysaccharide and protein together constitute a large molecule which may have more than one carbohydrate chain.

ii. Glycoproteins

These are defined as conjugated proteins containing one or more heterosaccharides with a relatively low number of sugar residues, lacking a serially repeating unit, and bound covalently to the polypeptide chain (Gottschalk, 1962). Different animal glycoproteins vary enormously in the number, composition, and size of their heterosaccharide groups, in the composition of the protein component, and in their carbohydrate content (usually lower than in polysaccharide-protein compounds but up to 80% in blood-group specific substances). Lack of a serially repeating unit and the low number of sugar units (2–20) in the heterosaccharide chains are the main features common to all glycoproteins. The types of sugar unit present are characteristic. In common with polysaccharide-protein compounds they possess N-acetyl-D-glucosamine and N-acetyl-D-galactosamine but uronic acids are absent. The hexose sugars mannose and galactose as well as fucose (a methyl pentose) are of common occurrence in glycoproteins. N-acetylneuraminic acid (NANA or sialic acid) is the most characteristic component; structurally it can be considered as being both a sugar and an amino acid. Its strongly acid carboxyl group (pK = 2·6) gives it acid properties through a wide range of pH. Sialic acid groups characteristically terminate the carbohydrate chains of glycoproteins at the ends remote from the protein moiety and in contact with the environment. Where their numbers are sufficient they impart their acidic character to the whole glycoprotein molecule.

(b) *Structure*. Much work remains to be done on the detailed structure of the carbohydrate-protein compounds of the ground substance. The following specific examples illustrate some of the types of structure found in this group of substances.

Hyaluronic acid, which occurs widely in connective tissues, but which is perhaps most easily isolated from synovial fluid and umbilical cord, seems to exist as a complex containing 25–30% of protein. This protein is probably loosely associated with the carbohydrate, as it can be removed, without causing marked reduction in the very high viscosity of synovial fluid (Gottschalk, 1966; Kent, 1967). The particle weight of hyaluronic acid is of the order of 1–4×10^6 (Rogers, 1961). The structure consists of a very long polysaccharide chain. This chain is not tightly rolled on itself because of mutual electrostatic repulsion between the negatively charged carboxyl groups on alternating glucuronic acid units. However, the molecule is too long, thin and flexible to form a rather rigid rod-like collagen, and is perhaps best pictured as a loose tangled skin or net in intimate contact with environmental water.

Chondroitin sulphate (Muir, 1961, 1964) from cartilage has a molecular weight of approximately 1–5×10^6, the molecule consisting of a protein core to which some 30–60 polysaccharide chains, each of molecular weight 50,000, are covalently attached (Mathews and Lozaityte, 1958; Partridge *et al.*, 1961). Mutual repulsion of the negatively charged groups on the carbohydrate chains gives the molecule a rigid character so that it behaves as a rod 3,700 Å in length. The polysaccharide chains are attached to serine units in the core protein by glycosidic bonds to xylose units, which, together with adjacent galactose units, are interposed between the repeating structure of the carbohydrate chain (Table 11) and the protein core (Rodén et al., 1963). This complex molecular assemblage is broken down by treatment with alkali, which attacks the glycoside links.

Bovine bone *sialoprotein*, the composition of which is given in Tables 6 and 7, has a molecular weight of 23,500. Structural studies suggest that it has a single, highly-branched, carbohydrate chain with *N*-acetylneuraminic acid units in the terminal positions. These are joined successively through galactose, hexosamine, and two other sugar units to a single glucosamine unit attached to the protein part of the molecule (Andrews and Herring, 1965). This structure is tentative only, but contrasts sharply with that of another glycoprotein from the ovine submaxillary gland which has a molecular weight of approximately 10^6 with 750 carbohydrate chains attached to the protein. Each of these consists of only two units, a terminal *N*-acetylneuraminic acid unit and an *N*-acetylgalactosamine unit, which is attached to the protein via the side chain hydroxyl group of serine (Gottschalk, 1966).

(*c*) *Behaviour and functions* in vitro *and* in vivo. At the present time it is not possible to account systematically for the behaviour of carbohydrate-protein compounds in tissues. This arises partly from their variety, the proportions of the various protein-polysaccharides differing greatly between tissues and even changing in the same tissue with age. Thus Meyer et al. (1956) have pointed out that adult human rib cartilage is rich in chondroitin sulphates A and B whereas chondroitin sulphate C and keratosulphate predominate in the cornea. Skin contains hyaluronic acid, chondroitin sulphate B and chondroitin sulphate C which successively predominate as the embryonic tissue grows older (Loewi, 1961). As human rib cartilage ages, chondroitin sulphate is replaced by keratosulphate (Kaplan and Meyer, 1959). The proportion of fibrous proteins relative to protein-polysaccharide also differs greatly in various connective tissues. Assuming collagen to be the major fibrous component and hexosamines to be almost universally distributed among the carbohydrate-protein compounds, the hydroxyproline: hexosamine ratio is a convenient index for comparison. Values of 2·8 for cartilage, 12·2 for skin and 30 for tendon have been obtained (Engel et al., 1960).

A further difficulty is that the constituents of the ground substance are not simple substances acting in isolation. They vary quantitatively in composition, molecular size and state of aggregation. In particular, the extent to which they are bound to soluble and insoluble proteins can vary widely. Schubert (1966) has pointed out that the characteristic macromolecular components of connective tissues are not simply present in, but are *built into* the tissues. Thus, even when they are known to be soluble when isolated, they are not necessarily readily extracted from the tissue. For example, although cartilage is the connective tissue which is richest in polysaccharide-protein compounds, very little of these can be extracted from the gross tissue with water. If the tissue is finely ground, which mechanically destroys its structure, some 60–80% of the total polysaccharide together with associated protein, can be extracted. A further part of the original carbohydrate content, however, remains firmly attached to the insoluble (collagenous) residue, from which it can be removed only by reagents sufficiently drastic to break chemical bonds. It is evident from this that the carbohydrate in connective tissue is not all in the same state, some being bound to macromolecular, but potentially soluble, protein, while other carbohydrate structures are firmly attached to the insoluble fibrous network. The binding of polysaccharide to protein thus tends to stabilize the polysaccharide, and anchor it in position. Similar differences in the extractability of polysaccharides have been reported for bovine heart valve tissue (Lowther et al., 1967), and about 25% of chondroitin sulphate B in skin has been found to be firmly bound to insoluble collagen (Toole and Lowther, 1966).

The primary function of the carbohydrate-protein group of compounds in connective tissues is to provide an extracellular milieu which permits the subsequent formation and maturation of fibres as tissue development proceeds. This function approximately coincides with the histological concept of the ground substance. New portions of tissues, whether embryonic or in healing wounds, have a smaller proportion of collagen fibres, larger amounts of carbohydrate and smaller amounts of protein, than older tissues.

Young tissues also have a higher water content than mature ones, and this provides a clue to those important properties of polysaccharide-proteins which enable them to form the initial extracellular milieu. Fessler (1960) subjected a soluble collagen gel to ultracentrifugation and obtained a compact pellet containing nearly all the collagen and a little water. When the experiment was repeated with the addition of a small proportion of hyaluronic acid to the collagen, a larger pellet with a higher water content was obtained. He suggested that the thin chains of the hyaluronic acid were surrounded by an envelope of water, of radius approximately 50 Å from which the collagen macromolecules were excluded by a process similar to gel filtration. Evidence in support of this "excluded volume effect" was obtained by Ogston and Phelps (1961), who found that hyaluronic acid was unable to diffuse through a Millipore filter with a pore size of 100 mμ. This supports the idea of the hyaluronic acid being in the form of very long thin chains, arranged as a loose tangled skein. When the hyaluronate solution was separated by a Millipore filter from an albumin solution, the albumin diffused through into the hyaluronate, although the final concentration of albumin reached in the hyaluronate was always less than that on the side of the membrane where albumin only was present. This was attributed to the albumin molecules being unable to penetrate the considerable excluded volume of water surrounding the hyaluronic acid chains. Schubert (1966) repeated Fessler's centrifugation experiment using chondroitin sulphate-core protein complex from cartilage instead of hyaluronic acid. A much greater effect was obtained, the wet weight of pellets containing added chondroitin sulphate complex being up to ten times more than those containing collagen alone. This indicated the possibility of mechanical entanglement of the fine chondroitin sulphate side chains with the collagen. Taken together these experiments show that the polysaccharide-protein compounds of connective tissue ground substance have properties which enable them to spread out in solution in net-like form, and further that they are closely associated with a large amount of water, from which other macromolecules are largely excluded. As a consequence of their open structures, these polysaccharide-proteins will hold a very large volume of water for a minimum weight of polymer, and hence are a biologically efficient and economical means of beginning the occupation and organization of extracellular space.

The diffusional movement of other macromolecules will be restricted to regions away from the individual strands of this hydrated net, with the result that such molecules are channelled either between adjacent sheets of nettings or through the larger holes in the network. This mechanism presumably has an important effect on the direction in which forming fibres are laid down. Various endogenous enzymes of the hyaluronidase group temporarily depolymerize some polysaccharide-proteins *in vivo*, facilitating the movement of both fluid and polysaccharide through the tissue spaces (Fessler, 1960). They thus act as "spreading" agents or factors for animal venoms or bacterial toxins in connective tissues.

Many of the properties of carbohydrate-protein compounds which enable them to have specific functions in connective tissues must result from their being polyelectrolytes as well as highly polymeric. They are, except in the rare cases of compounds with non-acetylated amino groups, exclusively anionic in character with weakly, moderately or strongly acidic properties due to uronic acid carboxyl, sialic acid carboxyl or sulphate groups, respectively. They therefore tend to associate with (or "bind") cations over an appropriate range of pH. These cations will be either small metal ions in solution, towards which polyelectrolytes will tend to behave like an ion exchange resin (Gordon and Eastoe, 1964) or positively-charged groups in large molecules such as proteins. Unfortunately the conditions prevailing within tissues are for the most part not sufficiently known (as regards, for example, pH and ionic concentration) for a simple physico-chemical treatment of processes such as ion-exchange to be usefully applied. As an example of this, it is known that the force of attraction increases with valency, and it would therefore be expected that (divalent) calcium ions would be associated preferentially with chondroitin sulphate compared with, say, sodium ions. However, this association has been used as an argument for chondroitin sulphate acting as (i) a promoter of calcification due to its ability to combine with calcium ions in mineralizing cartilage (Sobel, 1955) and (ii) an inhibitor of mineralization in soft tissues such as skin due to its reducing the concentration of free calcium ions in solution (Glimcher, 1959). Knowledge of the equilibrium involved and information about the concentration of free calcium ions in the tissue fluid, is needed to reconcile or decide between these two apparently contradictory hypotheses. It is clearly even more difficult to work out a rigorous quantitative treatment of the factors involved in the aggregation of collagen macromolecules into fibrils, a process sensitive to the ionic environment (Sections **IIIA** and **IVB**), and therefore inevitably influenced by the presence of macromolecular polyelectrolytes of another species with their retinue of smaller ions. Finally, the proximity of relatively small regions of different macromolecules may result in temporary local configurations of atoms, capable of bringing about specific processes. Again hypotheses based on such concepts are notoriously difficult to test experimentally, for example the role suggested for a chondroitin sulphate-collagen complex in initiating mineralization (Sobel and Burger, 1954).

2. Lipids

The lipids form a rather heterogeneous class of substances defined, from the point of view of chemical analysis, by their high solubility in such organic solvents as mixtures of chloroform and methanol, ether and certain other hydrocarbons. Histologically lipids are demonstrated by Sudan dyes, by other physical staining methods, and by histochemical techniques, provided that these can reach the immediate site. The main classes of lipid which have so far been identified in connective tissues are neutral fats, fatty acids, phospholipids and sterols, particularly cholesterol.

(a) *Lipids in soft connective tissues.* Comparatively few chemical investigations appear to have been made concerning the lipids of native soft connective tissues. Attention has been directed rather to lipids in connective tissue produced in response to implanted foreign bodies. Examples of these are (i) a synthetic sponge polymer, prepared from polyvinyl alcohol by a cross-linking reaction, and (ii) carrageenin, a sulphated polygalactose, extracted from the seaweed Irish moss (*Chondrus crispus*), which stimulates rapid growth of connective tissue granulomata when injected subcutaneously (Jackson, 1957).

High and variable results were obtained by Noble and Boucek (1955) for individual and total lipids in the connective tissue which grew into polyvinyl sponges implanted in the rat and rabbit. Substantially lower values were quoted by Boucek *et al.* (1955). They showed that approximately two-thirds of the phospholipid, cholesterol, neutral fat and total lipid content of rat and rabbit connective tissue is associated with the saline-soluble fraction, although significant amounts still remained with the insoluble fraction which also contained the collagen. It is possible that the type of loose connective tissue formed in polyvinyl sponges may not be representative of connective tissue generally. As a result of feeding experiments with C^{14}-labelled acetate, Noble and Boucek (1957) suggested that cells of connective tissue formed in sponge implants can synthesize cholesterol. Bole *et al.* (1962) have shown that polyvinyl sponge is not completely inert, but itself undergoes changes *in vivo* involving loss of weight and increasing solubility in the chloroform-methanol solvent used for lipid extraction. These findings may account for the variability of earlier results. These workers also suggested methods for minimizing errors from these sources, and emphasized the effects on the results of the site chosen for implantation. Interscapular implants gave high values due to contamination by adipose cells of the fibrous capsule that forms around the implant, the main component of which is neutral fat. Low dorso-lumbar implants were found to be free from this contamination.

TABLE 12

Cholesterol and phospholipid concentrations in rabbit subcutaneous connective tissue
(McCandless et al. 1960)

Age	Cholesterol mg/g	Phospholipid mg $P \times 25$/g			
		Total	Cephalin	Lecithin	Sphingomyelin
3 weeks	1·86	9·2	2·9	2·9	2·0
5 weeks	2·75	8·9	2·7	3·4	2·3

The cholesterol and phospholipid concentrations in carrageenin-stimulated subcutaneous connective tissue of rabbits have been determined by McCandless *et al.* (1960), values for the normal animals being shown in Table 12. When the animals were fed with cholesterol, the cholesterol content of the tissue increased eight-fold and the phospholipid content only slightly. Fat-filled cells, resembling macrophages, appeared but there were no related changes in collagen development. Levin and Head (1965) found that incorporation of C^{14}-labelled acetate into sterols in carrageenin-stimulated guinea pig granulomata was greater after three days, when leucocytes are present, than after eight days when fibroblasts and macrophages are the most numerous cells. A change in the composition of the lipid fraction suggested that in the later stages, lipid may have been produced by fibroblasts. Jackson (1964) has found that fibroblasts in healing wounds are capable of synthesizing a variety of lipids.

Bovine foetal dental pulp has been shown to contain 6% of its dry weight of phospholipids of which 80% are directly extractable, 10% more after treatment with EDTA and the final 10% in slightly acidified solvent (Shapiro and Wuthier, 1966). The types of phospholipid present were the same as those in mineralized dental tissues (Table 14). Unidentified lipids detected in pulp were considered to be similar to those in hard tissues, which may be responsible for Sudan black staining in zones undergoing mineralization. Melcher (1967a) has demonstrated the presence of lipid in the corium of monkey skin and gingiva by staining with Sudan black dissolved in acetone. This lipid appears to be strongly bound to collagen fibres, or material in their neighbourhood, since the staining is strikingly increased after extraction with acidified chloroform:methanol, although it is eventually abolished by increasing the time and temperature of extraction. In a parallel chemical and histological investigation, isolated rat tail tendons which have a high collagen content and which are relatively free from extraneous lipids, were examined for bound lipid (Melcher, 1967e). The isolated tendons were sectioned and extracted in changes of acidified chloroform:methanol, the second extract being found to contain small amounts of two unidentified substances which behaved like lipids on silica gel thin-layer chromatograms, but were not phospholipids. This small amount of lipid apparently bound to collagen, may bear some relation to the larger proportion reported in reticulin by Windrum et al. (1955), or the similar staining material in hard tissues. However, it is obvious that the problem requires extensive investigation.

(b) *Lipids in mineralized tissues.* Calcified connective tissues in general contain substantially smaller amounts of lipidic substances than soft tissues. However, such lipids as are present more nearly represent true connective tissue constituents, because gross portions of bone and dentine are readily separated manually from adventitious tissue elements which permeate softer tissues and from which they are more difficult to dissect. Leach (1958) showed that small amounts of various non-polar lipids and phospholipid are present in compact bone from bovine femora (Table 13). Wuthier and Irving (1964) have confirmed the presence of all these lipid fractions in developing calf bone which they divided into resting, proliferating and hypertrophic cartilage, primary spongiosa and cancellous bone. The non-polar lipid fraction of bone also included free fatty acids, and was two to three times more abundant than the phospholipids. The phospholipid group contained all those substances subsequently reported in dentine (Table 14), except cardiolipin, and in addition, four unidentified lipids.

Leopold et al. (1951) reported the presence of 0·024% of cholesterol in human dentine, partly as the sterol and partly in esterified form. They considered it to be bound to protein. Hess et al. (1956) extracted 0·36% of total lipids from dentine by means of ethanol followed by ether; these included 0·014% of phospholipids. A more detailed analysis of the major groups of non-polar lipids present in human dentine (Dirksen and Ikels, 1964) showed similar amounts to those in bone, except for a lower triglyceride content

(Table 13). Shapiro *et al.* (1966) found a total phospholipid content of 0·12% in bovine foetal dentine based on the weight of demineralized tissue. This corresponds to approximately 0·03% on whole dentine, which is appreciably higher than earlier values. Most of this could be extracted with chloroform-methanol before demineralization, but approximately one quarter was

TABLE 13

Lipids extracted from bone and dentine

	Ox bone (Leach, 1958) mineralized	Human dentine (Dirksen and Ikels, 1964) mineralized	demineralized
Total extracted	0·07	0·041	0·177
Free cholesterol	0·0089	0·003	0·007
Cholesterol esters	0·0011	0·003	0·004
Triglycerides	0·054	0·002	0·002
Diglycerides	—	0·001	0·001
Monoglycerides	—	0·0005	0·0008
Phospholipid (P ×25)	0·0015	0·002	0·005

Values are expressed as per cent by weight of mineralized tissue.

TABLE 14

Phospholipids of bovine foetal dentine and pulp (Shapiro et al. 1966, Shapiro and Wuthier, 1966)

		Dentine	Pulp
neutral phosphatides	Sphingomyelin	11·0	13·6
	Lecithin	56·0	38·9
	Phosphatidylethanolamine	17·5	17·5
acid phosphatides	Phosphatidylinositol	4·0	3·0
	Phosphatidylserine	9·0	20·9
	Phosphatidic acid	2·0	4·2
	Cardiolipin	1·0	1·3

Values for the total quantity of each phospholipid extracted are expressed as a percentage of total phospholipids.

extractable only after removal of the inorganic fraction. The presence of almost all the individual lipid substances previously reported in dentine by Dirksen (1963) was confirmed, and the relative proportions of the phospholipids determined (Table 14).

Irving (1958) has described a method for selectively staining with Sudan black those sites in bone and teeth, where mineralization is assumed to be taking place. A preliminary extraction with pyridine is necessary to unmask the substance to be stained. At first the material was thought to be a polysaccharide but, because of its eventual removal by prolonged extraction with appropriate solvents, it was subsequently considered to be a lipid which does not contain phosphorus, unsaturated bonds (Irving, 1963), sulphate, free amino groups or plasmologens, but may be acidic (Wuthier and Irving, 1964). Staining in the mineralization zones is extracellular, but Sudanophilic particles have also been observed in the intracellular granules of odontoblasts and the cells of epiphyseal cartilage. The possibility of this unidentified substance acting as a nucleating site for mineralization has been suggested on the basis of various lipids being known to associate with calcium or inorganic phosphate ions. The chemical nature of lipids specifically present in calcified tissues is currently being investigated (Shapiro, 1967).

IV. Dynamics of the Tissues of the Periodontium

A. ORIGIN OF CELLS RESPONSIBLE FOR SYNTHESIS AND REMOVAL OF CONNECTIVE TISSUES

It has been shown in Section **II** that highly specialized cells are responsible for the synthesis of all connective tissues, and for resorption of mineralized connective tissues. This section is concerned with the stem cells from which fibroblasts, osteoblasts, cementoblasts and osteoclasts are derived.

1. Fibroblasts

Embryologically, fibroblasts are derived from mesoderm. However, there is controversy over the identity of the cells which give rise to new fibroblasts required for mature connective tissues. This topic has recently been reviewed by Van Winkle (1967), who points out that two theories concerning their origin have been advanced. The first maintains that they originate from emigré blood-borne cells, and the second that they arise locally from cells in loose connective tissue, particularly those associated with blood vessels. The older evidence advanced by the protagonists of the two different views was based largely on morphological observations. More recently, information has been obtained from *in vitro* and *in vivo* cell culture, and by use of irradiation and radioautography. Nevertheless, the conflict has still not been resolved convincingly.

Blood cells have been cultured in a number of experiments, and the results of these have tended to suggest that at least some of the cells have the potential to modulate and produce a substance chemically or morphologically identifiable as collagen. However, Ross and Lillywhite (1965) have emphasized the importance of avoiding contamination of the blood sample by tissue fibro-blasts during the operative procedures. They have performed experiments in which steps were taken to obtain blood cells free of other connective tissue cells, and these have not supported the belief held by earlier workers that some blood cells have fibroblastic potential.

The radioautographic and irradiation experiments of workers such as MacDonald (1959) and Grillo and Potsaid (1961) also favour a local origin for the fibroblasts. Dunphy (1963), Grillo (1964), and Van Winkle (1967) all agree with this view, although Grillo admits the possibility that blood-borne cells may give rise to an insignificant proportion of the collagen-producing cells. However, Gillman and Wright (1966), on the basis of experiments in which H^3-thymidine was administered before making a skin wound, concluded that some blood-borne mononuclear cells may emigrate to the damaged tissue, undergo mitosis, and eventually become morphologically indistinguishable from fibroblasts. It is possible that these dividing cells could readily be confused with perivascular cells of the part if labelling with isotope is carried out post-operatively, as is usually the case. It has therefore not yet been proved beyond doubt that all fibroblasts involved in wound repair are derived from local sources. The possibility remains that at least some of them are derived from haematogenous stem cells which are able to become fibroblastic under appropriate conditions.

The role of fibrocytes is controversial. For example, Van Winkle (1967) concludes that they can play no further role in fibrogenesis, whereas Glücks-mann (1964) has found that they can take up radioactive sulphate, which suggests that they are capable of secreting ground substances. Messier and Leblond (1960) have shown that dermal fibrocytes of young rats and mice have a low turnover, and this observation has been supported by Glücksmann. It is clear that the behaviour of this cell is not nearly so well understood as its actively secreting precursor.

2. Osteoblasts and Cementoblasts

A cell may be called an osteoblast only at the time when it is synthesizing bone matrix (Bassett, 1964). For a number of years it has been believed that the several types of specialized bone cells are different functional states of the same cell (Bloom et al., 1941). However, the extent to which the various specialized cells are able to modulate from one functional state to another is open to question.

It seems to be accepted widely that osteoblasts are derived from the undiff-erentiated connective tissue cells which Heller et al. (1950) described as spindle-shaped. These cells have been called by a number of different names, but are possibly most frequently known as *undifferentiated mesenchymal cells*. Young (1963b) considers that this term confers upon them too wide a potential, and prefers to call them *osteoprogenitor cells.* However, as under certain circumstances, cells derived from populations which might be expected to give rise to bone, form cartilage or unmineralized connective tissue instead (for example, see Bassett, 1964), it might be wiser to retain the term *undifferentiated cell.* Owen (1963) has called them pre-osteoblasts, but perhaps this term, like that of osteoprogenitor cell, describes the cell once it is committed to a path of differentiation.

Little seems to have been written about the origin of the undifferentiated cell and it is apparently assumed that this cell is a local resident. Although cells associated with small vessels have been favoured as the font of these cells (Trueta, 1963), the controversy that surrounds the origin of fibroblasts does not seem to have been raised in relation to osteoblasts. Owen (1963) has found, at least in the developing long bone of rabbit, that fibroblasts do not make any significant contribution to the population of cells concerned in osteogenesis.

The transformation of undifferentiated cells into osteoblasts has been confirmed by tracer experiments using tritiated thymidine (Kember, 1960; Young, 1962a and Owen, 1963). The undifferentiated cells synthesize DNA and undergo mitosis, after which some of the daughter cells differentiate into osteoblasts, surround themselves with bone matrix and become transformed into osteocytes. However, not all the undifferentiated cells that take up thymidine divide (Owen and MacPherson, 1963) and, in addition, it has been shown that an exceedingly small proportion of osteoblasts will also take up thymidine (Tonna and Cronkite, 1961). It seems apparent that not all osteoblasts are incorporated into bone as osteocytes. Both Owen (1963) and Young (1963b) state that osteoblast death is rarely observed, and the latter author is of the opinion that many revert to the pool of undifferentiated cells.

Few investigations aimed directly at elucidating the origin of cementoblasts appear to have been carried out. However, morphological studies on developing teeth appear to suggest that they stem from undifferentiated cells in the periodontal ligament (Selvig, 1963).

3. Osteoclasts and Cementoclasts

Kölliker, according to Tonna (1963), proposed in 1873 that osteoclasts are formed by the fusion of osteoblasts. Since that time much argument has raged between those who believe that osteoclasts are the result of fusion of mononuclear cells, and those who believe that division of nuclei in the absence of cytoplasmic cleavage leads to the formation of multinucleated osteoclasts. Work using tritiated thymidine has shown unequivocally that osteoclast nuclei do not synthesize DNA and therefore do not divide (Kember, 1960; Tonna and Cronkite, 1961; Young, 1963b). This proof hinges on the fact that triated thymidine is available for incorporation into DNA for less than an hour after injection, and osteoclast nuclei are found to be labelled only after longer periods following injection, and frequently only one of the nuclei present in the cell is involved. This observation supports the view that osteoclasts are formed by fusion of mononucleated cells. However, it is of interest that Cameron et al. (1964) have not yet seen cells in the electron microscope that are in the process of fusing.

The next question to be answered is what type of cells fuse to form osteoclasts. Tonna and Cronkite (1961) and Tonna (1963) believe that preosteoblasts and osteoblasts may be involved. Kember (1960) thinks that the relevant cells are undifferentiated cells. In this he is supported by Young (1964), who points out that osteoblasts and osteoclasts synthesize very different substances. This means that the cytoplasmic components must be reorganized extensively before direct transition from the functional state of osteoblast to that of osteoclast can take place. Jee and Nolan (1963) claim to have produced evidence that osteoclasts can result from the fusion of histiocytes, but Tonna (1963) has disputed their conclusion and maintains that histiocytes are not the main contributors to osteoclasts and may not contribute at all. Tonna's view is supported by the experiments of Irving and Handelman (1963). In this connection, it is of interest that Fischman and Hay (1962) have shown that osteoclasts in newts form by fusion of mononucleated leukocytes, probably monocytes. This finding may of course be peculiar to the salamander. The available evidence in mammals certainly seems to implicate the undifferentiated cells as precursors of osteoclasts, but the possibility has not yet been excluded that other cells might also be involved. However, a recent electron microscopic investigation by Scott (1967) has opened up an entirely new aspect of the question. She claims to have shown that osteoblasts and osteoclasts are each derived from different, morphologically distinct, perivascular precursor cells.

Foreign body giant cells are similar in appearance to osteoclasts, although some differences in size and morphology have been described (Irving and Handelman, 1963; Mathews et al., 1967). Some of their oxidative and hydrolytic enzymes have been examined histochemically (Cabrini et al., 1962; Irving and Handelman, 1963). The latter investigators obtained a comparatively stronger reaction for acid phosphatase in osteoclasts. It is not yet clear whether the two types of giant cells are formed from identical precursor cells, but Irving and Handelman's system is one in which this problem might conceivably be investigated.

Before concluding this section, the concept propounded by Bloom et al. (1941), that the several types of cells found in and around bone are different functional states of the same cell, must be taken up. Recently, Tonna (1960) and Young (1964), on the basis of their studies with tritiated thymidine, have supported this belief. They are both of the opinion that osteoclasts can disassociate into apparently less specialized cells (osteoprogenitor cells of Young) which are then available once again for differentiation into either osteoblasts or osteoclasts. Mathews *et al.* (1967) believe that the arrangement of the centrioles in osteoclasts is related to their potential dissolution. On the other hand, as discussed on page 197, effete osteoclasts are frequently seen in organ culture. Young believes that there may be turnover of cells in osteoclasts, new cells differentiating and being incorporated, while constituent cells disassociate and return to the undifferentiated state. Young also believes that osteoblasts can "dedifferentiate" to less specialized cells which, if required, can then acquire osteoclastic characteristics. The morphological changes which take place in osteoblasts after administration of parathyroid extract described by Heller *et al.* (1950), and confirmed many times since, certainly lend support for this view. However, a great deal of direct evidence still needs to be obtained before the concept of Bloom *et al.* can be regarded as proven. The fate of osteocytes released from resorbed bone is particularly obscure.

The relationship between osteoclasts and the giant cells which are associated with resorption of cementum can, at present, only be assumed. The origin and fate of these cells does not appear, as yet, to have attracted much attention.

B. SYNTHESIS OF CONNECTIVE TISSUES

1. Soft Connective Tissues

(a) *Intracellular synthesis.* A consideration of the synthesis of soft connective tissues must take into account elaboration in the fibroblast of each of the extracellular constituents, their secretion by the fibroblast and, finally, their aggregation into the extracellular fabric. Osteoblasts and chondroblasts are able to produce similar substances, but synthesize and secrete them in different proportions. Indeed, the relative amounts required of collagen and protein-polysaccharides, and of the different protein-polysaccharides, varies in different soft connective tissues. Electron microscopic and biochemical investigations carried out in recent years have elucidated these processes considerably, but many problems remain and there is much that is still poorly understood. It should be mentioned that there is some evidence that collagen may be produced by cells other than those normally implicated in the process. Green and Goldberg (1965) have found that Hela cells, which are a long-standing strain of cultured cells originally explanted from a carcinoma, can produce small quantities of collagen *in vitro*. Furthermore, Hay and Revel (1963) believe that dermal epithelial cells of ambystoma can produce collagen, but their evidence is inconclusive, and Ross and Klebanoff (1967) have observed changes in smooth muscle cells which suggest that these might be able to produce collagen under certain circumstances.

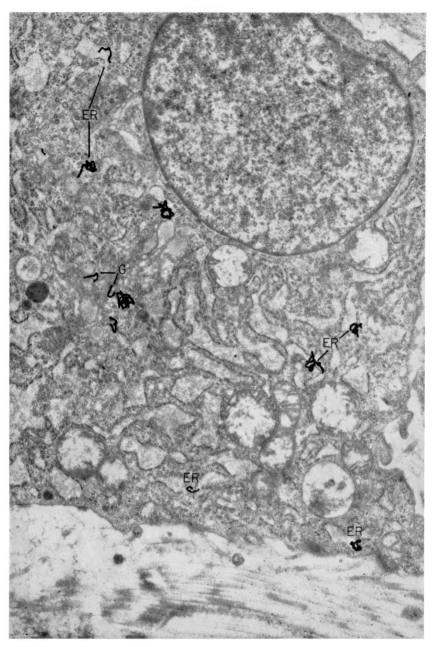

FIG. 60. Radioautograph of a portion of a 7-day wound 30 minutes after intraperitoneal administration of proline—H³. In this particular cell the silver grains can be seen to lie over both ergastoplasm (ER) and Golgi complex (G). The collagen fibrils in this area are not labelled. (× 10,000.) (Reproduced with permission from R. Ross and E. P. Benditt, *J. Cell Biol.* **27**, 83–106, 1965.)

As discussed earlier, there is considerable evidence that proteins, both collagenous and non-collagenous, are elaborated in the GER. The evidence for collagen synthesis is based largely on observations on the passage of H^3-proline into the cell, and its rapid localization in the Golgi complex and GER (Hay and Revel, 1963; Revel and Hay, 1963; Ross and Benditt, 1965) (Fig. 60). Unfortunately, this morphological evidence is necessarily circumstantial as it is as yet not possible to be certain that the proline is incorporated into collagen and not into other proteins. However, the biochemical analyses of Fitton Jackson (1958) and Lowther *et al.* (1961) point very strongly to the GER being the site at which collagen is synthesized. It is reasonable to assume that, in a tissue which is rapidly synthesizing collagen, a fair proportion of proline or glycine passing into the cell is destined for incorporation into that protein, and Ross and Benditt (1965) have found that fibroblasts do not store proline. It has been shown morphologically, at least in chondrogenesis, that proline passes from the GER to the Golgi vesicles (Revel and Hay, 1963). A detailed study of fibrogenesis in healing guinea-pig skin by Ross and Benditt (1965) has demonstrated that not all of the proline follows this path, and that some of it finds its way from the GER to the exterior by some other route. The belief in an alternative pathway has received support from Cooper and Prockop (1968), who have found in an *in vitro* study of cartilage that collagen macromolecules pass directly from the ground cytoplasm of the cell to the exterior. At present it is not possible to say whether the passage of collagen is restricted to any one pathway.

A number of questions now arise. These are concerned with synthesis of the collagen macromolecule, and the form in which, and means by which, it is secreted from the cell. Knowing that collagen is synthesized in the cell, what is the sequence of the synthetic process? It is conceivable that the three α chains might be synthesized individually, and then assembled in the characteristic triple helix. Alternatively, perhaps the triple helix is built as a single unit, the three α chains growing simultaneously *in situ*. Moreover, disregarding the method by which the macromolecule is built, are the α chains made by the addition of amino acids one at a time, or, are the amino acids assembled into sub-units, and these then aligned to form α chains. Unfortunately, as yet there is no answer to any of these questions.

The next question is whether final assembly of the collagen macromolecule occurs intracellularly, or whether it is secreted in parts which are assembled extracellularly. Lowther *et al.* (1961) have extracted from cellular fractions, material having an amino acid composition which is characteristic of collagen. Fitton Jackson (1965), however, has not been able to precipitate hydroxy-proline-rich material extracted from cellular fractions into electron microscopically identifiable collagen fibrils, a manoeuvre that can readily be performed successfully on extracts of extracellular connective tissue. The results of this experiment do not necessarily exclude the presence of macromolecular collagen intracellularly. They may alternatively, be interpreted as suggesting that collagen macromolecules undergo some change during secretion which allows them to aggregate to form fibrils. In general, opinions expressed in the literature, although not based on incontrovertible evidence, appear to favour intracellular synthesis of the whole macromolecule.

It has also been suggested that collagen fibrils are assembled intracellularly, but this is no longer widely held (Ross and Benditt, 1961; Fernando and Movat, 1963a; Goldberg and Green, 1964; Hancox and Boothroyd, 1965). There have been at least two reports of collagen fibrils, identifiable in the electron microscope, being observed intracellularly in membranous vesicles. In one case they were seen in cartilage from rabbits which had been given papain (Sheldon and Kimball, 1962), and in the other in specimens of pathological material (Welsh and Meyer, 1967).

The remaining question concerns the manner in which collagen is secreted by the cell. Some investigators have suggested that collagen is contained in fragments of cytoplasm shed by the fibroblast, that is by apocrine secretion, and that this process involves disruption of the cell membrane (Chapman, 1962). The weight of evidence now seems to favour the secretion of collagen being merocrine in nature, a process not involving disruption of the plasma membrane (Fernando and Movat 1963a; Goldberg and Green, 1964; Porter, 1964; Ross and Benditt, 1965). The disruption or discontinuity of the plasma membrane which is seen in electronmicrographs is possibly an artefact. How the collagen passes through the membrane is unknown, but Fitton Jackson (1964) has suggested that alkaline phosphatase, which may be located at or just within the cell membrane, may play some part. In this connection, it has long been known that connective tissue cells active in fibrogenesis exhibit a strong histochemical reaction for alkaline phosphatase (Fell and Danielli, 1943). Fitton Jackson (1956) found a strong reaction for the enzyme in the earliest intercellular spaces of developing avian tendon, and Gold and Gould (1951) have found that newly formed collagen fibres are rich in alkaline phosphatase, which they suggest might be absorbed from surrounding tissue fluids. A finding which may eventually prove to be of significance in understanding how collagen is secreted by the cell is that of Bhatnagar et al. (1968), who have shown that cartilage cells will not secrete collagen until proline and lysine have been hydroxylated.

The intracellular synthesis of protein-polysaccharide complexes must now be discussed. Early work carried out by Dziewiatkowsky et al. (1949) and Dziewiatkowsky (1951) showed that exogenous S^{35} is incorporated into chondroitin sulphates. Later, Grossfeld et al. (1956) showed that human skin and bone cells produce acid mucopolysaccharides, and Bélanger (1954) found that, in cartilage, S^{35} is taken up initially by the cells and then extruded into the extracellular matrix. Fewer et al. (1964) and Godman and Lane (1964) then demonstrated that S^{35} appears in the vesicles of the Golgi apparatus shortly after administration. It could not be detected in the GER, suggesting that this organelle plays no part in incorporating sulphate into polysaccharides. The isotope was then seen to migrate peripherally through the cytoplasm contained, according to Godman and Lane, in vesicles which lodged for relatively long periods in the cortex of the cell before discharging their contents into the extracellular milieu.

Peterson and Leblond (1964) have speculated on the sequence of events that occur in formation of glycoproteins. They suggest that after synthesis in the GER, the protein moiety is transferred to the vesicles of the Golgi zone. There monosaccharides become linked to one another and to proteins. Finally, the "packaged" glycoprotein migrates to the periphery of the cell where it is secreted into the extracellular environment. The available evidence appears to suggest the possibility that a similar pathway is taken by sulphated acid mucopolysaccharides. There is some evidence to suggest that proteins and polysaccharides are synthesized simultaneously (Gross et al., 1960; Dziewiatkowsky, 1964). Contrary to the earlier views however, Horwitz and Dorfman (1968) have concluded from a biochemical investigation that some hexosamine is added to the core-protein at the ribosome, and that other sugars are added in the GER.

It has been pointed out by Fitton Jackson (1960) that in each individual tissue the respective synthesizing cell must be assumed to be capable of producing both the fibrous protein and the other extracellular material of the matrix. As collagen and protein-polysaccharide complexes are found in such intimate relationship in the extracellular substance and, as has been discussed in Section III, the latter may influence the polymerization and orientation of the former, it might also be assumed that the synthesis and secretion of one may influence that of the other. However, Bhatnagar and Prockop (1966), using selective inhibitors, have shown that chondroblasts can synthesize and secrete collagen and sulphated mucopolysaccharides independently of one another.

Synthesis and secretion of the lipid component thought to be present in extracellular connective tissue remains to be discussed. Unfortunately, there is virtually no information available on this topic.

Finally, reference must be made to elastogenesis. It seems reasonable to suppose that fibroblasts produce elastin as well as the other extracellular components, but fibroblasts concerned with producing elastin-rich connective tissue do not exhibit any features which differ significantly from fibroblasts in other situations (Fahrenbach et al. 1966).

(b) *Extracellular synthesis* (see also Section III). There is a strong belief that initial aggregation of collagen macromolecules occurs at the cell surface (Fitton Jackson, 1956; Porter and Pappas, 1959; see Fitton Jackson, 1964). In this connection, it is of interest that Kallman and Grobstein (1965) have performed *in vitro* experiments which suggest that collagen secreted by connective tissue cells may aggregate at the surface of adjacent epithelial cells. *In vivo* and *in vitro* the first fibrils to appear in the developing connective tissue are too thin to exhibit the characteristic 640 Å periodicity of collagen fibrils (Section **II**), and either show no periodicity or a repeat period smaller than normal (Fitton Jackson, 1956; Goldberg and Green, 1964). Circumstantial evidence suggests that these fibrils are collagen, and this suggestion is supported by the work of Fitton Jackson and Smith (1957), who were able to detect protein-bound hydroxyproline in cultures of osteoblasts before they could identify typical collagen fibrils in the electron microscope. Eventually, thicker fibrils showing characteristic periodicity are found, and these become laid down in bundles. It is evident that aggregation of collagen macromolecules serves two distinct, tightly controlled, processes. The first of these is the establishment of new collagen fibrils, and the second, the thickening and lengthening of pre-existing fibrils by addition of new macromolecules. The former is evidently under direct control of the fibroblast, the latter less obviously so. The orderly nature of the process of fibre growth suggests however, that it is in some way controlled by cells. The close control exercised over these processes is shown by the remarkable uniform thickness of fibrils laid down in embryonic connective tissue (Fitton Jackson, 1956) and in connective tissue developing in healing wounds (Ross and Benditt, 1961; Fernando and Movat, 1963a), and by the exquisitely precise orientation of fibres in so many connective tissues. Both these pairs of workers have found that repairing connective tissue contains two populations of fibrils: one, of uniformly small diameter in the vicinity of the fibroblasts; the other, of uniformly thicker diameter occupying areas more remote from the fibroblasts.

As discussed in Section **III**, newly formed collagen macromolecules which are present in the extracellular milieu, but not yet tightly bound to other macromolecules, are readily soluble. The work of Gross (1958a,b) suggests that, in normally developing tissue, there is a slight lag between the time when the macromolecules are extruded from the cell and their being tightly crosslinked to other macromolecules. This is consistent with the view that they may be deposited on fibrils at a distance from the cell; the mechanism which determines the site of aggregation is unknown. Control may be effected by enzymatic processes directed by the cell.

Extracellular material, which probably contains acid mucopolysaccharides since it is metachromatic or stainable by alcian blue, can be identified in the light microscope at an earlier stage than developing collagen fibres (Fitton Jackson, 1956; Fernando and Movat, 1963a). The latter authors consider the granular interfibrillar material seen in the electron microscope to correspond with this material. Fitton Jackson reports that the earliest fibres are paS positive, which indicates that some form of neutral polysaccharide is intimately associated with them.

The developing collagen fibrils at first show no definite orientation

(Fernando and Movat, 1963a), but gradually are gathered into clearly identifiable bundles of varying shape and size. It is therefore conceivable that, as the fibrous architecture of the tissue is established, a constant re-modelling of collagen fibrils occurs. Fitton Jackson (1957a) has found that, in developing avian tendon, the controlled thickening of fibrils that occurs with age does so at the expense of the interfibrillar material, and that this process is accompanied by enlargement of the size of the fibril bundles. The control of fibril diameter extends to adult tissues, where the final dia-meter of the collagen fibrils and of the bundles into which they are gathered, is remarkably constant for any given tissue (Fitton Jackson, 1964).

When viewed in the light microscope, the earliest fibres seen in developing connective tissue which has been impregnated with silver, are very thin, argyrophilic, and arranged in a branched network. At a later stage of de-velopment, few of these fibres can be seen, but numerous, rather thicker, wavy fibres, which resemble mature collagen fibres, but which are still argyrophilic, are present. These fibres, unlike the branched fibres, are readily soluble in neutral or acid solvents (Jackson and Williams, 1956; Robb-Smith, 1957; Melcher, 1964). Later in development, mature connective tissue appears to comprise only non-argyrophilic collagen fibres. However, although difficult to see because of the overwhelming mass of collagen fibres, a net-work of the branched argyrophilic elements is present (Gross, 1961), and has been identified in skin (Kaye, 1929) and in gingiva (Melcher, 1964; 1965a) ensheathing the mature collagen fibres.

The terminology of argyrophilic fibres and their role in fibrogenesis has greatly confused microscopists (see Melcher, 1966b). The problems raised by this confusion are three-fold. Firstly, because the terminology is loose, it is often difficult to identify the type of argyrophilic structure being described. Secondly, there is still doubt about which structures seen in the electron microscope correspond with the two types of argyrophilic elements described by light microscopists. Finally, the presence of branched argyrophilic elements in both young developing and mature connective tissues, in contrast to the wavy argyrophilic fibres which are present in developing connective tissue only, has not yet been explained satisfactorily.

In an attempt to clarify the use of terms, we subscribe to the view of Robb-Smith (1957) that only the elements of the branched argyrophilic network should be called *reticulin*. The wavy argyrophilic fibres, which have the con-figuration of mature collagen fibres, and which are soluble, should be de-scribed quite differently, and we favour the term *argyrophilic developing collagen fibres*.

When seen in the electron microscope at an early stage of development, the extracellular substance comprises randomly orientated fibrils, which are unbanded or have the typical banding of collagen. The fibrils are distributed singly or in small bundles of different sizes, and are located in a mass of interfibrillar substance (Figs 61 and 62). The appearance of this complex given by Little and Kramer (1952) and Kramer and Little (1953) conforms to the description of the ultrastructure of reticulin isolated from parenchymatous organs (Section **III**). Material of similar appearance is also present in areas

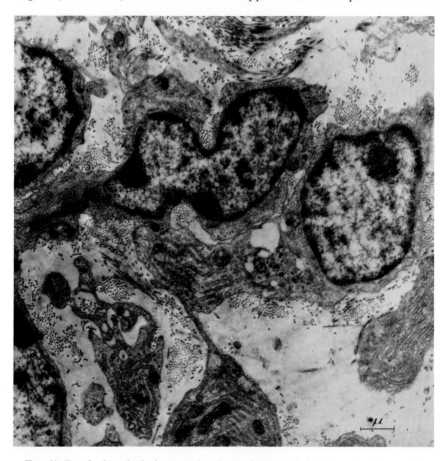

FIG. 61. Developing gingival connective tissue of mouse 18 days *in utero*. Young differentiating fibroblasts, and recently deposited intercellular substance comprising relatively few collagen fibrils and some unbanded thinner fibrils, and a large proportion of poorly defined interfibrillar material. Some of the collagen fibrils are randomly arranged, while others are gathered together in small bundles. The intercellular substance is believed to be reticulin.

corresponding to those seen in the light microscope to be occupied by reticulin networks, for example, the subepithelial reticulin of mature human gingiva and that between collagen fibres (Melcher, 1965a, Figs 63 and 64). One barrier to accepting that the two descriptions describe light and electron microscopic representations of the same structure is the obviously fibrous nature of the network when seen in the light microscope, in contrast to the amorphous, though fibril-containing material, which is seen in electron-micrographs. The explanation possibly lies in the very different circumstances under which they are viewed. The reticulin probably forms a continuum filling the spaces between the cells or, in some situations such as for

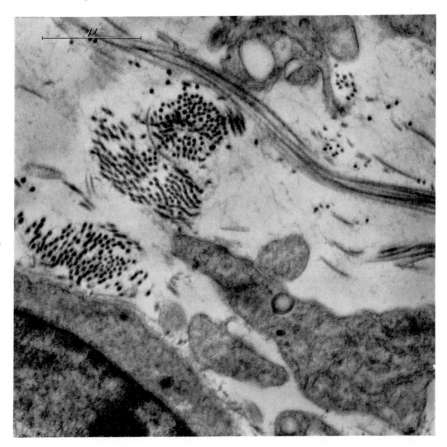

FIG. 62. Developing gingival connective tissue of mouse 18 days *in utero* at higher magnification than in Fig. 61. Some of the bundles of fibrils in the intercellular substance are sufficiently large to be resolved by the light microscope. Others, are not. The bundles are believed to be enlarging within the reticulin of which they are a part.

example beneath the epithelium of skin and gingiva or in the depths of the lamina propria, between cells and bundles of collagen fibrils. It is unlikely to be separated from the ground substance associated with the collagen fibres. This continuum, when viewed at the lower magnifications of the light microscope, will be seen to form a branched network and, as a result of the methods used to demonstrate it, will appear to comprise fibres. Stated in a different way, the light microscope reveals the contours of the whole structure, whereas the electron microscope reveals the fine components which go to make the elements of the structure. It is for this reason that we consider it unwise to refer to the elements seen in the light microscope as reticulin *fibres*.

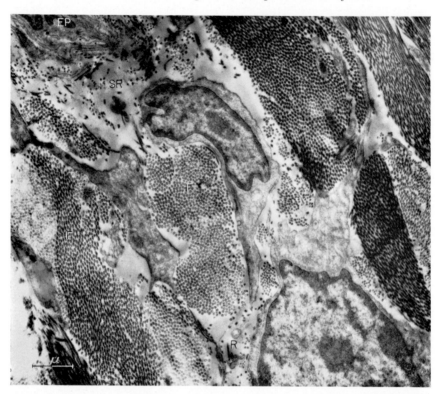

FIG. 63. Electron micrograph of connective tissue of attached gingiva from a mature monkey. Intercellular material, similar in appearance to the intercellular substance of young developing connective tissue, is present in sites corresponding to those where reticulin is seen at light microscopic magnifications; that is subepithelially and between collagen fibres. A small part of an epithelial cell (EP) is present in the upper left-hand quadrant. Between it and collagen fibres (F) is material believed to be subepithelial reticulin (SR). Small areas of material believed to be reticulin (R) are also present between collagen fibres and fibroblasts.

Three hypotheses have been offered to explain the role of argyrophilic fibres in developing and mature connective tissues. The first of these, offered by Maximow (1928), suggests that the reticulin network is transformed into collagen fibres as a result of traction exerted upon it by connective tissue cells. This hypothesis does not explain the presence of reticulin in mature connective tissues, and Robb-Smith (1957; 1958) has suggested that reticulin and argyrophilic developing collagen fibres are synthesized separately by fibroblasts, but that only the latter develop into mature collagen fibres. More recently, in an

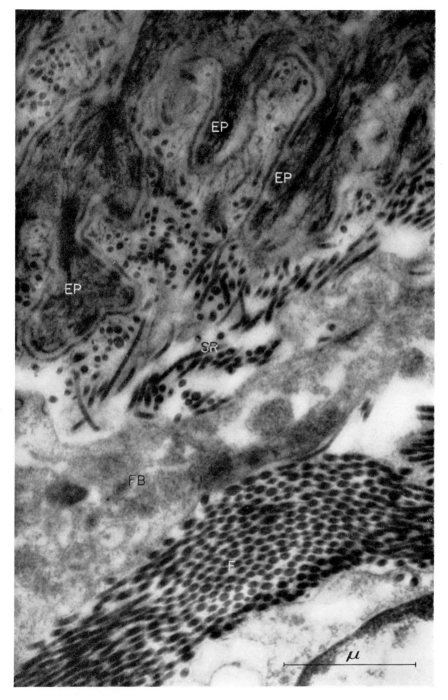

Fig. 64. Electron micrograph of connective tissue of attached gingiva from a mature monkey at higher magnification than in Fig. 63, contrasting the appearance of the sub-epithelial reticulin (SR) with a mature collagen fibre (F). Processes of an epithelial cell (EP) and part of a fibroblast (FB) are present. The lamina densa, and its related "hemi-desmosomes" and attachment filaments, can be seen.

attempt to reconcile the light and electron microscopic findings, Melcher (1966b) has suggested an alternative hypothesis. This proposes that reticulin which is secreted by the fibroblasts, provides the milieu in which collagen fibrils can be developed, and aggregated into collagen fibres, or in which collagen building blocks can be stored. This double role accounts for its presence in both young developing and mature connective tissues. Formation of collagen fibrils and fibres occurs within its substance and at its expense, and not by the transformation of reticulin *fibres* into collagen fibres. The reticulin present in mature connective tissues represents extracellular material which has not been colonized by collagen fibres. However, it is thought that under appropriate physiological and pathological stimuli this could occur, as for example in cirrhosis of the liver. The argyrophilic developing collagen fibres are thought to correspond to the bundles of collagen fibrils larger than 0.2μ in diameter that are present in, or at the periphery of, reticulin in actively developing connective tissue. They are therefore collagen fibres that are currently being thickened.

Very little is known about the forces which control the orientation of the collagen fibres in different connective tissues. However, the intimate relationship that exists between function and anatomy is exquisitely illustrated by the uniform arrangement of collagen fibres in a tendon, and also by the arrangement of the different groups of collagen fibres in the connective tissue of the gingiva. Elegant *in vitro* evidence is available which shows that tension plays a large part in orientating collagen fibres (Bassett, 1962).

Incorporation of protein-polysaccharide moieties into developing connective tissues has been studied largely in connective tissue being laid down in repair processes, and mostly by means of histochemical methods and light microscopy, or by biochemical techniques. Uptake of sulphate, and metachromasia, in a healing wound appears to reach a peak at a time that coincides with deposition of collagen fibres (Dunphy and Udupa, 1955; Kodicek and Loewi, 1956; Slack, 1957; Fernando and Movat, 1963b), and Bassett (1962) thinks that the paS-positive granules seen in osteoblasts may be associated with production of protein-polysaccharide substances. The metachromasia in developing tendon (Fitton Jackson, 1956) and in most other connective tissues, is gradually lost as the tissues mature. However, it must be remembered that inability to demonstrate acid mucopolysaccharides by histochemical methods does not necessarily mean that the substances are absent, but may result from the fact that they are tightly bound to other materials (for example, Toole and Lowther, 1966), and therefore cannot be stained by routine methods (Quintarelli, 1960a,b). Kent (1967) has reviewed some aspects of this topic and has pointed out that in the early stages of development the predominant acid mucopolysaccharide present is hyaluronic acid, whereas as the connective tissue matures, the balance shifts in favour of chondroitin sulphates. In contrast to metachromatic substances, the paS positive material, that is neutral and sialic acid-containing polysaccharide complexes, remains highly reactive in mature connective tissues developed in healing wounds (Dunphy and Udupa, 1955) and in other connective tissues.

Incorporation of lipid into developing connective tissue has received scant attention. There is some chemical and histological information concerning lipids laid down in forming connective tissues (Section III), and, a substance, thought on histological grounds to be lipid, appears to be bound in fibrous connective tissues as they mature (Melcher, 1967a).

The events which take place extracellularly in elastic fibrogenesis have only recently become the focus of systematic investigation. Much of the available information has been presented in Section IIA.

2. Osteogenesis and Cementogenesis

(a) *Intracellular synthesis.* The requirements for synthesis of hard connective tissues are organic matrix and mineral salts. Although there must, of necessity, be some quantitative and qualitative differences between the make-up of matrices of hard and soft connective tissues which allow mineralization of the former but not of the latter, the structure and function of the synthesizing osteoblast could reasonably be expected to resemble that of the functioning fibroblast. As discussed above, the structure of the osteoblast closely resembles that of the fibroblast. There is now adequate experimental evidence to confirm what has long been suspected, that osteoblasts synthesize the matrix of bone, and, furthermore, that osteocytes may also possess this capability (Dudley and Spiro, 1961; Young, 1962b; Bassett, 1962; page 319). The most striking difference between soft and hard connective tissues, the presence of mineral salts in the latter, might be assumed to be reflected in the cell structure. However, there is no evidence that this is so and, in fact, it looks very much as though the inorganic substances that take part in mineralization do not pass through the cell (Leblond *et al.*, 1950; Tonna and Pentel, 1967).

There does not appear to be any significant difference between the histochemical reaction of enzymes in osteoblasts and fibroblasts apparently involved in synthesis of extracellular matrix. Osteoblasts and the extracellular matrix, like fibroblasts and extracellular substance of soft connective tissue, give a positive histochemical reaction for alkaline phosphatase (Cabrini, 1961 and Fullmer, 1967). The latter author says that the role of this enzyme in bone formation is unknown, but Fitton Jackson (1964) has suggested a role for it in fibrogenesis (Section IVB) and Jeffree (1964) has found that there is a considerable degree of correlation between the alkaline phosphatase activity of whole bone and its rate of increase in weight. Histochemically demonstrable acid phosphatase has been described in osteoblasts (Cabrini, 1961; Ruyter, 1964) and in fibroblasts (Ruyter, 1964; Fullmer, 1965), but the role of this enzyme, if any, in synthesis of extracellular constituents of connective tissue is unknown.

One histochemically-demonstrable enzyme that does appear to play a significant role in synthesis of mineralized connective tissue is D (-) -β-hydroxybutyric dehydrogenase (Fullmer and Martin, 1964). However, as far as is known, these investigators have restricted their observations to hard connective tissues, but the results of their experiment are such as to suggest that the activity of the enzyme might also be related to synthesis of soft connective tissues.

It has recently been shown that osteogenesis follows a cyclic pattern. Simmons and Nichols (1966) have found that in rats osteogenesis is regulated diurnally, there being significantly greater activity in the environmental light period than in the environmental dark period.

(b) Extracellular synthesis. The early events in osteogenesis resemble those in soft connective tissue fibrogenesis. The organic matrix is characterized by randomly orientated collagen fibrils (Ascenzi, 1964). These eventually form bundles which gradually develop into layers having a criss-cross pattern (Fitton Jackson, 1957b; Dudley and Spiro, 1961; Cooper et al., 1966). The last pair of authors point out that the lamellar pattern of collagen fibrils in an Haversian system is established prior to mineralization. The diameter of the fibrils varies, but is generally reported to increase the further they are situated from the cell. For example, in bone obtained from developing chick, they have been found to range from between ~200 Å and ~400 Å to over 1200 Å (Dudley and Spiro, 1961; Decker, 1966). The fibrils eventually tend to be obscured by interfibrillar ground substance (Fitton Jackson, 1957b; Ascenzi, 1964) which the latter author has found to be hyaluronidase-labile. At the magnifications of the light microscope, this observation is paralleled by the fact that osteoid (like developing fibrous tissue) is metachromatic both in vivo (Johnson, 1964) and in vitro (Bassett, 1962).

It is evident from light microscopy, and particularly from electron microscopy, that a seam of organic matrix or osteoid is laid down prior to mineralization. Electron microscopy has shown that the mineralizing front in normally developing bone is always separated from the osteoblasts by a seam of osteoid. In addition to being metachromatic, the osteoid is paS reactive, being intensely so at the mineralizing front (Bevelander and Johnson, 1950; Heller-Steinberg, 1951; Cabrini, 1961). It might be mentioned that Moog and Wenger (1952) have suggested that there is a correlation between the presence of paS positive material and histochemically demonstrable alkaline phosphatase, but the precise significance of this observation does not appear yet to be clear. As has been discussed in Section IIIB, Irving (1963) has shown that the mineralizing front can be selectively stained by a special method for bound lipid and, furthermore, Johnson (1964) has pointed out that the junction between mineralized bone and osteoid is marked by a line that is strongly stained by haematoxylin and that there may be a correlation between these two observations.

There is some electron miscroscopic evidence to show that onset of mineralization occurs simultaneously with deposition of a mass of ground substance (Fitton Jackson, 1957b; Yaeger, 1961), and the light microscopic findings are not inconsistent with this belief. However, the precise location of the first deposited crystals of mineral salt is not resolved. Fitton Jackson and Randall (1956) and Fitton Jackson (1957b) have demonstrated that, at the start of mineralization of developing chick bone, small hydroxyapatite particles of less than 100 Å are deposited on the collagen fibrils, but not in the interfibrillar matrix. The particles were found to be localized in a ring almost exclusively between the d and ab bands of the main period of the fibril, but not to have a preferred orientation to the fibril axis. These observations have been supported by Dudley and Spiro (1961), who have described the presence of small dense mineral particles along the surface of the fibrils as well as within them, disposed in accordance with the periodicity of the fibril.

In contrast to these observations, some investigators claim that the first crystallites are not deposited in any particular relationship to the collagen fibrils (Ascenzi, 1964; Decker, 1966). However, in disagreement with Decker's views, Ascenzi believes that later in development the crystallites become orientated parallel to the fibres. Yaeger (1961), on the other hand, has found that in some areas of the specimen the inorganic particles were located both within the fibrils as well as between them. Contrary to the generally accepted view, Hancox and Boothroyd (1965) state that they have found the early deposits of inorganic crystallites to be randomly distributed in respect of the collagen fibrils; but they stress the fact that technical difficulties make precise observations on this problem difficult. They also found crystallites associated with cell processes, and postulate that cells may somehow influence the initiation of "seeding" of inorganic nuclei and so control the topography of mineralization. There are other indications that there is some relationship between collagen fibrils and inorganic matrix. Marino and Becker (1967) have claimed that there is a direct physical bond between apatite crystallites and collagen fibrils and, as mentioned earlier, Quigley and Hjørting-Hansen (1962) have shown that the inorganic framework of bone exhibits the electron microscopic periodicity of the collagen fibrils that have been removed.

The band of osteoid at the developing bone-face does not appear to show a gradient of mineralization (Dudley and Spiro, 1961). Usually, mineralization of a seam of osteoid appears to originate as isolated islands located near the mineralized surface, and these gradually coalesce (Yaeger, 1961; Ascenzi, 1964).

Sissons (1962) has clearly described the light microscopic and microradiographic appearance of forming bone. When stained with haematoxylin and eosin, the surface is covered by osteoblasts of active appearance separated

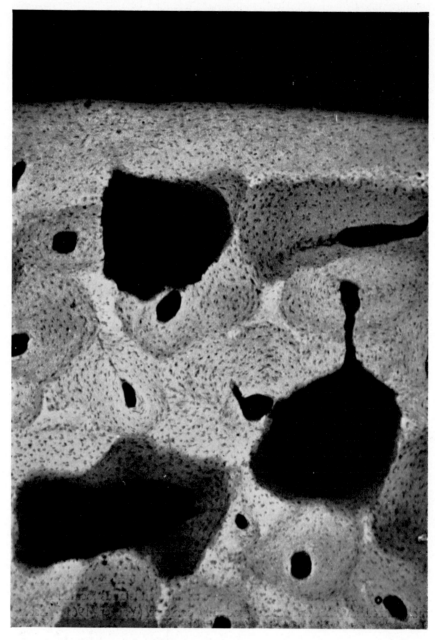

FIG. 65. Microradiograph of three developing osteons where the surfaces of bone formation are indicated by tissue of low mineral density. (×90.) (Reproduced with permission
from H. A. Sissons, In "Radioisotopes and Bone" (F. C. McLean, P. Lacroix and Ann
M. Budy, eds.), pp. 443–465, Blackwell Scientific Publications, Oxford, 1962.)

from more deeply stained bone by a thin layer of pale-staining osteoid. A developing surface appears in a microradiograph as incompletely mineralized bone, the density of which decreases as the surface is approached (Fig. 65). An inert bone surface is characterized by a narrow zone which stains intensely with haematoxylin and is covered by a rather sparse layer of flattened connective tissue cells. In microradiographs, an inert bone surface is characterized by a zone of increased mineral density that appears as a thin line (Fig. 66).

In general, the events involved in deposition of the matrix of cementum and its mineralization, appear to resemble those of bone (Albright and Flanagan, 1962; Selvig, 1965). Stern (1964) does not think that the zone of collagen fibrils approximately 250 Å in diameter that separates cells adjacent to cementum from the mineralized zone is cementoid. However, Selvig (1965) describes the precementum of human teeth as containing an irregular meshwork of single collagen fibrils and bundles of fibrils. Deposition of mineral salts in the precementum appears to occur first as islands separated from the cementum surface. The latter author, in another paper (Selvig, 1964), has described the mineralization of cementum in mouse molars. He found that here the crystallites were deposited first within and then on the surface of the fibrils, and later in the interfibrillar space. There is some evidence that, in mice, mineralization of organic matrix occurs more slowly in cementum than in alveolar bone (Carneiro and Moraes, 1966).

(*c*) *Mechanisms of mineralization.* The physico-chemical mechanisms by which mineralization of hard tissues occur are important in relation to the proper understanding of the formation, stability and destruction of bone, cementum and dentine. Mineralization of these collagenous hard tissues results in their eventually becoming impregnated with over two-thirds of their weight of numerous but very small hydroxyapatite crystallites. Only a brief account of the subject is given here as several reviews are available which cover particular aspects (Neuman and Neuman, 1953; Glimcher, 1959; Weidmann, 1959, 1963; Eastoe, 1967b, 1968).

The central problems of mineralization are the initiation and control of the phase transformation from calcium and phosphate ions in solution to solid apatite. There have been two main groups of ideas proposed to explain the initial formation of inorganic crystals; the "booster" or enzyme theory and the "target" or "epitactic" theory. The "booster" theory arose from the work of Robison (1923) who showed that zones in bone which were undergoing calcification contain a group of enzymes, the alkaline phosphatases, which catalyse the release of inorganic phosphate ions from organic phosphate compounds. He suggested that these alkaline phosphatases participate in mineralization, perhaps by acting upon a gradually accumulated local store of organic phosphate. This was presumed to result in an increased concentration of inorganic phosphate, leading to precipitation of solid

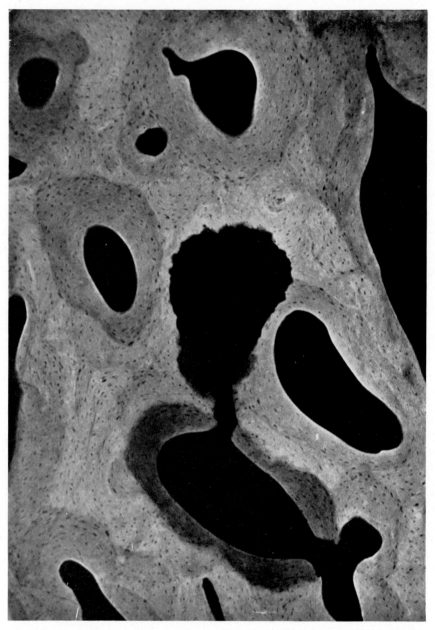

FIG. 66. Microradiograph of a resorption cavity present in the centre of the field. The surfaces of other osteons show the zone of increased mineral density which is an indication of inactivity. (×90.) (Reproduced with permission from H. A. Sissons, *In* "Radioisotopes and Bone" (F. C. McLean, P. Lacroix and Ann M. Budy, eds.), pp. 443–465, Blackwell Scientific Publications, Oxford, 1962.)

calcium phosphate. Realization that it is unnecessary to postulate any increase in phosphate ion concentration for ions to pass from solution to solid phase, caused the gradual abandonment of this idea. It has also become clear that the initiation of solid crystals of apatite involves more than a simple precipitation reaction, a concept which Robison himself recognized when he postulated a "second mechanism" necessary for smooth deposition of solid apatite.

The absolute concentrations of calcium and phosphate ions in the tissue fluid surrounding mineralizing bone are not easy to measure. The proportions of these ions which are in true solution are not known for certain, even in serum, as some are bound to proteins. However, there is a substantial body of evidence to suggest that the ionic product for calcium and phosphate in serum normally exceeds the solubility product for hydroxyapatite (Fleisch and Neuman, 1960). Hence ions would pass from solution to solid phase without any need for an increased concentration. This in fact happens experimentally in an artificial solution (prepared by dissolving calcium and phosphate in water to give the same concentrations as in plasma) provided that it is placed in contact with solid hydroxyapatite, the crystals of which grow in size at the expense of ions from solution. However, if such a solution is kept indefinitely out of contact with solid phosphate, a solid phase does not form even though the solubility product of hydroxyapatite is exceeded. It appears that hydroxyapatite crystals are not easily formed *de nouveau* and further, once formed, do not readily grow to a large size.

The "target" theory attempts to deal with the problem of the initiation of the first tiny crystal "seeds" in hard tissues. Neuman and Neuman (1953) have suggested that seeds are not formed in homogeneous solution because of the thermodynamic improbability of all eighteen ions which make up the apatite unit cell, colliding simultaneously. Glimcher (1959) considers that an aggregate of the size of a unit cell has no special significance, but that all groups of calcium and phosphate ions below a certain critical size are unstable and rapidly disintegrate into individual ions. This would account for the failure of homogeneous nucleation of apatite crystals in artificial solution, in plasma, and the tissue fluids generally. Mineralization is known to occur only in contact with a solid phase, for example the pre-formed matrix of those tissues which mineralize. It was therefore assumed that the organic matrix contains specific structures which form targets for calcium and phosphate ions from solution. Such structures probably consist of a spatial arrangement of charged groups on a polyelectrolyte which attract oppositely charged ions from solution, holding them in the relative positions of the apatite lattice. This mechanism is called *epitaxy* and it permits building up of aggregates of ions below the critical size, making them stable by means of the additional forces provided by the charged groups of the organic matrix. Once the aggregate has grown to the critical size it becomes stable and continues to grow, since its solubility product is exceeded in the tissue fluid.

It is now widely accepted that an epitactic mechanism of this general nature operates in mesodermal hard tissues. The constituent of the organic matrix which acts as target for nucleation is not yet entirely agreed by all investigators. Collagen is the obvious candidate for this role. Both collagen and the mineral crystallites are major constituents of bone. The crystals occur near, on the surface of, and possibly even within the fibrils. In addition, as already mentioned, the first signs of crystallization in developing embryonic bone appear at precise locations within the sub-banding of the 640 Å period (Fitton Jackson, 1957b). Glimcher (1959) has found that artificially reconstituted collagen is capable of epitactic nucleation of apatite from artificial solutions, but only when it is in the native form with 640 Å spacing.

Juxtaposition of charged groups on adjacent macromolecules within the fibril gives rise to the epitactic centres rather than the spacing itself, which is too large and serves only as an indicator of the appropriate state of aggregation. The holes within collagen fibrils, postulated by Hodge and Petruska (1962), provide a possible site both for epitactic centres and for the growth of crystals inside the fibril. Glimcher considers that the eventual size to which crystals grow may be limited by fibril parameters, but the nature of apatite itself may also influence this.

Complete acceptance of collagen as the epitactic agent of bone, cementum and dentine is obstructed by its widespread occurrence in other connective tissues which do not normally become mineralized. Either some controlling factor external to the fibril would need to operate or else there must be an intrinsic difference in the structure of collagen in hard and soft tissues. In many respects collagens from different tissues are remarkably similar, but there are sufficient indications of differences in stability and cross-linking in insoluble collagen to suggest that structural variations occur at the higher levels of organization. The state of bonding between collagen and the mucopolysaccharides of the ground substance may also be important in influencing the availability of epitactic centres. Glimcher (1959) has provided evidence to suggest that the higher proportion of polysaccharides, especially chondroitin sulphate, in skin compared with bone, prevents mineralization of skin by blocking the diffusion of ions to active sites on the collagen. On the other hand, chondroitin sulphate could conceivably act as a storage site for calcium ions, and Sobel (1955) considers that it acts in conjunction with collagen as a "local factor" in promoting mineralization.

If the body fluids generally are metastable (supersaturated) with respect to solid hydroxyapatite, the growth of apatite crystals in mineralized tissues will readily continue, without the need for a special mechanism to build up high concentrations of calcium and phosphate ions. However, this state of affairs appears to constitute a potential danger to the animal, in that equilibrium is poised in favour of the mineralization of tissues generally, including the blood itself. The first line of defence would seem to be the extreme difficulty of homogenous nucleation of hydroxyapatite, which ensures that crystals form only in special sites. This requires further that such crystals are mechanically retained in the mineralized tissues. In addition to this basic protection other controlling factors operate at various levels of biological organization. The possibility of the collagen-polysaccharide relationship controlling mineralization in different connective tissues has already been mentioned. It is also possible that the collagen of hard tissues may require activation by phosphorylation with adenosine triphosphate (ATP) before it is capable of acting as a nucleating agent (Weidmann, 1959, 1963). The existence of such a mechanism would provide a clear basis for the difference in behaviour between hard and soft tissue collagens. Another safety factor which may protect the tissues generally against the risk of mineralization is the widespread occurrence of inhibitory substances. Fleisch and Bisaz (1962) have shown that blood and urine both contain inorganic pyrophosphate ions which markedly inhibit mineralization. These may diffuse throughout the tissues but, at mineralization sites, a specific enzyme, pyrophosphatase, breaks them down to orthophosphate

$$H\,P_2O_7^{---} + H_2O \rightarrow 2\,HPO_4^{--} + H^+.$$

Since pyrophosphatase is a member of the alkaline phosphatase group of enzymes, these may still be regarded as possessing a primary role in mineralization by destroying a specific generalized inhibitor. Enzymes of this group may also be concerned in reactions providing energy for phosphorylation of collagen as well as in liberating inorganic orthophosphate ions for crystal growth.

The control mechanisms mentioned above operate at a molecular level throughout the tissues of the body. An additional level of control is present in the mineralized tissues themselves through drastic, but localized, changes in the overall activities of cells responsible for the laying down or resorption of mineralized matrix. The results of their activities are directly observable with the optical and electron microscopes. These cells in turn react to changes in local concentration of hormones (e.g. parathormone and calcitonin) and vitamins (especially vitamins A and D), so that their activities are affected by both the hormonal status and the diet of the individual.

C. RESORPTION OF CONNECTIVE TISSUES

1. Soft Connective Tissues

It is well-known that the extracellular constituents of soft connective tissues can be removed in physiological processes, such as for example in the path of erupting teeth, as well as in pathological processes. However, the cells that effect removal of fibres and ground substance are not readily identifiable, and there is no known counterpart of the multinucleated giant osteoclast responsible for removal of soft connective tissues. The only protease that can digest mature native collagen under physiological conditions is collagenase. If the collagen is denatured, then it can be digested by almost any protease. Bacterial collagenases were identified a number of years ago but, until recently, an animal collagenase had not been isolated. A number of enzymes purporting to fill this role were described, but the results of most of the experiments could be criticized because there was no convincing proof that the collagen substrate which they hydrolysed had not been denatured previously. This state of affairs led to the belief that collagen requiring removal *in vivo* must first be denatured, perhaps by a localized alteration in pH, and then digested by a non-specific protease.

Recently, however, what appears indisputably to be an animal collagenase has been identified by Gross and his colleagues, first in the metamorphosing tadpole tail (Gross and Lapiere, 1962), and then in mammalian soft connective tissues. The enzyme from tadpole tail has been found to differ in its action from the bacterial variety (Gross and Nagai, 1965); it is produced by epithelial cells (Eisen and Gross, 1965). However, this group of workers believe that the enzyme is not lysosomal in origin (but see Sections II and D below). A hyaluronidase is also produced in this system, but apparently by mesenchymal cells (Eisen and Gross, 1965). This work has opened the way to a search for collagenase and hyaluronidase in other systems. Collagenase activity has been demonstrated in inflamed, but sterile, gingival connective tissue (Beutner *et al.*, 1966; Fullmer and Gibson, 1966), and hyaluronidase activity in human gingiva (Goggins *et al.*, 1968).

Morphological studies have shown that the collagen fibres (Melcher, 1967b), the carbohydrate-containing complexes (Engel, 1953; Melcher, 1967b) and the bound lipids (Melcher, 1966c) of the extracellular substance are removed from gingival connective tissue into which erupting teeth are advancing. However, the nature of most of the enzymes involved in the process, and the identity of the cells that secrete them, is unknown, and a great deal of work remains to be done in this field.

2. Mineralized Connective Tissues

Considerable effort has been devoted to understanding the mechanisms by which mineralized connective tissues are resorbed and, although knowledge of these processes is far in advance of those which take place in soft connective tissues, some obscurity still prevails. Scant attention has been paid to the precise changes that take place during removal of cementum, so this discussion will be confined to resorption of bone.

The osteoclast is now clearly accepted as being the cell which effects removal of hard tissue from bone surfaces (Section IIA). It is also apparent that this cell either cannot remove osteoid *in vivo*, or else does so extremely inefficiently (Weinmann and Schour, 1945a; Irving and Handelman, 1963). The latter workers conclude from their experiments that osteoclasts can remove the organic matrix of bone, but only after it has been mineralized, and that this can occur even if the mineral salts are first removed experimentally. However, Goldhaber (1966) and Melcher and Hodges (1968) have found osteoclasts associated with osteoid *in vitro*. By contrast, although multinucleated giant cells have been found in contact with *in vivo* implants of the inorganic fraction of bone, this does not take place to any great extent (Melcher and Irving, 1963).

The question that now arises is whether osteoclasts remove all the constituents of bone simultaneously, or whether the inorganic and organic phases are removed separately, the one being removed first as an essential preliminary step to the removal of the other. Some morphological observations, for example those made by Dudley and Spiro (1961) and Gonzales and Karnovsky (1961), appeared to indicate that both phases disappear simultaneously. However, the views of Neuman et al. (1960) do not favour such a mechanism, as they have shown that proteolytic enzymes can attack the collagen of bone only after it has been demineralized first. Morphological support for this two-stage concept has come from Takuma (1962) and Hancox and Boothroyd (1963), who have demonstrated collagen fibrils denuded of mineral crystals in tissue being resorbed beneath multinucleated giant cells, and also from scanning electron microscopic observations by Boyde and Lester (1967). The first-mentioned observation was made on calcified cartilage, and the other two on bone. Hancox and Boothroyd believe that osteoclasis involves removal of mineral crystals to expose the underlying collagen fibrils, which are subsequently digested.

The means by which the mineral crystals are removed is not clear. Locally produced citrate (Neuman and Neuman, 1953; Neuman et al., 1956; Neuman et al., 1960; Goldhaber, 1963), lactate (Dowse et al., 1963; Nichols, 1963) and carbonate (Forscher and Cohn, 1963) have all been invoked as the agents responsible for dissolving the inorganic crystals. With regard to osteoclasis, some other mechanism may be operative because, as pointed out by Hancox and Boothroyd, all that may happen is that the crystals are loosened and then taken up by the osteoclasts, as has been shown by electron microscopy. The mechanism by which this occurs is not understood.

If osteoclasts are able to effect disintegration of the organic matrix of bone, they must be able to produce and secrete enzymes capable of disrupting the ground substance and collagen fibrils. As has been discussed earlier, a number of hydrolytic enzymes has been demonstrated in the giant cells, and certainly *in vitro*, these enzymes are believed to be able to break up the organic matrix of cartilage (Fell, 1964b). Although, as far as is known, there is no

11*

direct evidence that hydrolytic enzymes of osteoclasts attack protein-polysaccharide complexes, it would come as no surprise if they were shown unequivocally to do so. Indeed, Vaes (1967) has demonstrated hyaluronidase activity in cytoplasmic fractions, which he believes to be lysosomes, obtained from young bone. There is unfortunately, as yet, no evidence that the enzyme was obtained from osteoclasts. Woods and Nichols (1965a) have isolated a collagenase from rat bone cells but, unlike Gross and Lapiere (1962), they believe that the enzyme might be contained in lysosomes or similar bodies. However, they are uncertain that this is unique to bone cells, and suggest that it might be characteristic of remodelling connective tissues in general (Woods and Nichols, 1965b). Almost contemporaneously, Kaufman et al. (1965) showed that collagenolytic activity is produced in vitro by living bone during active resorption. Thus, while again there is still no direct evidence that the enzyme is released by osteoclasts, it has been demonstrated that there are cells in bone capable of producing a collagenase and that the enzyme is possibly lysosomal in origin. Before leaving this aspect of bone resorption, attention should be drawn to the fact that osteoclasis appears always to be accompanied by synthesis of connective tissue. Areas from which bone is resorbed are not left empty but are filled with soft connective tissue. This is an aspect of bone resorption to which little attention appears to have been paid. A surface being resorbed by osteoclasts shows an irregular outline in histological section. The same irregular surface is evident in microradiographs, and its limits are characterized by an abrupt change in mineral density (Sissons, 1962).

Despite the fact that there is a close association between bone resorption and multinucleated giant cells, there is considerable evidence that this is not the only mechanism whereby constituents are withdrawn from bone. For example, shortly after the administration of parathyroid extract, calcium, apparently derived from bone, is rapidly added to the blood (Young, 1963a), while oesteoclasts do not appear on bone surfaces for some hours (Heller et al., 1950; Cameron et al., 1967). MacGregor (1964) believes that, in the normal animal, exchange of some inorganic minerals between blood and bone may not be effected by osteoclasts, but rather by osteocytes. Frost et al. (1960) have suggested that, in hyperparathyroidism, some of the plasma calcium removed from bone may originate from perilacunar bone, and Bélanger (1965) believes that there is a relationship between osteocytic activity and the rapid passage of bone calcium into the blood.

There is now some evidence to support the belief that osteocytes may be able to resorb the bone surrounding their lacunae, a process which Bélanger (1965) has called *osteolysis*. Some years ago Rutishauser and Majno (1951) pointed out that, unlike osteoblasts, osteocytes do not give a positive reaction to histochemical tests for alkaline phosphatase, unless inhabiting enlarged lacunae. This finding suggests that osteocyte activity may vary, and also that the cells may be able to control the size of their lacunae. More recently, Baud (1962) has described two types of osteocyte; one small and surrounded by a smooth-surfaced bony wall, and the other large and located inside a lacuna with walls of rough contour suggesting that they have been the seat of a resorptive process. It is known, too, that under certain conditions osteocytes show a strong histochemical reaction for leucine amino peptidase (Lipp, 1959), and acid phosphatase (Susi et al., 1966), and Lipp (1954) has expressed the opinion that osteocytes are able to erode bone substance and to enlarge lacunae. Jowsey et al. (1964), using microradiographic techniques, have found that osteocyte lacunae are enlarged in diseases in which there is resorption of bone. They have also remarked on the enormous surface area which is provided by the walls of osteocyte lacunae; a readily available store of mineral salts if these can be resorbed into the plasma when required. Finally, it has been shown both that large osteocytes produce proteolytic enzymes which can hydrolyse gelatin, and that the matrix surrounding these osteocytes tends to be metachromatic and to stain with haematoxylin (Bélanger et al., 1963; Bélanger and Migicovsky, 1963; Bélanger, 1965). The evidence available certainly suggests that under appropriate conditions osteocytes are capable of synthesizing and removing bone matrix (see Baud, 1968), but that a great deal remains to be learnt about this process. It would also be interesting to determine whether cementocytes are capable of performing similar functions. (See also p. 433.)

D. Turnover of Connective Tissues

1. Turnover of Connective Tissues in General

Following consideration of the synthesis of connective tissues and their resorption, some general aspects of the overall problem of connective tissue turnover will be discussed. Knowledge of turnover is almost entirely confined to collagen. This protein was neglected by biologists for many years because it was regarded as being completely inert, forming merely a passive framework in the body. The earliest studies of the metabolic activity of collagen, based on the incorporation of $\alpha^{14}C$-glycine, showed that its turnover time could be measured, although this was considerably longer than for most body proteins (Neuberger et al., 1951, Neuberger and Slack, 1953). From these and later studies Harkness (1961) concluded that, although collagen is relatively inert metabolically, some breakdown and replacement occurs apart from that which is involved in growth.

Two different aspects of protein replacement need to be considered in connection with extracellular proteins in normal tissues. The first, which might be called *passive turnover*, involves breakdown of the older molecules and their replacement by identical but newly synthesized ones without any corresponding alteration in tissue structure. This process may largely be confined to the more soluble and less stable fractions of collagen. The second process, *remodelling*, is more complicated. It involves modification of shape and structure, as well as metabolism in response to perturbing factors or in accordance with regulating processes. These take place without impairment of function at any stage (Lapiere, 1967). In connective tissues these two mechanisms undoubtedly overlap and merge into one another, so that in any given tissue it is not possible separately to assess their quantitative effects. Similarly, in practice, the "normal" remodelling process will overlap, and be difficult to distinguish from, pathological changes of the same type where these occur in response to a mild, but persistent traumatic stimulus.

The more mature and less soluble "fibrous" forms of collagen are probably affected mainly by remodelling and little by turnover, because of their great chemical stability. Breakdown of these fibres involves the presence of highly specific proteolytic enzymes, the collagenases, which have only recently been demonstrated in mammalian soft and hard connective tissues (Lapiere, 1967). These vertebrate collagenases do not appear to be stored in the tissues, since they cannot easily be extracted after death, but they have been demonstrated as diffusing out of tissues growing in culture. It would seem that they are produced to meet immediate requirements in the vicinity of fibres about to be resorbed. Their action appears to be highly specific in initiating the breakdown process, the later stages of which are continued and completed by less specific acid hydrolases and cathepsins, probably of lysosomal origin.

There is a striking variation in the apparent rate of turnover of collagen in different tissues and organs. Thus dentine collagen, labelled with a radioactive amino acid and examined by radioautography, appears to remain stable for very long periods, indicating that its "half-life" is measured in years. This may also apply to those portions of bone which escape resorption, as Lapiere *et al.* (1965) have found times of this order for the oldest portions of bone. The total body collagen and skin collagen in the mouse on a protein-free diet have times of half-loss of 200 and 100 days respectively (Harkness *et al.*, 1958). The collagen of the uterus wall of spayed rats has a much quicker turnover with a half-loss in 20 days (Harkness *et al.*, 1956), whereas after parturition the rat uterus undergoes extremely rapid resorption, losing half of its collagen in approximately one day (Harkness and Moralee, 1956). Comparison of these turnover rates, determined by means of isotopic tracers, together with general consideration of the relative stability of these various tissues with time, as shown by changes in histology or gross morphology, suggests that differences in remodelling rather than passive turnover of collagen mainly account for the marked differences in the behaviour of collagen in different tissues. Nevertheless, there must also be differences in rates of passive turnover, since it must be slow in such a dense tissue as mature bone (where diffusion is minimal and the highly cross-linked collagen is locked in place by crystallites) compared with any young developing connective tissue with a high moisture content, where diffusion of macro-molecules can occur more readily.

The chemical identity of the labelled substance chosen to follow collagen turnover is important to ensure that it is the synthesis and breakdown of collagen which is measured specifically rather than that of any other protein. For chemical studies, the imino acid proline is the most appropriate substance to administer in isotopically-labelled form. It will be incorporated into most proteins in the form of proline residues but only in collagen will some of it be converted to hydroxyproline (Section IIIA). In order specifically to measure collagen synthesis, it is therefore essential to hydrolyse the protein, separate the hydroxyproline, and measure its radioactivity. An alternative would be to provide labelled lysine and isolate and measure hydroxylysine. However, this amino acid is unsuitable on grounds of expense and sensitivity. Hydroxy-lysine is also somewhat more difficult to separate than hydroxyproline. Identification of these amino acids in histological section is discussed in Section 2 below.

Specific isotopic labelling on these lines has made possible the study of rates of collagen synthesis or destruction in fractions of tissues which can be isolated by physical and chemical techniques. In order to study the earliest stages of the life cycle of collagen by this method, it is essential to investigate a tissue which is very rich in cells and actively engaged in collagen biosyn-thesis. In the early stages of development, granulomata produced in guinea pigs (Robertson, 1952) by subcutaneous injection of carrageenin contain loose granulation tissue similar to that found in healing wounds (Williams, 1957). Collagen synthesis takes place rapidly in these granulomata. This continues for a short time *in vitro* when the granuloma is removed, cut into slices, and incubated in a suitable medium. Lowther *et al.* (1961) found that various radioactive amino acids, including α-(^{14}C) proline, which had been added to the medium were incorporated into collagen in the granuloma cells. After incubation the tissue was disintegrated and homogenized in 0·25 M sucrose solution to break up the intact cells. Sub-cellular particles were then separated by differential centrifugation, the morphology of the various fractions being checked by electron microscopy. The collagen extracted from the nuclear, mitochondrial and microsomal fractions with neutral salt solution had a characteristic composition (Eastoe, 1961b). Hydroxyproline was separated from hydrolysates of the neutral salt soluble extracts of these sub-cellular fractions by paper chromatography, and its specific activity determined. This showed that the most newly-formed collagen was present in greatest proportion in the microsomes, suggesting that they are the main site for synthesis of collagen as for other proteins.

Eighty per cent of the collagen in the microsomal fraction was soluble in neutral salt solution, compared with much smaller proportions in the mito-chondrial and nuclear fractions. These observations support the evidence obtained by a number of workers that the neutral salt soluble fraction repre-sents the first collagen to be synthesized. In the earliest investigation of this fraction (Highberger et al., 1951; Harkness et al., 1954) it was extracted by means of slightly alkaline (pH9) phosphate solutions. The radioactivity of this alkali-soluble collagen rose to a maximum approximately 24 hours after administration of labelled glycine (Harkness et al., 1954). The phosphate solution also extracted a mixture of cellular and plasma proteins which incorporated the label even more quickly than the collagen fraction. Gross et al. (1955) subsequently found that an identical or similar fraction of col-lagen was soluble in a neutral solution of sodium chloride with less contami-nation from other proteins. The amount of neutral salt soluble collagen per unit weight of tissue is related to the rate of collagen production (Harkness, 1961), being greatly reduced in scurvy (Gross, 1958b) or when intake of food is restricted (Gross, 1958a). Neutral salt soluble collagen therefore represents collagen during the first day or so of its life and probably consists mainly of macromolecules in solution not yet affected by the cross-linking processes of maturation.

Nageotte (1927) found that a fraction of collagen is soluble in weak acids, while Fauré-Fremiet (1933) discovered that it could be precipitated in fibrous form by addition of chondroitin sulphate. The proportion of acid soluble collagen in any tissue is substantially higher than that of neutral salt soluble collagen. In fact dilute acid also dissolves all the neutral salt soluble fraction, which should therefore be removed in a preliminary extraction before the specifically acid soluble collagen is successfully extracted. The role of acid soluble collagen in collagen turnover is less clear than that of the neutral salt soluble fraction. Orekhovitch (1952) termed the acid soluble fraction, *pro-collagen*, believing it to be a precursor of insoluble collagen. Its participation in this role is less obvious than that of the neutral salt soluble fraction, in fact some of Orekhovitch's conclusions may have resulted from his failure to remove neutral salt soluble material before extracting with acid. The pro-portion of acid soluble collagen (10–20% of the collagen in the skins of young small mammals) is too high for all of it to be in solution. Its radioactivity increases and decreases more slowly than that of the neutral salt soluble collagen (Harkness et al., 1954). However, it seems unlikely that all of the collagen passes through the acid soluble phase before becoming insoluble, because the labelled isotope appears too rapidly, and in too large amounts, in the insoluble collagen for this to be possible (Harkness, 1961). Acid soluble collagen is not homogeneous since successive extracts from a labelled tissue have different activities. It may consist partially of recently formed fibrous collagen, probably on the outside of fibrils, and partially of collagen which is undergoing subsequent breakdown.

Lapiere (1967) has discussed how the rate of turnover of the entire colla-genous system of a tissue may be investigated. This involves measuring the changes with time of the incorporation *in vivo* of labelled amino acid into, and its subsequent departure from, various fractions of collagen. The results indicate its state of organization and degree of maturation. Such fractions can be separated from soft connective tissues on the basis of differences in their solubility. The least polymerized collagen extracted with neutral solutions of physiological ionic strength from the skin of growing rats had a turnover time measured in hours (Lapiere *et al.*, 1965). Somewhat more organized collagen obtained by subsequent extraction with salt solution of higher ionic strength, incorporated and lost its radioactivity more slowly, having a turnover time of the order of days. Collagen extracted at lower pH, which may have represented more highly aggregated collagen newly deposited in fibrils, turned over in weeks, while the most stable, heavily cross-linked fibrous collagen, which was insoluble under these conditions, took several months to gain and lose its label.

The technique was modified for bone by measuring the turnover time in four fractions of different density, because soluble collagens are not easily extracted from hard tissues. Herman and Richelle (1961) fractionated osteones according to their specific gravity and showed that the lightest fractions had the highest rate of exchange of calcium *in vitro*. These fractions (density 1·7–1·8) also showed a peak of incorporation of amino acid into the bone collagen within hours of the injection of a single dose of label. At the other end of the scale, those bone fractions with a density of 2·2–2·3 required a period of months or even years for the peak to be reached. Fractions of intermediate density turned over in days or weeks, respectively. These experiments with bone confirm that it is laid down locally in a moderately mineralized state and gradually becomes more mineralized, but at a decreasing rate as it becomes older. Further, should bone collagen ever be replaced other than by resorption and redeposition, this must occur at an extremely slow rate.

In the above experiments with normally growing rats, maturation of collagen proceeded similarly in soft and in hard tissues. Analysis of the quantitative data suggested that under conditions of normal growth only a small fraction of newly synthesized collagen ever reached the final aggregated and heavily cross-linked stage. Thus, though a wave of radioactivity passed through the various degrees of aggregation, its effect became progressively less marked as more and more mature fractions were reached. It could be concluded that degradative processes, which almost balanced the synthetic ones, were going on throughout the collagen. However, these processes affected mainly the unorganized and slightly organized or aggregated macromolecules which were in a state of continous flux, and left the more mature structures comparatively unaffected. Thus, when the tissues are in a steady state, much of the newly synthesized collagen becomes degraded before it is incorporated into the most ordered structures. By contrast, remodelling of collagen requires the degradation of mature collagen (Gross, 1964).

The newly-synthesized collagen would appear to act as a reserve pool to meet contingencies resulting from changes in the tissue environment (e.g. need for remodelling or reaction to injury). Under these conditions there is a greatly increased rate of incorporation of newly synthesized collagen into the insoluble fraction as new fibrils are formed. Simultaneously, there is an increase in neutral salt soluble collagen apparently derived from the insoluble collagen of fibrils undergoing breakdown (Lapiere, 1967). The state of any tissue can be regarded as resulting from a combination of passive turnover and remodelling, the relative contribution of each depending on the tissue site. The more dynamic aspects might be expected to play an important part in the connective tissue of the periodontium since it consists of a sandwich of soft tissue between two hard ones, one of which is subjected to intermittent forces resulting from mechanical impact. The periodontium thus acts as a shock absorber, within which considerable energy is dissipated. The forces thus brought into play may be expected to exert a profound effect on the maintenance of its structural integrity, as described in the next sub-section.

2. Turnover of the Connective Tissues in the Periodontium

Very little is known about the turnover of the connective tissues of the periodontium and of their respective constituents. In fact, only a handful of experiments aimed at elucidating this important aspect of the physiology of the organ has been reported. This is understandable, as techniques suitable for the purpose did not become available until comparatively recently.

Although of solid consistency, bone is strikingly plastic and the seat of intense remodelling processes. Rough guides to remodelling of mineralized connective tissue are provided by the presence within its substance of haematoxylin-stained cement lines, and by the contour of its surfaces. Unfortunately, soft connective tissue does not provide any such obvious clues to its history. Information on whether a particular piece of bone has ever been the seat of a resorptive process, and to what extent periods of apposition have been punctuated by periods of inactivity, is provided by a study of cement lines and bones surfaces. The cement lines, whose constituents, according to Philipson (1965), do not differ in any major way from those of the bone of osteones, mark the site of erstwhile surfaces. When straight, cement lines and bone surfaces indicate a pause at the end of a period of osteogenesis. When scalloped, they indicate a pause at the end of a period of resorption. Thus, cement lines mark the junction between two pieces of bone formed at different times (Amprino, 1963). They provide no indication of the rate of osteogenesis or osteoclasis, nor of the turnover of the individual constituents of the tissue. However, a measure of the rate of osteogenesis can be obtained experimentally by the use of markers that are incorporated into newly deposited bone, such as for example the tetracyclines. As elsewhere, the tell-tale pattern provided by cement lines is present in the bone of the alveolar process.

Bone surfaces are the seat of the varying phases of apposition and resorption that occur in response to outside stimuli. The periodontal aspect of alveolar bone is affected by stimuli from the teeth. For many years the simple dictum that pressure on bone causes resorption while tension leads to apposition, has been widely accepted. More recently the idea has emerged that the effects of strain on bone may be responsible for both phases of activity, local osteogenesis or osteoclasis occurring in response to the type of deformity suffered by the bone in that site (Epker and Frost, 1965). This suggestion is consistent with the growing evidence that one of the factors that may control osteogenesis or osteoclasis is electrical current generated by deformation of bone (see Becker et al., 1964; Bassett and Ruedi, 1966; Cochran et al., 1967). However, many different stimuli have been demonstrated in vivo and in vitro to have the capacity to influence deposition or resorption of bone. It therefore seems likely that formation or removal of bone occurs in response to a preponderance of favourable stimuli, rather than as a result of a single stimulus.

Resorption and deposition also occur within the body of bone. Enlow (1966) has pointed out that an increasing number of dead osteocytes, reflected by empty bone lacunae, are found in monkeys as they age. Osteocyte death possibly reflects local ischaemia (Jee, 1964), a situation that can be remedied by resorption of the affected area of bone and its replacement by vascular soft connective tissue which is subsequently recolonized by well nourished new osteones. In fact, the latter author believes that localized necrosis of bone due to ischaemia must be considered seriously as a factor that stimulates bone remodelling.

Published studies on turnover of constituents of the tissues of the periodontium have relied almost entirely on the use of radioactive substance and radioautography. The constituent that has been particularly singled out for investigation is collagen and, at the time of writing, information is lacking on the behaviour of the other organic and inorganic components. Unfortunately, investigation of collagen turnover by radioautography is dogged by many difficulties and pitfalls. A valid result is wholly dependent upon unequivocal histological identification of collagen. The imino acids unique to collagen, hydroxyproline and hydroxylysine, are derived intracellularly by hydroxylation of proline and lysine, and not from exogenous hydroxyproline and hydroxylysine (see Section IIIA). As a result, neither hydroxyproline nor hydroxylysine can be administered to label newly synthesized collagen. The concentration of hydroxylysine in collagen is so low that its histological detection by existing techniques is hardly practical. Consequently, for radioautographic studies of collagen synthesis and degradation, the most useful amino acids are radioactively-labelled proline or, alternatively, glycine which also forms a large part of the collagen macromolecule. However, both these amino acids are also incorporated into non-collagenous proteins. Experiments in which either of these amino acids are administered, and then traced by radioautography through collagen-synthesizing cells into collagen-rich extracellular substance, do not give reliable information about collagen synthesis, even if the extracellular location of the isotope is apparently in close association with collagen fibres. Indeed, Carneiro and Leblond (1966) have found recently that only about half of the H^3-proline and H^3-glycine secreted by mouse periodontal fibroblasts is incorporated in collagen. Therefore, radioautographic studies in which radioactive proline and glycine are used provide information on turnover of all proteins that contain these amino acids, and not only on collagen.

In an attempt to overcome this difficulty, some investigators have used collagenase. This enzyme digests collagen selectively, and removes the collagen-containing labelled amino acids. It is then theoretically possible to identify by negative means that which has been incorporated into collagen. Again, this method has pitfalls. Firstly, if the collagenase is contaminated by other proteases, non-collagenous proteins will be removed, and the proportion of labelled-collagen will be over-estimated. It is only comparatively recently that relatively pure collagenase has become available commercially; so, in assessing results of experiments in which collagenase has been used, the purity of the enzyme must be taken into consideration. Secondly, it is becoming increasingly apparent that protein-polysaccharide and perhaps protein-lipid complexes are tightly linked to extracellular collagen (for example, see Toole and Lowther, 1966). These proteins are not collagenous, but may contain significant quantities of proline or glycine. It is therefore conceivable that even when a pure collagenase is used, digestion of collagen fibrils will result in disruption of these closely associated protein complexes. A significant error could arise if these non-collagenous proteins were rich in labelled radioactive amino acids. A third difficulty encountered in assessing the turnover of specific proteins through labelled amino acids arises from degradation of tissue in other sites. This leads to release of previously-bound labelled amino acids which may then be reincorporated into tissue being synthesized at the experimental site (Tonna, 1965; Klein and Weiss, 1966; Tsurufuji and Nakagawa, 1967). Such an occurrence could lead to an erroneously depressed value for a tissue that is turning over rapidly. It should not be thought that these difficulties completely invalidate radioautographic investigations of collagen turnover. However, results should be examined bearing these pitfalls in mind, and even the most careful experiments should be seen as indicating trends rather than providing absolute data.

A number of investigators have examined collagen turnover in the periodontal ligaments of teeth of limited eruption; in the molars of mice, rats and hamsters (Stallard, 1963; Crumley, 1964; Carneiro, 1965; Carneiro and

Leblond, 1966; Carneiro and Moraes, 1966; Anderson, 1967). Of these, only Stallard and Carneiro have attempted to differentiate between collagenous and non-collagenous proteins. All these investigators have found a high turnover of protein in the periodontal ligament, and Carneiro and Leblond's investigation indicates that there is probably a high turnover of collagen. Protein turnover rate is not uniform throughout the ligament, and appears to be highest in the cervical and apical areas (Carneiro; Carneiro and Moraes) and in the alveolar aspect of the ligament (Stallard; Crumley; Anderson). The former finding is of interest when related firstly, to the belief that the greatest movement of teeth takes place in the extremities of the socket; secondly, to Pierce et al's (1967) conclusion that local factors probably exert an influence on collagen turnover; and thirdly to the observation that the integrity of the periodontal ligament appears to be related to function (Cohn, 1965; Eccles, 1965). The finding that turnover of the ligament is high in the vicinity of bone is of particular significance. It is compatible with other evidence that points to a higher turnover in monkeys of collagen in fibres in the bone aspect of the ligament than in the cemental aspect (Goldman, 1962). It is also striking that there does not appear to be a selectively high rate of turnover in the region of the "intermediate plexus", although Stallard has found that, like the peripheral part of the ligament, activity is higher here than in the part adjacent to cementum. How the turnover rate of collagen and other extracellular constituents in the periodontal ligament compares with that of other connective tissues in the body is unknown, but there is evidence that there are different rates of turnover of collagens in different tissues (Pierce et al., 1967).

There is very little information on the turnover rate of extracellular substance in gingiva. Claycomb and Summers (1965) have carried out a biochemical investigation on collagen in guinea pig tissue; the latter consisted of both palatal and gingival connective tissue. They concluded that the collagen in these tissues is metabolically highly active.

At the time of writing, there is a paucity of knowledge on the turnover of ground substance in periodontal connective tissues. Glücksmann (1964) among others, has shown that there is turnover of radioactive sulphate in connective tissues, that the rate varies from tissue to tissue, and that to some extent this may take place independently of fibrocytes. Baumhammers and Stallard (1968) have found that there is a rapid turnover of radioactive sulphate in the periodontal ligament, but not in bone and cementum of mice.

There is also very little information on the turnover of bone in the alveolar process, and of cementum. However, apposition of both these hard tissues appears to follow widening of the periodontal ligament occasioned by tooth movement (Stallard, 1963). It is probable that maintenance of alveolar bone is dependent upon the reception of stimuli from functioning teeth (Cohn, 1965; Eccles, 1965). There is some evidence that most of the proline incorporated into alveolar bone is contained in newly synthesized collagen (Carneiro and Leblond, 1966), in contrast to that of the periodontal ligament. Incorporation of radioactive proline, and therefore synthesis of new matrix, has been reported to be greater in the apical and crestal areas than elsewhere (Carneiro and Moraes, 1966). Information is needed however, on the turn-over rate of whole bone, and of its constituents in different parts of the alveolar process.

It has long been believed that cementum is deposited continuously through-out life (Kronfeld, 1938), and modern experimental techniques tend to con-firm this view (Carneiro and Moraes, 1966). Deposition appears to be greater apically than cervically (Zander and Hürzeler, 1958; Carneiro and Moraes, 1966), and there does not seem to be much turnover of protein once it has been incorporated (Carneiro and Moraes, 1966). A closer examination of the life-history of this tissue than has heretofore been possible should prove to be rewarding.

References

Albright, J. T. and Flanagan, J. B. (1962). 40th Meeting—*Int. Assoc. Dent. Res. Pr. Abstract.* No. 293, p. 77.

Amazawa, Y. (1963). *J. Nihon Univ. Sch. Dent.* **5**, 127–137.

Ames, W. H. (1952). *J. Sci. Fd. Agric.* **3**, 454–463.

Amprino, R. (1963). *Acta. anat.* **52**, 177–187.

Anderson, A. A. (1967). *J. Dent. Res.* **46**, 67–78.

Anderson, C. E. and Parker, Janet (1966). *J. Bone Jt Surg.* **48A**, 899–914.

Andrews, A. T. de B. and Herring, G. M. (1965). *Biochem. biophys. Acta* **101**, 239–241.

Annotation (1967). *Lancet* **1**, 1094–1095.

Anseth, A. (1965). *In* "Structure and Function of Connective and Skeletal Tissue" (S. Fitton Jackson, R. D. Harkness, S. M. Partridge and G. R. Tristram, eds). Pp. 506–507. Butterworths, London, England.

Araya, S., Saito, S., Nakanishi, S. and Kawanishi, Y. (1961). *Nature, Lond.* **192**, 758–759.

Arlinghaus, R., Shaeffer, J. and Schweet, R. (1964). *Proc. natn. Acad. Sci. Wash.* **51**, 1291–1299.

Arnold, J. S. and Jee, W. S. S. (1957). *Am. J. Anat.* **101**, 367–417.

Arnstein, H. R. V. (1965). *Br. med. Bull.* **21**, 217–222.

Arnum, S. S. and Hagerman, D. A. (1953). *J. Am-dent. Assoc.* **47**, 271–281.

Asboe-Hansen, G. and Levi, H. (1962). *Acta. Path. microbiol. scand.* **56**, 241–252.

Ascenzi, A. (1964). *In* "Bone and Tooth" (H. J. J. Blackwood, ed.), pp. 231–243. Pergamon Press, Oxford, England.

Astbury, W. T. (1940). *J. Soc. Leath. Trades Chem.* **24**, 69–92.

Ayer, J. P. (1964). *In* "International Review of Connective Tissue", Vol. 2 (D. A. Hall, ed.), pp. 33–100. Academic Press, London, England.

Barrington, E. P. and Meyer, J. (1966). *J. Periodont.* **37**, 453–467.

Bassett, C. A. L. (1962). *J. Bone Jt Surg.* **44A**, 1217–1244.

Bassett, C. A. L. (1964). *In* "Bone Biodynamics" (H. M. Frost, ed.), pp. 233–244. J. and A. Churchill, London, England.

Bassett, C. A. L. and Ruedi, T. P. (1966). *Nature.* **209**, 988–989.

Baud, C. A. (1962). *Acta. anat.* (*Basel*) **51**, 209–225.

Baud, C. A. (1968). *Clin. orthop.* **56**, 227–236.

Baumhammers, A. and Stallard, R. E. (1968). *J. Periodont. Res.* **3**, 187–193.

Bear, R. S. (1952). *Adv. Protein Chem.* **7**, 69–160.

Becker, R. O., Bassett, C. A. L. and Bachman, C. H. (1964). *In* "Bone Biodynamics" (H. M. Frost, ed.), pp. 209–232. J. and A. Churchill, London, England.

Bélanger, L. F. (1954). *Can. J. Biochem. Physiol.* **32**, 161–169.

Bélanger, L. F. (1965). *In* "The Parathyroid Glands" (P. J. Gaillard, R. V. Talmage and Ann M. Budy, eds.), pp. 137–143. The University of Chicago Press, Chicago, U.S.A.

Bélanger, L. F. and Migicovsky, B. B. (1963). *J. Histochem. Cytochem.* **11**, 734–737.

Bélanger, L. F., Robichon, J., Migicovsky, B. B., Copp, D. H. and Vincent, J. (1963). *In* "Mechanisms of Hard Tissue Destruction" (R. F. Sognnaes, ed.), pp. 531–556. American Association for the Advancement of Science, Washington, D.C., U.S.A.

Benditt, E. P. (1958). *Ann. N.Y. Acad. Sci.* **73**, 204–211.

Benditt, E. P. and Arase, Margaret (1959). *J. exp. Med.* **110**, 451–460.

Benditt, E. P., Wong, Ruth L., Arase, Margaret and Roeper, Elizabeth (1955). *Proc. Soc. exp. Biol. Med.* **90**, 303–304.

Benedetti, E. L., Bont, W. S. and Bloemendal, H. (1966). *Nature,* **210**, 1156–1157.

Bernier, J. (1952). *J. Am. dent. Assoc.* **45**, 4–15.

Beutner, E. H., Triftshauser, C. and Hazen, S. P. (1966). *Proc. Soc. exp. Biol. Med.* **121**, 1082–1085.

Bevelander, G., and Johnson, P. L. (1950). *Anat. Rec.* **108**, 1–22.

Bhatnagar, R. S. and Prockop, D. J. (1966). *Biochim. biophys. Acta* **130**, 383–392.

Bhatnagar, R. S., Kivirikko, K. I. and Prockop, D. J. (1968). *Biochim. biophys. Acta* **154**, 196–207.

Blenkinsopp, W. K. (1967). *Nature* **214**, 930–931.

Bloom, W., Bloom, M. A. and McLean, F. C. (1941). *Anat. Rec.* **81**, 443–475.

Blumenfeld, O. O. and Gallop, P. M. (1962). *Biochemistry* **1**, 947–959.

Bole, G. G., Roseman, S. and Lands, W. E. M. (1962). *J. Lab. clin. Med.* **59**, 730–740.

Bornstein, P. and Piez, K. A. (1964). *J. Clin. Invest.* **43**, 1813–1823.

Bornstein, P. and Piez, K. A. (1966). *Biochemistry* **5**, 3460–3473.

Boucek, R. J., Noble, N. L. and Kao, K-Y. T. (1955). *Circulation Res.* **3**, 519–524.

Bowers, G. M. (1963). *J. Period.* **34**, 210–209.

Bowes, J. H., Elliott, R. G. and Moss, J. A. (1955). *Biochem. J.* **61**, 143–150.

Boyde, A. and Lester, K. S. (1967). *Z. Zellforsch. mikrosk. Anat.* **83**, 538–548.

Breuer, C. B., Davies, M. C. and Florini, J. R. (1964). *Biochemistry* **3**, 1713–1719.

Brewer, D. B. (1957). *J. Path. Bact.* **74**, 371–385.

Budd, G. C., Darżynkiewicz, Z. and Barnard, E. A. (1967). *Nature* **213**, 1202–1203.

Burstone, M. S. (1960). *Ann. N.Y. Acad. Sci.* **85**, 431–444.

Burton, D., Hall, D. A., Keech, M. K., Reed, R., Saxl, H., Tunbridge, R. E. and Wood, M. J. (1955). *Nature, Lond.* **176**, 966–969.

Cabrini, R. L. (1961). *Int. Rev. Cytol.* **11**, 283–306.

Cabrini, R. L., Schajowicz, F. and Merea, C. (1962). *Experientia* **18**, 322–323.

Cahn, L. R. (1940). *J. Am. dent. Assoc.* **27**, 1056–1060.

Cameron, D. A. (1961). *J. biophys. biochem. Cytol.* **9**, 583–595.

Cameron, D. A. (1963). *Clin. Orthop.* **26**, 199–228.

Cameron, D. A. and Robinson, R. A. (1958). *J. Bone Jt Surg.* **40A,** 414–418.

Cameron, D. A., Paschall, H. A. and Robinson, R. A. (1964). *In* "Bone Biodynamics" (H. M. Frost, ed.), pp. 91–104. J. and A. Churchill, London, England.

Cameron, D. A., Paschall, H. A. and Robinson, R. A. (1967). *J. Cell Biol.* **33,** 1–14.

Campbell, P. N. (1960). *Biol. Revs. Cambridge Phil. Soc.* **35,** 413–458.

Carlström, D. and Engström, E. (1956). *In* "The Biochemistry and Physiology of Bone" (G. H. Bourne, ed.), pp. 149–178, Academic Press, N.Y., U.S.A.

Carmichael, G. G. and Fullmer, H. M. (1966). *J. Cell Biol.* **28,** 33–36.

Carneiro, J. (1965). *In* "The Use of Radioautography in Investigating Protein Synthesis" (C. P. Leblond and Katherine B. Warren, eds.), pp. 247–257. Academic Press, London, England.

Carneiro, J. and Leblond, C. P. (1966). *J. Histochem. Cytochem.* **14,** 334–344.

Carneiro J. and Moraes, F. Fava de (1966). *Archs. oral. Biol.* **10,** 833–845.

Caspersson, T., Farber, S., Foley, G. E. and Killander, D. (1963). *Exp. Cell. Res.* **32,** 529–552.

Cattoni, M. (1951). *J. dent. Res.* **30,** 627–637.

Chapman, J. A. (1961). *J. biophys. biochem. Cytol.* **9,** 639–651.

Chapman, J. A. (1962). *Br. med. Bull.* **18,** 233–237.

Chayen, J., Darracott, Sally and Kirby, W. W. (1966). *Nature* **209,** 887–888.

Ciancio, S. C., Neiders, M. E. and Hazen, S. P. (1967). *Periodontics* **5,** 76–81.

Claycomb, C. K. and Summers, G. W. (1965). *Archs. oral. Biol.* **10,** 319–322.

Cochran, G. V. B., Pawluk, R. J. and Bassett, C. A. L. (1967). *Archs. oral Biol.* **12,** 917–920.

Cohen, J. and Harris, W. H. (1958). *J. Bone Jt Surg.* **40A,** 419–434.

Cohn, S. A. (1965). *Archs. oral. Biol.* **10,** 909–919.

Combs, J. W. (1966). *J. Cell Biol.* **31,** 563–575.

Coolidge, E. D. (1937). *J. Am. dent. Assoc.* **24,** 1260–1270.

Cooper, G. W., and Prockop, D. J. (1968). *J. Cell Biol.* **38,** 523–537.

Cooper, R. R., Milgram, J. W. and Robinson, R. A. (1966). *J. Bone Jt Surg.* **48A,** 1239–1271.

Cox, R. W. and O'Dell, B. L. (1966). *Jl R. microsc. Soc.* **85,** 401–411.

Cox, R. W., Grant, R. A. and Horne, R. W. (1967). *Jl R. microsc. Soc.* **87,** 123–142; 143–155.

Crick, F. H. C. (1954). *J. chem. Phys.* **22,** 347–348.

Crick, F. H. C. (1967). *Proc. R. Soc.* B. **167,** 331–347.

Crumley, P. J. (1964). *Periodontics* **2,** 53–61.

Cunningham, L. W., Ford, J. D., Segrest, J. P. (1967). *J. biol. Chem.* **242,** 2570–2571.

Curran, R. C. and Kennedy, J. S. (1955). *J. Path. Bact.* **70,** 449–457.

Dallemagne, M. J. (1952). *Trans. 4th Josiah Macy Jr. Conf. Metabolic Interrelations,* p. 157.

Dallner, G., Siekevitz, P. and Palade, G. E. (1966). *J. Cell Biol.* **30,** 73–96.

Darżynkiewicz, Z. and Barnard, E. A. (1967). *Nature* **213,** 1198–1201.

Deakins, M. (1942). *J. dent. Res.* **21,** 429–435.

Decker, J. D. (1966). *Am. J. Anat.* **118,** 591–614.

de Jong, W. F. (1926). *Recl Trav. chim. Pays-Bas Belg.* **45,** 445.

Devis, Rosemary and James D. W. (1964). *J. Anat.* **98,** 63–68.

Dickens, F. (1940). *Chemy Ind.* **59,** 135.

Dickens, F. (1941). *Biochem, J.* **35,** 1011–1023.

Dirksen, T. R. (1963). *J. dent. Res.* **42,** 128–132.

Dirksen, T. R. and Ikels, K. G. (1964). *J. dent. Res.* **43,** 246–251.

Dische, Z., Danilczenko, A. and Zelmenis, G. (1958). *In* "Chemistry and Biology of Mucopolysaccharides" (G. E. W. Wostenholme and M. O'Connor, eds), pp. 116–136. Churchill, London, England.

Doty, P. and Nishihara, T. (1958). *In* "Recent Advances in Gelatin and Glue Research" (G. Stainsby, ed.), pp. 92–99. Pergamon Press, London, England.

Dowse, C. M., Neuman, M. W., Lane, K. and Neuman, W. F. (1963). *In* "Mechanisms of Hard Tissue Destruction" (R. F. Sognnaes, ed.), pp. 589–608. American Academy for the Advancement of Science, Washington D.C., U.S.A.

Dudley, H. R. and Spiro, D. (1961). *J. biophys. biochem. Cytol.* **11**, 627–649.

Dunphy, J. E. (1963). *New Engl. J. Med.* **268**, 1367–1377.

Dunphy, J. E. and Udupa, K. N. (1955). *New Engl. J. Med.* **253**, 847–851.

Dziewiatkowsky, D. D. (1951). *J. biol. Chem.* **189**, 187–190.

Dziewiatkowsky, D. D. (1964). *Biophys. J.* **4**, Suppl. 215–238.

Dziewiatkowsky, D. D., Benesch, Ruth and Benesch, R. E. (1949). *J. biol. Chem.* **178**, 931–938.

Eastoe, J. E. (1955). *Biochem. J.* **61**, 589–602.

Eastoe, J. E. (1956). *In* 'The Biochemistry and Phsyiology of Bone" (G. H. Bourne, ed.), pp. 81–105, Academic Press, New York, U.S.A.

Eastoe, J. E. (1961a). *In* "The Biochemists' Handbook" (C. Long, ed.), pp. 715–720. E. and F. N. Spon, London, England.

Eastoe, J. E. (1961b). *Biochem. J.* **79**, 648–652.

Eastoe, J. E. (1967a). *In* "Treatise on Collagen, Vol. 1: Chemistry of Collagen" (G. N. Ramachandran, ed.), pp. 1–72. Academic Press, London, England.

Eastoe, J. E. (1967b). *In* "Structural and Chemical Organization of Teeth" (A. E. W. Miles, ed.), Vol. II, pp. 279–315. Academic Press, New York, U.S.A.

Eastoe, J. E. (1968). *Calc. Tiss. Res.* **2**, 1–19.

Eastoe, J. E. and Eastoe, B. (1954). *Biochem J.* **57**, 453–459.

Eastoe, J. E. and Leach, A. A. (1958). *In* "Recent Advances in Gelatin and Glue Research" (G. Stainsby, ed.), pp. 173–178. Pergamon Press, London, England.

Eastoe, J. E., Long, J. E. and Willan, A. L. D. (1961). *Biochem. J.* **78**, 51–56.

Eccles, J. D. (1965). *J. dent. Res.* **44**, 860–868.

Ehrlich, P. (1877). *Arch. mikrosk. Anat. Entw-Mech.* **13**, 263–277.

Eisen, A. Z. and Gross, J. (1965). *Federation Proc.* **24**, 558.

Ende, N., Katayama, Y. and Auditore, J. V. (1964). *Nature* **201**, 1197–1198.

Engel, M. B. (1953). *J. dent. Res.* **32**, 779–784.

Engel, M. B., Joseph, N. R., Laskin, D. M. and Catchpole, H. R. (1960). *Ann. N. Y. Acad. Sci.* **85**, 399–420.

Enlow, D. H. (1966). *J. dent. Res.* **45**, 213.

Epker, B. N. and Frost, H. M. (1965). *J. dent. Res.* **44**, 33–41.

Fahrenbach, W. H., Sandberg, L. B. and Cleary, E. G. (1966). *Anat. Rec.* **155**, 563–576.

Farquhar, M. G. and Palade, G. E. (1963). *J. Cell. Biol.* **17**, 375–412.

Fauré-Fremiet, E. (1933). *C. r. Séanc. Soc. Biol.* **113**, 715–717.

Fawcett, D. W. (1955). *Anat. Rec.* **121**, 29–51.

Fawcett, D. W. (1961). *Lab. Invest.* **10**, 1162–1188.

Fawcett, D. W. (1962). *Circulation* **26**, 1105–1132.

Fell, Honor, B. (1964a). *In* "Bone Biodynamics" (H. M. Frost, ed.), pp. 189–207. J. and A. Churchill Ltd., London, England.

Fell, Honor B. (1964b). *In* "Bone and Tooth" (H. J. J. Blackwood, ed.), pp. 311–315. Pergamon Press, Oxford, England.

Fell, Honor, B. and Danielli, J. F. (1943). *Br. J. exp. Path.* **24**, 196–203.
Fernández-Madrid, F. (1967). *J. Cell Biol.* **33**, 27–42.
Fernando, N. V. P. and Movat, H. Z. (1963a). *Lab. Invest.* **12**, 214–229.
Fernando, N. V. P. and Movat, H. Z. (1963b). *Exp. molec. Path.* **2**, 450–463.
Fessler, J. H. (1960). *Biochem. J.* **76**, 124–132, 132–135.
Fewer, D., Threadgold, J. and Sheldon, H. (1964). *J. Ultrastruct. Res.* **11**, 166–172.
Fischman, D. A. and Hay, E. D. (1962). *Anat. Rec.* **143**, 329–334.
Fish, E. W. and Harris, L. J. (1935). *Br. dent. J.* **58**, 3–20.
Fitton Jackson, Sylvia (1955). *Nature* **175**, 39–40.
Fitton Jackson, Sylvia (1956). *Proc. R. Soc.* B. **44**, 556–572.
Fitton Jackson, Sylvia (1957a). *In* "Connective Tissue". (R. E. Tunbridge, Madeline Keech and J. F. Delafresnaye, eds.), pp. 77–85. Blackwell, Oxford, England.
Fitton Jackson, Sylvia (1957b). *Proc. R. Soc.* B. **146**, 270–280.
Fitton Jackson, Sylvia (1958). *In* "Microsomal Particles and Protein Synthesis" (R. B. Roberts, ed.), p. 121. Pergamon Press, New York, U.S.A.
Fitton Jackson, Sylvia (1960). *In* "Bone as Tissue" (K. Rodahl, J. T. Nicholson and E. M. Brown, eds.), pp. 165–185. McGraw-Hill, New York, U.S.A.
Fitton Jackson, Sylvia (1964). *In* "The Cell", Vol. VI (J. Brachet and A. E. Mirsky, eds.), pp. 387–520. Academic Press, London, England.
Fitton Jackson, Sylvia (1965). *In* "Structure and Function of Connective and Skeletal Tissue" (Sylvia Fitton Jackson, R. D. Harkness, S. M. Partridge and G. R. Tristram, eds.), pp. 277–281. Butterworths, London, England.
Fitton Jackson, Sylvia (1967). *In* "The Mechanisms of Tooth Support" (D. J. Anderson, J. E. Eastoe, A. H. Melcher, and D. C. A. Picton, eds.), pp. 1–4. John Wright, Bristol, England.
Fitton Jackson, Sylvia and Randall, J. T. (1956). *Nature* **178**, 798.
Fitton Jackson, Sylvia and Smith, R. H. (1957). *J. biophys. biochem. Cytol.* **3**, 897–911.
Fleisch, H. and Bisaz, S. (1962). *Nature, Lond.* **195**, 911.
Fleisch, H. and Bisaz, S. (1962). *Helvetia Physiol. acta* C52–C53.
Fleisch, H. and Neuman, W. F. (1960). *J. Am. chem. Soc.* **82**, 996–997.
Forscher, B. K. and Cohn, D. V. (1963). *In* "Mechanisms of Hard Tissue Destruction" (R. F. Sognnaes, ed.), pp. 577–588. American Academy for the Advancement of Science, Washington, D.C., U.S.A.
Frank, R. M. and Nalbandian, J. (1963). *J. dent. Res.* **42**, 422–437.
Frank, R. M., Lindemann, G. and Vedrine, J. (1958). *Revue fr. Odonto-Stomat.* **5**, 1507–1516.
Freeman, J. A. (1964). "Cellular Fine Structure", pp. 35–40. Blakiston Division, McGraw-Hill, London.
From, S. Hj. and Schultz-Haudt, S. D. (1963). *J. Periodont.* **34**, 216–222.
Frost, H. M., Villanueva, A. R. and Roth, H. (1960). *Halo Volume. Henry Ford Hosp. Med. Bull.* **8**, 228–238.
Fullmer, H. M. (1959a). Stain Technol. **34**, 81–84.
Fullmer, H. M. (1959b). *J. dent. Res.* **38**, 510–518.
Fullmer, H. M. (1960). *J. Histochem. Cytochem* **8**, 290–295.
Fullmer, H. M. (1965). *In* "International Review of Connective Tissue Research", Vol. III (D. A. Hall, ed.), pp. 1–76. Academic Press, London, England.
Fullmer, H. M. (1966). *J. dent. Res.* **45**, 469–477.
Fullmer, H. M. (1967). *In* "Structural and Chemical Organization of Teeth" (A. E. W. Miles, ed.), Vol. II, pp. 349–414, Academic Press, New York, U.S.A.
Fullmer, H. M. and Gibson, W. A. (1966). *Nature* **209**, 728–729.
Fullmer, H. M. and Lillie, R. D. (1956). *J. Histochem. Cytochem* **4**, 64–68.

Fullmer, H. M. and Lillie, R. D. (1957). *J. Histochem. Cytochem* **5**, 11–14.
Fullmer, H. M. and Lillie, R. D. (1958). *J. Histochem. Cytochem* **6**, 425–430.
Fullmer, H. M. and Martin, G. R. (1964). *Nature* **202**, 302.
Gersh, I. and Catchpole, H. R. (1949). *Am. J. Anat.* **85**, 457–522.
Gillman, T. and Wright, L. J. (1966). *Nature* **209**, 1086–1090.
Gillman, T., Penn, T., Bronks, D. and Roux, M. (1955a). *Arch. Path.* **59**, 733–749.
Gillman, T., Penn, J., Bronks, D. and Roux, M. (1955b). *Br. J. Cancer.* **9**, 277–283.
Ginsburg, H. and Lagunoff, D. (1967). *J. Cell Biol.* **35**, 685–697.
Glegg, R. E. and Eidinger, D. (1955). *Archs. Biochem. Biophys.* **55**, 19–24.
Glegg, R. E., Eidinger, D. and Leblond, C. P. (1954). *Science, N.Y.* **120**, 839–840.
Glenner, G. G. and Cohen, L. A. (1960). *Nature*, **185**, 846–847.
Glenner, G. G., Hopsu, V. K. and Cohen, L. A. (1962). *J. Histochem. Cytochem* **10**, 109–110.
Glick, D. and Hosoda, S. (1965). *Proc. Soc. exp. Biol. Med.* **119**, 52–56.
Glimcher, M. J. (1959). *Rev. mod. Phys.* **31**, 359–393.
Glimcher, M. J. (1960). *In* "Calcification in Biological Systems" (R. F. Sognnaes, ed.), pp. 421–487. American Association for the Advancement of Science, Washington, D.C., U.S.A.
Glimcher, M. J., Friberg, U. A. and Levine, P. T. (1964). *J. Ultrastruct. Res.* **10**, 76–88.
Glimcher, M. J., Katz, E. P. and Travis, D. F. (1965). *J. Ultrastruct Res.* **13**, 163–171.
Glücksmann, A. (1938). *Anat. Rec.* **72**, 97–114.
Glücksmann, A. (1941–1942). *J. Anat.* **76**, 231–239.
Glücksmann, A. (1964). *In* "Advances in Biology of Skin", Vol. V: Wound Healing (W. Montagna and R. E. Billingham, eds.), pp. 76–94. Pergamon Press, London, England.
Glücksmann, A., Howard, A. and Pelc, S. R. (1956). *J. Anat.* **90**, 478–485.
Godman, G. C. and Lane, N. (1964). *J. Cell Biol.* **21**, 353–366.
Godman, G. C. and Porter, K. R. (1960). *J. biophys. biochem. Cytol.* **8**, 719–760.
Goffman, W. (1966). *Nature* **212**, 449–452.
Goggins, J. F., Fullmer, H. M. and Steffek, A. J. (1968), *Arch. Path.* **85**, 272–274.
Gold, N. I. and Gould, B. S. (1951). *Archs. Biochem.* **33**, 155–163.
Goldberg, B. and Green, H. (1964). *J. Cell Biol.* **22**, 227–258.
Goldhaber, P. (1960). *In* "Calcification in Biological Systems" (R. F. Sognnaes, ed.), pp. 349–372. American Association for the Advancement of Science, Washington, D.C., U.S.A.
Goldhaber, P. (1961). *J. Bone Jt Surg.* **43B**, 180–181.
Goldhaber, P. (1963). *In* "Mechanisms of Hard Tissue Destruction" (R. F. Sognnaes ed.), pp. 609–636. American Academy for the Advancement of Science, Washington, D.C., U.S.A.
Goldhaber, P. (1965). *In* "The Parathyroid Glands" (P. J. Gaillard, R. V. Talmage and A. M. Budy, eds.), pp. 153–169. University of Chicago Press, Chicago, U.S.A.
Goldhaber, P. (1966). *J. Dent. Res.* **45**, 490–499.
Goldhaber, P. and Barrnett, R. (1960). *J. dent. Res.* **39**, 728.
Goldman, H. M. (1951). *J. dent. Res.* **30**, 331–336.
Goldman, H. M. (1962). *J. dent. Res.* **41**, 230–234.
Gömöri, G. (1937). *Am. J. Path.* **13**, 993–1002.
Gonzales, F. and Karnovsky, M. J. (1961). *J. biophys. biochem. Cytol.* **9**, 299–316.

Gordon, A. H. and Eastoe, J. E. (1964). "Practical Chromatographic Techniques," George Newnes, London, England.

Gordon, A. H. and Sweets, H. H. Jnr. (1936). *Am. J. Path.* **12**, 545–552.

Gottschalk, A. (1962). *Perspect Biol. Med.* **5**, 327–337.

Gottschalk, A. (1966). *In* "Glycoproteins, their Composition Structure and Function" (A. Gottschalk, ed.), pp. 20–28, 434–438. Elsevier, Amsterdam, Netherlands.

Gould, B. S. (1960). *Vitam. Horm.* **18**, 89–120.

Gould, B. S., Manner, G., Kretsinger, R. and Rich, A. (1965). *In* "Structure and Function of Connective and Skeletal Tissue" (Sylvia Fitton Jackson, R. D. Harkness, S. M. Partridge and G. R. Tristram, eds), pp. 281–287. Butterworths, London, England.

Grant, R. A., Horne, R. W. and Cox, R. W. (1965). *Nature, Lond.* **207**, 822–826.

Grassmann, W., Hannig, K. and Schleyer, M. (1960). *Hoppe-Seyler's Z. Physiol. Chem.* **322**, 71–95.

Green, H. and Goldberg, B. (1965). *Proc. natn. Acad. Sci.* **53**, 1360–1365.

Greenlee, T. K., Jnr., Ross, R. and Hartman, J. L. (1966). *J. Cell Biol.* **30**, 59–71.

Grillo, H. C. (1964). *Archs Surg.* **88**, 218–224.

Grillo, H. C. and Potsaid, M. S. (1961). *Ann. Surg.* **154**, 741–750.

Gross, J. (1958a). *J. exp. med.* **107**, 265–277.

Gross, J. (1958b). *Fedn. Proc. Fedn. Am. Socs. exp. Biol.* **17**, 62.

Gross, J. (1961). *In* "Structural Aspects of Ageing" (G. H. Bourne, ed.), p. 181. Pitman, London, England.

Gross, J. (1964). *Medicine (Baltimore)*, **43**, 291–303.

Gross, J. and Lapiere, C. M. (1962). *Proc. natn. Acad. Sci. U.S.A.* **48**, 1014–1022.

Gross, J. and Nagai, Y. (1965). *Proc. natn. Acad. Sci. U.S.A.* **54**, 1197–1204.

Gross, J., Highberger, J. H. and Schmitt, F. O. (1955). *Proc. natn. Acad. Sci. U.S.A.* **41**, 1–9.

Gross, J., Mathews, M. B. and Dorfman, A. (1960). *J. biol. Chem.* **235**, 2889–2892.

Grossfeld, H., Meyer, K. and Godman, G. C. (1956). *Anat. Rec.* **124**, 489 (abstract).

Guidotti, G. (1957). *Exptl. Cell. Res.* **12**, 659–661.

Gustafson, A.-G. and Persson, P. A. (1957). *Odont. Tidskr,* **65**, 457–463.

Gustafson, G. T. and Pihl, E. (1967a), *Acta Path microbiol. scand.* **69**, 393–403.

Gustafson, G. T. and Pihl, E. (1967b). *Nature, Lond.* **216**, 697–698.

Gustavson, K. H. (1958). *In* "Recent Advances in Gelatin and Glue Research" (G. Stainsby, ed.), pp. 253–254. Pergamon Press, London, England.

Hall, D. A. (1961). "The Chemistry of Connective Tissue", pp. 55–56. Charles C. Thomas, Springfield, Ill., U.S.A.

Hall, D. A., Lloyd, P. F., Saxl, H. and Happey, F. (1958). *Nature, Lond.* **181**, 470.

Hall, D. A., Happey, F., Lloyd, P. F. and Saxl, H. (1960). *Proc. R. Soc. B.* **151**, 497–516.

Hall, W. B. (1966). *Archs. oral Biol.* **11**, 1325–1336.

Ham, A. W. and Leeson, T. S. (1965). "Histology", 5th ed. Lippincott Company, London, England.

Han, S. S., Avery, J. K. and Hale, L. E. (1965). *Anat. Rec.* **153**, 187–210.

Hancox, N. M. (1956). *In* "The Biochemistry and Physiology of Bone" (G. H. Bourne, ed.), pp. 213–250. Academic Press, New York, U.S.A.

Hancox, N. M. (1965). *In* "Cells and Tissues in Culture", Vol. II (E. N. Willmer, ed.), pp. 261–272. Academic Press, London, England.

Hancox, N. M. and Boothroyd, B. (1961). *J. biophys. biochem. Cytol* **11**, 651–661.

Hancox, N. M. and Boothroyd, B. (1963). *In* "Mechanisms of Hard Tissue Destruction" (R. F. Sognnaes, ed.), pp. 497–514. The American Association for the Advancement of Science, Washington, D.C., U.S.A,

Hancox, N. M. and Boothroyd, B. (1964). *In* "Modern Trends in Orthopaedics" (ed. J. M. P. Clark), Vol. 4, pp. 26–52. Butterworths, London, England.

Hancox, N. M. and Boothroyd, B. (1965). *Clin. Orthopaed.* **40**, 153–161.

Hannig, K. and Nordwig, A. (1967). *In* "Treatise on Collagen. Vol. I. Chemistry of Collagen" (G. N. Ramachandran, ed.), pp. 73–101. Academic Press, London.

Harding, J. J. (1965). *Adv. Protein Chem.* **20**, 109–190.

Harkness, R. D. (1961). *Biol. Rev.* **36**, 399–463.

Harkness, R. D. and Moralee, B. E. (1956). *J. Physiol. Lond.* **132**, 502–508.

Harkness, R. D., Marko, A. M., Muir, H. M. and Neuberger, A. (1954). *Biochem. J.* **56**, 558–569.

Harkness, M. L. R., Harkness, R. D. and Moralee, B. E. (1956). *Quart. J. exp. Physiol.* **41**, 254–262.

Harkness, M. L. R., Harkness, R. D. and James, D. W. (1958). *J. Physiol. Lond.* **144**, 307–313.

Hartles, R. L. (1964). *Adv. oral Biol.* **1**, 225–253.

Hawk, P. B. and Gies, W. J. (1901). *Am. J. Physiol.* **5**, 387–425.

Hay, Elizabeth, D., and Revel, J. P. (1963). *Devel Biol.* **7**, 152–168.

Hedbom, A. and Snellman, O. (1955). *Expl. Cell Res.* **9**, 148–156.

Heller-Steinberg, M. (1951). *Am. J. Anat.* **89**, 347–380.

Heller, M., McLean, F. C. and Bloom, W. (1950). *Am. J. Anat.* **87**, 315–348.

Herman, H. and Richelle, L. J. (1961). *Bull. Soc. Chim. biol.* **43**, 273–282.

Herold, R. C. and Kaye, H. (1966). *Nature*, **210**, 108–109.

Herovici, C. (1963). *Stain Technol.* **38**, 204–205.

Herring, G. M. (1964a). *Clin. Orthop.* **36**, 169–183.

Herring, G. M. (1964b). *In* "Bone and Tooth" (H. J. J. Blackwood, ed.), pp. 263–268. Pergamon, Oxford, England.

Herring, G. M. (1964c). *Nature, Lond.* **201**, 709.

Herring, G. M. and Kent, P. W. (1963). *Biochem. J.* **89**, 405–414.

Hess, W. C., Lee, C. Y. and Peckham, S. C. (1956). *J. dent. Res.* **35**, 273–275.

Higginbotham, R. D., Dougherty, T. F. and Jee, W. S. S. (1956). *Proc. Soc. Expl. Biol. Med.* **92**, 256–261.

Highberger, J. H., Gross, J. and Schmitt, F. O. (1951). *Proc. natn. Acad. Sci. U.S.A.* **37**, 286–291.

Hisamura, H. (1938). *J. Biochem. Tokyo* **28**, 217–226, 473–478.

Hodge, A. J. and Petruska, J. A. (1962). *In* "Electron Microscopy", Proc. 5th Int. Congr. for Electron Microscopy, Philadelphia (S. S. Breese, ed.). Academic Press, New York, U.S.A.

Hodge, A. J. and Schmitt, F. O. (1960). *Proc. natn. Acad. Sci. U.S.A.* **46**, 186–206.

Hodge, A. J., Petruska, J. A. and Bailey, A. J. (1965). *In* "Structure and Function of Connective and Skeletal Tissue" (Sylvia Fitton Jackson, R. D. Harkness, S. M. Partridge and G. R. Tristram, eds), pp. 31–41. Butterworths, London, England.

Hodge, H. C. and McKay, H. (1933). *J. Am. dent. Assoc.* **20**, 227–233.

Hörmann, H. (1960). *Beitr. Silikosforsch.* **4**, 205.

Huggins, M. L. (1954). *J. Am. chem. Soc.* **76**, 4045–4046.

Horwitz, A. L., and Dorfman, A. (1968). *J. Cell Biol.* **38**, 358–368.

Hunt, T. E. and Hunt, Eleanor, A. (1957). *Proc. Soc. expl. Biol. Med.* **94**, 166–169.

Hutton, J. J., Tappel, A. L. and Udenfriend, S. (1967). *Archs Biochem. Biophys.* **118**, 231–240.

Irving, J. T. (1958). *Nature, Lond.* **181**, 704–705.

Irving, J. T. (1963). *Archs. oral Biol.* **8**, 735–745.

Irving, J. T. and Handelman, C. S. (1963). *In* "Mechanisms of Hard Tissue Destruction" (R. F. Sognnaes, ed.), pp. 515–530. American Association for the Advancement of Science, Washington, D.C., U.S.A.

Ishikawa, G., Yamamoto, H., Ito, K. and Masuda, M. (1964). *J. dent. Res.* **43**, 936–937 (abstract).

Ito, S. (1962). *In* "The interpretation of Ultrastructure" (R. J. C. Harris, ed.), pp. 129–148. Academic Press, New York, U.S.A.

Jackson, D. S. (1957). *Biochem. J.* **65**, 277–284.

Jackson, D. S. (1964). *In* "Advances in Biology of Skin", Vol. V: Wound Healing (W. Montagna and R. E. Billingham, eds.), pp. 30–38. Pergamon Press, London, England.

Jackson, D. S. and Williams, G. (1956). *Nature*, **178**, 915–916.

Jakus, Marie A. (1961). *In* "The Structure of the Eye" (E. K. Smelser, ed.). Academic Press, New York, U.S.A.

Jee, W. S. S. (1964). *In* "Bone Biodynamics" (W. H. Frost, ed.), pp. 259–277. J. and A. Churchill, London, England.

Jee, W. S. S. and Nolan, P. D. (1963). *Nature*, **200**, 225–226.

Jeffree, G. M. (1964). *In* "Bone and Teeth" (H. J. J. Blackwood, ed.), pp. 299–309. Pergamon Press, Oxford, England.

Johansen, E. and Parks, H. F. (1960). *J. biophys. biochem. Cytol.* **7**, 743–746.

Johns, P. (1967). "Some Recent Advances in Bone Research", R.P.P. **65**. The Gelatine and Glue Research Assoc., Birmingham, England.

Johnson, L. C. (1964). *In* "Bone Biodynamics" (H. M. Frost, ed.), pp. 543–654. J. and A. Churchill, London, England.

Jones, A. L. and Fawcett, D. W. (1966). *J. Histochem. Cytochem.* **14**, 215–232.

Jorpes, J. E., Holmgren, H. and Wilander, O. (1937). *Z. microskop.-anat. Forsch.* **42**, 279–301.

Jorpes, J. E., Odeblad, E. and Boström, H. (1953). *Acta. haemat.* **9**, 273–276.

Jowsey, J., Riggs, B. L. and Kelly, P. J. (1964). *Proc. Staff Meet. Mayo Clin.* **39**, 480–484.

Julén, Christina, Snellman, O. and Sylven, B. (1950). *Acta physiol. scand.* **19**, 289–305.

Juva, K., Prockop, D. J., Cooper, G. W. and Lash, J. W. (1966). *Science, N.Y.* **152**, 92–94.

Kajikawa, K., Tanii, T. and Hirono, R. (1959). *Acta. Path. Japan.* **9**, 61–80.

Kallman, F. and Grobstein, C. (1965). *Devel Biol.* **11**, 169–183.

Kang, A. H., Bornstein, P. and Piez, K. A. (1967). *Biochemistry* **6**, 788–795.

Kaplan, D. and Meyer, K. (1959). *Nature, Lond.* **183**, 1267–1268.

Karrer, H. E. (1960). *J. Ultrastruct. Res.* **4**, 420–454.

Kaufman, E. J., Glimcher, M. J., Mechanic, G. L. and Goldhaber, P. (1965). *Proc. Soc. expt. Biol. Med.* **120**, 632–637.

Kaye, Madge, (1929). *J. Soc. Leather Trades Chem.* **13**, 73–87; 118–154.

Keller, R. (1962). *Nature*, **196**, 281.

Kember, N. F. (1960). *J. Bone Jt. Surg.* **42B**, 824–839.

Kent, P. W. (1967). *In* "The Mechanisms of Tooth Support" (D. J. Anderson, J. E. Eastoe, A. H. Melcher and D. C. A. Picton, eds), pp. 5–13. John Wright, Bristol, England.

Kirby-Smith, H. T. (1933). *Am. J. Anat.* **53**, 377–402.

Kivirikko, K. I. and Prockop, D. J. (1967). *Biochem. J.* **102**, 432–442.

Klein, L. and Weiss, P. H. (1966). *Proc. natn. Acad. Sci. U.S.A.* **56**, 277–284.

Klement, R. (1929). *Hoppe-Seyler's Z. Physiol. Chem.* **184,** 132.

Kodicek, E. and Loewi, G. (1956). *Proc. R. Soc.* (*London*) B. **144,** 100–115.

Kramer, H. and Little, K. (1953). *In* "Nature and Structure of Collagen" (J. T. Randall, ed.), pp. 33–50. Butterworths, London, England.

Kramer, H. and Windrum, G. M. (1954). *J. Histochem. Cytochem.* **2,** 196–208.

Kraw, A. G. and Enlow, D. H. (1967). *Am. J. Anat.* **120,** 133–148.

Kretsinger, R. H., Manner, G., Gould, B. S. and Rich, A. (1964). *Nature* **202,** 438–441.

Kroner, T. D., Tabroff, W. and McGarr, J. J. (1955). *J. Am. chem. Soc.* **77,** 3356–3359.

Kronfeld, R. (1931). *J. Am. dent. Assoc.* **18,** 1242–1274.

Kronfeld, R. (1938). *J. Am. dent. Assoc.* **25,** 1451–1461.

Kroon, D. B. (1954). *Acta. Anat.* **21,** 1–18.

Lagunoff, D. and Benditt, E. P. (1961). *Nature,* **192,** 1198–1199.

Lagunoff, D., Phillips, M. and Benditt, E. P. (1961). *J. Histochem. Cytochem.* **9,** 534–541.

Lagunoff, D., Benditt, E. P. and Watts, R. M. (1962). *J. Histochem. Cytochem.* **10,** 672–673.

Lagunoff, D., Phillips, M. T., Iseri, O. A. and Benditt, E. P. (1964). *Lab. Invest.* **13,** 1331–1344.

Landucci, J. M., Pouradier, J. and Durante, M. (1958). *In* "Recent Advances in Gelatin and Glue Research" (G. Stainsby, ed.), pp. 62–67. Pergamon Press, London, England.

Lapiere, Ch. M. (1967). *In* "The Mechanisms of Tooth Support" (D. J. Anderson, J. E. Eastoe, A. H. Melcher and D. C. A. Picton, eds), pp. 20–24. John Wright, Bristol, England.

Lapiere, Ch. M. Onkelinx, C. and Richelle, L. J. (1965). *In* "Symposium International sur la Biochemie et la Physiologie du Tissu Conjonctif, Lyon".

Leach, A. A. (1958). *Biochem J.* **69,** 429–432.

Leaver, A. G., Triffitt, J. T. and Hartles, R. L. (1963). *Archs. Oral. Biol.* **8,** 23–26.

Leblond, C. P., Wilkinson, G. W., Bélanger, L. F. and Robichon, J. (1950). *Am. J. Anat.* **86,** 289–327.

Leblond, C. P., Glegg, T. E. and Eidinger, D. (1957). *J. Histochem. Cytochem.* **5,** 445–458.

Lehninger, A. L. (1964). "The Mitochondrion. Molecular Basis of Structure and Function." Benjamin Inc. New York, U.S.A.

Leopold, R. S., Hess, W. C. and Carter, W. J. (1951). *J. dent. Res.* **30,** 837–839.

Levene, C. I. and Gross, J. (1959). *J. exp. Med.* **110,** 771–790.

Levene, P. A. (1925). "Hexosamines and Mucoproteins." Longmans Green, London, England.

Levin, E. and Head, C. (1965). *J. Lab. clin. Med.* **66,** 750–757.

Lillie, R. D. (1954). "Histopathologic Technic and Practical Histochemistry." Blackiston Division, McGraw-Hill, New York, U.S.A.

Linghorne, W. J. (1954). *J. Can. dent. Assoc.* **20,** 672–678.

Lipp, W. (1954). *Acta Anat.* **20,** 162–200.

Lipp, W. (1959). *J. Histochem. Cytochem.* **7,** 205.

Listgarten, M. A. (1966). *Am. J. Anat.* **119,** 147–177.

Little, K. and Kramer, H. (1952). *Nature, Lond.* **170,** 499–500.

Little, K. and Windrum, G. M. (1954). *Nature, Lond.* **174,** 789.

Lloyd, A. G. (1965). *Postgrad. Med. J.* **41,** 382–391.

Loewi, G. (1961). *Biochem. biophys. Acta* **52,** 435–440.

Lowther, D. A. (1963). *In* "International Review of Connective Tissue Research" (D. A. Hall, ed.), Vol. 1, pp. 63–119. Academic Press, New York, U.S.A.

Lowther, D. A., Green, N. M. and Chapman, J. A. (1961). *J. biophys. biochem. Cytol.* **10**, 373–388.

Lowther, D. A., Toole, B. P. and Meyer, F. A. (1967). *Archs Biochem. Biophys.* **118**, 1–11.

MacDonald, R. A. (1959). *Surgery* **46**, 376–382.

MacGregor, J. (1964). *In* "Bone and Tooth" (H. J. J. Blackwood, ed.), pp. 351–355. Pergamon Press, Oxford, England.

Mancini, R. E., Paz, M. A., Vilar, O., Davidson, O. W. and Barquet, J. (1965a). *Proc. Soc. exp. Biol. Med.* **118**, 346–350.

Mancini, R. E., Barquet, J., Paz, M. A. and Vilar, O. (1965b). *Proc. Soc. exp. Biol. Med.* **119**, 656–660.

Manner, G. and Gould, B. S. (1965). *Nature* **205**, 670–671.

Manner, G., Kretsinger, R. H., Gould, B. S. and Rich, A. (1967). *Biochem. biophys. Acta* **134**, 411–429.

Manson, J. D. (1963). *Oral. Surg.* **16**, 432–438.

Maresch, R. (1905). *Zentbl. allg. Path. path. Anat.* **16**, 641–649.

Marino, A. A. and Becker, R. O. (1967). *Nature* **213**, 697–698.

Martin, G. R., Piez, K. A. and Lewis, M. S. (1963). *Biochem. biophys. Acta* **69**, 472–479.

Marwah, A. S., Dasler, W. and Meyer, J. (1963). *J. Periodont.* **34**, 142–144.

Masamune, H., Yoshizawa, Z. and Maki, M. (1951). *Tohoku J. exp. Med.* **53**, 237–241.

Mathews, J. L., Martin, J. H. M., Race, G. J. and Collins, E. J. (1967). *Science, N.Y.* **155**, 1423–1424.

Mathews, M. B. and Lozaityte, I. (1958). *Archs Biochem. Biophys.* **74**, 158–174.

Maximow, A. A. (1928). *Proc. Soc. exp. Biol. Med.* **25**, 439–442.

McCandless, E. L., Bailey, R. E. and Zilversmit, D. B. (1960). *Circulation Res.* **8**, 724–729.

McConnell, D. (1965). *Archs. oral Biol* **10**, 421–431.

McLean, F. C. and Bloom, W. (1941). *Arch. Path.* **32**, 315–333.

McPherson, A. (1967). *Proc. R. Soc. Med.* **60**, 847–849.

Mehmel, M. (1930). *Z. Kristallogr. Kristallgeom.* **75A**, 323–331.

Melcher, A. H. (1962). *Dent. Practit.* **12**, 461–462.

Melcher, A. H. (1964). *Archs. oral. Biol.* **9**, 111–125.

Melcher, A. H. (1965a). *Archs. oral. Biol.* **10**, 783–792.

Melcher, A. H. (1965b). *Dent. Practit.* **16**, 130–132.

Melcher, A. H. (1966a). *Archs. oral. Biol.* **11**, 219–224.

Melcher, A. H. (1966b). *J. dent. Res.* **45**, 426–439.

Melcher, A. H. (1966c). *J. Periodont. Res.* **1**, 237–244.

Melcher, A. H. (1967a). *Br. J. exp. Path.* **48**, 188–195.

Melcher, A. H. (1967b). *In* "The Mechanisms of Tooth Support" (D. J. Anderson, J. E. Eastoe, A. H. Melcher and D. C. A. Picton, eds), pp. 94–97. John Wright and Sons Ltd., Bristol, England.

Melcher, A. H. (1967c). *J. Periodont. Res.* **2**, 127–146.

Melcher, A. H. (1967d). *Archs. oral. Biol.* **12**, 1649–1651.

Melcher, A. H. (1967e). *Gerontologia.* (In press).

Melcher, A. H. and Irving, J. T. (1963). *J. Bone Jt. Surg.* **45B**, 162–175.

Melcher, A. H. and Hodges, G. M. (1968). *Nature* **219**, 301–302.

Messier, B. and Leblond, C. P. (1960). *Am. J. Anat.* **106**, 247–285.

Meyer, K., Davidson, E., Linker, A. and Hoffman, P. (1956). *Biochim. biophys. Acta* **21**, 506–518.

Michi, T., Imagawa, Y. and Araya, S. (1963). *J. dent. Res.* **42**, 756–757. (Abstract).

Miller, E. J., Martin, G. R. and Piez, K. A. (1964). *Biochem. biophys. Res. Commun.* **17,** 248–253.

Miller, J. J. III. and Cole, L. J. (1968). *Nature* **217,** 263–264.

Mills, B. G. and Bavetta, L. A. (1966). *J. Geront.* **21,** 449–454.

Mjör, I. A. (1962). *Anat. Rec.* **144,** 327–339.

Mjör, I. A. (1963). *Acta. Anat.* **53,** 259–267.

Moog, Florence and Wenger, E. L. (1952). *Am. J. Anat.* **90,** 339–371.

Moore, R. D. and Schoenberg, M. D. (1960). *Exp. Cell. Res.* **20,** 511–518.

Movat, H. Z. and Fernando, N.V. P. (1962). *Exp molec. Path.* **1,** 509–534.

Mühlemann, H. R. and Houglum, M. W. (1954). *Oral Surg.* **7,** 392–394.

Muir, Helen (1961). *Biochem. Soc. Symp.* **20,** 4–22.

Muir, Helen (1964). *Int. Rev. Connective Tissue* **2,** 101–154.

Nageotte, J. (1927). *C. r. hebd. Séanc. Soc. Biol.* **96,** 172–174.

Neuberger, A. and Slack, H. G. B. (1953). *Biochem. J.* **53,** 47–52.

Neuberger, A., Perrone, J. C. and Slack, H. G. B. (1951). *Biochem. J.* **49,** 199–204.

Neuman, W. F. and Neuman, M. W. (1953). *Chem. Rev.* **53,** 1–45.

Neuman, W. F., Firschein, H., Chen, P. S. Jnr, Mulryan, B. J. and Di Stefano, V. (1956). *J. Am. chem. Soc.* **78,** 3863.

Neuman, W. F., Mulryan, B. J. and Martin, G. R. (1960). *Clin. Orthop.* **17,** 124–134.

Newton, A. V. (1964). *Dent. Practit.* **14,** 289–292.

Nichols, G. Jr. (1963). *In* "Mechanisms of Hard Tissues Destruction" (R. F. Sognnaes, ed.), pp. 557–575. American Association for the Advancement of Science, Washington, D.C., U.S.A.

Noble, N. L. and Boucek, R. J. (1955). *Circulation Res.* **3,** 344–350.

Noble, N. L. and Boucek, R. J. (1957). *Circulation Res.* **5,** 573–578.

O'Dell, D. S. (1965). *In* "Structure and Function of Connective and Skeletal Tissue" (S. Fitton Jackson, R. D. Harkness, S. M. Partridge and G. R. Tristram, eds), pp. 412–417. Butterworths, London, England.

Ogle, J. D., Arlinghaus, R. and Logan, M. A. (1962). *J. biol. Chem.* **237,** 3667–3673.

Ogston, A. G. and Phelps, C. F. (1961). *Biochem. J.* **78,** 827–833.

Orekhovitch, B. V. (1952). *Proc. 2nd int. Congr. Biochem.* 106–128.

Owen, Maureen (1963). *J. Cell Biol.* **19,** 19–32.

Owen, Maureen (1967). *J. Cell Sci.* **2,** 39–56.

Owen, Maureen and MacPherson, Sheila (1963). *J. Cell Biol.* **19,** 33–44.

Palade, G. E. (1956). *J. biophys. biochem. Cytol* **2,** 417–422.

Palade, G. E. (1958a). *In* "Frontiers in Cytology" (L. Palay, ed.), pp. 293–294. Yale University Press, New Haven, U.S.A.

Palade, G. E. (1958b). *In* "Microsomal Particles and Protein synthesis" (R. B. Roberts, ed.), pp. 36–61. Pergamon, New York, U.S.A.

Palade, G. and Porter, K. R. (1967). *Science N.Y.* **156,** 106–110.

Palade, G. E. and Siekevitz, P. (1956a). *J. biophys. biochem. Cytol.* **2,** 171–200..

Palade, G. E. and Siekevitz, P. (1956b). *J. biophys. biochem. Cytol.* **2,** 671–690.

Parekh, A. C. and Glick, D. (1962). *J. biol. Chem.* **237,** 280–286.

Partridge, S. M. (1958). *In* "Recent Advances in Gelatin and Glue Research" (G. Stainsby, ed.), pp. 255–256. Pergamon Press, London, England.

Partridge, S. M. (1962). *Adv. Protein Chem.* **17,** 227–302.

Partridge, S. M. and Davis, H. F. (1955). *Biochem. J.* **61,** 21–30.

Partridge, S. M. and Davis, H. F. (1958). *Biochem, J.* **68,** 298–305.

Partridge, S. M., Davis, H. F. and Adair, G. S. (1955). *Biochem, J.* **61,** 11–21.

Partridge, S. M., Davis, H. F. and Adair, G. S. (1961). *Biochem. J.* **79,** 15–26.

Pauling, L. and Corey, R. B. (1951). *Proc. natn. Acad. Sci. U.S.A.* **37**, 272–281.
Paynter, K. J. and Pudy, G. (1958). *Anat. Rec.* **131**, 233–251.
Peach, R., Williams, G. and Chapman, J. A. (1961). *Am. J. Path.* **38**, 495–514.
Peterson, Marian and Leblond, C. P. (1964). *J. Cell Biol.* **21**, 143–148.
Philipson, B. (1965). *J. Histochem. Cytochem.* **13**, 270–281.
Pierce, J. A., Resnick, H., and Henry, P. H. (1967). *J. Lab. clin. Med.* **69**, 485–493.
Piez, K. A. (1963). *Ann. N.Y. Acad. Sci.* **109**, 256–268.
Piez, K. A. (1965). *Biochemistry* **4**, 2590–2596.
Piez, K. A. (1967). *In* "Treatise on Collagen, Vol. I: Chemistry of Collagen"
    (G. N. Ramachandran, ed.), pp. 207–252. Academic Press, London, England.
Piez, K. A. and Gross, J. (1960). *J. biol. Chem.* **235**, 995–998.
Piez, K. A. and Likins, R. C. (1957). *J. biol. Chem.* **229**, 101–109.
Piez, K. A. and Likins, R. C. (1960). *In* "Calcification in Biological Systems"
    (R. F. Sognnaes, ed.), p. 411. American Association for the Advancement of
    Science, Washington, D.C., U.S.A.
Piez, K. A., Weiss, E. and Lewis, M. S. (1960). *J. biol. Chem.* **235**, 1987–1991.
Piez, K. A., Eigner, E. A. and Lewis, M. S. (1963). *Biochemistry*, **2**, 58–66.
Piez, K. A., Martin, G. R., Kang, A. H. and Bornstein, P. (1966). *Biochemistry* **5**,
    3813–3820.
Porter, K. R. (1954). *J. Histochem. Cytochem.* **2**, 346–375.
Porter, K. R. (1964). *Biophys. J.* **4**, Supplement 167–196.
Porter, K. R. and Pappas, G. D. (1959). *J. biophys. biochem. Cytol.* **5**, 153–166.
Pritchard, J. J. (1952). *J. Anat.* **86**, 259–277.
Pritchard, J. J. (1956). *In* "The Biochemistry and Physiology of Bone" (G. H.
    Bourne, ed.), pp. 1–25. Academic Press Inc., New York, U.S.A.
Provenza, D. V. (1964). "Oral Histology. Inheritance and Development." Pitman,
    London, England.
Quigley, M. B. and Hjørting-Hansen, E. (1962). *Acta. odont. Scand.* **20**, 359–366.
Quintarelli, G. (1960a). *Archs. oral Biol.* **2**, 277–284.
Quintarelli, G. (1960b). *Archs. ital. Biol. Orale* **1**, 1–32.
Ramachandran, G. N. (1967). *In* "Treatise on Collagen. Vol. I: Chemistry of
    Collagen" (G. N. Ramachandran, ed.), pp. 103–183: Academic Press, London,
    England.
Ramachandran, G. N. and Kartha, G. (1954). *Nature, Lond.* **174**, 269–270.
Ramachandran, G. N. and Kartha, G. (1955). *Nature, Lond.* **176**, 593–595.
Rannie, I. (1963). *Trans. Eur. orthod. Soc.* **39**, 127–136.
Rautiola, C. A. and Craig, R. G. (1961). *J. Periodont.* **32**, 113–123.
Revel, J.-P. and Hay, Elizabeth, D. (1963). *Z. Zellforsch. mikrosk. Anat.* **61**, 110–144.
Rich, A. and Crick, F. H. C. (1955). *Nature, Lond.* **176**, 915–916.
Rich, A. and Crick, F. H. C. (1961). *J. Molec. Biol.* **3**, 483–506.
Riley, J. F. (1953). *J. Path. Bact.* **65**, 461–469.
Riley, J. F. and West, G. B. (1953). *J. Physiol.* **120**, 528–537.
Ritchey, Beryl and Orban, B. (1953). *J. Periodont.* **24**, 75–87.
Robb-Smith, A. H. T. (1945). *Lancet* ii. 362–368.
Robb-Smith, A. H. T. (1957). *In* "Connective Tissue" (R. E. Tunbridge, Madeline
    Keech and J. F. Delafresnaye, eds), pp. 177–184. Blackwell, Oxford, England.
Robb-Smith, A. H. T. (1958). *In* "Recent Advances in Gelatin and Glue Research"
    (G. Stainsby, ed.), pp. 38–44, Pergamon Press, London, England.
Robertson, W. Van B. (1952). *J. biol. Chem.* **196**, 403–408.
Robinson, R. A. (1952). *J. Bone Jt Surg.* **34A**, 389–435.
Robinson, R. A. and Watson, M. L. (1955). *Ann. N.Y. Acad. Sci.* **10**, 596–627.

Robison, R. (1923). *Biochem, J.* **17**, 286–293.
Rodén, L., Gregory, J. D. and Laurent, T. C. (1963). *Fedn. Proc. Fedn. Am. Socs. exp. Biol.* **22**, 413.
Rogers, H. J. (1951). *Biochem J.* **49**, xii–xiii.
Rogers, H. J. (1961). *Biochem. Soc. Symp.* **20**, 51–78.
Rogers, H. J., Weidmann, S. M. and Parkinson, A. (1952). *Biochem, J.* **50**, 537–542.
Rose, G. G. (1961). *J. biophys. biochem. Cytol.* **9**, 463–478.
Rose, G. G. and Pomerat, C. M. J. (1960). *J. biophys. biochem. Cytol.* **8**, 423–430.
Ross, R. and Benditt, E. P. (1961). *J. biophys. biochem. Cytol.* **11**, 677–700.
Ross, R. and Benditt, E. P. (1964). *J. Cell. Biol.* **22**, 365–390.
Ross, R. and Benditt, E. P. (1965). *J. Cell Biol.* **27**, 83–106.
Ross, R. and Greenlee, T. K. (Jnr.) (1966). *Science* **153**, 997–999.
Ross, R. and Klebanoff, S. J. (1967). *J. Cell Biol.* **32**, 155–167.
Ross, R. and Lillywhite, J. W. (1965). *Lab. Invest.* **14**, 1568–1585.
Rothbard, S. and Watson, R. F. (1962). *J. exp. Med.* **116**, 337–346.
Rothbard, S. and Watson, R. F. (1965). *J. exp. Med.* **122**, 441–453.
Rubin, A. L., Drake, M. P., Davison, P. F., Pfahl, D., Speakman, P. T. and Schmitt, F. O. (1965). *Biochemistry*, **4**, 181–190.
Rutishauser, E. and Majno, G. (1951). *Bull. Hosp. Jt Dis.* **12**, 468–490.
Ruyter, J. H. C. (1964). *Histochemie.* **3**, 521–537.
Salthouse, T. N. (1965). *J. Histochem. Cytochem.* **13**, 133–140.
Salthouse, T. N. (1966). *Nature, Lond.* **210**, 1277.
Sawicki, W. (1967a). *Experientia* **23**, 940–941.
Sawicki, W. (1967b). *Experientia* **23**, 460–461.
Schayer, R. W. (1956). *Am. J. Physiol.* **186**, 199–202.
Schiller, Sara and Dorfman, A. (1959). *Biochem. biophys. Acta* **31**, 278–280.
Schmitt, F. O. (1956). *Proc. Am. phil. Soc.* **100**, 476–486.
Schmitt, F. O. and Hodge, A. J. (1960). *J. Soc. Leath. Trades Chem.* **44**, 217–247.
Schmitt, F. O., Levine, L., Drake, M. P., Rubin, A. L., Pfahl, D. and Davison, P. F. (1964). *Proc. natn. Acad. Sci. U.S.A.* **51**, 493–497.
Schroeder, W. A., Kay, L. M., LeGette, J., Honnen, L. and Green, F. C. (1954). *J. Am. chem. Soc.* **76**, 3556–3564.
Schubert, M. (1966). *Fedn. Proc. Fedn. Am. Socs. exp. Biol.* **25**, 1047–1052.
Schultz-Haudt, S. D. (1958). *Odont. Tidskr.* **66**, 3–98.
Schultz-Haudt, S. D. (1965). *Int. Rev. Connective Tissue* **3**, 77–89.
Schultz-Haudt., S. D. and Aas, E. (1960). *Archs. oral. Biol* **2**, 131–142.
Schultz-Haudt, S. D., Paus, S. and Assev, S. (1961). *J. dent. Res.* **40**, 141–147.
Schultz-Haudt, S. D., From, S. Hj. and Nordbro, H. (1964). *Archs. oral. Biol.* **9**, 17–25.
Scott, Bronnetta, L. (1967). *J. Cell Biol.* **35**, 115–126.
Scott, Bronnetta, L. and Pease, D. C. (1956). *Anat. Rec.* **126**, 465–496.
Seifter, S. (1965). *In* "Structure and Function of Connective and Skeletal Tissue" (S. Fitton Jackson, R. D. Harkness, S. M. Partridge and G. R. Tristram, eds), pp. 417–418. Butterworths, London, England.
Selvig, K. A. (1963). *Acta. odont. Scand.* **21**, 175–186.
Selvig, K. A. (1964). *Acta. odont. Scand.* **22**, 105–120.
Selvig, K. A. (1965). *Acta. odont. Scand.* **23**, 423–441.
Selvig, K. A. (1966). *Acta. odont. Scand.* **24**, 459–500.
Selvig, K. A. and Selvig, S. K. (1962). *J. dent. Res.* **41**, 624–632.
Selye, H. (1965). "The Mast Cells." Butterworths Inc., Washington, D.C., U.S.A.
Selye, H. (1966). *Science N.Y.* **152**, 1371–1372.
Shapiro, I. M. (1967). *J. Bone Jt Surg.* B **49**, 381.

12

Shapiro, I. M. and Wuthier, R. E. (1966). *Archs. oral Biol.* **11,** 513–519.
Shapiro, I. M., Wuthier, R. E. and Irving, J. T. (1966). *Archs. oral Biol.* **11,** 501–512.
Sheldon, H. (1959). *Johns Hopkins Hosp. Bull.* **105,** 52.
Sheldon, H. and Kimball, F. B. (1962). *J. Cell Biol.* **12,** 599–613.
Sheldon, H. and Robinson, R. A. (1957). *J. biophys. biochem. Cytol.* **3,** 1011–1016.
Sicher, H. (1959). *Oral Surg.* **12,** 31–35.
Sicher, H. (1966). "Orban's Oral Histology and Embryology Mosby." Saint Louis, U.S.A.
Siekevitz, P. (1959). *Expl Cell Res. Supp.* **7,** 90–110.
Simmons, D. J. and Nichols, G. Jr. (1966). *Am. J. Physiol.* **210,** 411–418.
Sisson, S. H. A. (1962). *In* "Radioisotopes and Bone" (F. C. McLean, P. Lacroix and Ann M. Budy), pp. 443–465. Blackwell, Oxford, England.
Slack, H. G. B. (1957). *Biochem. J.* **65,** 459–464.
Smellie, R. M. S. (1965). *Br. med. Bull.* **21,** 195–202.
Smith, D. E. (1963). *In* "International Review of Cytology" Vol. 14 (G. H. Bourne and J. F. Danielli, eds), pp. 327–386. Academic Press, London.
Smith, D. E. and Lewis, Yvette, S. (1958). *Anat. Rec.* **132,** 93–112.
Smith, J. W. (1960). *J. Anat.* **94,** 329–344.
Smith, J. W. (1965). *Nature, Lond.* **205,** 356–358.
Smith, J. W., Peters, T. J. and Serafini-Fracassini, A. (1967). *J. Cell Sci.* **2,** 129–136.
Snellman, O. (1963). *Acta chem. scand.* **17,** 1049–1064.
Snellman, O. (1965). *In* "Structure and Function of Connective and Skeletal Tissue", pp. 319–334. Butterworths, London, England.
Sobel, A. E. (1955). *Ann. N.Y. Acad. Sci.* **60,** 713–732.
Sobel, A. E. and Burger, M. (1954). *Proc. Soc. exp. Biol. Med.* **87,** 7–13.
Sognnaes, R. F., Shaw, J. H. and Bogoroch, R. (1955). *Am. J. Physiol.* **180,** 408–420.
Stack, M. V. (1951). *Br. dent J.* **90,** 173–181.
Stallard, R. E. (1963). *Periodontics* **1,** 185–188.
Stearns, M. L. (1940a). *Am. J. Anat.* **66,** 133–176.
Stearns, M. L. (1940b). *Am. J. Anat.* **67,** 55–97.
Stenger, R. J. (1965). *Exp. molec. Biol.* **4,** 357–369.
Stern, I. B. (1964). *Am. J. Anat.* **115,** 377–410.
Stetten, M. R. and Schoenheimer, R. (1944). *J. biol. Chem.* **153,** 113–132.
Stones, H. H. (1934). *Br. dent. J.* **56,** 273–282.
Susi, F. R., Goldhaber, P. and Jennings, Joan, M. (1966). *Am. J. Physiol.* **211,** 959–962.
Sylven, B. (1951). *Expl Cell. Res.* **2,** 252–255.
Takuma, S. (1962). *J. dent. Res.* **41,** 883–889.
Tapley, D. F., Kimberg, D. V. and Buchanan, J. L. (1967). *New Engl. J. Med.* **276,** 1124–1137, 1182–1191.
Taylor, J. J. and Yeager, V. L. (1966). *Anat. Rec.* **156,** 129–142.
Termine, J. D. and Posner, A. S. (1967). *Calc. Tiss. Res.* **1,** 8–23.
Thomas, J., Elsden, D. F. and Partridge, S. M. (1963). *Nature, Lond.* **200,** 651–652.
Thonard, J. C. and Blustein, R. (1965). *J. dent. Res.* **44,** 379–382.
Thunberg, T. (1948). *Acta physiol. scand.* **15,** 38–46.
Tonna, E. A. (1960). *Anat. Rec.* **137,** 251–270.
Tonna, E. A. (1963). *Nature,* **200,** 226–227.
Tonna, E. A. (1965). *In* "The Use of Radioautography in Investigating Protein Synthesis" (C. P. Leblond and Katherine B. Warren, eds), pp. 215–245. Academic Press, London, England.
Tonna, E. A. and Cronkite, E. P. (1961). *Nature* **190,** 459–460.
Tonna, E. A. and Pental, L. (1967). *Archs. oral Biol.* **12,** 183–188.

Toole, B. P. and Lowther, D. A. (1966). *Biochim. biophys. Acta* **121**. 315–325.

Tristram, G. R. (1949). *Adv. Protein. Chem.* **5**, 83–153.

Tristram, G. R. and Smith, R. H. (1963). *Adv. Protein Chem.* **18**, 227–318.

Trott, J. R. (1962). *Acta Anat.* 313–328.

Trueta, J. (1963). *J. Bone Jt Surg.* **45B**, 402–418.

Trueta, J. (1964). *In* "Bone Biodynamics" (H. M. Frost, ed.), pp. 245–258. J. and A. Churchill, London, England.

Tsurufuji, S. and Nakagawa, H. (1967). *Biochem. biophys. Acta* **140**, 142–147.

Vaes, G. (1967). *Biochem. J.* **103**, 802–804.

Van Winkle, W. Jr. (1967). *Surgery Gynec. Obstet.* **124**, 369–386.

Veis, A. and Schlueter, R. J. (1963). *Nature, Lond.* **197**, 1204.

Veis, A. and Schlueter, R. J. (1964). *Biochemistry* **3**, 1650–1657; 1657–1665.

Veis, A., Anesey, J. and Mussell, S. (1967). *Nature, Lond.* **215**, 931–934.

Wainwright, W. W. (1952). *J. Periodont.* **23**, 95–102.

Wakely, C. (1953). "The Faber Medical Dictionary". Faber and Faber, London, England.

Walker, D. G. (1961). *Johns Hopkins Hosp. Bull.* **108**, 80–99.

Wassermann, F. and Yaeger, J. A. (1965). *Z. Zellforsch. mikrosk. Anat.* **67**, 636–652.

Watson, J. D. (1965). "The Molecular biology of the gene." Benjamin Inc. New York, U.S.A.

Watson, R. F., Rothbard, S. and Vanamee, P. (1954). *J. exp. Med.* **99**, 535–549.

Weidmann, S. M. (1959). *Archs. oral. Biol.* **1**, 259–264.

Weidmann, S. M. (1963). *Proc. 9th ORCA Congr. dent. Caries. Paris*, p. 79. Oxford: Pergamon Press.

Weinmann, J. P. and Schour, I. (1945a). *Am. J. Path.* **21**, 857–875.

Weinmann, J. P. and Schour, I. (1945b). *Am. J. Path.* **21**, 833–856.

Weinmann, J. P. and Sicher, H. (1955). "Bone and Bones," 2nd Edition, p. 50. Henry Kimpton, London, England.

Weinreb, M. M., Sharav, Y. and Ickowicz, M. (1967). *Transplantation* **5**, 379–389.

Weinstock, A. and Albright, J. T. (1967). *J. Ultrastr. Res.* **17**, 245–256.

Weiss, J. M. (1953). *J. exp. Med.* **98**, 607–617.

Welsh, R. A. and Meyer, Adele, T. (1967). *Archs. Path.* **84**, 354–367.

Williams, G. (1957). *J. Path. Bact.* **73**, 557–563.

Windrum, G. M., Kent, P. W. and Eastoe, J. E. (1955). *Br. J. exp. Path.* **36**, 49–59.

Woods, J. F. and Nichols, G. Jr. (1965a). *J. Cell Biol.* **26**, 747–757.

Woods, J. F. and Nichols, G. Jr. (1965b). *Nature, Lond.* **208**, 1325–1326.

Wuthier, R. E. and Irving, J. T. (1964). *J. dent. Res.* **43**, 814–815 (abstract).

Yaeger, J. A. (1961). *Archs. oral. Biol.* **5**, 224–235.

Young, R. W. (1962a). *J. biophys. biochem. Cytol.* **14**, 357–370.

Young, R. W. (1962b). *Anat. Rec.* **143**, 1–7.

Young, R. W. (1963a). *In* "Mechanisms of Hard Tissue Destruction" (R. F. Sognnaes, ed.), pp. 471–496. American Association for the Advancement of Science, Washington, D.C., U.S.A.

Young, R. W. (1963b). *Clin. Orthop.* **26**, 147–160.

Young, R. W. (1964). *In* "Bone Biodynamics" (H. M. Frost, ed.), pp. 117–139. J. and A. Churchill, London, England.

Zander, H. A. and Hürzeler, B. (1958). *J. dent. Res.* **37**, 1035–1044.

Zwarych, Phyllis, D. and Quigley, M. B. (1965). *J. dent. Res.* **44**, 383–391.

7 | Periodontal Sensory Mechanisms

D. J. ANDERSON

Department of Oral Biology, University of Bristol, Bristol, England

I. Introduction

To entitle a section "Periodontal Sensory Mechanisms" is to make an assumption where doubt still exists. It would seem to be reasonable to assume that sensations evoked by mechanical stimulation of teeth depend on periodontal receptors, yet evidence can be called upon to show that receptors in the pulp or dentine may be implicated. Even were the involvement of "intradental" receptors clearly disproved, the site of the "extradental" receptors can only be termed "periodontal" if the word is allowed to include periodontal ligament and adjacent bone. Endings have been demonstrated histologically in the periodontal ligament (Chapter 3) and electrophysiological experiments on animals have shown that endings of the mechanoreceptor class can be excited by mechanical stimulation of the teeth. It does not follow from existing evidence that the histological and electrophysiological studies are dealing with the same endings. Evidence from human subjects must needs be indirect and, at best, be derived only by comparative studies using various tests of tactile and discriminative ability before and during anaesthesia and with natural and artificial teeth. However, it will be shown that the results of experiments using anaesthesia still leave doubt as to the role of periodontal receptors. The value of experiments on subjects with artificial teeth is questionable considering the large changes associated with the removal and replacement of teeth. It is not justifiable to assume that the differences in sensory experience between subjects with normal and artificial dentitions are due solely to the absence of periodontal receptors in the latter group.

II. Observations and Experiments in Man

Common experience shows that humans are capable of detecting the presence of very small particles between the occlusal surfaces of the teeth, and of judging differences in thickness and hardness of materials held between the teeth. In addition, it is possible to feel very small forces applied to the teeth. It seems likely that receptors in the tooth-supporting structures, or even in the teeth themselves, contribute to the performance of these functions, but it is also possible that a contribution comes from proprioceptive endings in muscles, tendons and joints. Similarly, while the control of normal masticatory movements depends on information from muscle, tendon and joint receptors, it is also possible that periodontal receptors play a part. They may be involved too, in providing the sensory information which results in the sudden cessation of chewing when the teeth meet prematurely on a piece of bone. This is commonly accompanied by a sensation of pain, and this also might have its origin in periodontal receptors.

A. Touch Thresholds

There is a great deal of evidence showing the ability of human subjects to detect very small forces applied to the teeth. Stewart (1927) recorded sensory thresholds in human subjects and, with 260 teeth, found that thresholds ranged between 7–50 g mm². Of these teeth, 195 showed thresholds in the narrower range of 16–32 g mm² and one third of the total of 260 fell in the range 17–21 g mm². The few pulpless teeth examined by him did not show thresholds outside the range for normal teeth. Force was applied to the centre of the labial surface of incisors and canines.

Münch and Schriever are quoted by Adler (1947) as having performed similar experiments in 1931. According to Adler they found that a force of 1·5 g could be detected when applied to the teeth, but he did not mention the direction of the force. Vital and pulpless teeth showed equal sensibility. Adler attempted to obtain estimates of thresholds to loads applied to the teeth of his subjects. He maintained that a sensation of "load" was evoked by higher forces than evoked a sensation of touch, and by smaller forces than evoked pain. Certainly, the figures he obtained were higher than those of Münch and Schriever and others to be discussed below. If touch thresholds depend on periodontal receptors it seems likely that load thresholds might depend in addition on other receptors round the mouth, and even on receptors in the dentine or pulp. As expected, Adler's thresholds were high, reaching 4–6 kg with axial forces and 1–3 kg with lateral forces, with considerable individual variation. Surface anaesthesia of the gingiva resulted in a rise in the axial thresholds by 30% and in lateral thresholds by 100%. Adler assumed that the surface anaesthetic diffused into the marginal periodontal membrane and it is of interest to note that palatal gingival anaesthesia had no effect on thresholds.

These results, coupled with the observation that mandibular "conduction" anaesthesia did not completely abolish the ability to detect load, suggest various conclusions. First, the gingival tissue and underlying bone may contain receptors, excitation of which provides the afferent impulse pattern upon which thresholds depend. Picton (1965) has shown that with loads of less than 100 g applied laterally there is distortion of bone as well as movement of the tooth in its socket, and this distortion would therefore involve gingival and bone receptors in addition to those in the periodontal ligament. On the other hand, palatal gingival anaesthesia did not affect the thresholds and it seems unlikely that receptors in bone and gingiva would be confined to the buccal side as the failure of palatal anaesthesia seems to indicate. It is quite possible as Adler suggested, that the periodontal ligament was subjected to the anaesthetic by diffusion from the site of injection, and that the density and arrangement of the supporting bone on the palatal side might minimize diffusion into the periodontal tissues on that side. One conclusion can be reached with certainty from Adler's results. "Load thresholds" do not depend solely on periodontal receptors for, although local and mandibular block anaesthesia raised thresholds, they did not abolish sensation to this form of stimulation. Work by investigators since Adler produced his results has been confined to tactile rather than load thresholds.

Direct determinations were carried out on human subjects by Loewenstein and Rathkamp in 1955 and more recently by Wilkie (1964). The former paper deserves careful consideration because it reports rather surprising results. Threshold determinations were made using a specially made "spring aesthesiometer". The use of Von Frey's aesthesiometers was abandoned when it was found that the force they developed could vary by ±35% even with the most careful calibration. Tests were made by applying long-axial force to 155 normal teeth and thresholds varied between 0·945 g from 1st incisors to 4·533 g from 2nd molars in the maxilla. In the mandible the incisor threshold was lower at 0·768 g and the 2nd molar threshold was slightly higher at 4·740 g. In 21 pulpless teeth, the observed average thresholds were 75% above those for normal teeth. Furthermore, placing a metal cap on normal teeth raised the threshold on average by 127%±33%. Capping denervated teeth resulted in no alteration of their thresholds. The only possible conclusions from the results obtained on pulpless teeth are firstly, that there are intradental receptors which are destroyed when the pulp is removed, and secondly, that when the pulp is removed, the periodontal innervation is damaged. Results of experiments with capped teeth support the first conclusion, although it seems hard to believe that small forces applied to the teeth can cause sufficient distortion to be transmitted to dentine or pulp to excite receptors therein. Further discussion of this interesting problem is beyond the scope of this review, but the work of Robinson (1964), Korber and Korber (1967) and Picton and Davies (1967), provides additional reading.

Wilkie (1964) used a device similar to that of Loewenstein and Rathkamp. He found that, in 27 subjects, thresholds to axial forces were lowest in upper and lower central incisors, in the range 0·52–0·44 g; in lateral incisors the range was higher, from 0·78–0·66 g and in canines 1·32–1·26 g.

Tactile sensibility was investigated by Manly et al. (1952) on normal and artificial dentitions using long-axially and labially applied forces. With long-axial forces the thresholds ranged from about 1 g on anterior teeth to 8–10 g on first molars. With labially applied forces the thresholds were lower, ranging between 0·5 and 0·6 g on incisors and 1·8–2·4 g on first molars. The thresholds in denture wearers were very much higher. Five of the eight subjects were unable to feel 125 g.

B. Discriminative Ability

The remaining work on human subjects has dealt with discriminative ability using various thicknesses of foil, wire or plastic held between the teeth. Manly et al. determined sensory thresholds in a variety of ways using subjects with natural and artificial dentitions. The ability to judge differences in thickness was not found to be different in normal or artificial dentitions. Furthermore, the topical application of anaesthetics made no difference to thickness discrimination of denture wearers. Presumably, therefore, neither periodontal receptors in normal dentition, nor gingival receptors in denture wearers are concerned in this activity, and the evidence points to muscle, tendon and joint receptors. In hardness judgment, when soft rubber discs were used, there was no difference between the three groups described above. However, with harder material, both the anaesthetized and unanaesthetized denture wearers showed performance inferior to that of the normal dentition.

From these experiments it appears that the wearer of an artificial dentition is at no disadvantage when compared with a person possessing a normal dentition if the test involves different degrees of separation of the teeth, as presumably is possible when estimating the thickness of materials and their hardness (using soft rubber). However, with very hard materials, the teeth do not compress the material or move closer together, therefore estimates must be based on other evidence which, it seems, must spring from a firmly based normal dentition and possibly from periodontal receptors therein.

Tests similar to those of Manly *et al.* using materials of varying thickness held between the teeth to assess sensory thresholds have been used by Kawamura and Watanabe (1960), Tryde *et al.* (1962), and by Shrilä and Laine (1963). Tryde *et al.* and Shrilä and Laine used flat strips of metal foil. Kawamura and Watanabe used wires of various diameters. The experiments by Shrilä and Laine are the most significant from the point of view of periodontal receptors because the authors used anaesthesia to reduce the sensory information from the area. In the normal mouth, it was found that one third of the 36 subjects were unmistakably aware of the presence of 8–10 μ thick foil between their teeth. All but 3 felt foil which was 30 μ thick and without exception all the subjects detected foil 60 μ thick. There was no difference between incisors and molar teeth. During mandibular block anaesthesia there was surprisingly little diminution in the sensibility of two-thirds of the subjects, who could still detect 30 μ foil. Of all the subjects only two failed to detect 60 μ foil during mandibular anaesthesia. When the anaesthesia was extended to involve both jaws three-quarters of the subjects could detect 90 μ foil and only two of the total failed to detect 150 μ foil.

The approach of Kawamura and Watanabe (1960) was rather different in that they asked their subjects to discriminate between different thicknesses of wire held between the teeth. Tests were made on normal and artificial dentitions. It appeared that the ability to discriminate was greater with thinner than with thicker wires held between the incisor teeth, since with 2·0 mm or 3·0 mm radius wire, 100% success in discrimination was achieved when the difference in radius between two wires was 0·2 mm or more. When the radius was 4·0 mm or 5·0 mm 100% discrimination was achieved with differences of 0·3 mm or more. This was not so with the molars. Whatever the radius between 2·0 mm and 5·0 mm, a difference of 0·2 mm and greater could be detected. As might be expected, the performance of denture wearers was inferior. With wire of radius 2·0 mm, a difference in radius of 0·4 mm was the smallest that could be detected and, with the thicker wires of 3·0 mm and 4.0 mm and 5·0 mm radius, the detectable difference was 0·5 mm and above.

Discrimination of another type was tested by Manly *et al.* by giving their subjects a bland pudding to eat, to which various quantities of $CaCO_3$ had been added. In 10 normal subjects 9 were able to detect $CaCO_3$ in amounts of 2·9 g/100 g whereas 6 of the 10 denture wearers required over 9 g/100 g before they could detect its presence.

C. PAIN

Pain can be evoked during chewing if sudden contact is made between the teeth through the intervention of some hard object in the food. If an artificial crown or other restoration is not properly adjusted into the occlusal plane,

12*

then chewing on the restored tooth may cause pain. Inflammatory changes in the supporting tissues may result from the heavy loads taken by the tooth and, in their turn, these changes may cause even light pressure on the tooth to be painful. Clinical evidence as to the mechanism of "periodontal" pain is so sparse that it is not even certain that the origin of this pain is always in the periodontal tissues. It is possible when a small hard object is accidentally bitten, that the pain is dentinal or pulpal in origin, resulting from a splitting force transmitted through the tooth by the object as it lies in a fissure between cusps. That this is possible, was shown in an investigation by Robinson (1964) into the possible cause of pain following the insertion of large fillings. Robinson found that force applied to the lateral walls of a cavity in a tooth is sometimes painful, and in the conditions of his experiment this can only have been dentinal or pulpal in origin.

Indirect support for the idea that the pain of a "high" filling may not be periodontal but "intradental" in origin comes from the experiments of Anderson (1962 and 1967). In these experiments on human subjects, a molar tooth was fitted with a metal cap, the occlusal surface of which was an exact replica of the natural occlusal surface of that tooth. The effect of fitting the cap was to concentrate all the biting force on one tooth, but the areas of distribution of force between the surfaces of the cap and opposing teeth were no different from normal for those teeth. This is rather a different state of affairs from that existing between a normal tooth and a "high" crown or filling, where the load may be concentrated on a small area of tooth surface, with the possibility of a splitting force transmitted through enamel to dentine and pulp. It is suggested, that the pain from a "high" restoration may be dentinal or pulpal in origin. It appears that this is the only plausible explanation for the fact that while "high" restorations are commonly painful and call for urgent adjustment, yet in the series of experiments reported by Anderson (1962, 1967) caps of at least 0·5 mm in thickness were tolerated for many weeks without requiring removal because of pain. In those experiments, the pressure on the periodontal tissues during the early stages, when only the capped tooth and opponents made contact, must have been comparable with that in many of the clinical examples of high fillings which demand adjustment because of pain commonly assumed to be periodontal in origin.

The purpose of introducing this discussion was not to claim that pain can never originate in the periodontal tissue. Such a claim would be contrary to common experience, which shows that pain is caused when an instrument or sharp piece of food is introduced into the periodontal ligament at the gingival margin. The clinician concludes that the periodontal tissues are involved in inflammatory changes if the tooth seems to the patient to be raised in its socket and is painful when subjected to light tapping. It is said that the pain is different in quality from dentinal and pulpal pain, and that it can be temporarily relieved by sustained pressure on the tooth.

III. Animal Experiments

The first studies of the electrophysiology of the pulp and periodontium were made by Pfaffman (1939a) who recorded nerve impulses from dental nerves in anaesthetized cats. After removing the eye, he located the dental branches of the maxillary division of the trigeminal nerve as they crossed the floor of the orbit. Tactile thresholds were determined by applying a series of calibrated bristles to the tooth crown. In adult animals the thresholds on

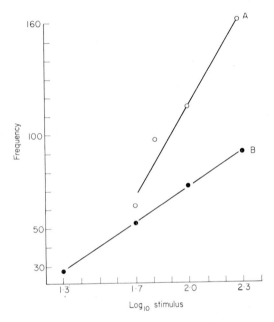

Fig. 1. The relation between the frequency of response and the log of the stimulus in two experiments A and B. The points on the lines are the frequencies during the first second of the response. (From Pfaffmann 1939a.)

canine teeth fell between 2·0 g and 3·0 g but in one young animal a lower figure of 0·5 g was recorded. Figure 1 shows the relationship between stimulus magnitude and impulse frequency, and the results from a small group of data indicated the existence of a logarithmic relationship between these two. Although the rate of application of the stimulus was not controlled, Pfaffman did observe that with rapid application he obtained higher impulse frequencies than with a slow rate of application, and he also noted that the maximum frequencies were higher than from soft tissue. The highest frequency achieved in all his experiments was 1200 i.p.s. maintained for only a few impulses at the beginning of the period of stimulation, but this very high figure is difficult to reconcile with present knowledge of the duration of the refractory period in nerve.

Fast and slowly adapting receptors were found, and in the second of the papers on this subject Pfaffman (1939b) reported that fast adapting receptors generally showed a higher stimulus threshold and a lower maximum frequency of discharge than slowly adapting units. He also found spontaneously discharging units which responded to stimulation, but afterwards became silent for a short period before returning gradually to their resting discharge rate. As to the site of the receptors and the route by which they are innervated, Pfaffman's conclusions, though probably correct, seem to have been arrived at erroneously. It is almost certain that he is correct in assuming that the receptors from which he was recording were in the periodontal ligament. However, it is not justifiable to conclude that, because removal of the pulp and destruction of the apical nerves left the response little changed, the fibres leave the ligament via the alveolar bone. If the fibres travelled apically through the periodontal ligament and joined pulpal fibres after the latter had emerged from the apex, they could well have escaped destruction by the techniques used by Pfaffman. In support of his contention, however, the histological studies of Levinsky and Stewart (1937) on the cat show that the majority of the periodontal ligament innervation leave by running laterally through the alveolar plate. Much of the work in the second paper by Pfaffman concerns the response of dental mechanoreceptors to vibratory stimuli, but while this work is of general physiological interest, its relevance in the context of this review is less than that of the first paper. It is of interest to observe in passing, that although single units were usually able to fire at upper frequency limits of 700–900 i.p.s. (exceptionally at 1200 i.p.s., see above), yet frequencies of vibratory stimulation of 1500 c.p.s. were followed in whole nerve preparations.

In 1954, Ness made a study of mechanoreceptors which could be excited by pressure applied to the mandibular incisor in the rabbit. The most important advance in this work was the careful investigation of the directional sensitivity of the receptors; a physiological characteristic to which Pfaffman made only brief reference. The general conclusion reached by Ness was that the nearer a stimulus is applied to the most sensitive direction of a receptor, the lower the threshold, the shorter will be the latency between stimulus and response, the greater the frequency of response and the longer the duration of the response. The maximum frequencies of impulse discharge were much lower than had been recorded by Pfaffman. With ordinary methods, 109 i.p.s. were recorded, but by twisting a flat instrument between the incisors (a procedure which in man would be extremely painful) the frequency of discharge reached 120 i.p.s.

Ness adopted the classification of "slowly adapting", "spontaneously discharging" and "fast adapting" receptors. The first two behaved in the same manner on stimulation but, as described by Pfaffman, the spontaneously discharging fibres fired steadily before stimulation; after the stimulus was removed, a period of silence ensued before the spontaneous rhythm was re-established.

Directionality was investigated by applying forces along axes determined accurately using a protractor. In Fig. 2 a composite plot is shown for all those receptor units which it was possible to study over the entire range of direction ±60° about the most sensitive direction. Ness concedes that the

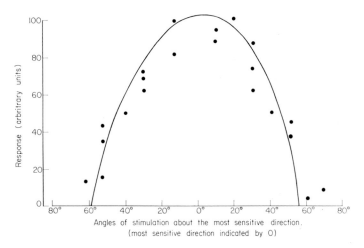

Angles of stimulation about the most sensitive direction.
(most sensitive direction indicated by O)

FIG. 2. Composite plot of the results of experiments to show the effect of varying the direction of stimulation over a range of ±60° about the most sensitive direction. (From Ness 1954.)

most sensitive direction was determined by eye, and it appears therefore that this is a point on which technique could be improved.

No direct evidence as to the location of the periodontal receptors is available from the work of Ness. He refers to preliminary histological investigations which have indicated that no nerve bundles pass into the labial aspect of the periodontal ligament, and has further reported that attempts to silence the receptors by means of a watch spring forced down the labial aspect of the periodontal ligament always failed. These two observations show that, in the rabbit, the main site of periodontal mechanoreceptors is on the lingual side of the tooth. Regarding directionality, this may be a property of the receptor itself. On the other hand, information about direction could be signalled by a system of non-directional receptors arranged in a set pattern rather than randomly in the periodontal ligament. This would appear to be unlikely, especially in continuously erupting teeth, if it is assumed that eruption is associated with continuous reorganization of the periodontal tissues. In the Pacinian corpuscle the axis of the receptor is a property of the receptor itself, but in less highly specialized receptors, the axis is likely to depend on the arrangement of the nerve endings in the connective tissue environment. Since there is no histological evidence for the existence of any highly specialized endings in the periodontal ligament, directionality would seem to be dependent on the position of the receptor and the state of the connective tissue environment.

During investigations of the functions of the trigeminal sensory nuclei Kruger and Michel (1962), Jerge (1963a,b) and others have described units which discharge when pressure is applied to the teeth and adjacent tissue. Kruger and Michel found fast and slowly adapting units which responded to light touch and heavy pressure to the teeth. Their method of applying the stimulus was manual, with no method for controlling the rate of application, magnitude or direction. They found no evidence to suggest that the neurones innervate more than one tooth and they reported that after the initial rapid discharge of impulses, maintained stimulation resulted in a "somewhat oscillatory slower rate". This may well have been caused by oscillations in the stimulating force, since this was applied manually, rather than a character-istic of the receptor. No subsequent investigator has reported an oscillating discharge. The record used by Kruger and Michel to illustrate this property shows the impulse frequency starting at zero, but returning rather slowly to zero after the stimulus is removed. Again, this finding has not been repro-duced by others in the field.

In the mesencephalic nucleus of the cat, Jerge found neurones which, in his view, innervate two distinct types of periodontal receptor. His Type I dental pressoreceptor showed thresholds with an average value of 1·8 g, ranging between 1 and 3 g. As described by others, these receptors respond with a minimum latency and magnitude of stimulation when the stimulus is applied in one direction and to both sides of this, up to 90°, the sensitivity fell away. Throughout the remaining 180° of the tooth's circumference the receptor would not respond, however great the stimulus might be. Jerge found fast and slowly adapting receptors represented in the mesencephalic nucleus. The very slowly adapting receptors described by Ness and Pfaffman were not represented there, but, according to Jerge, have been found in the Gasserian ganglion. Pressure on soft tissue around the gum margin excited a response from these Type I receptors. However, as a result of finding that electrical stimulation of the soft tissue and pressure stimulation over a small area of soft tissue failed to evoke a response, Jerge concluded that the re-ceptors were in the periodontal ligament, and could be excited if a sufficiently large disturbance applied to the soft tissue and bone were transmitted through these tissues to the periodontal ligament. In other words one neurone is not likely to supply both a periodontal and a gingival receptor.

The important distinguishing feature, however, of Type II units described by Jerge is their innervation of a complex peripheral field, presumably by branching axons. In respect of their adequate stimulus thresholds, latency, and adaptation, the difference between them and Type I units is small. In general, the thresholds were rather higher than were found in the single-tooth units; in the range 2–6 g. The claim that these receptors innervate more than one tooth, and sometimes adjacent soft tissue, cannot be substantiated in every instance. It is well established that pressure in one part of the dental arch or soft tissue may be transmitted to other areas. This was referred to by Jerge (1963a), and has been the subject of study by Picton (1965). However, it can hardly account for the observation by Jerge that light stimulation of soft tissue at some distance from the teeth evokes a response from units also excited by pressure on the teeth. His suggestion that this indicates branching of fibres to supply soft tissue and teeth therefore seems reasonable. However, there is still some doubt about multi-tooth receptors, especially in those circumstances in which a receptor is claimed to innervate several teeth with thresholds rising from tooth to tooth towards the back of the arch. This observation could also be due to transmission of the disturbance through bone, or through contact points between the teeth, to a single receptor in an anterior position in the mouth.

Kawamura and Nishiyama (1966) investigated the pontine bulbar projection of pressure afferents from the teeth in cats during manually applied force monitored by a strain gauge. The records were obtained with microelectrodes used in conjunction with stereotactic apparatus. It was found that most of the spots in the brain in which responses could be detected were excited by pressure on the teeth, whatever the direction of the pressure. Others were more specific in their directionality. This finding differs from those of Jerge (1963a), and others, who stress the fact that periodontal ligament receptors respond maximally to force applied in a particular direction, and show a marked decline in their response as the direction of force is changed.

Of 140 spots in the nuclei investigated by Kawamura and Nishiyama, 135 responded to stimulation of a single tooth. The remaining five corresponded to Jerge's Type II receptor in that they could be excited by stimulation of more than one tooth. However, the proportion of single and multi-tooth receptors differed markedly from that found by Jerge. He also used the cat, but found approximately equal numbers of the two kinds of receptor. Thresholds also differed markedly in the two sets of observations. The Type II receptors of Jerge were the less sensitive of the two groups, with thresholds at 6·0 g or below, whereas the range quoted by Kawamura was 2·0 to 300·0 g. Of the spots which responded to pressure on several teeth, one is quoted by Kawamura which could be activated by 50·0 g applied to incisor and canine and 250·0 g applied to a molar. It is quite possible that the receptor ending lay in the incisor-canine region and that heavy pressure applied to the molar excited this receptor by distortion transmitted through bone or teeth.

Spontaneously discharging receptors were described, but only 5 out of

140 fell into this category. One receptor deserves special mention because it behaved in a manner not described previously or subsequently. It fired while the force applied to the tooth rose from 5·0 g (the threshold value) to 70.0 g. Then it became silent although the force continued to rise, and did not fire again until the force fell through the range 70·0 to 5·0 g.

The most important recent advance in the study of dental mechanoreceptors has been the use, by Hannam (1967), of apparatus with which the forces applied to the teeth can be controlled in the rate of application, magnitude,

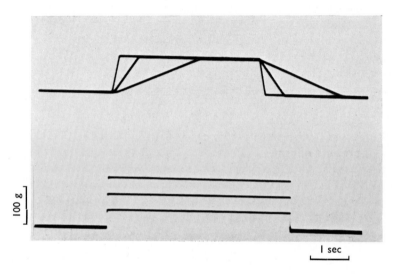

FIG. 3. Oscilloscope records from a transducer used to monitor force applied by a Pye-Ling vibrator to a tooth. Upper record; 100 g force applied and removed at three different rates. Records superimposed: Lower record; Forces of 50 g, 100 g and 150 g applied at the same rate. Records superimposed. (From Hannam, 1969).

duration and rate of removal. This is achieved with a Pye-Ling electro-magnetic force generator driven by controlled voltages. With this technique it has been possible to apply forces of constant magnitude at different rates, and forces at constant rate but of different magnitudes. These possibilities are illustrated by the force records shown in Fig. 3.

Although subsequent work suggests that classification of receptors may not be very helpful, Hannam (1967) accepted the classification adopted by Ness (1954) in which fast adapting, slowly adapting, and spontaneously discharging receptors were recognized. It was clearly shown earlier by Matthews (1965) and subsequently by Hannam (1967) that the spontaneously discharging receptors, which fire in the absence of any obvious external stimulus, behave as slowly adapting receptors during maintained stimulation. When the stimulus is removed, there is a sudden reduction of the impulse discharge, often resulting in a period of silence, followed by a gradual return to the resting frequency of discharge. This is illustrated in Fig. 4. Detailed study of this and other features of dental mechanoreceptors is complicated by the fact that they are located in a very narrow band of soft tissue between bone and teeth. For this reason it has so far been impossible to stimulate these receptors directly without the intervention of tissues which may modify the stimulus in transduction. It seems highly probable that spontaneous

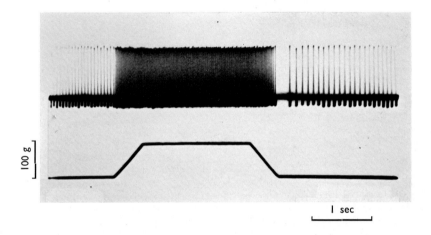

FIG. 4. The effect of stimulating a spontaneously discharging receptor. 100 g force applied in a lingual direction to a lower canine tooth in a dog. Upper record; Nerve action potentials: Lower record; Force record from transducer. Spontaneous activity prior to stimulation is augmented during stimulation. When the stimulus is removed a period of silence precedes the gradual restoration of the spontaneous frequency of impulse discharge. (From Hannam 1969).

activity merely indicates that a particular receptor, though basically no different from other slowly adapting receptors, is situated in a region under continuous pressure or tension, and is therefore subjected to continuous stimulation. Some support for this view is provided by the observation that it is possible, at least temporarily, to silence the receptor by pressing in the appropriate direction (Fig. 5). The silent period following stimulation may be the result of recoil of the tissues surrounding the receptor ending, thereby changing its environment. Further support for the view that spontaneous activity may be dependent on the environment, and is not a unique charac- teristic of the receptor, is given by the observation that a receptor initially silent, except during overt stimulation, may during the course of an experi- ment become spontaneously active. Conversely, spontaneously discharging receptors may cease to behave in this way, although still able to respond to external stimulation. Hannam (1967) found that the thresholds to mechanical stimulation of these receptors were always at the lower end of the range for dental mechanoreceptors. This is compatible with the hypothesis that spontaneous activity is due to a state of constant tension or pressure in the immediate environment of the receptors.

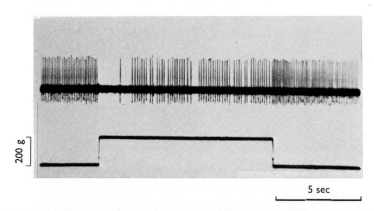

FIG. 5. Silencing of spontaneous activity by stimulation. Upper record; nerve action potentials: Lower record; Force record from transducer. Stimulation in an appropriate direction silences spontaneous activity, which resumes at a lower frequency than prior to stimulation. On removing the stimulus, there is a burst of high frequency activity before the resumption of the normal spontaneous frequency. (From Hannam. 1969).

In addition to the findings discussed already, Hannam (1967) has shown that the duration of the silent period depends on the magnitude of the stimulus and the rate at which it is removed. For example, as Fig. 6 shows, very slow removal of a stimulus will result in the restoration of spontaneous activity without any intervening silence.

Leaving the question of the mechanism of spontaneous activity still unanswered, it is worth giving some consideration to other important questions concerning dental mechanoreceptors. For example, what is the stimulus to these receptors, is it force or movement? The stimulus has its origin in the force generated during muscle contraction. However, the extent to which it is modified during transduction through the tooth and supporting tissues and whether it is the transmitted force or the resultant movement which excites the receptors, are questions yet to be answered. Dental mechanoreceptors pose a particularly difficult problem because of their inaccessibility to direct stimulation and, until this problem is solved, their properties will be imperfectly understood. However, this does not mean that their possible contribution to the control of masticatory function cannot be elucidated by methods already available. If they play such a role, then they are only one of various types of receptor in and around the mouth which are stimulated as a result of muscle activity, and which contribute towards the regulation of this activity via well established reflex pathways. Dental mechanoreceptors in their normal environment are excited only when force is applied to the teeth; therefore their function as part of a feedback system can only be studied by applying controlled forces to the teeth.

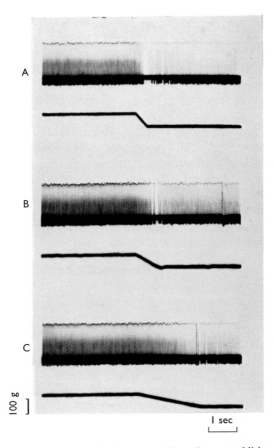

FIG. 6. The effect of rate of stimulus removal on the re-establishment of spontaneous activity. Record A. Stimulus of 100 g removed at rate of 200 g/sec. Note silent period. Record B; Stimulus of 100 g removed at rate of 100 g/sec: Record C; Stimulus of 100 g removed at rate of 40 g/sec. Note gradual decline in impulse frequency. (From Hannam 1969).

IV. The Physiological Role of Periodontal Receptors

In his classical paper on the decerebrate cat, entitled "The Pinna and other Reflexes", Sherrington (1917) demonstrated that the maintained jaw closure gives way to opening when pressure is applied to the teeth and neighbouring soft tissue.) When the pressure is released, the mandible snaps into the closed position. This, Sherrington postulated, provides the elementary neurological basis of rhythmic chewing. When the pressure is applied to teeth in the upper jaw, then there is little chance that opening depends on any receptors other than those in the periodontal tissue. It is a remarkable fact that although Kawamura and Fujimoto (1958) and others have confirmed certain observations made by Sherrington, a careful search of the literature reveals that only Harrison and Corbin (1941) have repeated the experiment of mechanically stimulating the teeth in decerebrate animals. In their experiments, which also included lightly anaesthetized animals, the response to light tapping of the teeth, especially the canines, was in some animals jaw opening and in others jaw closing. What was described as "blunt" pressure on the upper teeth or anterior part of the hard palate elicited jaw opening. Kawamura and Fujimoto (1958) determined the threshold values of electrical stimulation required to produce the opening reflex, and found that it was lowest on the dorsum of the tongue. They also used mechanical stimulation, but no reference was made in this paper to electrical or mechanical stimulation of the teeth. It therefore seems that the work of Harrison and Corbin represents the only attempt to confirm the findings of Sherrington concerning the teeth, and their results do not conclusively implicate periodontal receptors in what can be called the basic reflex mechanisms of chewing. Jerge (1964) states that

> "reflex opening is accomplished by the aggregate influence of receptors for touch and pressure in and adjacent to the mouth. The most obvious of these are the pressure receptors of the periodontal ligament . . .".

Clear cut evidence that periodontal mechanoreceptors can contribute to reflex jaw opening has recently been offered by Hannam and Matthews (1969) using anaesthetized cats. The method of stimulation made it possible to control the magnitude and duration of forces applied to the teeth and it was found that reflex jaw opening could only be produced by short duration stimuli. The force used was approximately 400 g and the threshold seemed to depend on the depth of anaesthesia. The fact that selective destruction of adjacent soft tissue and tooth pulp did not abolish the reflex whereas local anaesthesia did abolish it, supports the view that periodontal mechanoreceptors were responsible for the observed response.

Regarding the role of the spontaneously firing receptors, a quotation from Granit (1962) is appropriate. Granit says

> "In several cases it has been shown that spontaneous activity is most important for the maintenance of general excitability of the nervous centres. . . . We have evidence also for the belief that the spontaneous activity of the sense organs makes them one of the brain's most important 'energizers'."

References

Adler, P. (1947). *J. dent. Res.* **26**, 279–289.

Anderson, D. J. (1962). *Archs. oral Biol.* **7**, 7–15.

Anderson, D. J. (1967). *In* "The Mechanisms of Tooth Support" (D. J. Anderson, J. E. Eastoe, A. H. Melcher and D. C. A. Picton, eds), pp. 126–130. John Wright, Bristol.

Granit, R. (1962). "Receptors and Sensory Perception". Yale University Press, New Haven and London.

Hannam, A. G. (1967). *J. dent. Res.* (In press).

Hannam, A. G. (1969). *Archs. oral Biol.* (In press).

Hannam, A. G. and Matthews, B. (1969). *Archs. oral Biol.* **14**, 415–419.

Harrison, F. and Corbin, K. B. (1941). *Am. J. Physiol.* **135**, 439–445.

Jerge, C. R. (1963a). *J. Neurophysiol.* **26**, 379–392.

Jerge, C. R. (1963b). *J. Neurophysiol.* **26**, 393–402.

Jerge, C. R. (1964). *J. Prosth. Dent.* **14**, 667–681.

Kawamura, Y. and Fujimoto, J. (1958). *Med. J. Osaka Univ.* **9**, 377–387.

Kawamura, Y. and Nishiyama, T. (1966). *Jap. J. Physiol.* **16**, 584–597.

Kawamura, Y. and Watanabe, M. (1960). *Med. J. Osaka Univ.* **10**, 291–301.

Korber, K. H. and Korber, E. (1967). *In* "The Mechanisms of Tooth Support" (D. J. Anderson, J. E. Eastoe, A. H. Melcher and D. C. A. Picton, eds), pp. 157–161. John Wright, Bristol.

Kruger, L. and Michel F. (1962). *Archs. oral Biol.* **7**, 491–503.

Levinsky, W. and Stewart, D. (1937). *J. Anat.* **71**, 232–235.

Loewenstein, W. R. and Rathkamp, R. (1955). *J. dent. Res.* **34**, 287–294.

Manly, R. S., Pfaffman, C., Lathrop, D. D. and Keyser, J. (1952). *J. dent. Res.* **31**, 305–312.

Matthews, B. (1965). *J. dent. Res.* **44**, 1167.

Ness, A. R. (1954). *J. Physiol. Lond.* **126**, 475–493.

Pfaffman, C. (1939a). *J. Physiol. Lond.* **97**, 207–219.

Pfaffman, C. (1939b). *J. Physiol. Lond.* **97**, 220–239.

Picton, D. C. A. (1965). *Archs. oral Biol.* **10**, 945–955.

Picton, D. C. A. and Davies, W. I. R. (1967). *In* "The Mechanisms of Tooth Support" (D. J. Anderson, J. E. Eastoe, A. H. Melcher and D. C. A. Picton, eds), pp. 157–161. John Wright, Bristol.

Robinson, A. D. (1964). *Archs. oral Biol.* **9**, 281–286.

Sherrington, C. S. (1917). *J. Physiol. Lond.* **51**, 404–431.

Shrilä, H. S. and Laine, P. (1963). *Acta odont. scand.* **21**, 415–429.

Stewart, D. (1927). *Proc. R. Soc. Med.* **20**, 1675–1686.

Tryde, G., Frydenberg, O. and Brill, N. (1962). *Acta odont. scand.* **20**, 233–256.

Wilkie, J. K. (1964). *J. dent. Res.* **43**, 962.

8 | The Effect of External Forces on the Periodontium

D. C. A. PICTON

Department of Dentistry, University College Hospital Medical School, London, England

I. Origin and Character of External Forces

A. PERIORAL AND LINGUAL MUSCLES

For a large part of the day the muscles of mastication are relaxed and the mandible is said to be in the physiological rest position but, although the teeth are separated, forces are still acting on them. The soft tissues of the mouth, i.e. the lips and cheeks on the vestibular surface and the tongue on the lingual surface, are in contact with the teeth to a variable extent and for differing periods. The upper lip, for example, lies on the labial surface of upper incisors and canines in most individuals, leaving a zone usually a few millimetres wide at the incisive edge. When the lips are brought together the lower lip rests on the labial surfaces near the incisive edge also. The tongue probably contacts the lower incisors on the lingual side for a large fraction of the day but it may not reach the lingual surface of upper incisors, especially if there is a deep overbite. Acting indirectly, the soft tissues may exert force on the roots of teeth through the gingiva and the bone of the socket.

The magnitude of the forces from the oral musculature is a subject that has received attention recently (Winders 1962; Kydd *et al.*, 1963; Profitt *et al.*,

TABLE 1

Physiological forces from the tongue, lips and cheeks acting on the teeth

Reference	Exercise	Aspect measured	Vestibular force — Regions			Lingual force — Regions		Remarks
			Molars	Premolars	Incisors	Molars	Incisors	
Winders (1962)	Swallowing 2–3 ml water on command. Resting	Average maxima g/cm²	6̄5̄ / 65 ; 4·0 / 4·0 ; 4·0 / 4·0	6̄5̄ ; 4·0 ; 4·0	1̄ / 1̄ ; 11·4 / 6·2 ; 11·5 / 10·9	6̄5̄ / 65 ; 88·0 / 68·0 ; 9·0 / 8·9	1̄ / 1̄ ; 72·0 / 10·8 ; 10·1 / 6·5	11 white adult males, excellent occlusion
Kydd et al. (1963)	All types of swallowing	Average maxima g/cm²			70·0	6̄	123·0 ; 1̄	5 subjects × duration of force from lip: 1·64 tongue: 1·30
Profitt et al. (1964)	Involuntary swallow	Average maxima g/cm²			22·5	42·8	40·8	20 subjects
Gould and Picton (1964)	Sip-swallowing 10 ml water. Speaking "M". Resting force after swallowing	Average maxima g/cm²	6̄/ ; 6̄/ ; 89·4 / 39·5 ; 18·5 / 8·6 ; 21·1 / 7·1	4̄/ ; 4̄/ ; 135·3 / 156·9 ; 23·0 / 24·0 ; 21·3 / 26·2	1̄ ; 1̄ ; 61·6 / 61·2 ; 14·2 / 15·2 ; 18·1 / 7·5			10 white adult normal occlusion
Werner, 1964	Speaking "Mamma" and "Pappa"	Average maxima of M and P p/cm²	6̄ ; 6̄		1̄ ; 12 ; 77·6 ; 79·2	6̄		nine adults of both sexes with normal occlusion
	Resting force		16·2 / 15·7		19·0 / 16·2			fifteen subjects—normal occlusion
	Speech mixed words		23·6 / 34·1		36·9 / 34·0			ten subjects—normal occlusion
Lear et al. (1965b)	Speech, 1 word/sec	Average level (p/cm²) time (sec) average force (g) time (sec) at tooth surface 1 mm from tooth surface 2 mm from tooth surface	6̄ ; 7·5 ; 9·5	45 ; 1·23 ; 1·53	1̄ ; 1·60 ; 2·10	6̄ / 45 ; 7·5 / 1·23 ; 10·7 / 1·93	1̄ ; 1·60 ; 2·60	3 adult subjects for 45 data, on each for the other regions

1964; Lear *et al.*, 1965), but a clear picture of the magnitude, duration and distribution of the forces has not yet emerged. By means of transducers of force attached to the teeth (Gould and Picton, 1964) resting forces have been demonstrated on the vestibular surface of central incisors, first premolars and first molars. Peak forces recorded during speech and swallowing water indicate that there is more activity in the area covered by the modiolus, i.e. the upper canine and first premolar, in subjects with normal occlusion (Angle Class I), than elsewhere; lowest peak forces were located in the maxillary molar region. A summary of the estimates of force from different authors is given in Table 1. Estimation of force on the lingual side of the teeth has proved more difficult since transducers protruding more than 1 mm from the surface of the teeth may produce erroneously high readings (Gould and Picton, 1963, Lear *et al.*, 1965b). There seems little doubt, however, that the tongue exerts considerable intermittent force on the teeth, especially during swallowing (Winders, 1962), but the resting levels of force have not been established. It seems probable that the frequency and duration of these forces are of importance in determining the position of erupting teeth. This is because long-acting small forces, e.g. lip activity, may summate over a period of twenty-four hours and equal, in terms of average force per unit time, substantially larger forces which act for brief periods only. A further difficulty emerges in interpretation of the available data, since the transducers that have been used are flat and the force recorded from them is expressed as acting over the area of the transducers. It is not known, however, over what area of a tooth the tongue or cheeks act.

The activity of the lip musculature has been studied by Marx (1963 and 1965) using an electromyograph, and he found that the majority of subjects had some activity when the lips were in the habitual or "resting" posture. It is usually presumed that the increases in force recorded on the surface of teeth are due to contraction of the muscles in the tongue, lips or cheeks. However, Rushmer and Hendron (1951) and Faigenblum (1965) have shown that a sub-atmospheric pressure may develop over the dorsum of the tongue after swallowing. This lasts several seconds, and has been found to measure, on average, 9·7 mm Hg. Preliminary work (Gould *et al.*, 1967) indicates that the increase in force on the vestibular surfaces of teeth corresponds with an increase in pressure with speech; the increase in force produced during swallowing may be due, in part at least, to a sub-atmospheric pressure, produced by sucking in the lips and cheeks. This may gradually dwindle over many seconds.

B. FROM OTHER TEETH

1. Origin

(*a*) *Opposing teeth.* A number of studies have been made using cineradiography (Jankleson *et al.*, 1953) and miniature electric contacts in natural teeth or pontics (Anderson and Picton, 1957; Graf, 1962) from which it is evident that for some individuals, at least, the teeth are brought into contact with, their opponents during swallowing food or in idle swallowing. Direct observation of children indicates that fluids generally, and food in some individuals,

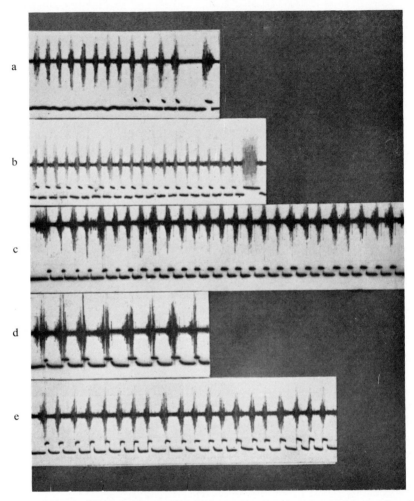

FIG. 1. Oscilloscope records of electrical activity in the masseter on the chewing side (upper tracing) and contact between the teeth on the opposite side. Tooth contact is shown by an elevation of the lower tracing. a, Subject 1. Biscuit: b, Subject 2. Carrot: c, Subject 6. Apple: d, Subject 8. Bread: e, Subject 10. Meat. (Reproduced with permission from D. J. Anderson and D. C. A. Picton (1957), *J. dent. Res.* **36**, 21–26.)

may be swallowed with the teeth apart (Rix, 1953). The contacts between opposing teeth may be made in the centric position or in excentric positions but little is known about the duration or the force exerted during contact. An illustration of the duration of contact on the non-working side of the mouth is shown in Fig. 1 but, depending on the substance between the teeth, force might be exerted prior to contact. Oscilloscope records fron a transducer of force in a lower molar are shown in Fig. 2. These illustrate the force developed

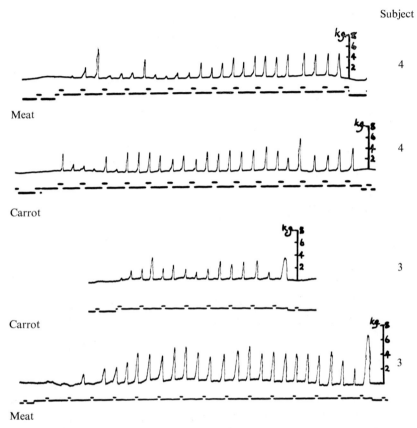

Fig. 2. Examples of oscilloscope records from the 2 subjects chewing carrot and meat. The upper tracing is the strain gauge response with a calibration scale included. The lower tracing is elevated at one-second intervals and is raised bodily for the duration of the chewing sequence. (Reproduced with permission from D. J. Anderson (1956), *J. dent. Res.* **35,** 671–673.)

on this tooth while swallowing food. Using cineradiography during mastication Ardran and Kemp (1960) found that there are two or three swallows for each mouthful. The frequency of swallowing food, fluids and saliva throughout the day, however, has been studied recently by Lear *et al.* (1965a) using an electronic recording device attached to the larynx. For young adult males an average of five hundred and eighty-five swallows per day was recorded (see Table 2).

A well-recognized behavioural condition, in which the patient grinds his teeth together, results in characteristic flat wear facets in enamel and dentine. These facets contrast with the concave facets that are produced by normal functional wear when food is between the teeth. These parafunctional facets can be found on one or more teeth which, in some people, may be opposed only on extreme excursion of the mandible. During a bout of grinding prolonged and heavy stressing of these particular teeth occurs (Glickman, 1964a) and, although a large axial component of force may be presumed, considerable lateral tipping of the teeth occurs.

TABLE 2

Frequency of deglutition (Lear et al. 1965a)
Hourly swallowing rates in 20 subjects studied over a 24-hour period
using a light pneumatic device attached to the larynx

	Mean rate	s.d.
Eating and drinking	180·0	55·0
Sleeping	5·3	1·7
Other activities	23·5	11·4
Overall rate/hour	24·4	8·7
Overall rate/day	585·0	

(b) *Mastication.* As the upper and lower dentitions are separated by 2 mm or more for a very large fraction of the day, the principal times when force is exerted by opposing teeth is during mastication. This process includes incision and separation of a fragment from the main item of food, together with the crushing and grinding necessary for deglutition. Incision of soft food consists of a relatively uncomplicated, though co-ordinated, sequence of muscular contractions in which the mandible is protruded and the incisors are brought together with small force. Biting tough food, however, may involve limb and neck muscles, so that the main portion is torn forcibly away from the fragment held between the anterior teeth. The magnitude and direction of the forces are quite different in the two cases.

Although it has been shown that there may be contact between opposing teeth during eating (Anderson and Picton, 1957; Graf, 1962), force is exerted on a tooth though the bolus with each chewing thrust in the absence of, or prior to, contact with the opposing teeth. Thus, when food was eaten under experimental conditions in which a force transducer was placed in a lower molar tooth 0·5 mm below the occlusal level so that it was not possible to touch the transducer with the opposing tooth, force was recorded with each thrust (Anderson and Picton, 1958). With a transducer of force at the normal occlusal level, Anderson (1956a,b) found that the magnitude of the force may increase as the chewing sequence progresses. There is no doubt that the texture of the food has a direct bearing on the pattern of the forces exerted on the teeth (see Table 3). Thus Dahlberg (1942) found that more thrusts were used when hardened gelatin was chewed than egg white, and that rubber

TABLE 3

Average peak loads recorded during mastication

Reference	Food	Force kg	Remarks
Yurkstas and Curby (1953)	Bread roll	1·8	Average peak load/tooth, transducers were placed in partial or full dentures in several subjects
	Tender steak	1·4	
	Carrot (raw)	1·3	
	Apple	0·7	
	Carrot (boiled)	0·4	
Anderson, 1956	Biscuit	0·61	Average peak pressure (kg/cm^2) on the transducer platform. Transducers placed in a lower first molar of four adult subjects
	Carrot	0·62	
	Meat	0·46	

TABLE 4

Average interval between chewing thrusts derived from the records of Anderson (1956) and Graf (1962)

Source	Subject	Food	Number of thrusts		Average interval (m Sec)
	1.	Biscuit	16		426
Anderson	2.	Biscuit	18		401
	2.	Meat	23		375
	3.	Biscuit	11		426
	3.	Carrot	24		427
	4.	Meat	21		442
				x̄	416
	R.H.	Bread	87		392
Graf	J.B.	Pea Nuts	61		351
	J.A.	Bread	30		467
				x̄	403
		Average time interval for all subjects			412

required most of all. Furthermore, it has been shown that the frequency of contact between opposing teeth differs depending on the nature of the food (Anderson and Picton, 1957) (Fig. 3). The activity of the masseter also gives a strong indication of the magnitude and character of the forces exerted on

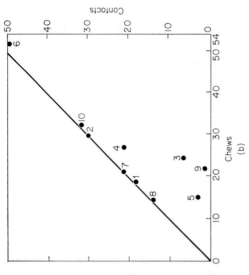

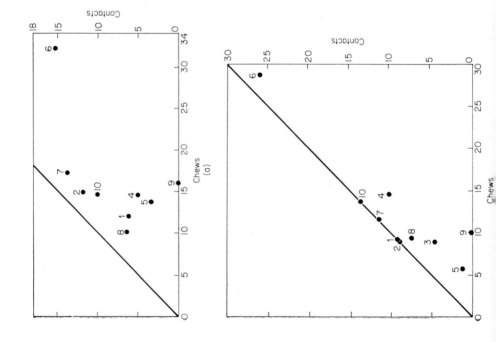

Fig. 3. The relation between the number of chewing movements and the number of contacts. The sloping line shows the direction which would be taken by the points if contact occurred with every chewing movement. The number with each point identifies the subject. (a) biscuit; (b) meat; (c) apple. (Reproduced with permission from D. J. Anderson and D. C. A. Picton (1957), *J. dent. Res.* **36**, 21–26.)

the teeth. When action potentials from this muscle were recorded, Kawamura (1964) found short abrupt discharges when peanuts were being chewed, but chewing gum produced bursts of activity which were less well defined and more protracted.

The removal of biting force from the teeth after a chewing thrust is abrupt; this is indicated by Anderson's oscilloscope records from the strain gauge dynamometer placed in a lower molar (Fig. 2). An estimate of the interval between thrusts is given in Table 4.

(c) *Adjacent teeth.* A tooth extracted from an intact arch usually shows facets of wear on the mesial and distal surfaces. These indicate the areas which had been in contact with adjacent teeth. These facets are a record of the mobility of adjacent teeth relative to each other in the bucco-lingual and axial directions. When biting force is applied to a tooth it is displaced in the alveolus and, if the force is not entirely axial, the tooth tilts. If there is a mesial or distal component to the force the tooth will tilt in that direction, so that the adjacent teeth will be displaced. Almost all teeth were found to tilt mesially under biting force in a group of young men (Picton 1962a). When these subjects bit on a posterior tooth the anterior teeth were found to tilt mesially, although no direct biting force was exerted on these teeth. This observation is consistent with the work of Osborn (1961) in which substantially more force was needed to pull out a fine steel strip from between adjacent posterior teeth when the jaws were clenched than when the mouth was open. Reverting to the previous study, when biting force was applied to anterior cheek teeth which had been shown to tilt mesially the posterior teeth were also found to tilt mesially; thus, they appeared to be pulled mesially. Furthermore, Mühlemann (1954) has found that anterior teeth are more mobile if the points of contact are removed. When taken together, these findings indicate that force applied to a tooth in contact with its neighbours tends to cause displacement of the adjacent teeth either by transmitting force directly at the contact areas or, perhaps, by traction on the transseptal fibre system.

2. Direction of Force

There have been several quantitative studies of masticatory force, but these have been made mostly with relatively large dynamometers of one type or another placed between opposing teeth; the form and limitations of the transducers have been discussed by Jenkins (1966). These studies have been primarily concerned with the measurement of maximum biting forces which may well greatly exceed normal masticatory loads. With regard to the more difficult problem of measuring the dynamic loads produced during eating it is convenient to resolve the force developed between opposing teeth into axial and horizontal components.

(a) *Axial force*. By far the most valuable studies on physiological masti-catory loads have been made using electronic devices built into dentures or natural teeth (Howell and Brudevold, 1950; Anderson, 1956). With these transducers dynamic records were obtained so that the magnitude, rate of application, and interval between thrusts could be assessed. (See Fig. 2 and Table 3.) The data from Anderson were obtained from young male adults eating small fragments of meat, carrot, biscuit and apple. Peanuts, coconut and raisins were used in experiments carried out by Howell and Brudevold.

As the platform receiving the forces in the studies just mentioned was, in each case, parallel to the occlusal plane, it may be taken that the forces were directed principally in the long axis of the teeth. However, posterior teeth in the majority of subjects are inclined with the long axes directed anteriorly relative to opposing teeth. Thus, when food is placed between the teeth, there is an anterior component of force tending to tilt the teeth forward. Similarly, many teeth are inclined lingually (e.g. lower molars), or labially (e.g. upper incisors), so that horizontal components of force must be con-sidered.

(b) *Horizontal components of force*. Practically no systematic attempt has been made to estimate horizontal components of force. Using the horizontal displacement of teeth as an indication of the presence of horizontal force, Schöhl (1960) and Picton (1961) have demonstrated that they exist with biting thrusts made in the bucco-lingual direction. Parfitt (1961) used an upper incisor to estimate the magnitude of force in the labial direction, while the subject ate celery and meat. The detection of mesial tilt of teeth under biting force illustrates that there may be a mesio-distal component as well; this has been mentioned in *1* (*c*).

Repeated tilting of teeth mesially has been suggested as a cause of mesial drift in man by a number of writers including Brodie (1934) and Dewell (1949). Drift is a phenomenon which in many mammals results in groups of neigh-bouring teeth migrating towards a common centre, so that contact with adjacent teeth is maintained as the approximal surfaces became worn away. Thus the cheek teeth of each quadrant in herbivores remain in contact as do the adjacent incisors of many animals. In each case the teeth at the ends of the row are inclined towards the centre of the row. In most intact human dental arches contact is maintained between adjacent teeth, and the long axis of most, if not all, teeth is inclined mesially. These observations *per se*, how-ever, do not prove that during mastication repeated tilting of teeth in the direction towards which they are inclined is the motive force causing migra-tion. Thus, collagen fibres resist forces of this type acting for a short time, and many teeth are aligned in other directions (e.g. the labial inclination of upper incisors, yet repeated biting forces do not result in migration labially). Recently a limited amount of experimental evidence in adult monkeys (*Macaca irus*) has demonstrated that mesial drift can occur in the absence of opposing teeth (Moss and Picton, 1967). Furthermore, it was suggested that the direction of migration is determined, in fully formed teeth, by the inclination of the long axis of the roots provided there is space for the teeth to drift.

(*c*) *Rotational Force*. In attempting to resolve the forces acting on a tooth during mastication there is a danger of over-simplifying the problem as the dynamic aspect must be considered. Since the movements of the mandible are not linear, but tend to be more or less complex arcs, it seems probable that the forces on a tooth cause rotational movements of the tooth in its alveolus. In addition, when biting force is applied to a fragment of food, a tooth close to the centre of the fragment will probably have more force acting on it than adjacent teeth; and, over the surface of individual teeth, there may be a gradient of force so that the path of movement into the socket may be a complex spiral.

Although it seems unlikely to occur in animals generally, in man and a few favoured pets, force from opposing teeth on opening the mouth when sticky foods are eaten may tend to extrude a tooth from its socket.

C. Gravity

It is unlikely that gravity has an important influence on the teeth of small animals. However, the supporting systems of heavier teeth such as the tusk or molars of the elephant, must compensate for this factor. The eruptive forces acting on lower teeth must overcome this effect whereas, in upper teeth, a substantial restraining mechanism must operate to counteract the weight of the tooth. Although the mass of these teeth changes slowly, the mesial end of each molar in the elephant is functional before the distal end is completed. Later, the tooth is progressively worn away from the mesial end until finally only a small fragment of the distal region is left. It seems probable, then, that mechanisms must exist in the periodontium of larger teeth to compensate for their weight, and that these mechanisms become modified as the mass changes. Little or no work has been carried out on the histology of the periodontium of larger animals. It would be interesting to know whether the periodontium of these animals is in any way modified to accommodate the greater weight of large teeth.

D. Miscellaneous Forces

A wide variety of objects and habits should be mentioned as having some influence on the teeth. Thus, habits such as digit sucking are widespread in young children and may be practiced frequently and for extended periods of the day. During this time the thumb, for example, may be in contact with and, therefore, may exert force upon the lingual surface of upper anterior teeth and

13

on the labial surface of lower anterior teeth. The teeth may be used occupationally (for example, as an extra hand by the shoe mender and the trapeze artist). The amount of force exerted on the teeth for these purposes may vary, but except in duration, it is probably not greatly different in character from that exerted by masticatory forces.

Pathological lesions in the mouth may also exert force on either the crowns or the roots of teeth. Continuous force is exerted on adjacent teeth by an expanding tumour in the alveolar process, but if the tumour is on the tongue the force is variable or intermittent. Normal force may be reduced abruptly, or removed, following the extraction of a tooth or excision of an organ previously in contact with the teeth. Posture, as in sleep, may be the source of extraoral forces acting on the labio-buccal surfaces of the teeth. These forces may operate over long periods, either directly or indirectly, via the intervening lips or cheeks (Werner, 1964).

E. DURATION OF ACTION OF THE FORCES

It is evident from the discussion so far that the periods over which intraoral forces act on a tooth may vary considerably. They range from a biting thrust, in the order of m sec to almost continuous action, such as the upper lip on maxillary incisors, or gravity. The duration of action has a direct bearing on the response produced in the tissues. The effect of continuous or semi-continuous force on soft tissues, as Ness (1967) has pointed out, is illustrated graphically by the gross distortion of the lips or ear lobes which is produced in some African tribes by placing foreign bodies of progressively increasing size in the tissues. The necks of "giraffe-women", and head flattening practiced by some American Indians, also demonstrate the effect on the body of continuous, though abnormal, external forces; the response here is more complex, since these disfigurements are started in childhood and affect the developing skeleton in addition to the soft tissues.

Less bizarre examples of the effect of continuous force are shown by orthodontic traction of teeth. Horizontal force applied to a point on the crown of a tooth causes the tooth to tilt; migration of a whole root through bone is produced if tubes or brackets are cemented to the crown so that tilting of the tooth is prevented.

Short acting forces are generally well resisted by the tissues. Thus a tendon transmits force from a muscle to the bone with very little temporary or permanent change in dimensions. Similarly, distortion of bone produced in the same way is transitory. Frequent repetition of the force will, if it is large relative to the previous experience of the tissues, tend to cause compensatory changes. Examples of these are strengthening of the tendon, and reinforcement of the bone architecture which exemplifies Wolff's law (Weinmann and Sicher, 1947).

This question arises; where is the dividing line between a semi-continuous force and a frequently repeated force of long duration? It may be that there is no absolute division, and that different tissues will respond differently and that the age of the tissues is an all important factor.

F. ALTERATION OF THE FORCES ACTING ON THE TEETH

1. Increase of Force

The range, in magnitude and character, of the forces acting on the teeth of a young adult are considerable during a given period, say twenty four-hours. Consecutive periods of twenty-four hours, however, would probably not show substantial differences in the overall pattern of force. In the young growing child the magnitude, at least, changes quite rapidly. Thus at six years, for example, the growth of masticatory muscles enables the child to exert more force on the deciduous teeth in mastication, but spacing of these teeth associated with growth of the dental arches removes the approximal support of adjacent teeth. Attrition of the teeth, especially of the labial segment, reduces the surface area over which the vestibular forces act. Meanwhile the eruption of the lower first permanent molar substantially alters the forces acting on the upper second deciduous molar, against which it partly occludes. Later the loss of periodontal support and, finally, shedding of deciduous incisors often results in the child "incising" with the deciduous canines.

This combination of growth in size of the jaws and soft tissues, associated with an increase in the forces exerted by these structures, is superimposed on an increasing number of erupted teeth and, due to passive eruption, a gradual increase in surface area of the clinical crowns over which the forces act. The patterns of activity of the soft tissues and the form of the occlusion become more settled when the second molars are fully formed, but measurements of maximum biting forces suggest that the forces of mastication generally tend to increase for some years (Worner and Anderson, 1944).

2. Decrease of Force

As an individual passes the "prime of life" there is a generalized loss of muscle activity and gradual atrophy of muscle fibres. It may be presumed that this phenomenon occurs in the mouth even though the dentition is still intact. Premature loss of attachment of the periodontal fibres in the cervical regions and elongation of the clinical crown results, in younger individuals, in a much increased surface area over which the forces may act, and a reduced area of support. Thus, a greatly increased leverage is produced. If attrition has been severe, however, the clinical crowns are small and, though occlusal drift may have resulted in a reduced area of root attachment, the leverage may not be unfavourable.

An abrupt reduction in the forces acting on a tooth follows the extraction of an opposing tooth. Interdigitation of opposing teeth determines that, in most occlusions, two opposing teeth have to be extracted for the forces of mastication to be removed. Although edentulous areas of the alveolar mucosa can be used to crush hard food, it is usual to find stagnation of food debris around unopposed teeth. This indicates that the latter have not been used for chewing. Tongue and cheek pressures may also change after a tooth has been extracted as the tongue tends to bulge into a small edentulous space. The soft tissues may adopt a new resting posture if a large number of teeth are removed and not replaced by a denture.

Numerous operative dental procedures may alter the forces acting on a tooth, orthodontic traction and insertion of a "high" restoration being perhaps the most common. The alteration of the forces acting on a tooth brought about by these manoeuvres may be abrupt and of an intermittent character, such as those from a high restoration; or they may be much smaller and more continuous, such as these from an orthodontic spring. A sudden increase in force to physiological levels follows restoration of occlusion to a tooth which has been unopposed as a result of extractions.

II. Effect on the Periodontium

The effects of the forces discussed above can usefully be examined by studying the physiology of the periodontium and the microscopic appearance of the periodontal tissues after known forces have been applied to a tooth for relatively long periods. Although the normal histology of the region has been described in detail in Chapter 6 it is of value here to emphasize a few salient structural features, as the ability of the periodontium to resist forces acting on the crown is intimately related to the morphology of the tissues.

A. STRUCTURE

1. Fibres

The collagen fibre bundles are arranged in groups which appear well aligned to resist by tension the forces acting on the crown of the tooth from axial and horizontal directions. In a mechanical concept these fibres are seen as inelastic ties uniting the root to the alveolus, but when the tooth is at rest they are relaxed and wavy. Small horizontal forces to the crown displace the root, and are said to straighten out the fibres on the side to which the force is applied but to cause an increased relaxation on the opposite side. The dense network of principal fibres might also provide a well packed cushion under compression.

Two features should be noted at this point. Firstly that individual fibre bundles do not cross uninterrupted from cementum to bone. The collagen fibres leave one bundle, spread out and blend with adjacent bundles, so forming a region of interlacing fibres sometimes called the *intermediate plexus* (Fig. 35, Chapter 6). The second point is that peripheral fibre groups are larger, and are separated by the foramina and grooves in the alveolus, whereas at the root surface, they are smaller and regularly distributed. This indicates that the fibres are likely to be of unequal length.

2. Blood Vessels

(see also Chapter 3, Section **VI**)

It was Joseph Fox in 1833 who suggested that the blood vessels in the periodontal ligament might act as a shock absorbing system. Detailed information on the vascular architecture in the human periodontium is sparse (Castelli, 1963; Provenza, 1966), mostly having been obtained from studies on the distribution of the blood vessels of molars of rat and monkey (Kindlová and Matena, 1962). The number of vessels in the periodontal tissues is high when it is remembered that the principal constituent is collagen fibres. Arteries enter the ligament mainly through the alveolar wall and fundus; the average diameter is 21 μ. They appear to be similar in structure to arteries elsewhere. The larger vessels, at least, pass mainly longitudinally between fibre bundles peripherally, or in grooves in the alveolus itself. Thus, when the fibre bundles are tensed or compressed, occlusion of the larger arteries is probably avoided.

At the alveolar margin there is an extensive network of arteriovenous loops or rete, while elsewhere fine vessels and capillaries can be seen passing close to the cementum and in amongst the fibre bundles. They drain into numerous veins, average diameter 28 μ, which mostly run longitudinally in the ligament towards the apex, where they link up to form an extensive venous network or rete. In multi-rooted teeth venous rete are found in the region of diversion of the roots. Blood leaves the venous network via small vessels passing though the alveolar wall where a further venous network is located. Glomera have been described in the human ligament by Provenza (1966). These may act as a shunt for blood to pass directly from arteries to veins.

The form and complexity of the vessels indicates that they play an important part in supporting the tooth against sudden stress rather in the manner of a hydraulic damping device or dashpot. Great significance has been attached to the form of the vessels by Bien (1966) and this will be discussed in Section VI. The initial displacement of the root is resisted by blood as it is squeezed out of the alveolus or from one region of the ligament to another. However, young teeth with an incompletely formed apex, or teeth having had the apical tissues removed surgically, are fully functional. Consequently, the presence of venous rete around the apex are not essential to normal tooth support.

3. Cells and Fluids

For the purposes of this discussion extracellular and intracellular fluids may be considered together. The high fibre content of the ligament results in a relatively small number of cells, principally fibroblasts, orientated with, and lying amongst, the collagen bundles. As fluids under pressure are incompressible, two changes may occur when pressure or tension is developed in a region of the ligament. The shape of the cells may change or the cells and fluid may be displaced from the region. Since the socket is extensively perforated there may be a tendency for cells and fluid to be extruded from the compressed region via these foramina. However, some degree of tilt of the root is produced by non-axial force, so that cells and fluid may tend to be displaced from a region of compression towards a region of tension.

4. Socket

The alveolus is a thin thimble of bone perforated by numerous obliquely directed foramina distributed mainly in the cervical and apical thirds (Birn, 1966). The inner and outer plates of compact bone are sometimes not separated by supporting bone trabeculae. However, in many teeth the alveolus consists of cancellous trabeculae. The periodontal fibre bundles are attached to one surface of these, and trabeculae of the supporting bone to the other, linking the socket either with neighbouring sockets or with the adjacent external bony plates.

5. Dimensions

The radius of the alveolus, taken at the fundus or in transverse section, is slightly greater than the corresponding dimension of the root. The ligament is narrowest in the middle third of the root so that the socket is somewhat dumb bell-shaped with regard to the root. In spite of this feature, the root surface of many teeth is parallel to the adjacent surface of the socket, so that with axial force the root can be visualized as sliding past the socket with little or no decrease in width of the periodontal space except at the apex or between the roots.

The dimensions of the periodontal space in man have been measured by various writers but the data from Coolidge (1937) are shown in Tables 5–11 and Fig. 4. It is evident from these measurements that teeth in heavy function, i.e. molars, and teeth in young adults, tend to have a wider ligament than newly erupted teeth, non-functional or old teeth.

TABLE 5

Thickness of periodontal membrane of 172 teeth from fifteen human jaws (Coolidge, 1937)

	Average of alveolar crest	Average of midroot	Average of apex	Average of tooth
Ages 11–16				
83 teeth from 4 jaws	0·23	0·17	0·24	0·21
Ages 32–50				
36 teeth from 5 jaws	0·20	0·14	0·19	0·18
Ages 51–67				
35 teeth from 5 jaws	0·17	0·12	0·16	0·15
Age 25 (1 case)				
18 teeth from 1 jaw	0·16	0·09	0·15	0·13

TABLE 6

Thickness of periodontal tissues in varying conditions of function

	Alveolar crest mm	Midroot mm	Apex mm	Average mm
Teeth in heavy function				
44 teeth from 8 jaws	0·20	0·14	0·19	0·18
Teeth not in function				
20 teeth from 12 jaws	0·14	0·11	0·15	0·13
Embedded teeth				
5 teeth from 12 jaws	0·09	0·17	0·18	0·08
Malposed and drifting teeth	0·22	0·16	0·18	0·19

TABLE 7

Comparison of thickness of periodontal membrane of four incisors and four molars (jaw 17, subject aged eleven years)

	Alveolar crest mm	Midroot mm	Apex mm	Average mm
Four lateral incisors	0·33	0·25	0·28	0·29
Four molars	0·22	0·15	0·26	0·21

TABLE 8

Comparison of thickness of periodontal membrane of molar in heavy occlusion and of molar without an antagonist (jaw 35, subject aged fifty-four)

	Alveolar crest mm	Midroot mm	Apex mm	Average mm
Lower left second molar				
in heavy occlusion	0·28	0·13	0·18	0·20
Lower right second molar				
without antagonist	0·14	0·09	0·08	0·10

TABLE 9

Comparison of thickness of periodontal membrane of erupted malposed molar and of completely embedded molar (jaw 47, subject aged thirty-eight)

	Alveolar crest mm	Midroot mm	Apex mm	Average mm
Erupted lower left third molar	0·33	0·13	0·11	0·19
Completely embedded lower right molar	0·13	0·13	0·13	0·13

TABLE 10

Comparison of periodontal membrane of molar in heavy occlusion and of two bicuspids in normal occlusion (jaw 52, subject aged fifty-one)

	Alveolar crest mm	Midroot mm	Apex mm	Average mm
Lower left third molar in heavy occlusion	0·24	0·19	0·21	0·21
Left first bicuspids in normal occlusion	0·18	0·13	0·17	0·16

TABLE 11

Comparison of periodontal membrane on labial and lingual sides and on mesial and distal sides in three crowded incisors (jaw 62, subject aged eleven)

	Mesial mm	Distal mm	Labial mm	Lingual mm
Upper right central incisor, mesial and labial drift	0·12	0·24	0·12	0·22
Upper left central incisor, no drift	0·21	0·19	0·24	0·24
Upper right lateral incisor, distal and labial drift	0·27	0·17	0·11	0·15

Tables 5–11 reproduced with permission E. D. Coolidge (1937). *J. Am. dent. Ass. dent. Cosmos.* **24**, 1260–1270.

It seems clear from the variations in the dimensions of the ligament, the number and thickness of the fibre bundles, the density and thickness of the alveolar wall and supporting trabeculae, that these tissues are closely concerned with supporting the tooth against the forces acting on it. Final proof is provided by the disappearance or remodelling of these tissues which follows the extraction of the tooth.

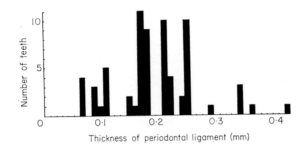

Fig. 4. Graphic representation of the thickness of periodontal ligament at the alveolar crest of a group of thirty-six teeth in Table 4 (ages 32–50 years). The figures on the horizontal line represent the thickness of the periodontal ligament in hundredths of millimetres; the figures on the vertical line represent the frequency with which the various measurements are found. The greatest number of measurements fall at 0·17 mm. The arithmetical average is 0·20 mm. The arithmetical average for all measurements of these thirty-six teeth as shown in Table 5 is 0·18 mm since the smaller measurements at the midroot reduce the total averages. (Reproduced with permission from E. D. Coolidge (1937), *J. Am. dent. Ass. dent. Cosmos.* **24**, 1260–1270.)

B. Physiology

For convenience the short term effects of forces acting on a tooth will be considered separately from the long term effects, although the latter may occur as a result of repeated short acting forces.

1. Short Term Effects

(*a*). *Change of Position.* The method of study almost invariably has been to measure *in vivo* or *in vitro* the change in position of a tooth produced by force of known magnitude. Various transducers of movement have been designed to reveal the displacement of the crown of the test tooth relative to one or more other teeth in the arch. The mechanical devices which were developed first were miniature dial gauges from which a pointer protruded to rest lightly on the tooth (Mühlemann, 1951). When force is applied the tooth is displaced, and the gauge indicates directly the distance the tooth has been moved. A wide variety of electronic devices are now in use. These include linear variable inductance transformers (Parfitt, 1960), strain gauges (Schöhl 1960; Picton, 1963), and capacitance devices (Körber, 1962). The important advantages of

13*

an electronic device are that a graphic record of the position of the tooth can be obtained throughout the application of the force and that the rate of application of the force can be very rapid.

Detailed knowledge of the amount of force being applied to the tooth at any instant can be obtained from a dynamometer incorporating an electronic device. In this way the simultaneous record of change in force and displacement of the tooth enables the relationships to be studied in detail. On the basis of the relationship between the characteristics of the force and tooth displacement, a considerable amount of information has been derived on the properties of the periodontal ligament.

i. Force and displacement

When light force is applied to a tooth it is displaced very readily, but as the force approaches 100 g the amount of movement for a given increase in force becomes substantially less. Mühlemann (1951) considers that two phases of "tooth mobility" were demonstrated in the horizontal direction: TM_1 being the phase of relatively free movement with force below 100 g, and TM_2 the phase of restricted displacement with force up to 1·5 kg, above which pain was produced. More recent work (Parfitt, 1961) in the axial direction, and in the horizontal direction (Körber and Körber, 1967) reveals a logarithmic relationship between force and movement of a tooth; this phenomenon is present when the duration and the frequency of application of the force differ widely, though the log value may change.

Mühlemann and Zander (1954) consider that the two parts to the tooth mobility curve are due to the root being moved in the alveolus with little restraint until the wavy collagen bundles are straightened (TM_1); above 100 g, tension in the bundles is developed so that the bone of the socket resists further displacement (that is, TM_2 is due to distortion of the alveolus). More recently it has been possible with electronic transducers to demonstrate that the *force : movement curve* is semi-logarithmic, and this relationship indicates that there is a gradual transition from one mechanism of support to another starting well below 100 g.

ii. Rate of application of force

Parfitt (1960) and Körber and Körber (1967) have demonstrated that when the force is applied rapidly substantially less displacement of the crown is produced than if it is applied slowly. It is difficult to reconcile this finding, and that the curves are of semi-logarithmic form, with the simple concept of inelastic collagen fibres straightening out and transmitting stress to the socket. A visco-elastic mechanism has been postulated by these writers to explain the findings.

iii. Recovery following the removal of force and the interval between thrusts.

When axial or horizontal force is removed the crown swiftly returns towards the starting position in a linear manner with time, but as it approaches the starting position a second and logarithmic recovery phase develops (Figs 5 & 6). The second phase is prevented by a small residual force (e.g. 15 g) on the

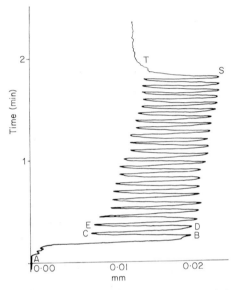

Fig. 5. The axial movement/time curve of an upper incisor tooth in the evening. A, The initial position; B, the position at 500-g peak force on the first application; C, the first return on removal of force; D, the position at 500-g peak force on the second application; S, the position at 500-g peak force on the twenty-second application; T, the return point after the final removal of force. (Reproduced with permission from G. J. Parfitt (1960), *J. dent. Res.* **39**, 608–618.)

tooth. Superficially, these characteristics are consistent with the bone of the socket recoiling in an elastic manner (recovery phase 1) and the collagen fibres gradually reverting to the wavy condition (recovery phase 2).

The interval between thrusts has a close bearing on the amount of tooth movement produced by a given level of force. Parfitt (1960) has noted that in a series of thrusts with intervals of a few seconds the amount of axial movement of the tooth was gradually reduced with each successive thrust (Fig. 5). Thus, the tooth returned fractionally less far after each successive thrust. The explanation of this phenomenon appears to be a gradual reduction of the displacement in the first or free phase of mobility. This work was subsequently confirmed (Fig. 7) (Picton, 1963), and a time lapse of approximately one to one and a half minutes was found to be necessary for a tooth to

return to the starting position. Parfitt has also noted that the tooth appeared
to be progressively intruded into the socket as the series of thrusts continued.
This observation could be explained using the concept of a tensional system
only if there was gradual slipping of the collagen units in the fibre bundles.

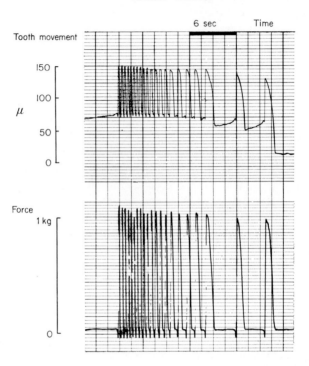

FIG. 6. A graphic record of bucco-lingual force, shown in the lower trace, applied to an
upper incisor and the resulting movement of the tooth recorded in the upper trace. The
record is read from right to left, chart speed 10 in. per min. The second thrust was applied
approximately 3 sec after the release of the first thrust. The interval between thrusts was
gradually reduced. Subject C.A. (Reproduced from D. C. A. Picton (1965), *Archs. Oral Biol.*
10, 945–955.)

When intervals greater than 1·5 min (2 mins), were used (Picton, 1964), the
amount of axial movement of a tooth gradually increased with successive
thrusts. This feature appeared to be due to a progressive extrusion of the
tooth between thrusts relative to the starting position; the change in amount
of movement occurred in the first phase of mobility (see Fig. 8). A constant
intrusive force to the tooth of approximately 3 g prevented the gradual increase
in mobility.

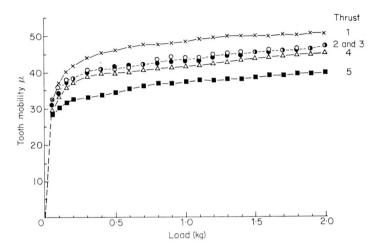

FIG. 7. Load/vertical mobility curves for five thrusts to a human upper central incisor with an interval of 5 sec. There is a progressive reduction in movement with each successive thrust as the tooth fails to return to the position at which the previous thrust was applied. The effect appears to be due to a progressive change in the mechanism resisting the initial one or two hundred grams force.

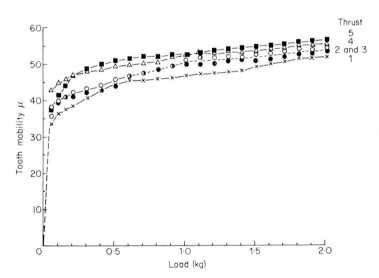

FIG. 8. Load/vertical mobility curves for five thrusts to the same tooth as in Fig. 9 with an interval of 2 min. There is a small but distinct increase in movement as the series progesses, which may be accounted for by changes in the resistance to the initial one hundred grams force. (Reproduced from D. C. A. Picton (1963), *Archs. Oral Biol.* **8**, 291–299.)

iv. The "state" of the periodontal ligament

A number of factors affect the mobility of a tooth. Himmel *et al.* (1957) found a gradual reduction in horizontal mobility during the day and, furthermore, that sleep restored the previous high values. This work has been confirmed by O'Leary *et al.* (1966). Parfitt (1961) found that teeth were also more mobile in the axial direction following sleep or lying down, and he considered that a progressive reduction in mobility with intrusion of the tooth occurred during eating and throughout the day. However, following heavy function, Mühlemann (1954) found that teeth were more mobile in the horizontal direction; he also found that subjects known to grind their teeth at night had greater mobility values on waking than when these parafunctional habits were corrected. These conflicting observations may be due to the methods of study or to differences in the horizontal and axial supporting systems of the teeth. More recently O'Leary *et al.* (1967) showed a significant reduction in horizontal mobility of anterior and posterior teeth in six subjects after eating bread rolls for ten minutes.

v. Pulsation of a tooth

When a tooth is "at rest" it can be shown to move rhythmically in the socket; that this pulsation is synchronous with the heart beat. Körber (1963) and Hofmann and Diemer (1966) considered that oscillations in the horizontal direction are due to pulsation of arteries in restricted areas of the periodontal ligament. Parfitt (1960) found pulsations of a similar character in the long axis of a tooth when a force of 0·5–4 g was applied axially. As this effect was obliterated when the force was increased to 15 g, he considered it to be due to occlusion of the arteries in the apical region of the socket. Although the vascular architecture around the rodent incisor is quite different from that in man, Taylor (1950), on viewing the pulp through a window of dentine, found that retraction of the tooth retarded or stopped the pulpal blood flow. However, when force of 200 g or 2 kg was applied axially to human incisors for five minutes, no change was noted in the amount of axial tooth movement immediately after the release of the thrust (Picton, 1964). Extrusion with an increase in mobility might have been expected to follow if the arteries in the periodontium had been occluded, since reactive hyperaemia of the tissues elsewhere in the body follows occlusion of the blood supply (Barsoum and Smirk, 1936). This finding is in accordance with the course of the arteries of the ligament between the fibre bundles or in grooves in the alveolar wall.

vi. Distortion of the tooth and alveolus

When horizontal force is applied to the crown of a tooth which is held rigidly at the apex a gradient of distortion can be demonstrated along the tooth (Savdir and Rateitschak, 1964). *In vivo*, however, with a similar force, the gradient of distortion may be presumed to be of more complex form. Körber (1963) has shown that deformation does occur *in vivo*. He inserted a long narrow piezo-electric crystal into a root canal; one end was cemented to the apical end of the canal and the other to the pulp chamber. A potential

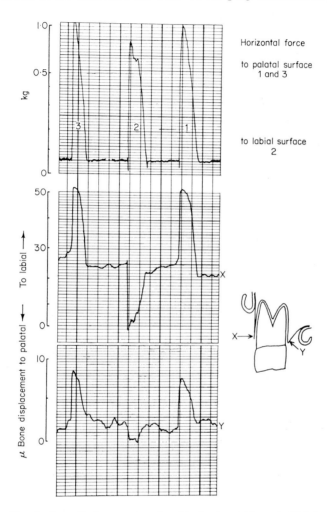

FIG. 9.—Alveolar bone displacement produced by horizontal force to PM₁ in a monkey. A graphic record of three thrusts to an upper premolar. Thrusts 1 and 3 were applied to the palatal surface, thrust 2 to the labial side of the tooth. The two transducers of movement rested on the alveolar margins at X = labial bone displacement and Y = palatal bone displacement. Deflection of the pens X and Y upwards was due to displacement of bone towards the labial side while downward movement indicated displacement palatally. The undulating base-line of Y corresponded with the heart beat and respiration. (Reproduced from D. C. A. Picton (1965), *Archs Oral Biol.* **10**, 945–955.)

difference was recorded from the crystal with each application and removal of force to the crown. Compression of extracted human teeth in the long axis has been studied by Neumann and Di Salvo (1957). Although the loads used were greatly in excess of masticatory loads, it may be concluded that a tooth is compressed two microns or less during mastication.

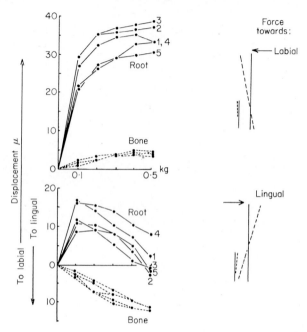

FIG. 10. Graph of horizontal root movement/force from an upper incisor of an adult monkey. Two transducers of movement were used. Through a small hole cut in the labial bone one transducer rested on the root while the other touched the bone at the edge of the hole. Five thrusts were applied to the crown towards the lips, upper graph, and towards the palate, lower graph; intervals of 1·5 minutes were used. With force towards the lips the root was displaced in the same direction and a greater distance than the adjacent bone, i.e. there was a decrease in width of the ligament. Force towards the palate caused the root to move labially while the bone was displaced lingually i.e. the root transducer was apical to the axis of rotation of the tooth. A schematic representation is given on the right to represent the displacement of the tooth and labial bone. (Reproduced from D. C. A. Picton and W. I. R. Davies (1967), *Archs. Oral Biol.* **12**, 1635–1643.)

The alveolar margin was first shown to be distorted by Mühlemann and Zander (1954). They placed a pointer on the labial bone of monkeys and found that it was displaced when horizontal force to the tooth exceeded 100 g. This observation was considered to support the concept that the second phase of mobility was due to tensed collagen bundles pulling on the alveolar wall. Subsequently it was found, also in monkeys (Picton 1965), that distortion of the labial and lingual alveolar plates of bone could be detected with horizontal or axial force to the tooth of 50 g or less, and that the displacement was of curvilinear form with a fast linear recovery. The margins of the socket were usually, but not invariably, displaced in the same direction as the force acting on the tooth, and to approximately the same extent, whether the force was

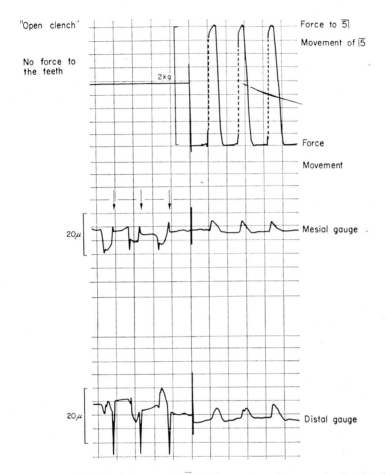

FIG. 11. A record of the movement of $\overline{/5}$ relative to the adjacent teeth. Reading from right to left three biting thrusts were applied to $\overline{5/}$. The dynamometer was then removed from the mouth and the "open clench" exercise (arrows) was repeated, three times in all. Force was recorded in the upper trace while distortion of the mesial and distal movement transducers was recorded in the lower two traces. (Chart speed 12 in/min.) (Reproduced from D. C. A. Picton (1962b), *Archs. Oral Biol.* **7**, 573–580.)

towards the palate or lips (Fig. 9). The socket margins were found to diverge when axial force was applied to anterior teeth. The margins of alveoli adjacent to the test tooth were found to be distorted in a similar manner but to a smaller extent; the distortion of bone in one region therefore appeared to spread to the neighbouring sockets. The soft tissues may exert force on the roots of teeth indirectly through the alveoli, since light finger pressure on the attached gingiva or gentle movement of the lip produces displacement of the alveolar margins and of the crowns of the teeth.

All the work described so far in this section has been concerned with measuring the mobility of the teeth or the alveolar bone, and inferring from these the changes occurring in the periodontal ligament. A direct approach has been made to measure, in monkeys, the dimensional changes in the ligament by recording simultaneously through a small hole cut in the labial bone the displacement of the root and of the bone at the margin of the hole (Picton and Davies, 1967). It was found that following application of horizontal force the root and adjacent bone were usually displaced in the same direction, but that in twenty per cent of instances the bone was displaced in the direction opposite to the root. This suggests that the labial bone did not necessarily follow the displacement of the underlying root but that it might have been distorted by a spread of stress from elsewhere in the alveolus (Fig. 10).

Force applied to a group of teeth, or even to one tooth, causes distortion of the adjacent bone, which tends to spread to the rest of the jaw (Fig. 11). This has been demonstrated by Jung (1952) and by McDowell and Regli (1961), who found adduction of contralateral pairs of posterior teeth when force was applied to the jaw. It seems probable that contraction of the muscles of mastication causes greater distortion of the mandible than the maxilla (Picton, 1962b).

vii. Effect of drugs, hormones, etc.

A limited amount of experimental work has been undertaken on the effect of drugs influencing the periodontal tissues. Thus Parfitt (1960) found that atropine given to the subject tended to decrease the axial movements of a tooth. Local anaesthetic solutions containing vaso-constrictors have been injected around upper human incisors in a preliminary and unreported series of tests by the writer. Unexpectedly, though ischaemia was produced over a wide area, there was no change in axial mobility. The effect of substances which act selectively on one tissue element in the ligament have been tested *in vitro* on the jaws of sheep preserved for some days (Parfitt, 1967). He reports that collagenase, and temperature changes known to affect collagen, altered the elastic characteristics of the *force : movement curves*, and concludes that collagen is at least partly responsible for the elastic properties of the ligament. Alterations in tonicity or acidity of the tissues affected the visco-elastic after-effect of intrusion under load or recovery. This implies that ground substance is concerned with this property of the supporting system. The gradual intrusion of a tooth which is produced by a small axial force maintained for some minutes can be markedly altered by factors affecting the tissue fluid content; drugs increasing blood pressure cause a tooth to rise in the socket so that it is displaced a greater distance when axial force is applied subsequently. This alteration appears to be independent of the elastic and visco-elastic properties, and may be in series with them. Clearly this is a promising line of study and of considerable importance; details of the results are awaited with interest.

The generalized effects on connective tissue of the hormonal changes during pregnancy are revealed in the mouth by changes in tooth mobility. Thus Mühlemann (1951) and Mühlemann *et al.* (1965) have reported a progressive increase in horizontal mobility of human teeth with advance in pregnancy. This was rapidly reduced to the previous level at full term or with premature loss of the foetus. (See Chapter 10, Section **IV**).

When investigating in man the cause of the increase in tooth mobility which occurs during sleep Himmel *et al.* (1957) tested the effect of ACTH on their subjects. They found that subjects who slept normally, but received ACTH, showed a smaller increase of mobility during the night than in the absence of the hormone. The mechanism of this effect has not been elucidated but is presumably due to the action of the hormone on the connective tissue elements in the ligament.

(b) Theories of action

i. Compression and/or tension

Although histological evidence favours the tensional concept, the limited experimental evidence suggests a combination of tension and compression in different regions of the periodontium. For example, when the direction of displacement of the alveolar margins on the labial and lingual sides of the test tooth in monkeys was used as the indicator of tension or compression (Picton, 1965), the average displacement was similar at 250 g horizontal force whether the force was directed labially or lingually; the direction of displacement was reversed when the direction of the force was reversed. Axial force appeared to be resisted by compression since the alveolar margins were diverged, whereas tension of the principal fibres would have caused convergence of the margins. On these limited experimental grounds, therefore, the justification for the use of the term "periodontal ligament" in preference to "periodontal membrane" is not clear.

The relatively simple concept of the wavy collagen fibres gradually straightening out as the force increases, and that they then act as inelastic strings transmitting tension to the alveolus, seems incompatible with the findings of Parfitt (1961, 1967). Parfitt's tripartite theory is that: (i) the elastic properties of the periodontium found with the application or release of short acting force are due to the stretching or distortion of collagen; (ii) the visco-elastic after-effect found to follow the elastic intrusive phase or recovery phase in (i) is due to the ground substance; (iii) the drift or creep produced by long-acting force in the axial direction (Parfitt, 1960) or horizontally (Mühlemann *et al.*, 1965) is due to changes in volume of the vascular elements of the periodontium. Bien and Ayers (1965) working on maxillary incisors of rats have advanced an hypothesis to explain their findings which is discussed in (v).

ii. Axial and horizontal mechanisms of support

Many of the characteristics of tooth mobility are common to the two directions of displacement and it would not be unreasonable, therefore, to assume that the mechanisms of support may be similar or even identical. However, a few features of difference are known. Thus, the repeated axial

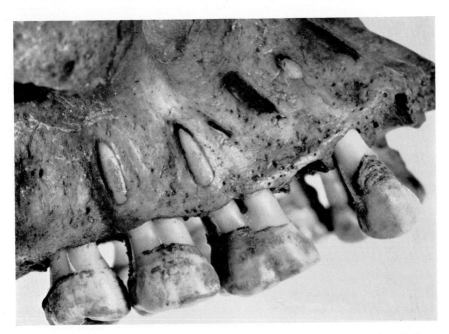

FIG. 12. The right side of the maxillary alveolar arch from a North American Indian. Multiple large defects or fenestrations in the alveolar bone were present over the buccal roots of the cheek teeth. These non-pathological features indicate the local nature of the mechanisms of tooth support.

thrusts during eating caused a progressive reduction in axial mobility with intrusion of the tooth (Parfitt, 1960), but chewing hazel nuts was shown by Mühlemann (1954) to increase horizontal mobility. As horizontal force tends to produce a tilting movement, localized regions of tension and of compression develop in the line of the force, but regions tangential to the force are not involved directly. Axial force, however, seems likely to affect the whole periodontium in a relatively uniform manner which, with the limited evidence available, seems to be under compression rather than tension.

iii. Generalized or localized mechanisms

Synge (1933), on mathematical grounds, considers that teeth are too tight in their sockets for the collagen fibres to straighten out. Gabel (1956) considers that the fibres at right angles to the force might support the tooth by resisting displacement of tissue elements from regions of compression. To test this hypothesis a narrow scalpel blade approximately 75 μ thick was pressed deeply into the periodontal ligament on the mesial and distal sides of the roots af anterior teeth of monkeys (Picton, 1967). This extensive trauma, however, produced surprisingly little increase in horizontal mobility in the bucco-lingual direction. It was concluded from these results that the integrity of the fibres in these regions is not of great importance in resisting horizontal force. Furthermore, structural defects in the labial wall of the alveolus known as fenestration and dehisence (Fig. 12), illustrate morphologically that a complete bony alveolus is not necessary for normal tooth support.

The conclusion that might be drawn from these observations, and the lack of disturbance to support which usually follows even extensive apicectomies, is that although compression within the ligament may be important in tooth support the effect must be localized to restricted areas of the alveolus. However, tension would not seem to be hampered by an incomplete alveolar wall.

iv. Gradients of axial movement

Although with horizontal force the cervical region of the root tends to compress the periodontal ligament, with axial force the change in width of the ligament is probably very small except in the apical or furcation areas. Reference to Fig. 13 reveals that axial displacement of the root of, say, 20 μ produces very little reduction in width coronal to X–X. As the distance the alveolus is displaced axially must be very small relative to the root movement, a gradient of displacement exists across the ligament. Thus, cells and blood vessels near to the root as well as collagen fibres will be carried apically perhaps 18 μ, whereas cells and vessels close to the alveolus will be displaced a few microns only. If this concept, which may be compared with plates of glass separated by a film of liquid, is close to reality then there will be little compression of blood vessels above X–X, except where collagen fibres on straightening out pinch small vessels entwined within the bundles. Apical to X–X, however, a decrease of 20 μ in the width of the ligament may be accounted for partly by compression of the vascular plexuses, and also by partial displacement of the tissue elements from this region into the area coronal to X–X.

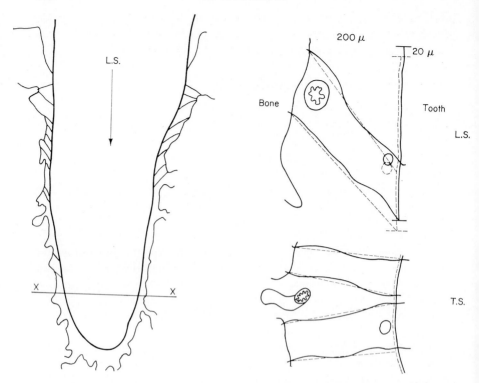

Fig. 13. The outline of a premolar root has been drawn *in situ*. Above X—X, axial intrusion of the tooth would produce very little reduction in width of the periodontal ligament. Below X—X, the width would be reduced by ten to twenty per cent under a load of five hundred grams. The change in dimensions of a small area of the periodontium above X—X is represented diagrammatically on the right, in longitudinal section above, and in transverse section below. An hypothetical force of a few hundred grams in the long axis of the tooth would have caused this change.

v. An haemodynamic theory of tooth support

The complexity of the vascular architecture of the periodontium has led a number of writers to conclude that it plays an important part in the suspension of the tooth. Bien and Ayers (1965) and Bien (1966) have re-examined this question in the light of experimental evidence gained from rats where intrusive movements of maxillary incisors have been studied before and after death of the animal. The oscillations of the test tooth were measured relative to the adjacent control tooth with a vernier micrometer eyepiece. Two phases of movement were noted under load and after removal of the force; in addition, the period and amplitude of intrusion and recovery were found to change significantly after the death of the rat (Fig. 14). In the curve representing oscillation of the tooth in the dead animal, as long as extracellular fluid remains within the periodontium, the curve is identical with that of the living animal. After the extracellular fluid is squeezed from the periodontium, the curve enters a second phase. In the living animal after the initial impulsive load is resisted by the squeeze film, further resistance to the load occurs because additional fluid is fed into the system, driven through the walls of cirsoid aneurysms formed when the smaller blood vessels are constricted

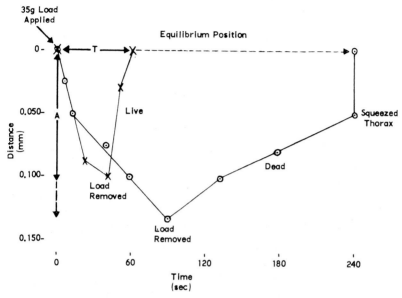

Fig. 14. The displacement of a rat maxillary incisor in its socket under a load. The plottings are diagrammatic representations of the intrusion of the tooth into its socket under a load, and its restoration to the equilibrium level after removal of the load. A complete cycle is the period T (abscissa) while the magnitude of the intrusion from the point of equilibrium is the amplitude A (ordinate). (Reproduced with permission from S. M. Bien (1966), *New York Acad. Sci.* **28**, 4, 496–499.)

by the periodontal fibres. During the restoring cycle in the dead animal, the tooth failed to return to the equilibrium position until after the thorax was squeezed. The difference between the cycles of the live and the recently sacrificed animals show that the periodontal fibres do not act as a suspensory system for the tooth. As in previous studies, these experiments indicate a combination of mechanisms which Bien (1966) has examined mathematically.

The analogy of a squeeze film is proposed as a result of calculation of the Reynold's ratio using the formula

$$R = \text{length of tooth} \times \frac{\dfrac{\text{period of oscillation}}{\text{amplitude of movement}}}{\text{Kinematic viscosity}}$$

The viscosity of the tissue was taken to be similar to that for whole blood (approximately 4 centistokes). The Reynold's ratio worked out in the range

2·5–7·6 × 10³ for light and heavy forces in living and dead animals. This is said to indicate that the mechanisms resisting tooth movement in the rat, both intrusive and recovery, are predominantly viscous in character. The suggested analogy is the squeeze film, which is a thin film of lubricant between load bearing surfaces in which the fluid under pressure is squeezed to the edges of the plates, in this case to the cervical and apical regions of the socket.

To explain the second part of the intrusive and recovery cycle after the squeeze film becomes exhausted, a second and slower mechanism is postulated to resist the continued movement of the tooth and dissipate kinetic energy. Bien and Ayers (1965) consider that calculation of the spring constant of the periodontal ligament of rats supports this concept.

Thus:

$$K = \text{mass} \left(\frac{2\pi}{\text{period of oscillation}}\right)^2$$

where mass is obtained from the gram-weight of the load. The range of estimates of K for the incisors of the living rats represents the flexibility of a soft spring, and was $4·2 \times 10^{-4}$ for 35 g force and $5·5 \times 10^{-4}$ with 183 g force. These were significantly greater than after sacrifice of the same animals, which indicates the importance of the intact blood supply in this phenomenon. The suggested form of this spring is that small blood vessels interweaving between the principal fibres become obstructed when the fibres are straightened. Ballooning of these vessels would occur, so that the resulting numerous flexible-walled sacs would act as minute springs and kinetic energy would be used up by forcing fluid through porosities in the walls.

Calculations based on data obtained from single rooted teeth should reveal whether these concepts can be extended to tooth support at large. The spring constant theory is developed further by Bien (1966) to explain the onset of resorption of alveolar bone by the action of minute gas bubbles resulting from occlusion of the capillary loops in the periodontium.

2. Long Term Effects of Force Acting on a Tooth

Long term effects of alteration in the pattern of force acting on a tooth are mediated through the short term changes discussed above. Thus the application of an orthodontic spring to a tooth, or the onset of a thumb sucking habit, would act in the first place in a manner similar to a steady experimental force of a few grams which causes horizontal creep or axial intrusion. The effect of these forces in terms of migration of a tooth is often easy to see in children; but quite drastic alterations in the pattern of force, such as follow wholesale extraction of adjacent and opposing teeth, may not result in any change in the position of a tooth in the adult. The resistance of the supporting tissues to the changed environment may be due to the greater density of the alveolar bone in the adult (Reitan, 1964), and to the resistance of the principal and transseptal fibres systems to displacement of the remaining teeth (Thompson *et al.*, 1958). Reitan (1959) found that collagen bundles in the gingiva remained stretched and tangential to incisors which had been rotated experimentally in dogs for periods up to two hundred and thirty-two days. Principal fibres were considered to have been realigned in twenty-eight to fifty-seven days. The factors concerned in the response to the change in environment include the magnitude, direction, duration and frequency of the additional force acting on a tooth, together with the architecture of the supporting tissues at the time of the change, and the ability of the tissue to respond to the change (Reitan, 1951). Occasionally, migration of a tooth may develop in an environment of oral forces which has not changed. Thus, a tooth may drift away from the side on which an inflammatory lesion of the periodontal ligament has developed; the explanation of this phenomenon is not certain, but movement may be due to pressure on the tooth exerted by granulation tissue in the lesion (Glickman, 1964b).

(*a*) *Migration due to unidirectional small horizontal force.* A considerable amount of research by various workers (Schwarz, 1932; Oppenheim, 1942; Reitan, 1951, 1956; Storey, 1955a,b) has shown the histological pattern produced by the application of continuous horizontal force to a tooth. Some of these studies have been made on animals, and most have involved standard orthodontic techniques for the application of the force. Extrapolation of the results to the unencumbered human mouth must therefore be made with caution. Within twenty-four hours, structural changes can be demonstrated on the side towards which the tooth is being displaced; on the other side changes develop more slowly and are less marked. As horizontal force tends to tilt a tooth, a region of compression develops between the root and the cervical one third of the alveolus on the side remote from the point of application of the force (to be called the compression zone), and a region of tension forms on the other side (the tension zone). In the apical region the sides of tension and compression are reversed (Fig. 15). The axis of rotation is said to be approximately in the apical one third of the root but the axis probably depends on the magnitude of the force and the anatomy of the root in question. In all cases, however, there will tend to be a gradation of effect from a maximum, close to the alveolar margin, to no effect at the level of the axis of rotation. The nature of the changes produced in the supporting tissues depends on the magnitude of the force acting on the tooth. There is no clear evidence, however, as to what constitutes a small or large force. The area over which the force acts is of importance; thus, tilting force to a lower incisor will act over a small area of a small root, whereas horizontal bodily-displacing force to a first molar will be spread over a much larger root area.

After the application of a force of a few grams for several hours the tooth is seen in longitudinal section to be tilted away from the force. The collagen fibres are straightened out in the tension zone, with the blood vessels appearing flattened; in the compression zone the collagen bundles are more wavy than usual, and the blood vessels are round and dilated. Dale *et al.* (1964), using tritiated thymidine in rats, found that cells in the tension zone, but not in the compression zone, were synthesizing DNA a few hours after elastic bands had been placed between the molar teeth.

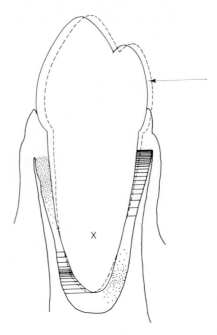

FIG. 15. Diagrammatic representation of the effect of horizontal force to the crown of a premolar. X, axis rotation; ⬤, zone of compression; ≡, zone of tension.

Cellular changes become more evident as the force continues. In the compression zone osteoclasts appear within two or three days along the radicular surface of the alveolus and begin to remove bone. In the tension zone osteoblastic activity can be distinguished on the inner surface of the alveolus and bundle bone is laid down along the course of the straightened collagen fibre bundles of the periodontal ligament. These two processes tend to restore the width of the periodontal ligament to previous dimensions. Other changes in the bone trabeculae may be seen; apposition of new bone is found on the external surface of the alveolar wall where resorption has started, so that the previous thickness of the wall of the socket is also restored.

If horizontal force of 20 g or more is used the tissues in the compression zone are subject to greater destruction. Around the coronal one third of the root the periodontal ligament is disrupted, and hyalinization of the cells and fibres occurs (Figs 16–19). Resorption of the necrotic bone occurs on the

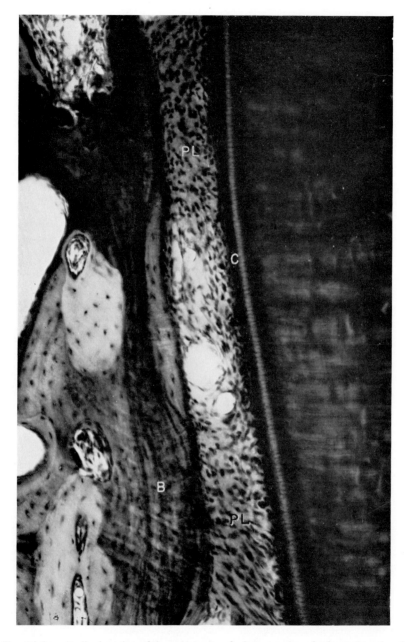

Fig. 16. Longitudinal section of the root *in situ* of a lower canine of a ferret. B = bundle bone; C = cementum; PL = periodontal ligament. Haematoxylin, eosin and Biebrich's scarlet. (×250).

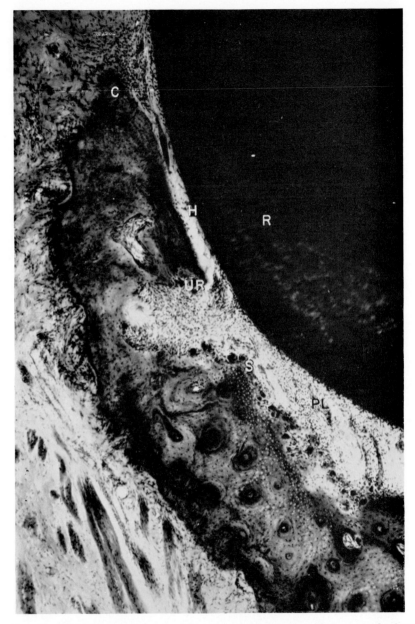

FIG. 17a. Zone of compression in oblique longitudinal section of the root of a lower canine at the alveolar crest ten days after the insertion of an upper metal appliance with anterior inclined plane producing heavy intermittent biting force on the lower canines (ferret). C, crest of alveolus; R, root; H, hyalinization of ligament; UR, undermining resorption; S, surface resorption; PL, periodontal ligament. Haematoxylin, eosin and Biebrich's scarlet. (× 100.)

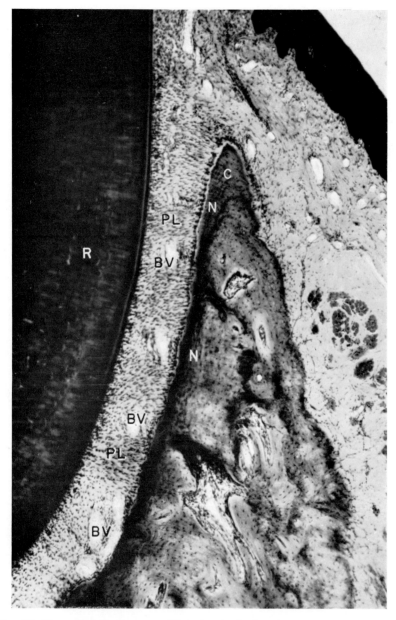

Fig. 17b. Zone of tension in same oblique longitudinal section as Fig. 17a. C, crest of alveolus; N, new bone; PL, periodontal ligament; BV, blood vessels. Haematoxylin, eosin and Biebrich's scarlet. (×100.)

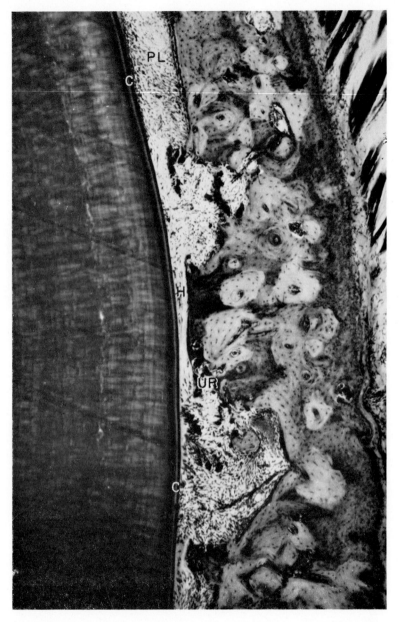

FIG. 18a. Zone of compression in longitudinal section of the root of a lower canine *in situ*
six weeks after the insertion of an appliance producing heavy intermittent biting forces on
the lower canines (ferret). PL, periodontal ligament; C, cementum; H, hyalinization of the
ligament; UR, undermining resorption. Haematoxylin, eosin and Bierbrich's scarlet. ($\times$ 100.)

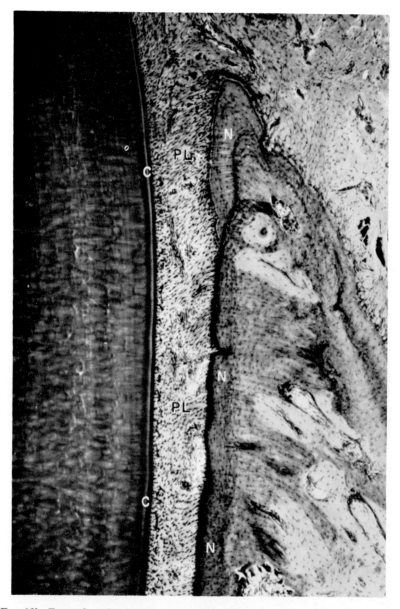

FIG. 18b. Zone of tension in same longitudinal section as Fig. 18a. N, new bone; PL, periodontal ligament; C, cementum. Haematoxylin, eosin and Biebrich's scarlet. (×100.)

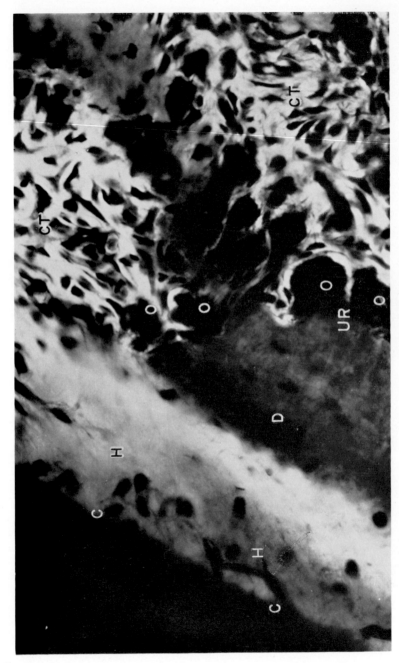

FIG. 19. High magnification of the area of necrosis of the periodontal ligament from Fig. 18 showing undermining resorption. C = cementum, CT = connective tissue, D = dead bone, H = hyalinization of the ligament, O = osteoclasts, UR = undermining resorption. Haematoxylin, eosin and Biebrich's scarlet. (×600.) Figs 16–19 reproduced with permission from J. P. Moss.

side of compression, but not from the internal surface, as osteoclasts cannot reach the bone through the necrotic and avascular region. Osteoclasts appear however, on the alveolar bone at the margins of the necrotic zone and on the external surface of trabeculae forming the wall of the alveolus; this "under-mining resorption" removes the dead trabeculae of bone. In this way the

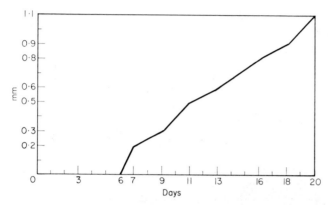

FIG. 20. The appliance remained completely passive during the first six days and no perceptible tooth movement took place. Guttapercha was then added to the appliance. Tooth movement by intermittent functional forces was produced by the contact created between appliance and root surface. The tooth was moved 1·1 mm during the remaining 14 days. 70–100 g intermittent force. (Reproduced with permission from K. Reitan (1956), *Eur. Orthodont. Soc. Tr.* **32**, 108–126.)

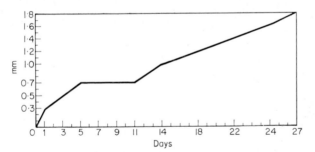

FIG. 21. A cell free area, interrupting tooth movement, existed from the fifth to the eleventh day. The tooth was moved 1·8 mm during 27 days. 70–100 g intermittent force. (Reproduced with permission from K. Reitan (1956), *Eur. Orthodont. Soc. Tr.* **32**, 108–126.)

compression in this region of the ligament is relieved; vascularization and cellular invasion of the necrotic periodontal tissue is followed by reformation of the normal architecture of the ligament and alveolus. According to Reitan (1956), if the migration of the tooth is measured each day, a period of no movement indicates the presence of a zone of necrosis (Figs 20–23). No further migration can occur until the necrotic alveolar bone is removed. The histological changes in the tension zone are less dramatic, although some necrosis

14

may develop prior to the deposition of bundle bone. The character and rate at which this new bone forms is also related to the magnitude of the force on the tooth (Storey, 1955a). Larger orthodontic forces often produce resorption of

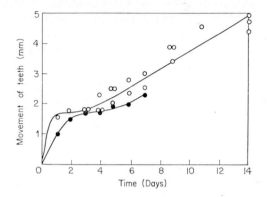

FIG. 22. The relation of tooth movement to time for 21 guinea pigs and 7 rats. The tooth movement was measured from the histological sections at the level of the gingival attachment between the two incisor teeth. ○ Guinea pig; ● Rat. (Reproduced with permission from E. Storey (1955), *Aust. J. dent.* **59,** 209–219.)

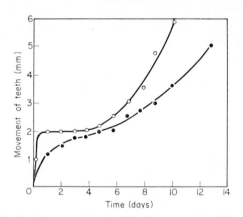

FIG. 23. The difference in tooth movement between a heavy (100 g) and a light force (25 g). Note that with heavy forces after an initially greater tooth movement there is cessation of tooth movement for some days. The relatively sudden increase in rate of tooth movement with heavy forces is associated with the removal of the lateral alveolar bone by a process of "undermining resorption." ● Initial force 25 g; ○ initial force 100 g. (Reproduced with permission from E. Storey (1955), *Aust. J. dent.* **59,** 209–219.)

the root in the compression zone and the apical region (Oppenheim, 1942). It seems quite possible that small areas of resorption also occur under physiological conditions.

The changes just described have mainly been studied experimentally by placing orthodontic springs in contact with the test tooth so that a known constant or intermittent force is applied. It is generally accepted that small intermittent forces produce the least destructive changes. Under physiological conditions it seems likely that similar histological changes develop to those noted for small orthodontic forces. Thus, for example, Coolidge (1937) found similar cellular changes around a child's teeth which were drifting in the horizontal direction (see Table 11). It may be of interest to note that the photomicrographs in Figs 20–23 are of teeth from ferrets subjected to intermittent force, as the lower canine bit against a metal appliance.

The actual mechanisms by which these cellular changes are effected is not clear. The usual explanation, which is an over-simplification, is that as the tooth is tilted in the socket an increase in tissue pressure is produced in the compression zone, and that this is the stimulus for the differentation of osteoclasts along the alveolar wall. Gradual resorption of bone restores the tissue pressure to its previous level and the osteoclasts then disappear. In the tension zone, it is said, traction on the collagen fibre bundles acts as the stimulus for the deposition of bundle bone along the course of these fibres. Other points must be considered however. For example, in the absence of necrosis, resorption of bone in the compression zone results in loss of Sharpey's fibres. Whether the principal fibres detached as a result become trapped in osteoid laid down by newly differentiated osteoblasts after osteoclasia has ceased, or whether new collagen fibres are secreted for the re-establishment of the anchorage, is not clear. It is not easy to understand why bone should be resorbed easily, whereas resorption of adjacent cementum is relatively infrequent and of slight extent. The explanation usually given for the latter (Orban, 1936) is that cementum is always covered by a layer of precementum, and osteoclasts will not remove this.

It seems of value here to try to fit together the findings from studies of tooth mobility with those from use of long acting forces, in order to understand the tissue changes in the latter. Thus Mühlemann et al. (1965) noted creep with horizontal force maintained for eight hundred seconds, and Parfitt (1967) found that axial force for ten minutes could produce a displacement of 1 mm or more under experimental conditions without altering the elastic characteristics of tooth support. Both Bien (1966) and Parfitt consider that gradual intrusion is due to hydrodynamic effects associated with displacement of tissue fluid. It seems possible, then, that when continuous light horizontal force causes the tooth to tilt, although the collagen units on the side of tension transmit force to the alveolar bone, they also gradually slip and the fibre lengths, therefore, increase. Morgan (1960) found that raw collagen of skin did not obey Hook's law, and that thin short fibres were extended relatively more than thick long fibres under the same force. Tissue fluid on the side of compression is displaced, and the collagen fibres may shorten to some extent by an increase in the cross linkages. An explanation for the appearance of osteoclasts and osteoblasts within a few hours, when these conditions are maintained, has been put forward recently on the basis of the piezo-electric properties of living bone (Gold, 1967). In this concept a distorted trabeculum of bone develops a negative charge along the surface rendered concave and a positive charge along the convex surface. The negative charge is believed to be the stimulus for the appearance of osteoblasts, and the osteoclasts differentiate due to the positive charge. Following the respective activities of these cells, and the reformation of the trabeculum, the imbalance in potential between the surfaces is corrected and the cellular

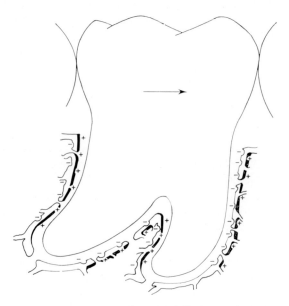

FIG. 24. A schematic representation of mesial drift. Resorption occurs on the mesial surface of the alveolus while bundle bone is laid down along the principal fibres on the distal surface.

activity ceases. It this hypothesis is extended to the alveolus, then the polarity in the compression zone would be positive and in the tension zone negative. Distortion of the root would be minimal under these conditions relative to a trabeculum of bone, so that changes in polarity at the root surface would be too small to initiate osteoclastic or cementoblastic responses. However, there is at the moment no experimental evidence to support these changes in the socket.

(b) *Mesial drift.* The forces which may produce this phenomenon in man have been discussed on page 371. The cellular changes by which the alterations in tooth position are effected are similar to those described for a small continuous horizontal force in (a) above, since mesial drift is but one aspect of the same question. There appears to be some uncertainty in the literature as to whether there is bodily horizontal movement only, or a large element of tilt in addition. Inspection of heavily worn human teeth *in situ* often reveals much greater attrition of the occlusal surface distally than mesially. This suggests that there has been a considerable element of tipping mesially to maintain approximal contact. With extreme degrees of attrition, such as occur when the whole crown is worn away, mesial drift may not compensate sufficiently and spaces develop between roots interproximally. The histological changes in the ligament and alveolus with normal approximal wear are summarized diagrammatically in Fig. 24, but as normal masticatory function must be maintained these changes probably occur over small areas of the alveolar wall at any one time (Fig. 25). Orban (1929) demonstrated that a record of the previous position of a tooth may be revealed by the location of the epithelial debris of Malassez which, on the distal side of the root, may be left some distance behind as the root migrates mesially.

It is a common clinical observation that extraction of a tooth often results in the adjacent tooth tilting mesially. In addition to the changes in the pattern of muscular and masticatory forces, and the removal of mesial support, a suggested explanation of this tilting is that the collagen in the damaged circumferential and transseptal fibre systems contracts and so tends to approximate the two teeth adjacent to the socket (Scott and Symons, 1964).

(*c*) *Extrusive movement or occlusal drift.* In heavily worn human dentitions the whole of the anatomical crown of teeth may be lost. In herbivores much greater loss of tooth substance due to attrition is quite normal, yet the teeth remain in occlusion. The process whereby the teeth migrate or drift occlusally to compensate for occlusal loss is not fully understood and may be a continuation of the earlier prefunctional phase of eruption (see Chapter 4).

The structural changes can be seen readily histologically following the experimental extraction of opposing teeth in animals. There is an increase in thickness of cementum especially around the apex, and between the roots of multi-rooted teeth, and a deposition of bundle bone at corresponding sites in the alveolus (Fig. 26). It is not clear, however, whether this deposition is the cause of the migration, tending to force the tooth occlusally, or a result of this movement. The latter appears more likely to be the case, since a persistent increase in pressure within a soft connective tissue in contact with bone is generally considered to cause resorption rather than deposition of bone. The changes in the principal fibres which must recur as the root drifts occlusally are not clarified either. It seems possible, in part at least, that as adjustments between collagen units at molecular level can take place very swiftly (as for example as occurs during eruption), there is "resplicing" of the fibres as the root moves past the alveolar bone, rather than the fibres being detached and then re-attached to bone and cementum.

(*d*) *Intrusive movement.* Minor adjustments in the position of a tooth probably occur routinely after a large filling has been inserted. When the

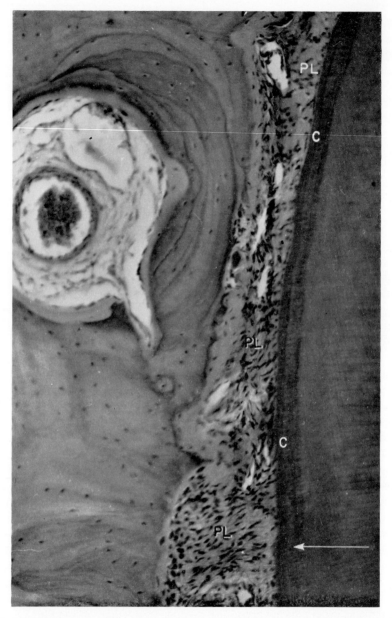

FIG. 25a. Transverse section of palatal root (mesial side) *in situ* of maxillary second molar of a monkey. Experimental mesial drift was permitted by removing the contact with the first molar four months previously. The direction of migration is shown by an arrow. PL, periodontal ligament; C, cementum. Haematoxylin, eosin and Biebrich's scarlet. (×250.)

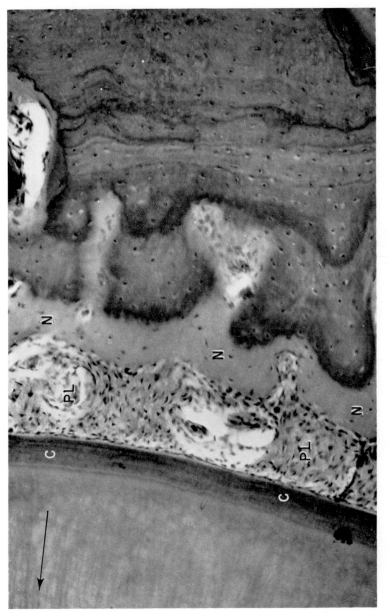

Fig. 25b. Transverse section of same palatal root as Fig. 25a (distal side). PL, periodontal ligament; C, cementum; N, new bone. Haematoxylin, eosin and Biebrich's scarlet. (×250.)

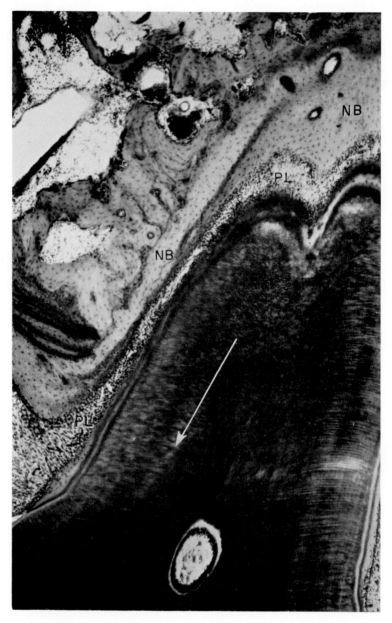

FIG. 26. Longitudinal section of a maxillary molar of a ferret which had been out of occlusion for two months. Occlusal drift of the tooth was accompanied by formation of alveolar bone and cementum, together with a marked reduction in width of the periodontal ligament. Haematoxylin, eosin and Biebrich's scarlet. (× 250.) (Reproduced with permission from J. P. Moss.)

restoration is noticeably "high" mild inflammation may develop in the periodontal ligament with the result that the tooth becomes tender to bite on. (See Chapter 7). Adjustments in the alveolus usually result in resolution of the discomfort within a few days. The insertion of small cap splints or bite planes, in children at least, causes separation of the teeth concerned while the remaining teeth come into occlusion. Some of these adjustments may be in the horizontal plane so that the teeth tilt away from the obstruction, but intrusive movement into the alveolus is probably an important part of this adjustment.

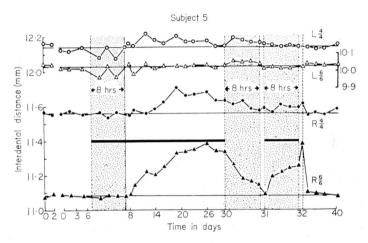

FIG. 27. Graph of interdental distances in millimetres plotted against time in days. The period during which the bite-raising cap was worn on $\overline{6|}$ is shown by the heavy horizontal line between vertical dotted lines, preceded by a control period and followed by a recovery period. The mean control values are shown by thin horizontal lines throughout the records and 2× standard deviations of these means are shown by shaded areas in the control period. Measurements were taken at 2 hourly intervals for 8 hour periods following the first insertion, the removal and reinsertion of the cap. These periods are shown by shaded columns. (Reproduced with permission from D. J. Anderson (1962), *Archs. Oral Biol.* **7**, 7–15.)

Experimentally, Anderson (1962, 1967) probably produced intrusion in eight young adult humans by fitting a gold cap to one lower first molar so that all the other teeth in the mouth were separated by approximately 0·5 mm. Within two or three weeks the occlusion of the other teeth was re-established although the cap was still in position. The likely explanation of these changes is that eruption of the other teeth was combined with intrusion of the capped tooth and its opponents (Fig. 27). Histological evidence of intrusion has been demonstrated under rather similar conditions in animals (Gottlieb and Orban, 1931; Glickman *et al.*, 1961; Waerhaug and Hansen 1966). It is clear from these studies that the changes that take place in the fundus of the alveolus and in the furcation region are very similar to those changes which occur in the zone of compression when a force of 20 g or more is applied to a

14*

tooth in the horizontal direction. Thus, there are early indications of tissue damage. Within 24 hours, areas of thrombosis and hyalinization are present in the apical region and perhaps throughout the ligament. This is followed by osteoclastic resorption of bone and root, and reformation of the tissue elements extending over many weeks. If the changes induced are similar to those in the zone of compression from horizontal force (see (*a*) p. 397), an important association is present between the effects of continuous horizontal force and infrequently applied force from opposing teeth. Physiological evidence from short term tooth mobility studies suggests that teeth become progressively displaced axially with continuous or repeated small loads, due to a change in the physical characteristics of the soft tissue of the periodontium (Parfitt, 1967). Histological evidence indicates that some degree of tissue damage is induced in the ligament before substantial adjustments in the position of a tooth occurs.

(*e*) *Increasing function.* The effect on a tooth of forces of different magnitude has been studied in human material and experimentally in animals, by several writers. Thus, Coolidge (1937) compared the width of the periodontal ligament around teeth in heavy function, such as a bridge-abutment tooth carrying an artificial occlusal surface in addition to its own. He found that the width was substantially greater than for teeth in normal function in the same mouth (in the order of 50 %); in addition, the thickness of the principal fibre bundles was much greater. Kronfield (1936) demonstrated that the supporting trabeculae of the alveolus were more numerous, and wider, and the wall of the socket itself was thicker around teeth in heavy function.

These structural differences develop as a result of the greater stresses encountered by the periodontium at the onset of the increased function. Thus, a tooth carrying a new bridge pontic might have to carry double the masticatory loads previously encountered. With each chewing thrust the tooth will be intruded into the alveolus appreciably further than prior to the insertion of the bridge. The extra tension in the fibre bundles and alveolar wall is probably the stimulus for increased activity of fibroblasts and osteoblasts, and the formation of larger fibre bundles and thicker bone trabeculae. The increased width of the ligament is less easy to account for, but may be due to the bowing in of localized areas of the alveolar wall towards the root. Over these areas of convexity, osteoclasts could appear and begin to resorb the radicular surface of the socket, while osteoblasts differentiate and form new bone on the outer surface.

In extreme experimental conditions in children where "jiggling" of a tooth has been produced by means of an obtrusive gold inlay in the opposing tooth, Mühlemann and Herzog (1961) have shown histologically a greatly increased width of the ligament (four times the width of the control ligament) as a result of osteoclastic activity. The ligament seems quite able to adjust to substantially increased forces imposed on the tooth provided the change is not too abrupt and the tissues are relatively "young". If these restrictions are not observed then destructive change predominate as in (*d*).

(*f*) *Decrease in function.* Gradual reduction in function results in changes in the supporting tissues which are the exact opposite of those described in (*e*). Thus, the ligament becomes narrower, the fibre bundles decrease in number

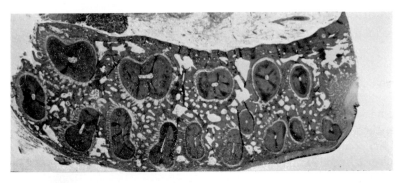

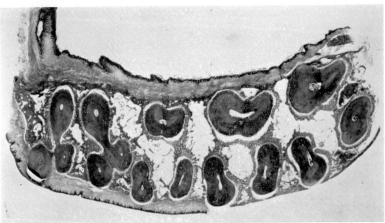

Fig. 28. Horizontal section through the maxilla of an adult monkey three months after the extraction of the mandibular cheek teeth from the left side. The effect of function can be seen on the distribution, thickness and density of the bony trabeculae. Haematoxylin, eosin and Biebrich's scarlet. (×2.)

and thickness, the bone of the alveolus and supporting trabeculae becomes reduced in thickness, and the number of trabeculae is substantially decreased (Figs 26 and 28).

Extraction of opposing teeth dramatically reduces the masticatory loads reaching a tooth. As the result, the tooth is not intruded into the alveolus to any marked extent and the collagen bundles, alveolus and supporting trabeculae are stressed to only a small fraction of the previous extent. The precise mechanism of the changes which follow is not known, but it can be presumed that fewer new collagen units are laid down than are removed, and that the trabeculae are reduced by osteoclastic action in conformity with Wolff's law. A certain minimum level of stress seems to be necessary for the preservation of trabeculae generally and, without this, resorption occurs until the remaining bone is stressed to this level. The reduction in width of the ligament is due mainly to deposition of cementum on the root rather than additional bundle bone to the socket; Kellner (1928) found non-functioning teeth had more cementum than functioning teeth in the same jaw in the proportions of 3 : 2.

(g) *Absence of function.* It is unlikely that a tooth erupted into the mouth can be truly devoid of forces acting upon it. The principal constituents of the normal periodontium can be seen in unerupted teeth and tooth germs transplanted into skin (Hoffman, 1961). The main differences between these and normal controls are the greatly reduced width of the ligament (Tables 6 and 8) and the orientation of the relatively few and slim collagen bundles many of which are aligned parallel to the root surface in the intermediate zone (Chapters 4 and 6). Hoffman considers that the ligament of the transplanted tooth germ shows structural pre-adaptation of the tissue elements in readiness for the advent of intraoral forces as soon as the tooth erupts. Cohn's work on rats (1965) shows that the absence of substantial forces on the tooth for long periods in the ageing individual may result in obliteration of the ligament. In these unopposed rat molars the cementum was found to be united with the alveolus without intervening soft connective tissue. However, in man at least, teeth unopposed for many years do not become ankylosed, nor do the roots of teeth which remain unerupted. Kronfield (1936) demonstrated that fat replaces the normal architecture of the ligament in embedded teeth or teeth out of occlusion for many years.

References

Anderson, D. J. (1956a). *J. dent. Res.* **35,** 664–670.
Anderson, D. J. (1956b). *J. dent. Res.* **35,** 671–673.
Anderson, D. J. (1962). *Archs. oral Biol.* **7,** 7–15.
Anderson, D. J. (1967). *In* "Mechanisms of Tooth Support. A Symposium" (D. J. Anderson, J. E. Eastoe, A. H. Melcher and D. C. Picton, eds). John Wright and Sons, Bristol, England.
Anderson, D. J. and Picton, D. C. A. (1957). *J. dent. Res.* **36,** 21–26.
Anderson, D. J. and Picton, D. C. A. (1958). *J. dent. Res.* **37,** 312–317.
Ardran, G. M. and Kemp, F. H. (1960). *Dent. Practit.* **11,** 23–26.
Barsoum, G. S. and Smirk, F. H. (1936). *Clin. Sci.* **2,** 337–352.
Bien, S. M. (1966). *In* "Advances in Oral Biology II", p. 173–199. (P. H. Staple ed.). Academic Press, New York, U.S.A.
Bien, S. M. and Ayers, H. D. (1965). *J. dent. Res.* **44,** 517–520.
Birn, H. (1966). *J. Periodont. Res.* **1,** 51–68.

Brodie, A. G. (1934). *Angle Orthod.* **4**, 335–348.
Castelli, W. (1963). *J. dent. Res.* **42**, 786–792.
Cohn, S. A. (1965). *Archs. Oral Biol.* **10**, 909–919.
Coolidge, E. D. (1937). *J. Am. dent. Ass. dent. Cosmos.* **24**, 1260–1270.
Dahlberg, B. (1942). *Acta med. scand. Supp.* **139**.
Dale, J. G., Hunt, A. M. and Hamilton, M. (1964). *J. dent. Res.* **43**, 830–831.
Dewell, B. F. (1949). *Am. J. Orthod.* **35**, 98–105.
Faigenblum, M. J. (1965). *Dent. Practit.* **16**, 214–216.
Fox, J. (1833). Natural History and Diseases of Human Teeth, 3rd edn. E. Cox, London.
Gabel, A. B. (1956). *J. Periodont.* **27**, 191–198.
Glickman, I. (1964a). Clinical Periodontology, 3rd edn. W. B. Saunders, Philadelphia, U.S.A.
Glickman, I. (1964b). Clinical Periodontology, 3rd edn. W. B. Saunders, London, England.
Glickman, I., Sheldon, R. and Smulow, J. (1961). *J. dent. Res.* **40**, 709.
Gold, P. (1967). *J. Periodont.* **38**, 119–123.
Gottlieb, B. and Orban, B. (1931). *J. dent. Res.* **11**, 505–510.
Gould, M. S. E. and Picton, D. C. A. (1963). *Brit. Dent. J.* **114**, 175–180.
Gould, M. S. E. and Picton, D. C. A. (1964). *Archs. Oral Biol.* **9**, 469–478.
Gould, M. S. E., Drake, J. and Picton, D. C. A. (1967). *J. dent. Res.* (In press.)
Graf, H. (1962). "Occlusal Contact Patterns in Mastication." M.S. Thesis, University of Rochester, New York, U.S.A.
Himmel, G. K., Marthaler, T. M., Mühlemann, H. R. and Rateitschak, K. H. (1957). *Helv. Odont. Acta.* **1**, 16–18.
Hoffmann, R. L. (1961). *J. dent. Res.* **39**, 781–798.
Hofmann, M. and Diemer, R. (1966). *Deutsch Zahnaerztl* **21**, 707–718.
Howell, A. H. and Brudevold, F. (1950). *J. dent. Res.* **29**, 133–141.
Jankleson, B., Hoffman, G. M. and Hendron, J. A. (1953). *J. dent. Res.* **36**, 21–26.
Jenkins, N. (1966). "The Physiology of the Mouth", 3rd ed. Blackwell Scientific Publications, Oxford, England.
Jung, F. (1952). *Stoma* **5**, 74–81.
Kawamura, Y. (1964). *In*, "Advances in Oral Biology" (P. H. Staple, ed.), I, p. 77. Academic Press, New York.
Kellner, E. (1928). *Z. f. Stomatol.* **26**, 271–282.
Kindlová, M., and Matena, V. (1962). *J. dent. Res.* **41**, 650–660.
Körber, K. H. (1962). *Deutsch Zahnaerztl* **17**, 1585–1595.
Körber, K. H. (1963). *Deutsch Zahnaerztl* **18**, 576–584.
Körber, K. H., and Körber, E. (1967). *In* "Mechanisms of tooth support. A symposium" (J. E. Eastoe, A. H. Melcher and D. C. A. Picton, eds), p. 148. John Wright and Sons, Bristol, England.
Kronfeld, R. (1936). *New York J. Dent.* **6**, 112–122.
Kydd, W. L., Akamine, J. S., Mendel, R. A. and Kraus, B. S. (1963). *J. dent. Res.* **42**, 858–866.
Lear, C. S. C., Flanagan, J. B. and Moorrees, C. F. A. (1965a). *Archs. Oral Biol.* **10**, 83–99.
Lear, C. S. C., Grossman, R. C., Flanagan, J. B. and Moorrees, C. F. A. (1965b). *Archs. Oral Biol.* **10**, 669–689.
Marx, R. (1963). *Eur. Orthod. Soc. Tr.* **39**, 318–328.
Marx, R. (1965). *Eur. Orthod. Soc. Tr.* **41**, 187–201.
McDowell, J. A. and Regli, C. P. (1961). *J. dent. Res.* **40**, 1183–1185.
Morgan, F. R. (1960). *J. Soc. Leath. Trades Chem.* **44**, 170–181.

418   D. C. A. PICTON

Moss, J. P. and Picton, D. C. A. (1967). *Archs. Oral Biol.* (In press.)
Mühlemann, H. R. (1951). *Oral Surg.* **4,** 1220–1233.
Mühlemann, H. R. (1954). *J. Periodont.* **25,** 125–129.
Mühlemann, H. R. and Herzog, R. L. (1961). *Helv. Odont. Acta* **5,** 33–39.
Mühlemann, H. R. and Zander, H. A. (1954). *J. Periodont.* **25,** 128–137.
Mühlemann, H. R., Savdir, S. and Rateitschak, K. H. (1965). *J. Periodont.* **36,** 148–153.
Ness, A. R. (1967). *In* "Mechanisms of tooth support. A symposium" (D. J. Anderson, J. E. Eastoe, A. H. Melcher and D. C. A. Picton, eds), p. 84. John Wright and Sons, Bristol. England.
Neumann, H. H. and Di Salvo, N. A. (1957). *J. dent. Res.* **36,** 286–290.
O'Leary, T. J., Rudd, K. D. and Nabers, C. L. (1966). *Periodontics.* **4,** 308–315.
O'Leary, T. J., Rudd, K. D., Nabers, C. L. and Stumpf, A. J. (1967). *Periodontics.* **5,** 26–28.
Oppenheim, A. (1942). *Oral Surg.* **28,** 263–301.
Orban, B. (1929). *J. Am. dent. Assoc.* **16,** 405–415.
Orban, B. (1936). *J. Am. dent. Assoc.* **23,** 1849–1870.
Osborn, J. W. (1961). *Archs. Oral Biol.* **5,** 202–211.
Parfitt, G. J. (1960). *J. dent. Res.* **39,** 608–618.
Parfitt, G. J. (1961). *J. Periodont.* **32,** 102–107.
Parfitt, G. J. (1967). *In* "Mechanisms of Tooth Support. A Symposium" (D. J. Anderson, J. E. Eastoe, A. H. Melcher and D. C. A. Picton, eds). John Wright and Sons, Bristol, England.
Picton, D. C. A. (1961). "An Experimental Study of Tooth Mobility in Man." Ph.D. Thesis, University of London.
Picton, D. C. A. (1962a). *Archs. Oral Biol.* **7,** 151–159.
Picton, D. C. A. (1962b). *Archs. Oral Biol.* **7,** 573–580.
Picton, D. C. A. (1963). *Archs. Oral Biol.* **8,** 291–299.
Picton, D. C. A. (1964). *Archs. Oral Biol.* **9,** 55–63.
Picton, D. C. A. (1965). *Archs. Oral Biol.* **10,** 945–955.
Picton, D. C. A. (1967). *Helv. Odont. Acta.* **11,** 105–112.
Picton, D. C. A. and Davies, W. I. R. (1967). *Archs. Oral Biol.* (In press.)
Profitt, W. R., Kydd, W. L., Wilskie, G. H. and Taylor, D. T. (1964). *J. dent. Res.* **43,** 555–562.
Provenza, D. V. (1966). "Oral Histology, Inheritance and Development." J. B. Lippincott Co., Philadelphia.
Reitan, K. (1951). *Acta. Odont. scand.* **9,** Supp. 6.
Reitan, K. (1956). *Eur. Orthod. Soc. Tr.* **32,** 108–126.
Reitan, K. (1959). *Angle Orthod.* **29,** 105–113.
Reitan, K. (1964). *Angle Orthod.* **34,** 244–255.
Rix, R. E. (1953). *Eur. Orthod. Soc. Tr.* **29,** 191–202.
Rushmer, R. F. and Hendron, J. A. (1951). *J. appl. Physiol.* **3,** 622–630.
Savdir, S. and Rateitschak, K. H. (1964). *Paradontologie* **18,** 125–136.
Schöhl, H. (1960). *Deutsch. Zahnaerztl* **15,** 1185–1191.
Schwarz, A. M. (1932). *Ortho. Oral. Surg. Rad. Int. Jnl.* **18,** 331–352.
Scott, J. H. and Symons, N. B. B. (1964). "Introduction to Dental Anatomy", 4th ed. E. and S. Livingstone Ltd., London.
Storey, E. (1955a). *Aust. J. Dent.* **59,** 147–161.
Storey, E. (1955b). *Aust. J. Dent.* **59,** 209–219.
Synge, J. L. (1933). *Phil. Mag.* **15,** 969–974.
Taylor, A. C. (1950). *Science III,* **40.**

Thompson, H. E., Myers, H. I., Waterman, J. M. and Flanagan, V. D. (1958). *Am. J. Orthodont.* **44**, 485–497.

Waerhaug, J. and Hansen, E. R. (1966). *Acta Odont. scand.* **24**, 91–105.

Weinmann, J. P. and Sicher, H. (1947). "Bone and Bones", p. 154. H. Kimpton, London.

Werner, H. (1964). *Acta Odont. Scand.* **22**, *Supp.* 40.

Winders, R. V. (1962). *Angle Orthod.* **32**, 38–43.

Worner, H. K. and Anderson, M. N. (1944). *Aust. J. Dent.* **48**, 1–11.

Yurkstas, A. and Curby, W. A. (1953). *J. Prosth. Dent.* **3**, 82–88.

9 | Effect of Nutrition on the Periodontium

H. W. FERGUSON

School of Dental Surgery, University of Liverpool, Liverpool, England

I. Introduction

Nutrition may be defined as the sum of the processes by which an animal or plant takes in and utilizes food substances. In the case of animals this involves ingestion, digestion, absorption and assimilation.

Although the art of nutrition is as old as man himself it is only in the last sixty years or so that its study has become universally accepted as a scientific pursuit. None the less, in this relatively short space of time, the science of nutrition has established beyond all doubt that the ingestion of certain food constituents is essential to the well-being of every living organism. Prior to the beginning of the present century workers in the field of nutrition were mainly concerned with investigating the nature and metabolism of the principal food elements, proteins, carbohydrates and fats. Many years before this, however, it had been realized that certain diseases could be prevented or cured by including in the diet specific food items, the classic example, of course, being the prevention of scurvy by dietary supplements of fresh fruit and/or vegetables. It was, however, not until the first decade of the present century that the nature of some of these accessory food factors was discovered. It was found that certain natural unrefined foods contained minute quantities of hitherto unrecognized substances essential for life. To emphasize their vital importance, they were named vitamins.

The discovery of vitamins undoubtedly revolutionized both dietetics and the study of disease. In short, the concept of deficiency disease was evolved, since a number of workers had demonstrated conclusively that certain pathological conditions were not caused primarily by infection or toxins, but by a deficiency of one or more of these essential nutrients. In the early 1930s the first synthetic vitamin preparations became available for clinical trial, and their introduction ushered in the heyday of vitamin therapy—a heyday which was to last for almost two decades. During this period many of these preparations were often used indiscriminately in vain attempts to prevent or cure all manner of pathological states, including those which afflict the oral cavity. However, the disappointing results frequently obtained by the use of synthetic vitamin preparations have now relegated their use to a more realistic position in the table of effective therapeutic agents.

Whilst many workers were at this time devoting their energies to vitamin research, a small number had begun to investigate the metabolism of certain inorganic elements in relation to a variety of bodily functions. Of these, by far the most exhaustively studied over the years have been calcium and phosphorus; phosphorus because of its ubiquitous distribution throughout animal and plant organisms and its essential role in almost every cell-regulating process, and calcium because of its essential role in the formation and maintenance of skeletal structure and as an essential component of the blood.

A vast amount of research is still carried out into every aspect of calcium and phosphorus metabolism, and particularly into the interrelationships which are now known to exist between these elements and certain of the vitamins, notably vitamins A and D. However, increasing attention has been paid in recent years to certain other elements which, although present in tissues in much smaller amounts, have nevertheless been shown in certain instances to be essential for life. These include fluorine, iron, zinc, magnesium and molybdenum.

From what has already been said, it is clear that the scope of nutritional research is immense. In fact, the results of such research now constitute a considerable proportion of available scientific literature. The task which faces the present reviewer, however, is to decide how much of the evidence gleaned from general nutritional studies is applicable to the structures which comprise the periodontium. It is undoubtedly true that the components of the periodontium consist of structural units identical to those found in other tissues; it is also apparent that their peculiar anatomical and functional relationships appear to modify their response to various forms of nutritional and other stress. Again, particularly in the case of man, the periodontium is unique in that it is constantly being influenced by a large number of complicating local factors. These include plaque, calculus, occlusal disharmonies, improperly designed dental restorations, and orthodontic and prosthetic appliances. Indeed, there is at the present time a considerable body of well-informed opinion which believes that, as more of these local factors and their mode of action are discovered, the need to invoke any systemic nutritional factor in the etiology of periodontal disease becomes unnecessary. The justification for this viewpoint apparently rests on the results of relatively few field investigations. The results of these suggest that no strong correlation can be shown to exist between any specific nutrient deficiency and the onset of periodontal deterioration.

In contrast to the investigations on man, there is now an abundance of well-documented evidence derived from animal experiments which demonstrates conclusively that nutritional factors, both local and systemic, can greatly influence the health of the periodontium. However, the dangers of an extrapolation of the results of animal experiments to man cannot be too strongly emphasized. For example, the composition of many of the diets used in these experiments is grossly abnormal. It is extremely unlikely that similar human dietary regimes exist in any part of the world, even in the most underdeveloped countries. Furthermore, there is the question of complicating local factors operating in man. These, in general, do not apply to animal studies. Nevertheless, while the obvious difficulties of carrying out definitive nutritional studies in man remain, and they are likely to remain for a long time to come, data must continue to be obtained from well-designed animal experiments. In the chapter that follows, an attempt will be made to acquaint the reader with the evidence obtained from both human and animal studies which shows that nutritional factors, either local or systemic, contribute to the health or otherwise of the periodontium.

II. The Physical Characteristics of the Diet

A number of local factors operating in the oral cavity have already been mentioned as almost certainly playing an important role in the causation of periodontal disease. Amongst these is the local effect which diet itself has on the periodontal structures.

The local effect of nutrition may be considered under two headings:

Diet consistency

Diet composition

A. DIET CONSISTENCY

Studies so far reported on this particular aspect of nutrition have been concerned mainly with the effects of the physical consistency of the diet, particularly the effects of hard and soft diets. Although definitive studies of this nature do not appear to have been carried out in man, a number of investigations have been carried out in animals. For example, Burswasser and Hill (1939) found that a hard diet helped to maintain gingival health in dogs. Similar results were reported by Krasse and Brill (1960). On the other hand, studies by Cohen (1960), Baer and White (1960), and Persson (1961) showed that rats maintained on hard granular diets develop more extensive periodontal lesions than those maintained on a soft diet.

Egelberg (1965), reviewing the literature, is of the opinion that earlier investigations of this nature suffer from the weakness that there was no objective and quantitative method available for measuring the degree of inflammatory change. In an attempt to overcome this, he assessed the degree of gingival inflammation by measuring the amount of exudate using paper strips soaked in ninhydrin. Furthermore, he compared colour photographs of teeth stained with basic fuchsin. This provided a guide to the amount of plaque developed. These experiments were carried out on groups of dogs maintained on either a hard or soft diet for periods of up to thirty-five days. Egelberg's results indicated that the animals developed more bacterial plaque and more gingivitis when they were fed a soft diet.

Similar results were reported by Ferguson (1967a) using cats. He found that animals which had been maintained for varying periods (6 months to 2 years) on a commercial diet, nutritionally adequate but of soft consistency, developed severe periodontal lesions. When the animals were transferred to a hard diet devised by Scott (1960) there was a marked improvement in the periodontal condition.

It seems reasonable to conclude from these experiments that the beneficial effects obtained from a hard diet are mainly due to the mechanical cleansing effect on the teeth and adjacent soft tissues. On the other hand, the conflicting results reported in rats suggest that the degree of "hardness" may be an important factor in determining the extent of such beneficial results.

B. DIET COMPOSITION

Studies of periodontal disease in the Syrian hamster by a number of workers including Keyes and Likins (1946), Klingsberg and Butcher (1959), and Keyes and Jordan (1964) showed that animals kept on a soft, high carbohydrate diet developed severe periodontal lesions. Shaw and Griffiths (1961) reported similar results in the rice rat, an animal very susceptible to periodontal disease. In this last study, when the sucrose of the diet was replaced by lard, there was a striking reduction in the periodontal syndrome.

On the other hand, Carlsson and Egelberg (1965) reported that the addition of sucrose to a basic protein-fat diet, of hard or soft consistency, did not affect the formation of plaque, or the development of gingival inflammation in dogs. In an attempt to explain their conflicting results Carlsson and Egelberg suggested two possibilities: (a) differences in the oral bacterial flora between species, and (b) differences in eating habits.

There thus seems little doubt from these animal experiments that the local effects of diet, and particularly that of consistency, are quite likely to be important factors in the causation of periodontal deterioration. On the other hand, we have at the present time only a number of subjective clinical observations to support the results of animal experiments. It is obvious that well-designed clinical trials and field surveys are necessary before any conclusion can be applied to man.

III. The Vitamins

Vitamins may be defined as organic substances which are essential for the nutrition of vertebrates, some invertebrates, and many micro-organisms. They act in minute quantities in the regulation of various metabolic processes. Vitamins are present in small amounts in various natural foodstuffs and are sometimes produced within the body, but not usually in sufficient quantities to maintain health. As a result, they must be obtained from the diet or as synthetic preparations.

It has been customary to divide the vitamins into two groups on the basis of their solubility. Thus vitamins A, D, E and K are found associated with lipids and are termed *fat-soluble vitamins*. They are absorbed along with dietary fats and are not normally excreted in the urine to any degree. Because of this they can be stored in the body in moderate amounts, and consequently bodily reserves are not quickly exhausted. In contrast, the *water-soluble vitamins* B-complex and C are not stored in the body in appreciable quantities, and a constant dietary supply is essential to avoid their depletion.

Most of the water-soluble vitamins have been proved to be components of essential enzyme systems.

A. VITAMIN A

Vitamin A is found only in foods of animal origin, the principal source being fish-liver oils. Animals obtain the vitamin from its precursor or provitamin present in plants, principally as the pigment β carotene. Conversion of the carotenoids to vitamin A in the body of man or fish occurs after hydrolysis. This yields one or two molecules of vitamin A per carotenoid molecule.

1. Vitamin A Deficiency

Although according to Davidson et al. (1959) it is likely that vitamin A is necessary for the metabolism of all human cells, its precise biochemical action has so far been explained in one structure only, the retina. Deficiency of vitamin A in both man and animals results in hemeralopia (night blindness). It has further been established that the vitamin is essential for the integrity of epithelial tissues. Deficiency results in atrophy of the normal epithelial cell layer. This is followed by proliferation of the basal cells, and metaplasia of other epithelia to stratified keratinized epithelium.

Moore (1960), in a comprehensive review of the pathological conditions associated with vitamin A deficiency, listed three basic lesions:

(a) Hemeralopia
(b) Keratinization of many membranes
(c) Bone changes during growth.

For a detailed description of the specific functions of vitamin A in the retina the reader is referred to a recent review by Masek (1962). It has further been suggested that both man and animals deprived of vitamin A develop an increased susceptibility to infection. However, this so-called anti-infection role of the vitamin has not been proved since there is at present no evidence that it has any effect either on pathogens or on the immune response. However, if lack of the vitamin reduces the integrity of mucous membranes, then the organism will be more liable to infection.

Mellanby (1931) was the first to report bone changes in dogs maintained on diets deficient in vitamin A. He observed incoordination of movement in these animals, and related this to lesions of the central nervous system caused by overgrowth of the skull bones. Since this first report, bone dysplasia has been produced in many species of animal. Mellanby (1944) considers the bone changes resulting from vitamin A deficiency to be due principally to alterations in the position and activity of oesteoblasts and osteoclasts. On the other hand, Wolbach (1946) considered the primary effect of vitamin A deficiency to be on endochondral growth.

A number of experiments on various species of animal have shown that a deficiency of vitamin A can affect one or more of the periodontal components. Thus Mellanby (1941) found that dogs maintained on a diet deficient in vitamin A developed hyperplasia of the gingival epithelium with accompanying atrophy of the alveolar bone.

Glickman and Stoller (1948) showed that vitamin A-deficient albino rats developed deeper periodontal pockets than adequately nourished controls, but stressed that this occurred only in the presence of a local irritating factor, food debris. They could find no change in the fibres of the periodontal ligament or the alveolar bone. On the other hand, Miglani (1959), also using albino rats, found almost all the components of the periodontium to be severely affected by deficiency of vitamin A. The changes included hyperkeratosis and hyperplasia of the gingiva, atrophy of alveolar bone, and excessive resorption of cementum.

Hirschi (1950) extracted teeth in vitamin A-deficient hamsters and found a decreased amount of new bone in the healing sockets of the deficient animals. The effect of hypovitaminosis A on alveolar bone healing in rats following extraction of molar teeth was also studied by Frandsen (1963). He observed that formation of immature bone in the sockets was retarded. Osteoblastic activity was considerably suppressed, and there was also a complete lack of resorption. He concluded that it was the latter fault which was responsible for the changes seen in bone in vitamin A deficiency. These conclusions are, however, in conflict with an earlier study reported by Irving (1949) who observed the effect of vitamin A deficiency on the alveolar bone of the rat incisor. He concluded that the main change was an excess of osteoblastic activity, and that the reaction of the osteoclasts was secondary. These results were substantially in agreement with the early reports by Mellanby.

There seems no doubt that a lack of vitamin A causes general alteration in both epithelium and bone. The evidence that vitamin A deficiency can cause similar changes in the same components of the periodontium is less well-documented. Much more evidence is required before any real assessment can be made.

2. Hypervitaminosis A

The feeding of excessive doses of vitamin A to both man and animals results in a toxicity syndrome characterized partly by excessive bone fragility, deep bone pain and dry scaly skin. Of these, by far the most extensively studied, have been the bone changes.

Collazo and Rodriguez (1933) reported skeletal rarefaction and fragility of the long bones of rats given large quantities of vitamin A in the form of a fish oil concentrate. Similar results were reported by Wolbach and Bessey (1942). Wolbach (1946) attributed the changes to an acceleration of "epiphyseal cartilage sequences, preliminary to endochondral bone formation", but Stewart (1965) considered that the bone changes seen in cases of hypervitaminosis A were probably due to a partial reversal of osteoclastic and osteoblastic activity.

Little attention appears to have been paid to the effect of excess dosage of vitamin A on the periodontium. Wolbach and Bessey (1942) reported briefly that the alveolar bone of rats showed marked resorption and a lack of repair.

The effect of large doses of vitamin A acid on the bones and teeth of young rats was studied by Leaver and Triffitt (1964). They found that although the serum calcium levels were normal, there was a severe depression of serum citrate. Ferguson (1967b) studied the histological and microradiographic changes in the jaws of this same group of animals. Although resorption of alveolar bone was evident, this was not excessive. The molar crevicular epithelium appeared thinner than in the controls. Cementum was unaffected.

B. VITAMIN D

Of the several sterol compounds that have been isolated, two are chemically well-characterized and are of prime importance for the adequate nutrition of both man and animals. Vitamin D_2 or calciferol is obtained by ultraviolet irradiation of the plant sterol, ergosterol. Vitamin D_3 is similar, and is formed in the human skin from 7-dehydrocholesterol on exposure to sunlight or ultraviolet light.

The main nutritional dietary sources of vitamin D are the fish liver oils. Egg yolk contains substantial amounts and so does milk. Since, however, the levels of the vitamin in these natural sources are seasonably variable, the requirements for vitamin D are met by artificial supplementation of certain foodstuffs and by pharmaceutical preparations.

Despite intensive research into the functions of vitamin D over the years, its mode of action at the cellular level is still not known. Nevertheless, there is no dispute regarding at least two of its essential roles, *viz.* the maintenance of the normal serum calcium level of the blood and the proper mineralization of bones and teeth. Its close interrelationship with parathormone is also now well-documented, and McLean and Urist (1961) state that "the functional activities of the two substances are so closely interrelated that they must be considered as component parts of an integrated system".

1. *Vitamin D Deficiency*

In man and certain species of animal deficiency of vitamin D in the young causes rickets. The complementary disease state in the adult is osteomalacia. The essential pathological lesion in both conditions is a failure of osteoid tissue to mineralize. Although rickets as a disease has been recognized for many centuries, it was McCollum *et al.* (1922) who first demonstrated that the condition could be cured by supplements of vitamin D.

It is now universally accepted that vitamin D acts by promoting the absorption of calcium from the intestine. Deficiency of the vitamin results in changes in the composition of the blood plasma, particularly in the levels of calcium and phosphorus. Kramer and Howland (1921) have shown that active rickets is present when the product of the serum calcium and serum phosphate, expressed as mg/per cent, is less than 30. This rule, though admittedly empirical, has stood the test of time and is still of considerable value to clinicians (Nordin, 1960). In addition to the action of vitamin D in aiding absorption of calcium from the gut, it has been speculated in recent years that the vitamin has a local or peripheral action on bone. The evidence for and against this concept is admirably reviewed by McLean and Budy (1963).

In man there is, as far as the writer can ascertain, an almost total lack of information regarding the state of the periodontium in reported cases of rickets and osteomalacia. Thoma and Goldman (1960) have reported a case of rickets in a female child aged 12 years. The clinical photograph shows marked deformity of the maxilla and mandible, with severe malocclusion. The gingiva were greatly enlarged but no histological details are given.

In the main, two species of animal, the dog and rat have been used in the study of experimental rickets. According to Scott (1960) it is apparent that, as distinct from the dog, the cat's requirement for vitamin D is small. Attempts have been made by Ferguson (1965) to induce vitamin D deficiency in a number of kittens but, without success.

Becks and Weber (1931), using dogs, reported osteoporosis of the alveolar bone with replacement of bone by fibro-osteoid tissue. The periodontal ligament also became obliterated due, according to these workers, to the continued deposition of osteoid at the margins of the alveolar bone.

By far the greatest amount of work on experimental rickets has been done using the rat, but there is a divergence of opinion as to whether or not a simple lack of vitamin D produces rickets. On the one hand Freeman and McLean (1941) and Harrison *et al.* (1958) state that there is an increased production of osteoid tissue and disturbances in the calcium and phosphorus levels of the blood in young rats deprived of vitamin D. In contrast to this, Ferguson and Hartles (1963) have shown that a simple lack of vitamin D in young rats causes no demonstrable histological or biochemical changes in either the bones, including alveolar bone, or cementum. They have found, however, as did Coleman *et al.* (1950), that moderately severe rickets could be produced within a few weeks if the phosphorus content of the diet was reduced. Nevertheless, there was no doubt in Ferguson and Hartles' study, that the rachitic condition was greatly exacerbated if vitamin D as well as phosphorus was excluded from the diet (Figs 1a and b).

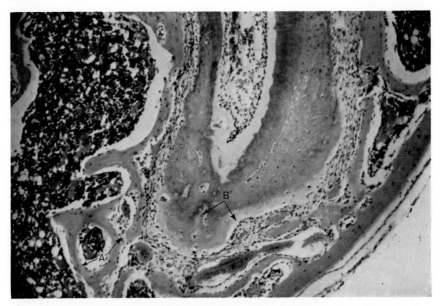

FIG. 1a. Decalcified section of part of molar root and surrounding alveolar bone of young rat deprived of phosphorus. Note areas of osteoid (A) and cementoid (B) tissue. Haematoxylin and Eosin. (×60.)

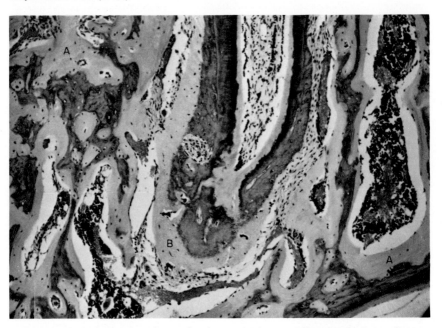

FIG. 1b. Decalcified section of part of molar root and surrounding alveolar bone of young rat deprived of both phosphorus and vitamin D. Note great increase in amount of osteoid and cementoid tissue compared with that shown in Fig. 1a. Haematoxylin and Eosin. (×60.)

Weinnman and Schour (1945a,b) fed young rats a diet with a high calcium/phosphorus ratio but deficient in vitamin D. They reported that the rate of cementum formation was normal, but that its calcification was defective. A similar situation was found in the alveolar bone, which showed large areas of osteoid tissue. These workers also reported compression of the periodontal ligament leading in some instances to hyaline degeneration of the connective tissue, and occasionally to a complete obliteration of the periodontal ligament. Similar results were reported by Coleman *et al.* (1953) and confirmed by Ferguson and Hartles (1964).

2. Hypervitaminosis D

It has been known for a number of years that vitamin D given in large doses to both humans and animals produces a well-defined toxicity syndrome. This is characterized by, amongst other features, bone changes, ectopic calcifications in several soft tissues, notably the heart and large arteries, and hypercalcaemia. The clinical relevance of this particular action of vitamin D lies in the frequency with which many patients overdose themselves in attempts to cure certain conditions, notably arthritis. For example, although the recommended daily intake of vitamin D should not exceed approximately 500 IU, Gershoff (1966) has reported that a number of adults have received as much as 100,000 IU daily for several months. All developed serious side effects with symptoms similar to those observed in atherosclerosis. As far as changes in the periodontium of humans is concerned, only one report can be traced. Dawson (1937) observed thinning of the alveolar bone and rarefaction of the roots of the molar teeth in a girl aged 4 years after overdosage with vitamin D.

On the other hand, there is a considerable literature relating to oral changes induced in various species of animal by excessive doses of the vitamin. There are, however, considerable contradictions in the earlier literature regarding the type of alveolar bone change produced. Some workers consider the bone to be rachitic, others osteoporotic, and yet others osteosclerotic. For a comprehensive review of these earlier studies the reader is referred to the paper by Becks (1942). Weinnman and Sicher (1955) commenting on the conflicting bone findings in hypervitaminosis D suggest that the type of bone change produced depends on the degree of kidney damage. These authors consider that as long as the dosage is not greatly excessive, the histological picture will be that of an exaggeration of the normal effect of vitamin D, namely, an enhanced osteogenesis. If, however, the intake of the vitamin is grossly excessive, and kidney damage occurs, the parathyroid glands will hypertrophy. This will result in bone changes indistinguishable from those observed in hyper-parathyroidism; namely, osteoclasis with fibrous tissue replacement. McLean and Budy (1963) state emphatically that large doses of vitamin D have a direct effect on bone, promoting its resorption in a manner similar to the effects of parathormone.

In a recent study on the effects of hypervitaminosis D on the periodontium of the hamster, Fahmy *et al.* (1961) report the following features: calcified deposits in the periodontal ligament, cemental spurs, calcification of the

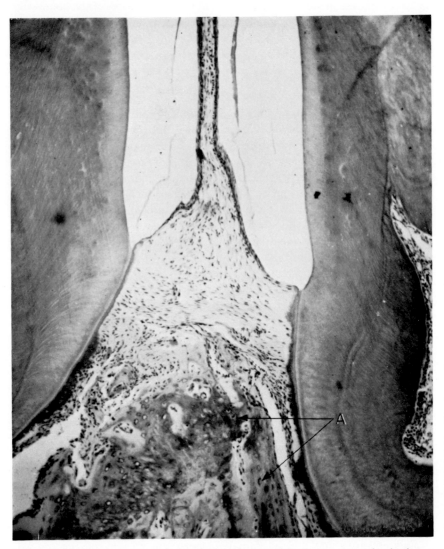

FIG. 2. Decalcified section of septum between M1 and M2 of young rat maintained on a diet containing 250×normal intake of vitamin D. Note large size of osteocyte lacunae (A) in alveolar crest. There is an increase in the number of connective tissue fibres of the periodontal ligament causing enlargement of the interdental papilla. Haematoxylin and Eosin. (×90.)

principal periodontal fibres, and resorption of alveolar bone. Ferguson (1967b) placed young rats on a diet which contained × 250 the normal amount of vitamin D. Histological examination of the jaws revealed that, although the alveolar bone showed some evidence of resorption, the outstanding feature was the presence of large numbers of enlarged osteocytes apparently engaged in lacunar resorption (see Chapter 6, page 318). The bone was immature, indicating a high rate of turnover. The cementocytes were also greatly enlarged, and some cementoid was present. The connective tissue fibres of the periodontium were increased in amount, and this resulted in an enlargement of the interdental papillae (Fig. 2).

C. VITAMIN E

Although it is well-recognized that a deficiency of vitamin E in rats results in sterility and muscular dystrophy these findings have not been confirmed in man. As far as the writer can ascertain no findings of relevance to the periodontium have been demonstrated in either man or animals as a result of vitamin E deficiency.

D. VITAMIN K

Despite the fact that an association between vitamin K and blood coagulation is well established its mechanism is not understood. According to Gershoff (1966) there is considerable evidence to suggest that vitamin K is associated with electron transport and oxidative phosphorylation. Macdonald and Gibbons (1962) found vitamin K compounds to be required for the growth of *Bacteroides melaninogenicus*, which may be associated with periodontal disease.

E. ASCORBIC ACID (VITAMIN C)

Ascorbic acid is a water soluble, crystalline compound present in varying amounts in fresh fruits and most vegetables. Most mammals are able to synthesize the vitamin but man, the ape and the guinea pig are unable to do so. Although many organs, particularly the liver, contain relatively high concentrations of the vitamin, they do not appear to act as storage centres. Consequently, ascorbic acid must be supplied to the body regularly.

The classic disease associated with a deficiency of ascorbic acid is, of course, scurvy, of which the characteristic oral manifestations are swelling and extreme friability of the gingiva and loosening of the teeth. The guinea pig has been the animal most used in the study of experimental scurvy. In 1926 Wolbach and Howe, using this animal, embarked on a series of classic experiments which culminated in 1952. These workers showed conclusively that the essential lesion in ascorbic acid deficiency is an inability of the supporting tissues to produce and maintain intercellular substances. The tissues affected in this manner are fibrous connective tissue, bone, cartilage and dentine. For a comprehensive description of their findings the reader is referred to the excellent review by Wolbach (1953). (The nature of the metabolic defect that results from deficiency of ascorbic acid is described in Chapter 6, page 261).

A number of studies in the guinea pig have been directed towards investigating the effects of ascorbic acid deficiency on the periodontium. For example, Boyle et al. (1937) reported destruction of the periodontal fibres, disturbance in alveolar bone formation and an increase in bone resorption. Similar changes were reported by Glickman and Stoller (1948). Waerhaug (1960) found that monkeys on a vitamin C deficient diet developed clinical signs of scurvy after ninety days. Histological examination of the periodontium revealed a widening of the periodontal ligament with an almost complete breakdown of the collagen fibres. However, the principal fibres adjacent to the epithelial cuff remained intact. Although the alveolar bone height appeared to be within normal limits there was some resorption of the inside of the alveolar wall. Waerhaug concluded that, although the microscopic findings were in many respects similar to those found in human scurvy, certain important differences were present and therefore the two conditions could not be considered synonymous.

In a comprehensive study, Hunt and Paynter (1959) maintained young guinea pigs on a diet either completely lacking in vitamin C, or containing 0·4 mg/day, or containing 5 mg/day. Those on 5 mg showed no microscopic alterations in any of the periodontal tissues. Those on 0·4 mg showed mild alterations in the normal pattern of bone deposition and resorption in the jaws. Those on zero intake showed very severe changes, including haemorrhage in the periodontal ligament, failure of collagen formation, alveolar bone and cementum.

Thus, there seems little doubt that in the guinea pig and monkey ascorbic acid deficiency, provided it is severe enough, can produce profound changes in most of the periodontal structures. As far as man is concerned, however, opinion is much less unanimous. Thomas et al. (1962) examined alveolar bone height in two groups of dental students, one of which received no ascorbic acid for twelve months, the other orange juice supplements. They found a 0·3% greater loss of alveolar bone in the deprived group. Extrapolation of their results to age 50 revealed 50% alveolar bone loss in the deprived group, compared to 25% in the supplemented group. By contrast, Glickman (1964) does not accept that a lack of ascorbic acid per se can affect the periodontium. He believes that local irritation is the prime factor, but concedes that a concomitant deficiency of ascorbic acid in the presence of local irritation will exacerbate periodontal destruction. Since 1958 Russell and his co-workers have carried out extensive clinical and biochemical investigations into the possible relationships between nutritional status and the condition of the periodontium in large population samples in various parts of the world. In no case was any association found between the state of the periodontium and ascorbic acid deficiency (Russell, 1963).

Ingestion of massive doses of ascorbic acid are harmless to both man and animals. This is because the body is unable to store the vitamin in appreciable quantities, and it is therefore rapidly excreted in the urine.

The relationship between ascorbic acid and wound healing as it affects the periodontium will be discussed later.

F. THE B COMPLEX VITAMINS

A number of substances form the B complex group of vitamins. These include thiamine (vitamin B_1), riboflavin (vitamin B_2), nicotinic acid, choline, pantothenic acid, pyridoxine (vitamin B_6), folic acid, and vitamin B_{12}. Although the vitamins of this group differ substantially in their chemical composition, ranging from substances of low molecular weight (choline) to that of high molecular weight (vitamin B_{12}), they all have certain features in common. These substances are believed to be distributed universally in all living cells. Williams *et al.* (1950) defined the B group of vitamins as

" organic substances which act catalytically in all living cells and which function nutritionally for at least some of the higher mammals".

Although it is well known that certain specific deficiency diseases are due to lack of individual vitamins of the B group, for example, beri-beri due to a deficiency of thiamine, it is unlikely that oral manifestations are due to a deficiency of only one of these substances. Almost certainly the deficiency is, in most human cases, multiple. As with the other vitamins a number of investigations using various species of animal have attributed certain changes in the periodontium to a deficiency of one or more of the B group of vitamins. A selection of these studies will now be briefly reviewed.

1. Thiamine

There is at present no evidence that a deficiency of this vitamin causes alteration in any of the periodontal structures.

2. Riboflavin

Severe lesions of the gingiva, periodontal fibres and alveolar bone have been reported in monkeys deprived of this vitamin (Topping and Fraser, 1939; Chapman and Harris, 1941). In man the most prominent features of riboflavin deficiency are angular chelitis, stomatitis and glossitis. Although Ross (1944) reported loss of alveolar bone, observed radiologically, in a group of patients suffering from riboflavin deficiency, his findings have not yet been confirmed.

3. Nicotinic Acid

Deficiency of this vitamin in man results in pellagra. Kirkland (1936) considers the main oral changes in this disease to include gingivitis of varying degrees of severity, a finding confirmed by Dreizen (1966). King (1940) suggests that there is a close aetiological relationship between nicotinic acid deficiency and Vincent's infection. Some observers appear to have used nicotinic acid successfully in the treatment of Vincent's infection while others have found it ineffective (Dreizen, 1966).

Few animal experiments appear to have been carried out to determine the effect of nicotinic acid deficiency on the periodontium. One such study is that of Becks et al. (1943) who maintained young dogs on a diet deficient in nicotinic acid for three years. They reported severe inflammatory changes in the whole of the oral mucosa, including the crevicular epithelium, and atrophy of the alveolar bone.

4. Folic Acid

A deficiency of this vitamin in man results in a macrocytic anaemia. The oral manifestations are similar to those found in the other B complex deficiencies, and include a generalized stomatitis and glossitis.

Although there is at present no evidence that a pure folic acid deficiency affects the human periodontium, several studies in animals have shown that severe periodontal lesions can be produced. Pindborg (1949) fed young rats a diet containing methyl folic acid, a substance antagonistic to folic acid. Histological examination revealed severe non-inflammatory destruction of all the components of the periodontium. Day et al. (1937) reported severe gingivitis and necrosis of oral and gingival mucosa in monkeys maintained on a folic acid deficient diet, and similar results were reported by Shaw and Griffiths (1962) using the capuchin monkey.

5. Pantothenic Acid

No oral manifestations of pantothenic acid deficiency have been reported in man. However, Levy (1949) studied the effect of pantothenic acid deficiency on the periodontium of young mice. After the animals had been on the deficient diet for two weeks there was a reduction in height of the alveolar crest, widening of the periodontal ligament, alteration in the shape of the osteoblasts and proliferation of epithelial cell rests. After four weeks there was downward proliferation of epithelium along the roots of the teeth but no necrosis of epithelium. Further resorption of the alveolar bone occurred with the accumulation of some osteoid. At no stage of the experiment were inflammatory changes observed.

6. Pyridoxine

No periodontal changes associated with pyridoxine deficiency have been reported in man. Levy (1950) studied the effect of such a deficiency on the periodontal structures of young mice. He reported resorption of the alveolar bone and ulceration of the epithelium of the interdental papillae. He stressed that the chief difference in the histological findings between pantothenic acid deficiency and pyridoxine deficiency was the inflammatory nature of the response in the latter.

7. Vitamin B_{12}

A deficiency of this vitamin causes pernicious anaemia in man. The principal oral manifestation is a glossodynia.

IV. Proteins

There is little doubt that protein-calorie deficiency is the major nutritional disease affecting much of the world's population at the present time. Protein depletion results in numerous pathological changes which can affect almost all tissues. It is hardly surprising, therefore, that a vast literature now exists dealing with this one nutritional topic. It is, however, beyond the scope of this chapter to discuss the effects of protein deficiency in general terms. Many excellent reviews are available for the interested reader, one of particular value being that of Miller and Nizel (1966).

The effect of protein deprivation on the periodontium of animals has been studied by a number of workers in recent years. Chawla and Glickman (1951) fed a protein deficient diet to young rats for eight weeks. They reported degeneration of the connective tissue of the gingiva and periodontal ligament, osteoporosis of the alveolar bone and retardation in the deposition of cementum. The osteoporotic changes seen in the alveolar bone were identical to those observed in the femur. Similar results were reported by Frandsen et al. (1953) who, in addition, observed a loss of integrity of the interdental papillae. Goldman (1954) studied the effect of protein deficiency in young and old rats and in spider monkeys. His findings were in agreement with those reported above. Of considerable interest was his observation that the old rats were much less severely affected than the young. This finding is in agreement with the view expressed by McCance and Widdowson (1962) that the age at which protein deprivation occurs is of importance.

Stahl et al. (1958) used the golden hamster in their study. They reported oteoporosis of the alveolar bone with a reduction in the cellularity of the periodontal ligament. Platt and Stewart (1962) fed young pigs a protein-deficient diet. They reported oral changes which included osteoporosis of the

15

jaw bones, and retardation in the growth of the mandible with consequent malocclusion.

Thus, there seems no doubt that well-defined changes occur in the periodontium of various species of animal maintained on diets lacking protein, the changes being much more severe when the deficiency state is induced in the young, actively growing animal. One might expect, therefore, that reports of similar changes in the periodontium of humans would be available. As far as the writer can ascertain, however, no such studies appear to have been conducted. Thus, confirmation of these interesting animal experiments must await future investigation in man.

V. Carbohydrates

Although the relationship of refined carbohydrate to the development of dental caries has received a great deal of attention over the years, much less has been paid to the effect of this particular food constituent on the periodontium. Two interesting studies have been carried out on Tristan da Cunha islanders. In 1938 Sognnaes examined the population when the sugar consumption was nil. He reported that 10% of the adult population had advanced periodontal disease, which included alveolar bone loss and gingival recession (Sognnaes, 1954). The population was again examined by Holloway et al. (1963), by which time the sugar consumption had risen to 1 lb per person per week. These workers reported that 32% of the population were affected by periodontal lesions of varying severity. On the other hand, Shannon and Gibson (1964) studied a group of healthy young males with slight periodontal lesions. They used as their index of comparison the oral glucose tolerance test. They could find no correlation between the test and periodontal status.

Rice rats fed a diet containing 67% sucrose were found by Auskaps et al. (1957) to develop more severe periodontal lesions than those fed a diet with reduced carbohydrate but increased lard content. Miller (1966), commenting on the results of experiments conducted by Frandsen et al. (1953) and Stahl (1962; 1963a,b) who were investigating the effects of low protein diets on rats, but whose diets in fact contained a high carbohydrate content, concluded that the results (severe periodontal destruction) were due to a dual dietary aberration, in which both lack of protein and excess carbohydrate played a part in the development of the lesions. Devising deficient diets of this type, which at the same time are adequate enough to keep the animals alive during the experimental period is, of course, a constant source of difficulty for the investigator in nutritional research. Although Miller's hypothesis is an attractive one, obviously a great deal more work will have to be done on both animals and humans before the true relationship between carbohydrates and periodontal status can be ascertained with any degree of certainty.

VI. Fats

Although a considerable literature now exists dealing with the nutritional importance of fats for the organism as a whole, knowledge concerning the effect of this nutrient on the periodontium is very sparse. As far as can be ascertained no studies have been carried out in man.

Rao *et al.* (1965) fed groups of young rats a fat-free diet, as well as one containing excess fat, for seven weeks. The following changes were noted in the fat-free group; increased cellularity of the periodontal ligament, with slight resorption of alveolar bone and cementum. Those fed a high fat diet showed degenerative changes in all the components of the periodontium. The well defined differences obtained by these workers using low and high fat diets is of considerable interest. Further study is warranted, particularly in view of the increasing concern of nutritionalists, and others, with the deleterious effects of excess fat-intake on the general health of substantial numbers of people in the Western hemisphere. (The relationship between intake of fat and plaque formation is dealt with in Chapter II.)

VII. The Inorganic Elements

About fourteen inorganic elements are known to be essential for life. Three of these are present in the body in macro-quantities, calcium, phosphorous and magnesium.

A. CALCIUM

An adequate intake of this element is necessary for maintenance of a number of essential bodily functions. These include calcification of bones and teeth, maintenance of the normal serum calcium level of the blood, control of muscle and nerve tissue, blood clotting, and activation of some enzymes. For a general discussion of the complex metabolic functions of calcium metabolism the reader is referred to the excellent reviews by Irving (1957) and Harris (1966).

1. Calcium Deficiency

Osteoporosis is one of the most serious and puzzling of bone diseases. Nordin (1960) has defined this condition as a

" disorder or group of disorders in which there is a reduced amount of bone present in the skeleton; the ash content of such bone is, however, normal and osteoid borders are small or absent".

Opinion is still sharply divided on whether lack of dietary calcium, or some interference with the absorption of calcium from the gut, are important factors in the causation of osteoporosis. Nicolaysen (1960) has stated that a calcium-deficiency disease has never been established. However, Nordin (1960), in an extensive review of calcium deficiency, considers that a lack of dietary calcium and/or malabsorption could explain some forms of the disease. A number of animal studies would seem to lend support to Nordin's views. For example, Harrison and Fraser (1960) fed young rats a well-defined diet deficient only in calcium. They reported that the long bones became extremely porotic, but that there was no evidence of rachitic changes. These results were

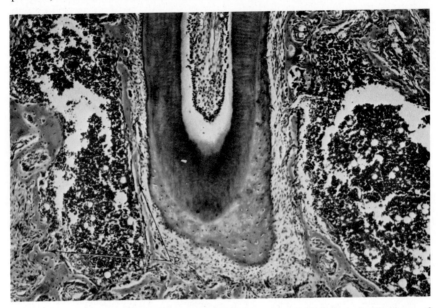

FIG. 3. Decalcified section of portion of molar root and surrounding alveolar bone of young rat deprived of dietary calcium. Note extensive porosis of alveolar bone. There is no excess of osteoid tissue and the secondary cementum, although reduced in amount, is well mineralized. Haematoxylin and Eosin. (×60.)

confirmed by Ferguson and Hartles (1963) also using young rats. Sognnaes (1961), in a comprehensive review of the dental aspects of mineral metabolism, considered that the alveolar bone enjoyed a certain priority in regard to the availability of minerals, including calcium, in certain deficiency states. Ferguson and Hartles (1964a,b) studied the effects of a diet, with a calcium/phosphorus ratio of about 1/20, on certain of the periodontal components in young rats. They reported that both the incisor and molar alveolar bone became porotic, more so than the long bones. The secondary cementum, although reduced in amount, was well mineralized (Fig. 3).

In a later study Ferguson and Hartles (1966) placed mature rats on a diet similar to that used in the study on young rats described above. After fourteen weeks on the diet only slight porotic changes were observed in the incisor alveolar bone. The molar alveolar bone appeared to be unaffected, as was the secondary cementum (Figs 4a,b). Ferguson (1967a) placed young cats on a

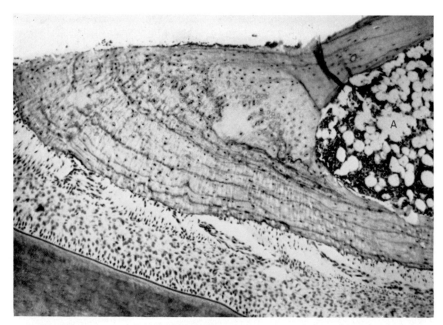

Fig. 4a. Decalcified section of portion of incisor alveolar bone of mature rat deprived of dietary calcium. A large cavity is shown in a portion of the bone (at A) but the remainder appears normal. Haematoxylin and Eosin. (×60.)

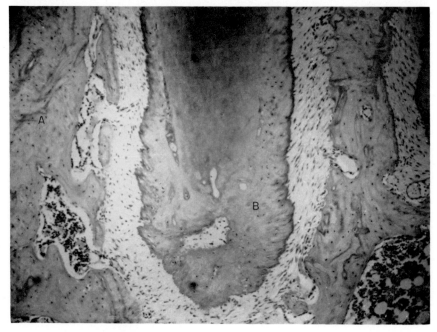

Fig. 4b. Decalcified section of portion of molar root and surrounding alveolar bone of mature rat deprived of dietary calcium. Neither the secondary cementum B nor the alveolar bone A appear to have been affected. Haematoxylin and Eosin. (×60.)

diet of minced ox heart which has a very low calcium content. As in the case of the young rats, severe porosis of the alveolar bone developed. There were no changes in the cementum (Fig. 5). Oliver (1967) confirmed the changes in the alveolar bone of young rats deprived of calcium. In addition, however, he observed a reduction in size and number of many of the periodontal fibres.

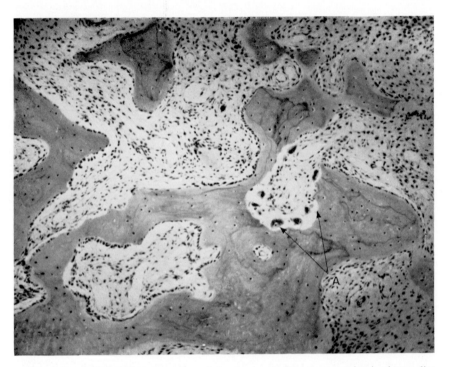

FIG. 5. Decalcified section of portion of alveolar bone of young cat maintained on a diet deficient in calcium. The bone is extremely porotic and a number of osteoclasts are seen in an area of active resorption (A). Haematoxylin and Eosin. ($\times$70.)

These results indicate that an adequate dietary intake of calcium is much more important for the proper mineralization of bone and cementum of the young, actively growing animal than when the animal is mature. The results do not appear to support the view expressed by Sognnaes that alveolar bone has any degree of priority over other bones for acquiring available calcium during periods of stress.

In humans, Radusch (1947) reported an increase in alveolar bone resorption and loss of lamina dura in patients suffering from achlorhydria, a condition associated with defective absorption of calcium.

As far as animal experiments are concerned, therefore, there seems little doubt that a deficiency of dietary calcium in the young causes marked porosis of the bones including the alveolar bone. The evidence for similar disturbances occurring in humans, due to calcium deficiency, is still controversial.

B. Phosphorus

As well as being necessary for the proper mineralization of bones and teeth, phosphorus plays an essential role in almost every cell-regulating process in the body. It is thus, like calcium, essential for life. This element is, however, so widely distributed throughout all animal and plant tissues that it is extremely unlikely that a pure phosphorus deficiency can occur in man. Malabsorption or inadequate utilization of phosphorus, from whatever cause will have effects similar to that of a pure deficiency syndrome. If this occurs, then it is skeletal tissue that suffers first.

1. Phosphorus Deficiency

In the young human, rickets results from a deficiency of vitamin D, but in the rat there is now well-documented evidence that the diet must be deficient in phosphorus before rachitic changes become manifest (Coleman *et al.*, 1950; Ferguson and Hartles, 1963). A study of the effects of phosphorus deficiency on the cementum and alveolar bone of young rats was carried out by Ferguson and Hartles (1964). They reported that the alveolar bone showed moderate rachitic changes. The mineralization of secondary cementum was also disturbed, as shown by fairly wide cementoid seams. In a later study Ferguson and Hartles (1966) maintained mature rats on a phosphorus-deficient diet for fourteen weeks. Slight osteomalacic changes were observed in the incisor alveolar bone, but the alveolar bone supporting the molar teeth appeared to be unaffected.

C. Magnesium

The amount of magnesium present in the body ranks third after calcium and phosphorus. Like calcium and phosphorus, the greater part of the magnesium content of the body is located in the bones and teeth.

Magnesium functions chiefly as an activator for various enzyme systems, particularly those which split and transfer phosphate groups. It also has been established that magnesium is essential for the normal growth of most animals. For example, rats deprived of magnesium die within three weeks. Although it is likely that magnesium plays many important, and even essential, metabolic roles, it is unlikely, according to Davidson *et al.* (1959), that a simple deficiency can occur in man. A deficiency could arise if some metabolic abnormality prevented the absorption of the element. As might be expected, there have been no reports of the effects of magnesium deficiency on the periodontium of man.

Although some experiments have been carried out on the effects of magnesium deficiency on dentine and enamel structure in rats, notably by Irving (1940) and Bernick and Hungerford (1965), no information appears to be available concerning the effects of such deficiency on the periodontium. The main difficulty in studying the effects of experimental magnesium deficiency lies in preparing a synthetic diet free from the element, since most of the constituents used in the preparation of such diets contain some traces of magnesium.

D. FLUORINE AND OTHER MICRO-ELEMENTS

In the last two decades or so, the role of fluorine in protecting tooth structure from dental caries has generated a vast amount of interest amongst dental research workers. As a result of these studies there seems little doubt that the addition of fluorine to domestic water supplies of the order of 1 p.p.m. significantly reduces the incidence of caries. Nevertheless, despite this overwhelming evidence, there is still a large body of opinion which opposes the addition of this element to the water supplies. Their antagonism appears to rest on the well-known fact that fluorine in large amounts is toxic to both humans and animals. The clinical manifestations of fluoride poisoning include spondylosis deformans, characterized by progressive osteosclerosis, ectopic ossification of tendons and ligaments, and spinal rigidity. It should be noted, however, that there is well-documented evidence to show that, in order for such changes to occur, the amount of fluoride ingested by food and/or water would have to be multiplied by a factor of approximately 100.

A number of studies, both human and animal, have been carried out to investigate the effect of fluoride on the periodontium. The results of animal studies are conflicting. McClendon and Gershon-Cohen (1954) fed rats a fluoride-free diet. They observed that periodontal disease was more prevalent and destructive than in control animals receiving a similar diet to which traces of fluoride were added. In contrast to this, Ramseyer et al. (1957) has found that albino rats maintained on a diet containing approximately 20 p.p.m fluoride show increased periodontal disease when compared with controls fed a diet containing 1 p.p.m. fluoride. Yet again, Costich et al. (1957), using guinea pigs, reported decreased periodontal disease in animals drinking water containing 40 p.p.m. fluoride when compared to a control group drinking distilled water.

An interesting study was carried out by Likins et al. (1963). These workers observed the effect of fluoride and tetracycline on the alveolar bone of rats maintained on an oat-flour diet which is known to cause alveolar bone resorption. No increase in absorption of alveolar bone was observed in the group of rats whose diet contained fluoride. There was, however, a reduction in the amount of alveolar resorption in the group fed tetracycline, and the authors attribute the result to a diminished inflammatory response. Since it is known that this particular antibiotic is incorporated directly into developing bone, an equally valid explanation could be that the bone-tetracycline complex is less susceptible to resorption.

A different approach was adopted by Zipkin *et al.* (1965). These workers induced alveolar bone resorption in young rats by injection of hydrocortisone. Half the animals were then fed a diet containing 17 p.p.m. fluoride; the control group did not receive added fluoride. Animals receiving the fluoride supplement exhibited less alveolar bone resorption than the controls.

Russell and White (1960) have reviewed the results of studies carried out in humans to ascertain the efficacy of dietary fluoride supplements on periodontal health. They are of the opinion that such studies have failed to reveal any association between the level of ingested fluoride and the health or otherwise of the periodontium.

The conflicting results reported above obviously indicate that more definitive studies in both humans and animals are required before any true assessment of the effect of fluoride on the periodontium can be evaluated.

Because of its proven importance in the maintenance of dental health, particularly caries prevention, it has been convenient to discuss fluorine under a separate heading. It should be noted, however, that this element is properly classified as one of the micro or trace elements. A large number of these are known to be present in both animal and plant tissues in minute quantities, and several have been shown to be essential to life. The term "trace-element" is losing its popularity in favour of the term "micro-element" since it has been shown that although the concentration in the body of these as a whole may be small, they may be present in some tissues in relatively high concentrations, e.g. the iodine content of the thyroid gland.

According to Harris (1966) it is difficult to establish how essential many of these elements are for the adequate nutrition of human beings, since they are so widely distributed in animal and plant tissues. Consequently, it is very difficult to devise a diet deficient in one or more of them. However, a number of animal studies have suggested quite clearly that at least several are essential for the well-being of man. Unlike the macro-elements calcium, phosphorus and magnesium, micro-elements have no structural function. Many are intimately concerned in a number of enzyme reactions. They function as components of catalytic systems which control biochemical and physiological processes in cells (Harris, 1966).

Some of these micro-elements have been investigated in attempts to establish a relationship to dental caries. These include Fe, Cd, Zn, Co, and Mn. As far as can be ascertained no definitive studies regarding the effect of these elements on the periodontium of man have been carried out, and the few results obtained in animal studies are so contradictory that there seems little point in discussing them at the present time. It is to be hoped that the newer

15*

and more refined biological techniques currently being developed will be utilized to obtain essential information concerning the true role of these elements for the nutrition of man. Until such information is forthcoming it is useless to speculate.

VIII. The Interactions of Calcium, Phosphorus and Vitamin D

The roles of these three substances in the nutrition of both man and animals have already been discussed individually. It is now proposed to deal very briefly with some interactions which have been established between them.

One of the principal actions of vitamin D is to promote the absorption of calcium from the intestine. It is also known that vitamin D given in large doses results in a raising of the serum calcium level of the blood. McLean (1941) suggests that raising the serum calcium level by this means could not be adequately explained by improvement in absorption alone. He considers that this "calcaemic" effect is due to a mobilization of bone salt; the inference being that vitamin D is capable in some way of acting on bone directly at the cellular level. This hypothesis has received support from the work of Carlsson and Lindquist (1955) who have shown that 10 units of vitamin D given to rachitic rats on a low calcium diet produces maximal absorption of [45]calcium, with a significant rise in serum calcium. With increased doses of 100 and 1000 units the serum calcium continued to rise but there was no further increase in absorption of calcium.

In a series of studies on young rats Ferguson and Hartles (1963; 1964a,b) have shown that the serum calcium levels of animals maintained on a diet deficient in calcium are significantly raised, although not restored to normal, when vitamin D is added to the diet. Vitamin D had a similar effect on the serum phosphate levels of animals maintained on a phosphate-deficient diet. Histological investigation of the alveolar bone of these groups of animals revealed that there was a greater amount of osteoid tissue present in both the low calcium and low phosphate animals when vitamin D was excluded from the diet. These workers have concluded that this is presumptive evidence that vitamin D in some way mobilizes bone salt.

According to Irving (1964), it is unlikely that vitamin D has any direct effect on the intestinal absorption of phosphorus. There have been some suggestions, however, that vitamin D can deprive the soft tissues of phosphorus when the dietary phosphorus is insufficient for the skeletal requirements of the animal, and that this released phosphorus is taken up by bone (Schneider and Steenbock, 1939).

Although a number of cause and effect relationships have undoubtedly been established between calcium, phosphorus and vitamin D, the actual mechanisms by which these functions are carried out at the cellular level remain obscure.

IX. The Relationship of Certain Nutrients to Healing of the Periodontium

It is now generally recognized that the failure of a wound to heal normally is due primarily to a deficiency of collagen production. The essential role of ascorbic acid in the healing of wounds, and in maintaining the integrity of the healed scar, has been known for many years. One of the earliest reports describing scurvy (Walter, 1748) made mention of the fact that wounds that had been healed for years broke down if the patient became scorbutic. This association between ascorbic acid deficiency and wound healing has received much attention over the years, and a comprehensive review of the subject is given by Gould (1966). Dunphy (1960), in an excellent review on the nature of the healing of wounds, considers that two nutrients are of prime importance, ascorbic acid and protein. He maintains that in ascorbic acid deficiency there is a reduction in the amount of sulphated mucopolysaccharide formed, and that this results in blocking the formation of collagen fibres.

Udupa et al. (1956) consider that although protein deficiency results in a slowing of all phases of wound repair, as does ascorbic acid deficiency, there is an essential difference between the two. In the latter, collagen which is produced is normal; a situation never found in ascorbic acid deficiency.

A number of animal studies support the view that both ascorbic acid deficiency and protein deficiency delay the healing of gingival wounds. Turesky and Glickman (1954) have evaluated gingival healing in normal and scorbutic guinea pigs. They report that there is prolonged local inflammation, impaired formation and maturation of basement membrane, reduction in the amount of ground substance and, consequently, in the amount and quality of collagen formed.

Cabrini and Carranza (1963) have studied the distribution of alkaline and acid phosphatase in gingival wounds made in guinea pigs subjected to partial and total ascorbic acid deficiency. A reduction in the level of alkaline phosphatase was observed in the scorbutic group in areas of fibroblastic proliferation, i.e. young, immature healing connective tissue. No difference in the reactivity of acid phosphatase was found between the two groups.

The gingival healing response following experimental wounding in rats fed a protein-free diet has been studied by Stahl (1962). He has reported a delay in connective tissue and alveolar bone repair. In a later study Stahl (1963a,b) experimentally wounded the gingiva of groups of young and mature rats, again maintained on a protein-free diet. Observations suggested a delay in osteogenesis and persistent inflammation, but age did not appear to induce histological differences in the healing sequence.

There seems to be no doubt, therefore, that a deficiency of ascorbic acid, or protein, can delay the healing of wounds, including those inflicted on the gingiva. It follows that an accurate assessment of the dietary intake of these two nutrients should be carried out in patients in whom periodontal surgery is contemplated. However, further studies in both humans and animals will be necessary before a true assessment of their fundamental roles in wound healing can be ascertained with certainty.

A recent study by Pories *et al.* (1967) has shown that zinc compounds have a beneficial but poorly understood, effect on wound healing. A series of young adults requiring excision of pilonidal sinus tracts was divided into two groups. Half were given oral zinc sulphate medication during the period of wound healing, the remainder acted as controls. Measurements of the rate of wound healing, by estimating the wound volumes at intervals, showed that the group receiving the zinc sulphate medication had a 43% decrease in the time taken for the wounds to heal completely. No toxic side effects were noticed. This study is of importance to those undertaking periodontal surgical procedures.

X. Concluding Remarks

An attempt has been made in the preceding pages to acquaint the reader, albeit briefly, with the main lines of investigation which have been undertaken in recent years to try and ascertain the relationship between nutritional factors and the state of the periodontium.

From the information currently available two conclusions appear to emerge with some degree of clarity. Firstly, animal experimentation has demonstrated conclusively that when a large number of nutrients are either withheld from the diet, or ingested in excessive amounts, a deleterious effect on one or more of the periodontal components may be observed. Secondly, the evidence that similar changes occur in the periodontium of man is very much less convincing.

Definitive nutritional experiments in man will, as far as one can foresee, always present the investigator with severe problems. It is nevertheless this reviewer's opinion that such studies are essential before any truly valid assessment of the role of nutrition in the maintenance of periodontal health can be completely evaluated.

References

Auskaps, A. M. Gupta, O. P. and Shaw, J. H. (1957). *J. Nutr.* **63**, 325–343.
Baer, P. N. and White, C. L. (1960). *J. Periodont.* **31**, 27–30.
Becks, H. (1942). *J. Am. dent. Ass.* **29**, 1947–1968.
Becks, H., Wainright, W. W. and Morgan, A. F. (1943). *Am. J. Orthodont.* **29**, 183–207.
Becks, H. and Weber, M. (1931). *J. Am. dent. Ass.* **18**, 197–264.
Bernick, S. and Hungerford, G. F. (1965). *J. dent. Res.* **44**, 1317–1324.
Boyle, P. E. (1937). *Harv. dent. Rec.* **11**, 5–9.
Burswasser, P. and Hill, T. J. (1939). *J. dent. Res.* **18**, 389–393.
Cabrini, R. L. and Carranza, F. A. (1963). *J. Periodont.* **34**, 74–79.
Carlsson, A. and Lindquist, B. (1955). *Acta physiol. scand.* **35**, 53–55.

Carlsson, J. and Egelberg, J. (1965). *Odont. Rev.* **16,** 42–49.

Chapman, O. D. and Harris, A. E. (1941). *J. infect. Dis.* **69,** 7–17.

Chawla, T. N. and Glickmann, I. (1951). *Oral Surg.* **4,** 578–602.

Cohen, B. (1960). *Proc. R. Soc. Med.* **53,** 275–280.

Coleman, R. D., Becks, H., Copp, D. A. and Frandsen, A. M. (1953). *Oral Surg.* **6,** 756–764.

Coleman, R. D., Becks, H., Kohl, F. V. N. and Copp, D. H. (1950). *Archs. Path.* **50,** 209–232.

Collazo, J. A. and Rodriguez, S. (1933). *Klin. Wschr.* **12,** 1768–1771.

Costich, E. R., Hein, J. W., Hodge, H. C. and Shourie, K. L. (1957). *J. Am. dent. Ass.* **55,** 617–619.

Davidson, S. D., Meiklejohn, A. P. and Passmore, R. (1959). "Human Nutrition and Dietetics." E. and S. Livingstone, Edinburgh and London.

Dawson, A. R. (1937). *J. Calif. dent. Ass.* **13,** 188–189.

Day, P. L., Darby, W. J. and Langston, W. C. (1937). *J. Nutr.* **13,** 389–399.

Dreizen, S. (1966). *In* "The Science of Nutrition and its Application in Clinical Dentistry" (A. E. Nizel ed.), pp. 146–168. W. B. Saunders Company, Philadelphia and London.

Dunphy, J. E. (1960). *Ann. Roy. Coll Surg. Engl.* **26,** 69–87.

Egelberg, J. (1965). *Odont. Rev.* **16,** 31–41.

Fahmy, H., Rogers, W. E., Mitchell, D. F. and Brewer, H. E. (1961). *J. dent. Res.* **40,** 870–877.

Ferguson, H. W. (1967a,b). Unpublished.

Ferguson, H. W. (1967). *J. dent. Res.* (*Abst.*) (In press).

Ferguson, H. W. and Hartles, R. L. (1963). *Archs. oral Biol.* **8,** 407–418.

Ferguson, H. W. and Hartles, R. L. (1964a). *Archs. oral Biol.* **9,** 447–460.

Ferguson, H. W. and Hartles, R. L. (1964b.) *Archs. oral Biol.* **9,** 647-658.

Ferguson, H. W. and Hartles, R. L. (1966). *Archs. oral Biol.* **11,** 1345–1364.

Frandsen, A. M. (1963). *Acta odont. scand.* **21,** 19–34.

Frandsen, A. M., Becks, H., Nelson, M. M. and Evans, H. M. (1953). *J. Periodont.* **24,** 135–142.

Freeman, S. and McLean, F. C. (1941). *Archs. Path.* **32,** 387–408.

Gershoff, S. N. (1966) *In* "The Science of Nutrition and its Application in Clinical Dentistry" (A. E. Nizel, ed.), pp. 125–145. W. B. Saunders Company, Philadelphia and London.

Glickman, I. (1964). "Clinical Periodontology", 3rd edn. W. B. Saunders Company, Philadelphia and London.

Glickman, I. and Stoller, M. (1948). *J. dent. Res.* (*Abst.*), **27,** 758.

Goldman, H. M. (1954). *J. Periodont.* **25,** 87–96.

Gould, B. S. (1966). *In* "The Science of Nutrition and its Application in Clinical Dentistry" (A. E. Nizel, ed.). W. B. Saunders Company, Philadelphia and London.

Harris, R. S. (1966). *In* "The Science of Nutrition and its Application in Clinical Dentistry" (A. E. Nizel, ed.), pp. 67–110. W. B. Saunders Company, Philadelphia and London.

Harrison, H. C., Harrison, F. H. E. and Park, E. G. (1958). *Am. J. Physiol.* **192,** 432–436.

Harrison, M. and Fraser, R. (1960). *J. Endocr.* **21,** 197–205.

Hirschi, R. G. (1950). *J. oral Surg.* **8,** 3–11.

Holloway, P. J., James, P. M. C. and Slack, G. L. (1963). *Brit. dent. J.* **115,** 19–25.

Howland, J. and Kramer, B. (1921). *Am. J. Dis. Child.* **22,** 105–119.

Hunt, A. M. and Paynter, K. J. (1959). *J. dent. Res.* **38,** 232–243.

Irving, J. T. (1940). *J. Physiol.* **99**, 8–17.
Irving, J. T. (1949). *J. Physiol.* **108**, 92–101.
Irving, J. T. (1957). "Calcium Metabolism." Methuen and Co. Ltd., London.
Irving, J. T. (1964). *In* "Mineral Metabolism", Vol. 2, Part A (C. L. Comar and F. Bronner, eds), pp. 249–313. Academic Press, New York and London.
Keyes, P. H. and Jordan, H. V. (1964). *Archs. oral Biol.* **9**, 377–397.
Keyes, P. H. and Likins, R. C. (1946). *J. dent. Res. (Abst.),* **25**, 166–167.
King, J. D. (1940). *Lancet* **2**, 32–35.
Kirkland, O. (1936). *Am. J. Orthodont.* **22**, 1172–1176.
Klingsberg, J. and Butcher, E. O. (1959). *J. dent. Res.* **38**, 421.
Krasse, B. and Brill, N. (1960). *Odont. Rev.* **11**, 152–165.
Leaver, A. G. and Triffitt, J. T. (1964). *J. dent. Res. (Abst.),* **43**, 957.
Levy, B. M. (1949). *J. Am. dent. Ass.* **38**, 215–223.
Levy, B. M. (1950). *J. dent. Res.* **29**, 349–357.
Likins, R. C., Pakis, G. and McClune, F. J. (1963). *J. dent. Res.* **42**, 1532.
Macdonald, J. B. and Gibbons, R. J. (1962). *J. dent. Res.* **41**, 320–326.
Masek, J. (1962). *In* "World Review of Nutrition and Dietetics" (J. A. Bourne, ed.), Vol. 3, pp. 149–194. Pitman Medical Publishing Co., London.
McCance, R. A. and Widdowson, E. M. (1962). *Proc. R. Soc.* B. **156**, 326–337.
McCollum, E. V., Simmonds, N., Becker, J. E. and Shipley, P. G. (1922). *J. biol. Chem.* **53**, 293–312.
McLean, F. C. (1941). *J. Am. dent. Ass.* **117**, 609–619.
McLean, F. C. and Urist, M. R. (1961). "Bone", pp. 114–127. University of Chicago Press, Chicago.
McLean, F. C. and Budy, A. M. (1963). *In* "Vitamins and Hormones", vol. 21. (R. S. Harris, I. G. Wool and J. A. Loraine, eds), pp. 51–66. Academic Press, New York and London.
McClendon, J. F. and Gershon-Cohen, J. (1954). *Am. J. Roentg.* **71**, 1017–1020.
Mellanby, E. (1931). *Brain,* **54**, 247–290.
Mellanby, E. (1944). *Proc. R. Soc.* B. **132**, 28–46.
Mellanby, M. (1941). *J. dent. Res.,* **20**, 489–509.
Miglani, D. C. (1959). *Oral Surg.* **12**, 1372–1386.
Miller, S. A. (1966). *In* "The Science of Nutrition and its Application in Clinical Dentistry" (A. E. Nizel, ed.) pp. 25–37. W. B. Saunders and Company, Philadelphia and London.
Miller, S. A. and Nizel, A. E. (1966). *In* "The Science of Nutrition and its Application in Clinical Dentistry" (A. E. Nizel, ed.) pp. 45–57. W. B. Saunders Company, Philadelphia and London.
Moore, T. (1960). *In* "Vitamins and Hormones", Vol. 18 (R. S. Harris and D. J. Ingle, eds), pp. 499–512. Academic Press, New York and London.
Nicolaysen, R. (1960). *Clin. Orthop.* **17**, 226–234.
Nordin, B. E. C. (1960). *Clin. Orthop.* **17**, 235–258.
Oliver, W. M. (1967). M.D.S. Thesis, University of Liverpool.
Persson, P. A. (1961). *J. Periodont.* **32**, 308–311.
Pindborg, J. J. (1949). *Oral Surg.* **2**, 1485–1496.
Platt, B. S. and Stewart, R. J. C. (1962). *Br. J. Nutr.* **16**, 483–495.
Pories, W. J., Henzel, J. H., Rob, C. G. and Strain, W. H. (1967). *Lancet* **1**, 121–124.
Radusch, D. F. (1947). *J. Periodont* **18**, 110–111.
Ramsøyer, W. F., Smith, A. H. and McCay, C. M. (1957). *J. Geront.* **12**, 14–19.
Rao, S. S., Shourie, K. L. and Shankwalker, G. B. (1965). *Periodontics,* **3**, 66–76.
Ross, J. A. (1944). *Br. J. Radiol.* **17**, 247.
Russell, A. L. (1963). *J. dent. Res.,* 42, 233–244.

Russell, A. L. and White, C. L. (1960). *In* "Fluorine and Dental Health" (J. C. Muhler and M. K. Hine, eds.), pp. 115–127. Staples Press, London.

Schneider, H. and Steenbock, H. (1939). *J. biol. Chem.* **128**, 159–171.

Scott, P. P. (1960). *In* "British Small Animal Veterinary Association Congress Proceedings", pp. 84–90. Pergamon Press, Oxford.

Shannon, L. L. and Gibson, W. A. (1964). *Periodontics*, **2**, 292–297.

Shaw, J. H. (1962). *J. dent. Res.* **41**, 264–274.

Shipley, P. G., Park, E. A., McCollum, E. V. and Simmonds, N. (1922). *Am. J. Dis. Child.* **23**, 91–106.

Sognnaes, R. F. (1954). "Oral Health Survey of Tristan da Cunha." Det. Norske. Videnskaps-Academi, Oslo.

Sognnaes, R. F. (1961). *In* "Mineral Metabolism", Vol. 1, B. (C. L. Comar and F. Bronner, eds), pp. 678–733. Academic Press, New York and London.

Stahl, S. S. (1962). *Archs. oral Biol.* **7**, 551–556.

Stahl, S. S. (1963a). *J. dent. Res.* **42**, 1511–1516.

Stahl, S. S. (1963b). *Periodontics*, **1**, 142–146.

Stahl, S. S., Miller, S. C. and Goldsmith, E. D. (1958). *J. dent. Res. (Abst.)*, **37**, 984.

Stewart, R. J. C. (1965). *In* "World Review of Nutrition and Dietetics", Vol. 5, pp. 275–337. S. Karger, Basel/New York.

Thoma, K. H. and Goldman, H. M. (1960). "Oral Pathology." The C. V. Mosby Company, St. Louis.

Thomas, A. E., Busby, M. C. Jr., Ringsdorf, W. M. Jr. and Cheraskin, E. (1962). *Oral Surg.* **15**, 555–565.

Topping, N. H. and Fraser, H. F. (1939). *Pub. Hlth. Rep.* **54**, 416–431.

Turesky, S. and Glickmann, I. (1954). *J. dent. Res.* **33**, 273–280.

Udupa, K. N., Woessner, J. F. and Dunphy, J. E. (1956). *Surgery Gynec. Obstet.* **102**, 639–645.

Waerhaug, J. (1960). *J. dent. Res. (Abst.)*, **39**, 1089.

Walter, R. (1746). "A Voyage Round the World", J. and P. Knapton, London, cited by Gould, S. B. (1966) in "The Science of Nutrition and its Application in Clinical Dentistry" (A. E. Nizel, ed.), pp. 169–182. W. B. Saunders Company, Philadelphia and London.

Weinmann, J. P. and Schour, I. (1945a). *Am. J. Path.* **21**, 821–831.

Weinmann, J. P. and Schour, I. (1945b). *Am. J. Path.* **21**, 833–855.

Weinmann, J. P. and Sicher, H. (1955). "Bone and Bones." C. V. Mosby Company, St. Louis.

Wolbach, S. B. (1946). *Inst. Med. Chic.* **16**, 118–145.

Wolbach, S. B. (1953). *Br. J. Nutr.* **12**, 247–255.

Wolbach, S. B. and Bessey, O. A. (1942). *Physiol. Rev.* **22**, 233–289.

Wolbach, S. B. and Howe, P. R. (1926). *Archs. Path.* **1**, 1–24.

Williams, R. J., Eakin, R. E., Beerstecher, E. Jr. and Shive, W. (1950). "The Biochemistry of the B Vitamins." Reinhold Publishing Corporation, New York.

Zipkin, I., Bernick, S. and Menezel, J. (1965). *Periodontics*, **3**, 111–114.

10 | Effects of Endocrine Secretions on the Periodontium and its Constituent Tissues

J. P. WATERHOUSE

Department of Oral Pathology, College of Dentistry, University of Illinois, Chicago, U.S.A.

I. Hormones and Metabolism

A. INTRODUCTION

The endocrine and nervous systems together form a complex unit of great flexibility which enables transient or long-lasting adjustments in metabolism to be made in response to internal bodily or external environmental changes. The interaction between the endocrine system and both the central and peripheral parts of the nervous system is a very close one. For example, the hypothalamus, part of the central nervous system, controls the anterior pituitary, which itself controls many of the other endocrines. Furthermore, the hormone noradrenaline, which is secreted by the adrenal medulla, acts as the post-ganglionic nerve transmitter substance. A consequence of this close interaction between systems is that changes due to functional demands or disease in either will cause compensatory, or if extreme, pathological, changes in the other.

The effects of hormones are not limited to specific organs. Some hormones affect all cells and tissues more or less directly. For example, insulin and somatotrophic hormone (STH) influence all cells and much of the inter-cellular material of the body.

Responses are frequently produced within the endocrine system by related sequences of events rather than by direct actions. For example, regulation of secretion of the anterior pituitary often occurs in response to systemic stimuli. These stimuli often do not act directly on the cells of the pituitary, but may act indirectly via the blood stream on other brain centres (Section H). Secretion by endocrine glands other than the pituitary depends to a large degree on circulatory levels of pituitary regulatory hormones such as thyro-trophic hormone (TSH) or adrenocorticotrophic hormone (ACTH), and gonadotrophic hormones. The output by the anterior pituitary of such trophic hormones is controlled by a feed-back mechanism, in addition to the central nervous system. Falling levels of circulatory adrenal corticosteroids stimulate the anterior pituitary directly or indirectly through the hypothalamus, and a higher level of secretion of ACTH results. Follicle-stimulating hormone (FSH) stimulates the ovary to produce oestrogen. As oestrogen blood level rises, further FSH production is depressed, and the anterior pituitary is stimulated to release luteinizing hormone (LH). External stimuli, such as the duration of daylight, also affect the liberation of gonadotrophins by the anterior pituitary in some animals by activating the nerve centres in the hypothalamus.

The effects of the sex hormones, adrenal corticosteroids, adrenaline (epinephrine) and noradrenaline, insulin, thyroid and parathyroid hormones, and anterior pituitary hormones, will be discussed in this chapter. Some hormones in these groups are known to affect the periodontium of man and animals to a significant degree, and they have been placed in order of import-ance of known effect upon the organ.

Numerous comprehensive texts on endocrinology are available and in this section, therefore, the hormones are discussed in quite general terms. For more detailed information the reader is referred to excellent accounts by Williams (1962), Pincus *et al.* (1964), and Gray and Bacharach (1967).

B. SEX HORMONES

1. Androgens

These are substances capable of stimulating the development of male secondary sexual characteristics and organs. Testosterone, the most active natural androgen, is secreted mainly by the interstitial (Leydig) cells of the testis under the influence of anterior pituitary gonadotrophins, particularly (LH) and to a lesser degree by the adrenal cortex under the stimulation of adrenocorticotrophic hormone (ACTH). The less potent androgens, androsterone and dehydroepiandrosterone (DHA), are found in the urine. These are closely related structurally to testosterone, and are steroids like the oestrogens and corticosteroids. In addition to their masculinizing effects, androgens cause retention of nitrogen, phosphorus and potassium, and stimulate protein formation. That is, they are anabolic agents and therefore promote growth of muscle and deposition of bone.

2. Oestrogens

Oestrogens play a major role in the maturation and maintenance of activity of the female sex organs. They are produced mainly by the cells lining the follicles in the ovary. The placenta, especially late in pregnancy is a major source; the adrenal cortex also produces oestrogenic hormones, but only in small amounts and usually only under pathological conditions. The three principal naturally occurring oestrogens in the human are oestrone, oestradiol-17β, and oestriol, and of these, oestradiol-17β is the most potent. Numerous other oestrogenic substances have been isolated from the urine of man and other species, and a number of synthetic oestrogens are active orally and are in therapeutic use. Oestrogens also have widespread anabolic effects, probably in almost all mammalian tissues (Hechter and Halkerston, 1964). They promote nitrogen retention and protein synthesis, water retention in connective tissues, and deposition of glycogen.

3. Progesterone

Progesterone, a hormone secreted by the corpus luteum of the ovary, renders the endometrium ready for implantation of a fertilized ovum. That is, it promotes the changes of the secretory phase of the endometrial cycle, and in this it acts in concert with oestrogens. The effects of progesterone are no confined to the endometrium. It is also an important metabolic intermediary in the synthesis in the mammalian body of androgens, oestrogens and cortico-steroids from cholesterol.

4. Relaxin

Relaxin is produced by the ovary, and in some species also by the uterus and placenta. Blood levels of the hormone rise steeply during pregnancy, reaching a peak at or just before parturition, and decline rapidly in the few hours thereafter. Relaxin appears either to enhance the effect of oestrogen, or else to render certain tissues more responsive to its action. Relaxin seems to cause depolymerization of connective tissue fibres, and this is seen particu-larly in the ligaments of the pelvis immediately before parturition.

C. ADRENAL CORTICOSTEROIDS

The steroid hormones of the adrenal cortex are secreted under the influence of the regulatory hormone ACTH of the anterior pituitary. Corticosteroids influence greatly the balance of electrolytes in the body, the metabolism of carbohydrate, and the function of the sex organs. The distinction drawn between what have been termed mineralocorticoids (i.e. steroids affecting electrolyte balance), such as aldosterone, and glucocorticoids (i.e. steroids affecting carbohydrate metabolism), such as cortisol, is not a completely satisfactory one, since many steroids affect both sets of processes.

Cortisone and its metabolic product, cortisol (hydrocortisone), have an important inhibitory effect upon the inflammatory process. Cortisol acts to stabilize the lysosomal and possibly the other lipoprotein membranes of the cell. In organ culture it inhibits the breakdown of cells, whether this is caused by inadequate culture conditions, vitamin A, or antiserum (Fell, 1964). Further, the capacity of each of a variety of steroids to release beta-glucuroni-dase and acid phosphatase from preparations of rabbit liver lysosomes was tested by Weissmann and Thomas (1964). Their results indicate that anti-inflammatory agents such as cortisol or cortisone protect, while certain inflammation-promoting steroids such as etiocholanolone disrupt lysosomal membranes. The mechanism whereby cortisol and related substances stabilizes membranes is not clear despite active investigation of the problem. Gershfeld and Heftmann (1963) found that a variety of steroids including cortisol became non-specifically adsorbed at the monolayer-water interface of monomolecular lipid films, but did not find evidence that they penetrated the lipid films. Munck (1957) pointed out that steroids are adsorbed with a horizontal orientation at interfaces between a polar and a non-polar medium such as a water-heptane interface. This evidence suggests that cortisol localizes at, but does not penetrate surfaces of simple lipid films. Inferences from these observations cannot, however, be extrapolated to the situation of membranes *in vivo*. The view that steroids may regulate surface phenomena by preventing penetration of lipid membranes by agents such as vitamin A, is suggested by Weissmann and Thomas (1964).

A unifying theory of some glucocorticoid actions has been presented by Schayer (1967). He draws attention to the apparent antagonism between the effects of histamine, which acts as an intrinsic dilator of the vessels of the microcirculation, and glucocorticoids. The latter tend to close microvascular sphincters. The effects of glucocorticoids upon inflammation would thus be related to the prevention of early hyperaemia. This theory, while attractive, requires confirmation. In addition to their anti-inflammatory effect, glucocorticoids influence enzymes of carbohydrate, lipid and protein metabolism (Weissmann and Thomas, 1964).

D. ADRENAL MEDULLARY HORMONES

Adrenaline (epinephrine) is synthesized and stored in the chromaffin cells of the body. These cells stain with dichromate salts and occur in the adrenal medulla, peripheral sympathetic ganglia and other organs. Noradrenaline is found in post-ganglionic sympathetic nerve fibres and is the post-ganglionic nerve transmitter substance of the sympathetic part of the autonomic nervous system. The effects of injected adrenaline and noradrenaline mimic the effects of stimulation of the sympathetic nervous system. Receptors on which this system acts are divided, on the basis of inhibition by pharmacological agents, into what are termed alpha- and beta-receptors. Adrenaline affects both types, while noradrenaline predominantly affects alpha-receptors. The alpha-receptors are involved mostly in excitatory actions such as peripheral vaso-constriction, while the beta-receptors predominantly mediate inhibitory action such as bronchiolar dilation and dilation of the arterioles supplying muscle beds. The outstanding exception to this generalization is the excitatory cardiac receptor (A–V node) which is a beta-receptor.

E. INSULIN

Insulin is secreted by the beta cells of the Islets of Langerhans in the pancreas. It directly affects carbohydrate, fat and protein metabolism. In carbohydrate metabolism, insulin increases the rate of utilization of glucose by tissues, modifying the initial reaction in the synthesis of glycogen from glucose, in which glucose and a molecule of ATP are converted into glucose-6-phosphate and a molecule of ADP.

Insulin affects fat metabolism by increasing the building of glucose residues into fat and by preventing mobilization of lipid from deposits of fat. By promoting the incorporation of aminoacids into peptides, it has an anabolic effect on protein metabolism.

F. Thyroid Hormones

Thyroxine, the major hormone of the thyroid follicles, is formed by a series of reactions involving iodination of tyrosine to form di-iodotyrosine, and the subsequent reaction of two molecules of di-iodotyrosine to form thryoxine. The thyroxine is stored in protein-bound form in the colloid within the follicles as thyroglobulin, the molecular weight of which is about 650,000. Both the uptake and turnover of iodine are stimulated by the thyroid stimulating hormone (TSH) of the anterior pituitary. Thyroxine, on release from the thyroglobulin in the colloid, crosses the follicular epithelium to reach the thyroid capillaries and circulates in the blood bound to plasma proteins.

The effects of thyroxine-like hormones, which include other iodinated derivatives of tyrosine other than thyroxine, may be considered together and are varied and fundamental. Thyroxine increases oxygen consumption in animals. One indicator of bodily metabolism is the basal metabolic rate (BMR). The BMR is nearly constant in many species over a wide range in size (Rall et al., 1964), and it is increased in hyperthyroidism and reduced in hypothyroidism (Best and Taylor, 1961). Thyroxine increases the rate of development of animals. It also stimulates protein synthesis, possibly by controlling the availability of messenger RNA. This possibility is suggested by the antagonism between thyroid hormones and actinomycin D, which substance inhibits protein synthesis by suppressing the formation of messenger RNA (Butt, 1967).

Thyrocalcitonin and calcitonin are believed to be identical (Gudmundsson et al., 1966). The term thyrocalcitonin will be used in this account. Thyrocalcitonin is a hormone which lowers plasma calcium levels in man (Foster et al., 1966) and dog. A potent preparation can be obtained from the thyroid of almost all mammals (MacIntyre, 1968). A single injection does not change soft tissue calcium, but infusion over twelve hours reduces cardiac muscle calcium. It is inferred (Gudmundsson et al., 1966) that the hormone acts upon bone.

The secretion of thyrocalcitonin by the C cells of the thyroid is very strongly suggested by the work of Foster et al. (1964), Pearse (1966) and Bussolati and Pearse (1967). Foster et al. (1964) showed good evidence for the secretion of thyrocalcitonin by certain cells of the dog thyroid which were rich in mitochondria. These investigators found that in dog thyroid glands perfused with high calcium blood an increase in acid phosphatase occurred in the mitochondrion-rich cells although no difference was found between control glands and those perfused with low calcium blood. Pearse (1966) demonstrated by electron microscopy that the cytoplasm of the C cells of the dog thyroid contained many vesicles 1500–2000 Å in diameter, and showed that the C cells responded to high calcium levels by increased secretion of the product contained in the vesicles. Finally, Bussolati and Pearse (1967) demonstrated by immunofluorescent techniques, using an antibody made in guinea pig to pig thyrocalcitonin, that the C cells of the thyroid of the pig and the dog contain thyrocalcitonin.

The effect of thyrocalcitonin in man was investigated by Foster *et al.* (1966). They showed that thyrocalcitonin from pig thyroid lowered serum calcium in three hypercalcaemic patients and in one normal volunteer subject. Parathormone and thyrocalcitonin together provide a powerful hormonal mechanism which in health maintains the plasma calcium level within very narrow limits. The role of thyrocalcitonin in calcium homoeostasis is discussed in Section VB of this chapter.

G. PARATHYROID HORMONE

In purifying the parathyroid hormone, Rassmussen and Craig (1962) obtained by gel filtration six polypeptides each with phosphaturic and calcium mobilizing activity. These may have resulted from hydrolysis of a larger molecule. Parathyroid hormone causes these effects by promoting the release of calcium from bone, increased excretion of phosphate by the kidney and increased absorption of calcium by the gut (Levine, 1964).

A unified statement of the mechanism of its action cannot yet be made and other sites of activity than those mentioned have been demonstrated including the lactating mammary gland. In promoting calcium absorption from the gut parathormone acts in concert with vitamin D (Butt, 1967). Convincing evidence of the indirect mode of action of the parathyroids upon bone has been obtained from experiments in which calcification of cartilage from a rachitic rat was obtained by incubating it in serum from a dog given parathyroid extract intravenously. The effect of the administration of the parathyroid extract was to cause the serum calcium (and serum phosphorus) to rise and the serum of blood withdrawn from the dog during the hypercalcaemic period, caused calcification of the rachitic cartilage incubated in it. Serum from blood withdrawn before or after the hypercalcaemic period did not cause calcification of the rachitic cartilage (McLean, *et al.*, 1946). In addition to its indirect actions mentioned above in which it exerts its effect via calcium homoeostasis, parathormone has a direct local effect on bone, as may be demonstrated by the procedure of transplanting parathyroid glands into direct contact with bone. It causes local resorption, probably by stimulating formation of osteoclasts. Bone resorption by osteoclasts is discussed in Chapter 6.

H. ANTERIOR PITUITARY HORMONES

1. Introduction

The principal hormones of the anterior pituitary are: growth or somatotrophic hormone (STH), adrenocorticotrophic hormone (ACTH), thyroid stimulating or thyrotrophic hormone (TSH), and the pituitary gonadotrophins. The pituitary gonadotrophins consist of follicle stimulating hormone (FSH), luteinizing hormone (LH) and prolactin. Luteinizing hormone is sometimes termed interstitial cell stimulating hormone (ICSH). Basophil cells of the anterior pituitary secrete FSH, LH, TSH and probably ACTH, while acidophil cells secrete STH. The controlling influence of the hypothalamus upon the anterior pituitary is probably mediated by the release from nerve tracts in the hypothalamus of individual releasing factors for ACTH, LH and TSH into a portal system running down the pituitary stalk.

2. Somatotrophic (Growth) Hormone (STH).

This hormone is secreted by acidophil cells in the anterior pituitary and, in man and monkey, probably by the placenta (Jasmovich and Maclaren, 1962; Kaplan and Grunbach, 1964). It causes visceral and skeletal growth and probably affects all cells in the body. Its effect is an anabolic one and it stimulates formation of protein and retention of nitrogen, probably through control of RNA synthesis (Korner, 1964).

3. Adrenocorticotrophic Hormone (ACTH)

ACTH is probably secreted by basophil cells in the anterior pituitary, and has, in addition to its principal stimulating effect on the adrenal cortex a general fat-mobilizing effect.

4. Thyroid Stimulating Hormone (TSH)

This hormone is secreted by basophil cells of the anterior pituitary and controls the activity of the thyroid acinar cells. A second thyroid stimulating hormone, the long-acting thyroid stimulator (LATS), may be mentioned here, although it does not arise in the pituitary. It is an immunoglobulin, and may be an autoantibody. It is found in the blood of patients with hyperthyroidism.

5. Gonadotrophins and Prolactin

The gonadotrophins produced by the anterior pituitary are follicle stimulating hormone (FSH) and luteinizing hormone (LH). FSH stimulates growth of the ovarian follicle, the cells of which secrete oestrogen. An important effect of this is to cause thickening of the endometrium. In the later stages of the menstrual cycle the secretion of LH by the basophil cells of the anterior pituitary mediates ripening and rupture of the follicle. The ovum is released and a corpus luteum develops from the ruptured follicle. The corpus luteum secretes progesterone and some oestrogen, and these cause the secretory phase of the endometrium.

In the male the action of FSH is to promote spermatogenesis, and of LH to promote secretion of androgen by the interstitial or Leydig cells of the testis.

Prolactin in man stimulates enlargement of mammary glands and lactation. In some species, it may delay atrophy of the corpus luteum.

II. The Development of the Periodontium and Endocrine Secretions

The phrase "development of the periodontium" will be used to describe adaptation of the periodontium up to and including eruption and occlusion of the permanent teeth.

The susceptibility of animals, including man, to changes in circulating levels of any hormone is not the same throughout life, and the effects of administering a particular hormone to an animal during development are thus not the same as they are later in life. These differences are no doubt partly due to variations with age in levels of other hormones which themselves affect organs or systems.

A. SEX HORMONES

Definitive and detailed evidence of the effect of endocrine imbalance upon the periodontium of the child is scanty. The changes in circulating levels of male and female sex hormones, which occur with puberty in both sexes, are however widely believed to affect the gingiva. The effects of these changes are seen in the gingivitis arising as an apparently increased reaction to local irritants in the majority of boys and girls about the age of puberty (Cohen, 1955). This author has found that gingival enlargements in the presence of local irritation is more marked in children around puberty than in children aged 8–10 years or in late adolescence. The changes tend to regress some years later (Glickman, 1964).

Excess production of androgenic hormones occurs in the young of both sexes and in adult women in the commonest form of the *Adrenogenital Syndrome*. This syndrome may be the result of a defect in the C_{11}- or C_{21}-hydroxylating enzymes active in steroid biosynthesis, with consequent defect in cortisol formation and resulting hypersecretion of ACTH by the anterior pituitary (Robbins, 1967). It may also result from hyperplasia or tumour of the adrenal cortex. Greatly accelerated precocious growth, maturation of the skeleton (Weinmann and Sicher, 1955), and premature eruption of teeth may occur in the syndrome.

Nutlay *et al.* (1954) found that oestrogen administered to neonatal mice caused bone sclerosis in the alveolar processes due to endosteal bone deposition with a resulting reduction in marrow spaces. The marrow in these spaces became fibrous. These effects were not observed in adult mice. The effects, by contrast, of low oestrogen levels were investigated by Glickman and Quintarelli (1960) who carried out oöphorectomy on rats aged 4–6 weeks. They obtained a retardation in the rate of formation of alveolar bone and cementum and a reduction in the activity, indicated by fibre density and cellularity, of the periodontal ligament. The changes became more marked as time progressed. However, animals operated on at one year of age were not affected, which may indicate a reduced sensitivity to the hormones with increasing age of the tissues.

It should be noted, in interpreting the results of such experiments, that administration of oestrogen causes a reduction in secretion of FSH and probably of other hormones, by the anterior pituitary. This reduction in turn causes reduced secretion of oestrogen by the ovarian follicle. The ovaries remain intact. Oöphorectomy, however, removes the main source of oestrogen, and secondarily stimulates the basophil FSH-secreting cells of the anterior pituitary. Oöphorectomy and administration of oestrogen do not, therefore, have diametrically opposed effects.

B. OTHER HORMONES

Insulin facilitates the entry and utilization of glucose in cells of many tissues of the body. In the absence of sufficient amounts of effective insulin for normal metabolism, as in diabetes mellitus, the carbohydrate and hence the fat and protein metabolism of many of the organs of the body is disturbed. Its effects on the periodontium are believed to be an enhanced susceptibility to infection of the periodontal tissues, and not the initiation of a specific periodontal disease as such. The juvenile diabetic, particularly if his diabetes is uncontrolled, exhibits more bone loss due to periodontitis than a non-diabetic child with local gingival irritation of a similar degree (Goldman and Cohen, 1957).

The initial periodontal lesion in diabetics may be microvascular, and may precede the grosser vascular and other changes (McMullen et al., 1967). These authors demonstrated microangiopathy, which is characteristic of diabetes. This comprises deposition of periodic acid-Schiff-reactive material subendothelially in the walls of capillaries and other small vessels. These changes were observed in the gingiva of most diabetics and "genetic prediabetics" examined.

Effects of pituitary hormones upon the periodontal ligament may be observed in patients suffering from hypopituitarism. Eruption of the teeth is delayed in these children (Schour and Massler, 1943; Rushton, 1952).

III. The Influence of Endocrine Secretions on Gingiva

A. THE GINGIVA CONSIDERED AS A WHOLE

1. Sex Hormones

The specific stimulating effect of oestrogens and androgens is exerted particularly upon those target organs which mediate the development of the male or female sex characteristics. These are however not the only effects of sex hormones, and generalized anabolic effects also occur. Mucosa and skin, at least in old people, is thickened by oestrogens (Goldzieher et al., 1952), and androgens promote cell division in epidermis in several animal species (Bullough, 1962). An increase in mitotic rate could provide thickening or hyperplasia of mucosa, if other factors such as desquamation and cell adhesion in the superficial layers were not affected. This effect may account in part for the hyperplasia of the gingiva in males and females associated with inflammation around the age of puberty. (Section II). In old age, however, other factors must operate; although in the elderly androgen levels are not as high as in the young and the mucosa becomes relatively atrophic, the mitotic rate is raised not lowered (Meyer et al., 1956).

The effects of change in sex hormone balance upon the gingiva in man have been described repeatedly from clinical observations. However, the value of evidence from such observations depends greatly upon the use of epidemiological sampling methods and indices of periodontal health. Among such indices the PMA Index (Massler et al., 1950), the Periodontal Index (Russell, 1956), Periodontal Index (Ramfjord, 1959) and the Gingival Index (Löe and Silness, 1963) have proved valuable in investigations in this field.

Observations on the gingiva of women during pregnancy and the menses indicate the effects of oestrogens and other sex hormones. Early reports of the prevalence of gingivitis in pregnancy give percentages ranging from 30 to over 70% (Ziskin et al., 1936; Maier and Orban, 1949; and Ringsdorf et al., 1962). More recently Löe and Silness (1963) and Löe (1963) found gingivitis to be present in 100% of 121 pregnant women. They found, moreover, that the prevalence and severity of gingival inflammation was significantly higher in pregnant women than in women post-partum. The mean rating for gingivitis using the Gingival Index (Löe and Silness, 1963) and the Periodontal Index (Russell, 1956) reached a maximum during the eighth month of pregnancy, and decreased thereafter until the mean rating post-partum was similar to that in the second month of pregnancy. The prevalence of the localized hyperplasia of the gingiva during pregnancy, termed pregnancy epulis or pregnancy tumour, has been reported as 0·5% (Maier and Orban, 1949) and 0·8% (Löe and Silness, 1963). Such localized lesions may develop and grow rapidly during pregnancy, regressing only partially after parturition (Ziskin and Nesse, 1947).

The physico-chemical state of the ground substance of gingival connective tissue in pregnant women has been discussed by Engel (1950). He has shown that gingiva inflamed during pregnancy contains increased glyoprotein (Engel, 1952a), and that, furthermore, changes in the electrical properties of the gingiva indicate a decreased density of glycoprotein in the early months of pregnancy (Section IIID). Gingivitis in pregnant women responds, however, to removal of local irritants (Löe, 1963). After parturition, the state of the gingiva of a woman resembles that which prevailed before her pregnancy.

Permanent periodontal damage from gingivitis during pregnancy was not detected by Löe and Silness (1963). Hormonal imbalance, of this kind at least, therefore influences the severity of periodontal inflammation but, as Nuki and Löe (1966) have suggested, does not initiate it.

Some of the effects of puberty and pregnancy upon the gingiva can be explained by the suggested action of hormones upon epithelium and connective tissue ground substance, although each of these tissues is markedly affected by the reaction of the other (Chapter 2). The influence of bacterial plaque, the accumulation of which is favoured by loss of gingival contour, is also important.

2. Other Hormones

There is little doubt that in some patients diabetes mellitus causes increased susceptibility to gingivitis leading to periodontitis with bone loss, and a tendency for periodontal abscess formation. The relationship between diabetes mellitus and periodontal disease is not, however, a simple one, and it has been well reviewed by Glickman (1964) and Benveniste et al. (1967). Available evidence supports a correlation between gingival disease and the glucose tolerance of patients (Cheraskin and Ringsdorf, 1965). Glickman (1964), however, supports the widely held view that periodontal disease in diabetics does not differ from that of non-diabetics. The higher prevalence and severity of periodontal disease in diabetic patients is thus probably related to their impaired reaction to infection. It is likely that the vascular changes observed by McMullen et al. (1967) in the gingival tissues of four out of five diabetics and in nine out of ten pre-diabetics play a part in this impairment. In an investigation of 189 patients with diabetes mellitus and 64 control subjects, Finestone and Boorujy (1967) adduced evidence to show that the prevalence and severity of periodontal disease are increased in diabetics and that the Periodontal Index (Russell, 1956) on the one hand, and the duration of known diabetes or variation of blood sugar levels on the other, could be correlated. Benveniste et al. (1967), however, found that gingivitis and pocket depth did not, in their group of subjects, differ significantly between treated diabetics and non-diabetics.

B. Epithelium

1. Sex Hormones

(a) Man. The general anabolic effect of androgens and oestrogens has been noted above. The effects of sex hormones on gingival epithelium are, however, difficult to determine precisely. For example, stagnation and consequent inflammation and inflammatory hyperplasia are promoted by the loss of gingival contour which results from hyperplasia from many causes.

A type of desquamative gingivitis related to the menses has been described by Mühlemann (1948) as *Gingivitis Intermenstrualis*. However, Trott (1957) was unable to find satisfactory evidence for cyclical changes in keratinization of the gingiva during the menstrual cycle although inflammation of human gingiva is associated with reduced keratinization and an increased deposition of intracellular glycogen (Weiss, *et al.*, 1959).

Atrophic gingivitis and atrophy, with loss of suppleness of the mucosa, which are found in some humans after natural or surgical menopause, have been linked with the loss of ovarian secretions. The gingiva present red or eroded areas with thinned epithelium and increased vascularity. The principal symptoms are a burning or pricking sensation with sensitivity to heat, and the gingiva bleed easily. Low oestrogen levels, together with some possible degree of vitamin B complex deficiency, are likely causes (Massler, 1951 and 1956). Histologically, atrophy and reduced keratinization are seen (Trott, 1957). However, these findings are not common (Glickman, 1964), and it is likely that additional features such as anaemia and other nutritional deficiencies play a contributory part. Investigation of patients to whom hormones are being administered provides a further source of information. Gingival biopsies from humans receiving testosterone propionate show more marked keratinization than normal, epithelial hyperplasia and increased mitotic activity (Ziskin, 1947a,b).

(*b*) *Laboratory animals.* When interpreting the clinical or experimental results of administering hormones to an intact animal, it is important to note the relationship between the anterior pituitary and its target endocrine organs. Secretion by the anterior pituitary is largely controlled by a feed-back mechanism effected by the levels of circulating hormones of the target organs, i.e. the gonads, thyroid, adrenals and placenta.

The effects of oestrogens upon the gingiva have been investigated experimentally in several species. Oestrogens given to oöphorectomized monkeys, in whom the administration of follicle-stimulating hormone (FSH) had been accompanied by gingivitis, caused keratinization and an apparent increase in resistance of the gingiva to infection by oral micro-organisms (Ziskin *et al.*, 1936). Oestrogens cause a thickening of stratified squamous epithelium. Nutlay *et al.* (1954) have reported that injections or subcutaneous implantation of pellets of α oestradiol benzoate in older mice cause increased downgrowth of the epithelial attachment and hyperplasia of the epithelium of the interdental papilla between molar teeth. Conversely, castration of female rhesus monkeys results in atrophy of the epithelium of gingival and alveolar mucosa. Castration of male monkeys causes hyperkeratinization (Ziskin and Blackberg, 1946). This effect seems likely to be due to stimulation of the pituitary by castration. Furthermore, an androgen (testosterone propionate) produces more marked keratinization in keratinized epithelium, and some keratinization in non-keratinized epithelia of normal and castrated male monkeys and normal female monkeys (Ziskin, 1947a,b).

Rushton (1952) has found no increase in keratinization, nor in thickness of oral epithelium, in weanling golden hamsters given methyl testosterone orally up to the age of 9 months. However, the downgrowth of the attachment epithelium over the root cementum was retarded, and the animals gained less weight than controls, probably due to a depression of anterior pituitary function.

2. Other Hormones

(a) Man. Glucocorticoids inhibit mitosis in epidermis, and indeed atrophy of human epidermis can follow the topical application of corticosteroids (Zachariae, 1966). Adrenaline is one of the most active substances known in this respect and possibly plays a part in the mechanism whereby the daily cycle of mitotic activity is initiated (Bullough, 1962) (Chapter 5). Mitosis in the body is thus probably normally under the inhibiting effect of the pituitary-adrenal axis. Changes, possibly associated with hormones, occur in the oral mucosa with age. The mitotic rate in human gingiva (Meyer et al., 1956) and rat tongue and buccal epithelium (Hansen, 1966) has been shown to be higher in older than in younger age groups.

(b) Laboratory animals. Information is available from experimental investigations on the effects of hormones, other than sex hormones, on the periodontium. Glucocorticoids cause atrophy (thinning of both epidermis and dermis) of rat skin after topical application for up to 180 days (Castor and Baker, 1950). Surgically induced myxoedema in rabbits causes hyperpara-keratosis and keratosis in gingival epithelium (Rosenberg et al., 1961). Follicle stimulating hormone (FSH) given to oöphorectomized monkeys causes, or allows, inflammatory changes in the gingiva to become marked, the tissues becoming susceptible to infection by the oral flora (Ziskin et al. 1936).

Hypophysectomy in female monkeys causes atrophy of the gingiva and other parts of the oral mucosa (Ziskin and Blackberg, 1946). This may result from loss of sex hormones due to absence of pituitary stimulation of gonads and adrenals. Schour (1934) has reported that in the hypophysecto-mized rat, the epithelial attachment fails to maintain its integrity during development and function, and that the epithelium is atrophic or missing in areas between connective tissue and enamel in the molar teeth.

C. CONNECTIVE TISSUE CELLS

1. Sex Hormones

The general anabolic effects of androgens and oestrogens manifest them-selves in connective tissues by an increase in rate of formation of the elements of the connective tissue. The connective tissue of the gingiva of monkeys or

human beings receiving testosterone propionate experimentally or thera-
peutically undergoes hyperplasia. Increases in collagen and in cellularity are
found (Ziskin, 1947a). Administration of oestrogen causes an increase in
acid mucopolysaccharides in the ground substance of the connective tissue
of human oral mucosa, and correlated changes in the tissue mast cells (Schiff
and Burn, 1961).

2. Other Hormones

By contrast with sex hormones, glucocorticoids reduce activity of connective tissue cells. In an *in vitro* investigation, Castor (1965) has shown that
glucocorticoids including cortisol in excess, cause important changes in
function in cultured connective tissue cell strains derived from human knee-
joint-synovium. These include accelerated proliferation, reduced cell volume,
reduced rate of hyaluronate formation and decreased deposition of collagen.
All modifications of cell function are reversible on withdrawal of the hormone
after approximately three months of continuous exposure. Prednisolone and
methyl-prednisolone essentially duplicate these effects of cortisol.

Corticosteroids inhibit formation of fibrous connective tissue if applied
topically (Zachariae, 1966). One injection of a physiological dose of cortisol
(3 mg per kg) in normal rats causes a decrease in dermal concentration of
saline-soluble hexosamine and collagen, together with an increase in the
dermal concentration of acid-soluble collagen. This response is not found in
phenytoin-treated rats (Houck and Jacob, 1963).

Thyroid hormones have been reported to affect fibroblasts. The fibroblasts
in granulation tissue in normal guinea pigs to which thyroxine was administered showed reduced nuclear chromatin (Jörgensen, 1963) and therefore
their nuclei stained less intensely with haematoxylin and eosin. The amount of
collagen and ground substance produced by the fibroblasts was not altered.

The effects of sex and other hormones on cultured connective tissue cells
originating in the periodontium do not appear to have been studied. Some
inferences can be drawn from what is known of connective tissue cells
elsewhere in the body. However, the behaviour of those in the gingiva may be
affected by the presence of bacterial plaque in the adjacent crevice, and by a
collagenase in the gingiva (Gibson and Fullmer, 1966) (See Chapter 6).

D. FIBROUS ELEMENTS

Maibenco (1960) investigated the tissue changes and the alterations in
tissue constituents in the rat uterus at different stages of the oestrous cycle,
pregnancy and the puerperium. Uterine growth in pregnancy comprises
muscular hypertrophy and a concurrent marked increase in connective tissue
ground substance as well as an increase in fibrillar elements. There is little
evidence of muscular hyperplasia. A basis for the increase in connective

tissue was suggested by the observation of fibroblasts containing granules of ground substance or its precursory materials. Thus connective tissue and muscle increase under this stimulus and regress post-partum.

Thyroid hormones have been reported to affect the gingiva in experimental animals. Changes classed as degenerative in the gingiva in thyroidectomized rhesus monkeys, including oedema and fragmentation of collagen fibres in the connective tissue were reported by Ziskin and Stein (1942).

Surgically induced hypothyroidism in rabbits caused oedema and disorganization of the collagen of gingival connective tissue (Rosenberg et al., 1961).

Cortisone and DOCA both cause a decrease in ground substance and hydroxyproline/nitrogen and hexosamine/nitrogen ratios in the skin in young rats, but not in aged rats. In aged rats both cortisone and DOCA resulted in an increase in ground substance (Sethi et al., 1961). This is a further example of the changes in susceptibility of organs to hormones with development or with age.

E. THE GROUND SUBSTANCE

The ground substance of connective tissue is organized as a two-phase system (water-rich and colloid-rich), the effective equilibrium of which is influenced by acute inflammation and by hormones which alter the degree of aggregation of macromolecules in ground substance. This degree of aggregation controls the water and ionic content of the ground substance (Gersh and Catchpole, 1960). An influence of female sex hormones upon enzymatic activity in gingival connective tissue, moreover, is suggested by the predominance of females in reported series of patients with desquamative gingivitis, in which the connective tissue ground substance contains increased quantities of water-soluble glycoproteins (Engel, 1950).

The properties of the connective tissue, including tensile strength and consistency, are altered by hormones (Gersh and Catchpole, 1949; Catchpole, 1966). Examples include the effect of androgen to increase the turgor of the capon comb and of oestrogen to increase the turgor of skin of primates. The physical basis for the change includes alteration in colloidal charge and increased solubility of ground substance components including glycoproteins, associated with depolymerization of high molecular weight constituents of connective tissue ground substance (Catchpole, 1966). The effect upon the symphysis pubis in the guinea pig of oestrogen and relaxin (Perl and Catchpole, 1950) may be quoted. The ground substance became more reactive to the periodic acid-Schiff reaction and more water-soluble. Intravenously given Evans blue became localized in the region. The cartilage of the pubic joint of the mouse is similarly transformed into fibrous connective tissue under the influence of estrogens and relaxin. When measured biochemically, local acid phosphatase activity was found to be increased (Steinetz and Manning, 1967).

The accumulation of ions in connective tissues is generally determined by the net density of colloidal charge in the tissue, and at physiological pH the constituents carry a net negative colloidal charge neutralized by diffusible electrolytes from the blood (Catchpole *et al.*, 1966). The type of connective

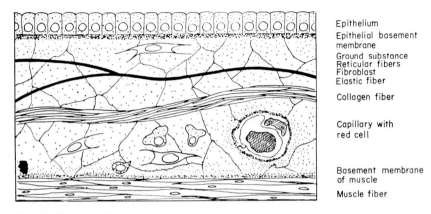

Epithelium
Epithelial basement membrane
Ground substance
Reticular fibers
Fibroblast
Elastic fiber

Collagen fiber

Capillary with red cell

Basement membrane of muscle

Muscle fiber

FIG. 1. Diagram of relations of connective tissue ground substance (light stipple) to cells, fibres and a blood vessel. The heavier stipple represents basement membrane of epithelium, muscle and endothelium of a small blood vessel (capillary). (After Gersh and Catchpole, *Perspect. Biol. Med.* 1960, **3**, 282–319.)

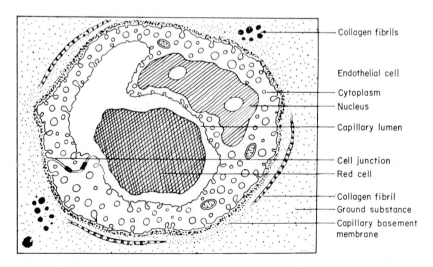

Collagen fibrils

Endothelial cell

Cytoplasm
Nucleus

Capillary lumen

Cell junction
Red cell

Collagen fibril
Ground substance
Capillary basement membrane

FIG. 2. Diagram of an endothelial cell in cross section of capillary wall. Impression drawn from electron micrograph of a cutaneous capillary. (Courtesy of Dr. H. H. Friederici and the publishers.) (After H. R. Catchpole, in Physiology and Biophysics (1965) 617, 643, Saunders, Philadelphia.)

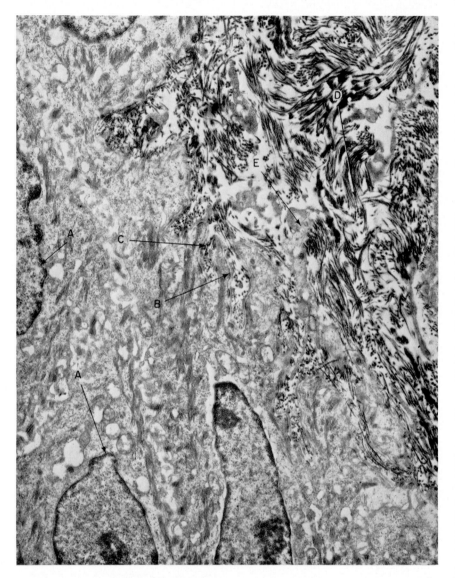

FIG. 3. Electron micrograph of the junction between epithelium and connective tissue. Palate, rat. Fixation, buffered glutaraldehyde and osmium tetroxide. A. Nuclei of epithelial basal cell. B. Hemidesmosome. C. Lamina densa. D. Collagen fibres in dermis. E. Fibroblast process. (×17,100.) Stain, lead citrate and uranyl acetate. (Drs. Meyer, Waterhouse, Ma, Kraucunas.)

tissue varies in different sites of the body (Chapter 6). Nevertheless, the muco-proteins of gingiva might be expected to have similarities with those in other tissues. A detailed analysis of the factors controlling the fluid content of tissues, particularly the capillary venous and lymphatic vessels, is given by Catchpole (1965) (Figs 1, 2 and 3). Altered carbohydrate metabolism and insulin affect the polysaccharide components of ground substance (Schultz-Haudt and Aas, 1962; Brunish, 1966).

F. GINGIVAL WOUNDS

Abnormal levels of circulating hormones do not, so far as can be judged, constitute an important threat to the healing of gingival wounds. The writer concludes this in the knowledge that much work utilizing experimentally high blood levels in animals has been carried out as has been discussed by Douglas (1963). Abnormally high or low levels may, of course, be due to disease of an endocrine organ, or to treatment of disease by systemic adminis-tration of hormones.

The possible effects of the high local levels of hormone attainable by topical application of, for example, corticosteroids will be considered later in this chapter. Alterations in systemic levels of hormones probably do not affect wound healing significantly. Hypophysectomy does not appreciably influence wound healing, and physiological and near-physiological doses of anterior pituitary extract do not delay wound healing. The same considerations apply to thyroidectomy and the thyroid hormones, and gonadectomy and the sex hormones, although healing of oral wounds has been reported to be accelerated by castration in males although not in females (Butcher and Klingsberg, 1961). However, progesterone has been shown by Lindhe *et al.*, (1968) to promote development of inflammation in the submucosa adjacent to a small wound in the hamster cheek pouch.

The effects of cortisone upon body weight and the tensile strength of healing wounds in the rat and guinea pig was investigated by Rehder and Enquist (1967). Even large doses (25 mg/kg) of cortisone did not affect the tensile strength of a healing surgical wound in either species. DiPasquale and Stein-etz (1964) reported that low doses of cortisone interfered with the healing of standardized skin wounds in rats, but only by producing anorexia; the effect was duplicated by food restriction without drugs. Large doses of steroid impaired wound healing but also induced a drastic loss of body weight. These effects were not reproduced by food restriction alone. The use of experi-mentally large doses of adrenal cortical hormones is not relevant to the treatment of humans. Poor wound healing has not been observed in patients recovering from adrenalectomy for malignant disease, although they receive as a rule the equivalent of some 50 milligrams of cortisone daily post-operatively (Douglas, 1963).

An experimental assessment of the local effects of corticosteroids upon organizing peritoneal wounds has been performed by Glucksman and Warren (1966). They reported some effect in limiting the early exudative phase of fibrin formation. Such observations are relevant to the topical application of preparations containing corticosteroids to wounds. The use in oral surgery of glucocorticoid corticosteroids has been reviewed by Saad and Swenson (1965) who investigated the topical effect of flurandrenolone (Cordran) ointment applied post-operatively under a dressing to gingivectomy wounds in a double-blind controlled study. Statistically significant differences in the rates of formation of granulation tissue, oedema, pain and rates of wound healing were not, however, obtained. Costicosteroids can protect cells from damage by bacterial toxins through a stabilizing effect upon lysosomal membranes (Weissmann and Thomas, 1964), but a beneficial effect upon the healing of infected or non-infected wounds has not, however, been demonstrated.

The effects of hormones upon granulation tissue formation in man and experimental animals are reviewed and discussed in some detail by Taubenhaus (1957). He states that hydrocortisone, oestradiol and testosterone in large doses inhibit granulation tissue formation, the last two by depressing STH secretion by the anterior pituitary. Aldosterone, the physiological mineralocorticoid, has in large doses a stimulating local action upon granulation tissue. Of the pituitary hormones, STH stimulates the formation of granulation tissue, while ACTH, as would be expected, depresses it. Administration of ACTH does not, however, seem to have an effect upon the tensile strength of clean wounds (Taubenhaus, 1957). Jörgenson (1963) showed that thyroxine reduced the amount of granulation tissue produced by a chronic surgical wound in normal guinea pigs. In scorbutic guinea pigs, however, the amount of granulation formed and its water content were reduced by thyroxine. The formation of granulation tissue is but one stage in the healing of certain types of wound. Thus the effects upon granulation tissue formation of given doses or concentrations of hormones must not be extrapolated, nor necessarily taken to infer effects on other aspects of wound healing. In conclusion, some inhibitory action by high concentrations of topical corticosteroids upon fibrin formation and upon connective tissue in healing wounds is, therefore, to be expected in man, but hormones systemically administered upon medical grounds are unlikely to affect the healing of gingival wounds.

IV. The Influence of Endocrine Secretions on the Periodontal Ligament

Alterations in levels of a variety of hormones have been shown to affect the periodontal ligament in man and animals. An early quantitative investigation of the effects of changes in hormone levels upon the periodontal ligament in man was that of Mühlemann (1951) who, using his periodontometric technique, noted an increase in tooth mobility during pregnancy. (Chapter 7.) It is possible that this increase in mobility is caused by raised blood levels of relaxin.

Oestrogen administered to six-week-old mice for five weeks caused increased cellularity in the periodontal ligament, although a ten-week period of administration caused a reduction in cellularity and numbers of collagen bundles (Shklar and Glickman, 1956), possibly because of depressed secretion of, at least, FSH by the anterior pituitary.

Although adrenalectomy caused marked reduction in osteoblastic activity in the interdental septum in two-month old albino rats, changes in the collagen fibres of the periodontal ligament were not observed (Shklar, 1965). Bissada et al. (1966) have reported that alloxan diabetes in the rat causes infrequent fragmentation of bundles of fibres of the periodontal ligament. Local irritation from wire ligatures placed around the necks of the teeth of these animals caused marked degeneration and loss of periodontal ligament fibres and the development of advanced periodontitis with occasional abscess formation. The wire ligaments caused only mild early periodontitis in non-diabetic animals. Untreated diabetes thus increases the susceptibility of the periodontal tissues of these animals to injury. (See Section **V**.)

Hyperthyroidism induced by large doses of thyroxin in guinea pigs increases vascularity of the periodontal ligament, and resorption and osteoporosis of the periodontal bone were noted (Goldman, 1943). Increased vascularity and widening of the periodontal ligament was produced in guinea pigs by Goldman (1943) by administering oral thyroxine. Thyroidectomy in the new born rat causes reduction in cellularity of the periodontal ligament of the incisors, an effect which can be reversed by subsequent administration of thyroxin or STH (Baume et al., 1954a). Surgically induced hypothyroidism in rabbits causes degeneration and fragmentation of fibres of the periodontal ligament (Rosenberg et al., 1961).

Hypopituitarism arising in childhood causes general retardation in growth of the skeleton, the body remaining well proportioned (Schour and Massler, 1943). Hypophysectomy in the rat causes retardation of eruption and a slowing in rate of deposition of cementum (Schour and Massler, 1943). To restore nearly to normal the enamel organ and the eruption rate in the hypophysectomized rat, both thyroxine and STH were needed (Baume et al., 1954b). It should be pointed out that the part played by the periodontal ligament in changes due to endocrine alteration in the eruption rate of the rat incisor is a permissive one. The measured rate of eruption of the continuously growing incisor of the rodent is an indication primarily of attrition and the opposed rat or rabbit incisor erupts only as fast as attrition allows. By contrast the unopposed or amputated incisor erupts at the full rate of which it is capable, which is more than twice the "opposed" eruption rate (Taylor and Butcher, 1951; Ness, 1956). The effects of local excess of STH, produced by injections of the hormone into the mucobuccal fold, on the periodontal ligament in the rat were investigated by Stahl and Joly (1958). An increase in cellularity of the periodontal ligament was observed.

V. The Influence of Endocrine Secretions on Bone and Cementum

A. Sex Hormones

The effects of hormones upon the physiology of bone depend upon the age of the individual. For example, long bones lose their capacity to respond by increase in length to STH after closure of the epiphyses. By contrast, the condyle of the mandible retains into early middle age a fibrocartilaginous cap from which growth in length can occur. Consequently, the ascending ramus of the acromegalic in whom excess STH is secreted after closure of bony epiphyses, is lengthened. Conversely, he develops thickening but not lengthening of his long bones, including the bones of his fingers (Weinmann and Sicher, 1955).

It may be inferred from the lengthened limbs and immature skeletal form of the eunuchoid individual of either sex that in the normal individual the circulating levels of pubertal and postpubertal sex hormones promote the development of the adult bone form characteristic of the male or the female. Further, through a probable depression of the secretion of STH by the anterior pituitary, sexual maturation initiates the termination of bodily growth (Weinmann and Sicher, 1955).

In man much information is available on the effects of deficiency and excess of sex hormones. Numerous clinical and laboratory observations on both sexes have been made and discussed (Albright et al., 1941b; Weinmann and Sicher, 1955; Bennett, 1966). Hypergonadism in man accompanies some hyperplasias or tumours of endocrine glands (see Adrenogenital Syndrome, Section II of this chapter). Absolute or relative hypogonadism results from congenital defect, removal of the gonads or from old age. Removal of the gonads before puberty, and congenital hypogonadism, cause, in man, postponement of maturity of the skeleton and suppression of secondary sex characteristics. Thus epiphyses of long bones remain open leading to great length of the limbs. The jaws become prominent. The pelvis retains the juvenile form characteristic of childhood (Weinmann and Sicher, 1955). The hypogonadal condition of post-menopausal osteoporosis resembles closely that found in younger women who have undergone oöphorectomy (Albright et al., 1940). The term osteoporosis describes a number of diseases in which bone deposition is faulty; this is in contrast to osteomalacia, in which mineralization is deficient (Albright et al., 1941a). Endocrine-mediated causes of osteoporosis of importance in man are discussed by Albright et al. (1941a) and include senility, the post-menopausal state (surgical or natural), and Cushing's syndrome (a clinical syndrome usually associated with ACTH-excess and adrenal cortical hyperplasia, in which excessive quantities of corticosteroids, particularly cortisol, are secreted). Individual bones of the skeleton have particular patterns of growth and function, and the jaws exemplify this. Bone of normal density in the jaws including the lamina dura of the teeth, as shown by radiography, persists in the presence of osteoporosis due to senility, post-menopausal state, or Cushing's syndrome affecting other parts of the skeleton (Albright et al., 1941a).

Sex hormones affect different species in different ways and to different degrees. Mice, especially, and rats are susceptible to sex hormones while hamsters, guinea pigs and other species are relatively unreactive (Weinmann and Sicher, 1955). Nevertheless, the effects of an increase or decrease in circulating levels of sex hormones in animals resemble in a general way those in man; they tend to bring epiphyseal bone growth to an end while stimulating bone deposition. The bone sclerosis resulting from endosteal deposition under the influence of oestrogen in the female might be regarded as the storage of mineral against the demands of a foetus and of lactation. The effects of oöphorectomy on the jaws, as might be expected, differ with the age of the animal. Piroshaw and Glickman (1957) showed that oöphorectomy results in osteoporosis of the jaws in young mice aged 4–6 weeks but not in older mice aged 1 year. They deduced that bone is maintained with a structure normal for the age of the animal by lower circulating levels of oestrogen in the older than in the younger group. This observation illustrates the anabolic effects of oestrogens. Mice oöphorectomized at 4–6 weeks were found by Glickman and Quintarelli (1960) (as detailed in Section II) to show a retarded rate of formation of periodontal bone, by contrast with those operated upon at one year.

The effects of oöphorectomy may be contrasted with those of the administration of oestrogen, although the effects of the two procedures are not in every respect opposed. Oöphorectomy prevents the feed-back mechanism by which the anterior pituitary and the ovary together control oestrogen levels, whereas the administration of oestrogen to the intact animal does not. Oestrogen administered to one and four month-old male rats causes inhibition of growth and sclerosis of the bone of the subepiphyseal zone of long bones (Pindborg, 1945). The effect of moderate doses of oestrogen upon long bones in the rat was later characterized by Budy et al. (1952) as interference with resorption of the spongy bone of the metaphysis, and this was confirmed by Bernick and Ershoff (1963). The effects of injections of oestrogen upon the alveolar bone of male and female mice were investigated by Stahl et al. (1950) who noted sclerosis of the bone with endosteal apposition of new bone with a probable high mineral content. A dose of 2 mg weekly of alpha oestradiol benzoate produced the maximum effect. A species difference of significance emerged, in that the molar area of jaws of the rat was not affected significantly. Thus oestrogen administered for five weeks to young (6 weeks old) mice caused increased deposition of endosteal alveolar bone. Administration for ten weeks caused, however, an inhibition of bone deposition along the alveolar periosteal surfaces (Shklar and Glickman, 1956). The latter result probably stemmed from pituitary depression. Nutlay, *et al.* (1954) reported bone resorption around infrabony pockets in aging mice who had received injections or subcutaneous implants of alpha-oestradiol benzoate. The bone resorption was however probably not caused primarily by the oestrogen but associated with developing periodontitis secondary to the epithelial hyperplasia caused by the oestrogen.

Androgens, in general, have powerful anabolic effects. Kowalewski (1958) demonstrated that 17-ethyl-19 nortestosterone, a powerful synthetic anabolic hormone, caused an increased ^{35}S sulphate-uptake in growing bone in young cockerels. A similar effect was not demonstrated with doses of testosterone. Testosterone as demonstrated by Budy *et al.* (1952) has little or no effect upon the growth of bone in the immature rat. The effects of testosterone on bone thus differ from those of oestrogen.

B. OTHER HORMONES

The catabolic effects on protein metabolism of glucocorticoids have been described earlier, and osteoporosis is a well recognized side effect of long-term administration of cortisone or other glucocorticoids. For example, Kowalewski and Gort (1959) found that cortisone reduced incorporation of radiosulphur into healing bone, a finding which indicated reduced synthesis of ground substance. Applebaum and Seelig (1955) found osteoporosis of the alveolar processes of the jaws in two to three month-old rats after daily subcutaneous injections of 2·5 mg cortisone for one or two months. Similar effects were incidentally noted when the adrenals were removed experimentally. The effect of adrenalectomy is a retardation of bone growth and deposition, rather than a catabolic one. The effects of administration of cortisone on the jaws of mice are similar to those in the rat, the mouse being more susceptible to the effects of the hormone. Glickman *et al.* (1951) and Glickman (1952) reported a reduction in alveolar bone height and osteoporosis of the jaws in white mice receiving injections of 0·5 mg cortisone daily for periods up to 6 weeks. Shklar (1965) however, showed that 30 days after bilateral adrenalectomy there was decreased osteoblastic activity and an absence of osteoid seams in the bone of the interdental alveolar septum of the molar area of 2-month old albino rats. The animals were maintained upon a low-protein diet with physiological saline supplements. Daily subcutaneous administration of 0·25 mg cortisone acetate restored normal osteoblastic activity as assessed histologically. Cementoblasts were not affected to nearly the same degree by adrenalectomy as were osteoblasts. Osteoporosis experimentally produced by glucocorticoids can be reversed by the administration of a substance having an anabolic effect, such as oestrogen (Glickman and Shklar, 1955), or by fluoride (Zipkin et al., 1965). The effect of fluoride might possibly be to render the apatite of bone mineral less labile. Since, during resorption of bone both mineral and matrix are removed, it is of interest that fluoride, which could be expected to interfere with the development of osteomalacia, is capable of interfering with the development of osteoporosis.

Glickman (1946) reported osteoporosis of the alveolar bone as part of generalized skeletal osteoporosis in experimentally induced (Alloxan) diabetes and Glickman et al. (1966) demonstrated that trauma from occlusion due to excessive occlusal forces was more severe and more long lasting in rats with alloxan diabetes than in controls. Osteoporotic changes in molar alveolar bone, with fewer osteoblasts than in control animals, were observed in 4 to 5-month old rats rendered diabetic by alloxan (Bissada et al., 1966). These osteoporotic changes moreover, were disproportionately marked in diabetic animals in whom a local periodontitis had been produced by wire ligatures. The cementum of the diabetic animals in which there had been no experimental interference with the jaws showed some localized resorption, while those with diabetes and periodontitis showed marked localized resorption of cementum. Thus, diabetes in these animals increases the susceptibility of the periodontal tissues to local injury (Section IV).

Levels of thyroid hormones within a particular range are necessary for normal growth and structure of the skeleton. The skeleton of the cretin shows delayed or arrested growth and maturation. The patient manifesting hyperthyroidism often shows osteoporosis of the skeleton probably secondary to increased renal loss of calcium and phosphorus. The jaws are not commonly affected, but may show osteoporotic changes if the disease has remained untreated for a number of years. Gingivitis and periodontal bone loss in "pyorrhea" were reported by Hulton (1936) to be common in adult patients with myxoedema. He believed that the association was not a direct one. This early report does not appear to have been confirmed in more recent times. Thyroidectomy in rats on the first day of life causes sclerosis of the bone surrounding the incisors, and fibrosis of the marrow with a reduction in cellularity and in remodelling. These effects were largely eliminated by the administration of thyroxine after thyroidectomy (Baume et al., 1954a). Thiouracil-induced hypothyroidism causes reduced alveolar bone deposition with a closer arrangement of appositional lines than normal (Glickman and Pruzansky, 1947) in the rat, and bone with smaller Haversian systems in the dog (English, 1949). In animals with alveolar oesteoporosis due to tryptophan deficiency (600 mg or less of dl-tryptophan per kg of diet), thyroid feeding caused an accentuation of the osteoporotic bone changes (Baveta et al., 1957).

The effects of experimental hyperthyroidism were investigated by Goldman (1943). He administered thyroid extract orally to guinea pigs for up to four

16*

months, and noted osteoporosis and fibrosis of the bone marrow. Thyrocalcitonin (Section IE) plays an important part in calcium homoeostasis and because of the importance of this topic in bone physiology, developments in knowledge of the role in it of thyrocalcitonin will be briefly outlined.

The regulation of plasma calcium by a feed-back mechanism controlling the rate of secretion of parathormone was proposed by McLean and Urist (1961). In supplementation of this mechanism the existence of a hitherto unknown serum-calcium-lowering hormone was first postulated by Copp et al. (1962) who termed the hormone calcitonin, and believed that it was produced by the parathyroid glands. In 1963 Hirsch et al. described a calcium-lowering substance in crude extracts of rat thyroid and produced evidence that this substance was not derived from the parathyroids in that species.

The mode of action by which calcitonin lowers the plasma calcium is indicated by the experiments of Gudmundsson et al. (1966) (see above) and of Martin et al. (1966). The latter administered calcitonin by infusion to the rat for periods of up to ten hours in all. From a fall in urinary hydroxyproline, which is derived from the collagen of bone, the investigators inferred that calcitonin probably inhibits bone breakdown, lowering thereby the level of plasma calcium. Wase et al. (1966) administered thyrocalcitonin to male rats and found that it enhanced the incorporation of isotopic calcium into the skeleton causing a more positive calcium balance.

The principal effect on bone of primary hyperparathyroidism in man (Teng and Nathan, 1960) is the development of generalized osteoporosis and circumscribed resorptive lesions. Functionally, there is a close relationship between parathormone and vitamin D. (See Chapter 9.)

The effects of parathormone upon developing bone resemble in general those upon mature bone; that is, stimulation of bone resorption and mobilization of skeletal calcium. Elzay (1964) has found that the bone resorption associated with administration of parathormone to 4-week mice was enhanced when the animals received oestrogen in addition. Generalized osteoporosis was produced experimentally in guinea pigs by Jaffe et al. (1931) by the administration of parathormone. Narrowing of bone trabeculae with osteoclastic resorption, and fibrosis of bone marrow were found histologically. Weinmann and Schour (1945) found that large doses of parathormone caused bone resorption and replacement by fibrous tissue in the alveolar process of the maxilla of the rat; the molar area was more affected by resorption and showed more growth than the incisor area. In human jaws hyperparathyroidism frequently results in the loss of the radiographic lamina dura, the apparently dense bone lining the tooth sockets. This is in contrast to the persistence of the lamina dura which is seen in osteoporosis associated with changes in secretion of sex hormones.

Hypophysectomy produces changes in every organ. It eliminates at once the source of the trophic hormones of the anterior pituitary including

somatotrophic hormone (STH), thyrotrophic (TSH) and adrenocorticotrophic hormones (ACTH). It simultaneously reduces the output of specific
hormones such as cortisol from target endocrine organs rendered atrophic by
reduction in circulating levels of, for example, ACTH. Hypopituitarism in
childhood causes, in addition to delayed eruption of teeth, an immature pattern of a retardation of development of teeth and thin cementum (Schour and
Massler, 1943). Effects of hypophysectomy on the jaws include the known results of deprivation of STH. Schour (1934) found a great reduction in growth
rate in a developing rat. Bone resorption early and net deposition late after
hypophysectomy were accompanied by slowing but not cessation of bone
remodelling with a suggestion of a mosaic pattern. Marrow spaces were
reduced and fibrosis of marrow occurred. Schour and Van Dyke (1932)
reported that hypophysectomy increased the thickness of the cementum five-
fold of the continuously growing incisor of the young rat. In explanation of
the apparent discrepancy between the generalized reduction in cellular
activity caused by hypophysectomy and the deposition of a thicker layer of
cementum than usual, Schour (1934) points out that eruption in the hypophysectomized rat is disproportionately slow. Cementum, although slowly
deposited, therefore accumulates.

Acromegaly, a disease usually due to hypersecretion of STH by a benign
tumour of the anterior pituitary gland arising after the epiphyses have closed,
causes overgrowth of the bones of the face and particularly of the mandible,
the ramus of which continues to grow after normal growth has ceased
(Section VA.) The disease also causes on occasions, overgrowth of dental
cementum (Schour and Massler, 1943). The effects of local excess of STH
upon the alveolar bone of the jaws of the rat were investigated by Stahl and
Joly (1958) who administered STH into the mucobuccal fold thrice weekly
for six weeks. They noted an increase in endosteal alveolar bone deposition.

VI. Conclusion

The periodontium functions as an organ. Nevertheless, its constituent
tissues are diverse. The presence of keratinizing, and non-keratinized epithelium and mineralized and non-mineralized connective tissue allow it to
respond to altered levels of diverse hormones. These include the hormones
such as insulin and somatotrophic hormone which affect directly the metabolism of all cells and of some intercellular substance, and those such as parathormone which have a major effect on a limited part of the periodontium.
Oestrogens and androgens occupy an intermediate position as they affect
essentially all tissues, but to markedly different degrees. Tissue sensitivities to
hormones vary, moreover, at different periods of life.

Despite the numerous potential effects of hormones upon the periodontium
it is clear from human and animal studies that once development in the

presence of normal levels of hormones is complete, the main effects of practical importance in man are those of puberty, of pregnancy, of the menopause, and of diabetes mellitus. The changes found in these conditions represent a failure of the biological adaptation mechanism of the periodontium to accommodate completely to altered metabolic conditions. Irreversible effects on the periodontium can be minimized by appropriate clinical treatment. The effects of diabetes mellitus are exerted in several ways including changes in microvasculature and a reduced ability of the periodontium to respond defensively to the bacteria of the plaque and to minor infections. The periodontal changes in pregnancy, and to a lesser degree those in diabetes mellitus, illustrate the fact that epithelium and connective tissue elements interact closely. No change of any magnitude in one can take place without corresponding changes in the others.

References

Albright, F., Bloomberg, Esther and Smith, Patricia H. (1940). *Trans. Ass. Am. Physns.* **55**, 298–305.

Albright, F., Burnett, C. H., Cope, O. and Parson, W. (1941a). *J. clin. Endocrinol.* **1**, 711–716.

Albright, F., Smith, P. H. and Richardson, A. M. (1941b). *J. Am. med. Ass.* **116**, 2465–2474.

Applebaum, E. and Seelig, A. (1955). *Oral Surg.* **8**, 881–891.

Baume, L. J., Becks, H. and Evans, H. M. (1954a). *J. dent. Res.* **33**, 80–90.

Baume, L. J., Becks, H., Ray, J. D. and Evans, H. M. (1954b). *J. dent. Res.* **33**, 91–114.

Bavetta, L. A., Bernick, S. and Ershoff, B. H. (1957). *J. dent Res.* **36**, 13–20.

Bennett, G. A. (1966). *In* "Pathology" (W. A. D. Anderson, ed.), Vol. 2, pp. 1293–1294. C. V. Mosby, St. Louis, Mo., U.S.A.

Beneveniste, R., Bixler, D. and Conneally, P. M. (1967). *J. Peridont.* **38**, 271–279.

Bernick, S. and Ershoff, B. H. (1963). *J. dent. Res.* **42**, 981–989.

Best, C. H. and Taylor, N. B. (1961). "The physiological basis of medical practice", 7th edn., pp. 764, 767. Williams and Wilkins, Baltimore, U.S.A.

Bissada, N. F., Schaffer, E. M. and Lazarow, A. (1966). *Periodontics* **4**, 233–240.

Brunish, R. (1966). *In* "Hormones and Connective Tissue" (G. Asboe-Hansen, ed.), p. 25. Munksgaard, Copenhagen.

Budy, Ann M., Urist, M. R. and McLean, F. C. (1952). *Am. J. Path.* **28**, 1143–1167.

Bullough, W. S. (1962). *Biol. Rev.* **37**, 307–342.

Bussolati, G. and Pearse, A. G. E. (1967). *J. Endocr.* **37**, 205–210.

Butcher, E. D. and Klingsberg, J. (1961). *J. dent Res.* **40**, 694–695.

Butt, W. R. (1967). "Hormone Chemistry", pp. 167, 325. D. Van Nostrand Company, Ltd., London, England.

Castor, C. W. (1965). *J. Lab. clin. Med.* **65**, 490–499.

Castor, C. W. and Baker, B. L. (1950). *Endocrinology* **47**, 234–241.

Catchpole, H. R. (1965). *In* "Physiology and Biophysics" (E. J. Ruch and F. L. Patton, eds), pp. 617–643. Saunders, Philadelphia, U.S.A.

Catchpole, H. R. (1966). *Fedn Proc. fedn Am. Socs exp. Biol.* **25**, 1144–1145.

Catchpole, H. R., Joseph, N. R. and Engel, M. B. (1966). *Fedn Proc. fedn Am. Socs exp. Biol.* **25**, 1124–1126.

Cheraskin, E. and Ringsdorf, W. M. (1965). *J. dent. Res.* **44,** 480–486.
Cohen, M. (1955). *J. dent. Res.* **34,** 679.
Copp, D. H., Cameron, E. C., Cheney, B. A., Davidson, A. G. F. and Henze, K. G. (1962). *Endocrinology* **70,** 638–649.
DiPasquale, G. and Steinetz, B. G. (1964.) *Proc. Soc. exp. Biol. Med.* **117,** 118–121.
Douglas, D. M. (1963). "Wound Healing and Management", pp. 54–56. Livingstone, Edinburgh.
Elzay, R. P. (1964). *J. dent. Res.* **43,** 331–345.
Engel, M. B. (1950). *J. Periodont.* **21,** 145–146.
Engel, M. B. (1952). *J. Am. dent. Ass.* **44,** 691.
Engel, M. B. and Catchpole, H. R. (1953). *Proc. Soc. exp. Biol. Med.* **84,** 336–338.
English, J. A. (1949). *J. dent. Res.* **28,** 172–194.
Fell, Honor B. (1964). *Vitams. Horms.* **22,** 81–127.
Finestone, A. J. and Boorujy, S. R. (1967). *Diabetes* **16,** 336–340.
Foster, G. V., MacIntyre, I. and Pearse, A. G. E. (1964). *Nature, Lond.* **203,** 1029–1030.
Foster, G. V., Joplin, G. F., MacIntyre, I., Melvin, K. E. W. and Slack, E. (1966). *Lancet* **1,** 107–109.
Gersh, I. and Catchpole, H. R. (1949). *Am. J. Anat.* **85,** 457–521.
Gersh, I. and Catchpole, H. R. (1960). *Perspect. Biol. Med.* **3,** 282–319.
Gershfeld, N. L. and Heftmann, E. (1963). *Experientia* **19,** 2.
Gibson, W. A. and Fullmer, H. M. (1966). *J. dent. Res.* **45,** 1225.
Glickman, I. (1946). *N.Y. J. Dent.* **16,** 226–251.
Glickman, I. (1952). *J. Am. dent. Ass.* **45,** 422–429.
Glickman, I. (1964). "Clinical Periodontology", 3rd edn., pp. 127, 134, 340. Saunders, Philadelphia, U.S.A.
Glickman, I. and Pruzansky, S. (1947). *J. dent. Res.* **26,** 471.
Glickman, I. and Quintarelli, G. (1960). *J. Periodont.* **31,** 31–37.
Glickman, I. and Shklar, G. (1955). *Oral Surg.* **8,** 1179–1191.
Glickman, I., Stone, I. C. and Chawla, T. N. (1951). *J. dent. Res.* **30,** 461.
Glickman, I., Smulow, J. B. and Moreau, J. (1966). *J. Periodont.* **37,** 146–155.
Glucksman, D. L. and Warren, W. D. (1966). *Surgery, St. Louis* **60,** 352–360.
Goldman, H. M. (1943). *Am. J. Orthodont.* **29,** 665–681.
Goldman, H. M. and Cohen, D. W. (1957). "Periodontia", 4th edn., pp. 29, 57. C. V. Mosby, St. Louis, Mo., U.S.A.
Goldzieher, J. W., Roberts, I. S., Rawls, W. B. and Goldzieher, M. A. (1952). *Archs. Derm.* **66,** 304–315.
Gray, C. H. and Bacharach, A. L. (1967). "Hormones in Blood", 2nd edn., Vols. 1 and 2, Academic Press, London, England.
Gudmundsson, T. V., MacIntyre, I. and Soliman, H. A. (1966). *Proc. R. Soc.* B **146,** 460–477.
Hansen, E. F. (1966). *Odont. T.* **74,** 196–201.
Hechter, O. and Halkerston, I. D. K. (1964). *In* "The Hormones" (G. Pincus, K. V. Thimann and E. B. Astwood, eds), Vol. 5, p. 787. Academic Press, New York, U.S.A.
Hirsch, P. F., Gauthier, G. F. and Munson, P. L. (1963). *Endocrinology* **73,** 244–252.
Houck, J. C. and Jacob, R. A. (1963). *Proc. Soc. exp. Biol. Med.* **113,** 692–694.
Hulton, J. H. (1936). *J. Am. dent. Ass.* **23,** 227–236.
Jaffe, H. L., Bodansky, A. and Blair, J. E. (1931). *Archs Path.* **11,** 207–228.
Jasmovich, J. B. and Maclaren, J. A. (1962). *Endocrinology* **71,** 209–220.
Jörgensen, O. (1963). *Acta Path. Microbiol. Scand.* **59,** 325–334.
Kaplan, S. L. and Grunbach, M. M. (1964). *J. clin. Endocr.* **24,** 80–100.

Korner, A. (1964). *Biochem. J.* **92,** 449–456.
Kowalewski, K. (1958a). *Endocrinology* **63,** 759–764.
Kowalewski, K. and Gort, J. (1959). *Acta Endocrinol.* **30,** 273–276.
Levine, Rachmiel (1964). *In* "The Hormones" (G. Pincus, K. V. Thimann and E. B. Astwood, eds), p. 844. Academic Press, London, England.
Lindhe, J., Branemark, P-I. and Birch, J. (1968). *J. Periodont. Res.* **3,** 180–186.
Löe, H. (1963). *J. Periodont.* **36,** 209–217.
Löe, H. and Silness, J. (1963). *Acta odont. Scand.* **21,** 533–551.
MacIntyre, I. (1968) *In* "The Scientific Basis of Medicine Annual Reviews" (J. McMichael, ed.), pp. 242-253, University of London, Athlone Press, London, England.
Maibenco, Helen. (1960). *Anat. Rec.* **136,** 59–71.
Maier, A. W. and Orban, B. (1949). *Oral Surg.* **2,** 334–373.
Martin, T. J., Robinson, C. J., and MacIntyre, I. (1966). *Lancet* **1,** 900–902.
Massler, M. (1951). *Oral Surg.* **4,** 1234–1243.
Massler, M. (1956). *Oral Surg.* **9,** 1185–1196.
Massler, M., Schour, I. and Chopra, B. (1950). *J. Periodont.* **21,** 146–165.
McLean, F. C. and Urist, M. R. (1961). "Bone", 2nd edn., pp. 118, 119, 123. University of Chicago Press, Chicago, U.S.A.
McLean, F. C., Lipton, M. A., Bloom, W. and Barron, E. S. G. (1946). *Trans. Confs Josiah Macy jr fdn* **14,** 9–19 and 34.
McMullen, J. A., Legg, Merle, Gottsegen, R. and Camerini-Davalos, R. (1967). *Periodontics* **5,** 61–69.
Meyer, Julia, Marwah, A. S. and Weinmann, J. P. (1956). *J. invest. Derm.* **27,** 237–247.
Mühlemann, H. R. (1948). *Schweiz. Mschr. Zahnheilk* **58,** 865–885.
Mühlemann, H. R. (1951). *Oral Surg.* **4,** 1220–1233.
Munck, A. (1957). *Biochim. biophys. Acta* **24,** 507–514.
Ness, A. R. (1956). *Proc. R. Soc.* B. **146,** 129–154.
Nuki, K. and Löe, H. (1966). *Dent. Practit.* **16,** 435–440.
Nutlay, A. G., Bhaskar, S. M., Weinmann, J. P. and Budy, A. M. (1954). *J. dent. Res.* **33,** 115–127.
Pearse, A. G. E. (1966). *Proc. R. Soc.* B. **164,** 478–487.
Perl, E. and Catchpole, H. R. (1950). *Archs Path.* **50,** 233–239.
Pincus, G., Thimann, K. V. and Astwood, E. B. (1964). "The Hormones, Physiology, Chemistry and Applications", Vols. I–V. Academic Press, New York, U.S.A.
Pindborg, J. J. (1945). *Acta Path. Microbiol. Scand.* **22,** 290–299.
Piroshaw, N. A. and Glickman, I. (1957). *Oral Surg.* **10,** 133–147.
Rall, J. E., Robbins, J. and Lewallen, C. G. (1964). *In* "The Hormones" (G. Pincus, K. V. Thimann and E. B. Astwood, eds), Vol. 5, p. 353. Academic Press, New York, U.S.A.
Ramfjord, S. P. (1959). *J. Periodont.* **30,** 51–59.
Rassmussen, H. and Craig, L. C. (1962). *Recent Prog. Horm. Res.* **18,** 269–295.
Rehder, E. and Enquist, I. F. (1967). *Archs Surg.* **94,** 74–78.
Ringsdorf, W. M., Ringsdorf, Jr., W. M., Powell, B. J., Knight, L. A. and Cheraskin E. (1962). *Ann. J. Obstet. Gynec.* **83,** 258–263.
Robbins, S. L. (1967). "Pathology", p. 1224. Saunders, London, England.
Rosenberg, M. M., Goldman, H. M. and Garber, E. (1961). *J. dent. Res.* **40,** 708–709.
Rushton, M. A. (1952). *Br. dent. J.* **93,** 27–31.
Russell, A. L. (1956). *J. dent. Res.* **35,** 350–359.
Saad, L. and Swenson, H. M. (1965). *J. Periodont.* **36,** 407–412.

Schayer, R. W. (1967). *Perspect. Biol. Med.* **10**, 409–418.
Schiff, M. and Burn, Helen F. (1961). *Archs Otolar.* **71**, 765–780.
Schour, I. (1934). *J. Periodont.* **5**, 15–24.
Schour, I. and Massler, M. (1943). *J. Am. dent. Ass.* **30**, 595–603, 764–773, 937–944.
Schour, I. and Van Dyke, H. B. (1932). *Am. J. Anat.* **50**, 397–434.
Schultz-Haudt, S. D. and Aas, E. (1962). *Odont. Tidskr.* **70**, 397–428.
Sethi, P., Ramey, E. R. and Houck, J. C. (1961). *Proc. Soc. exp. Biol. Med.* **108**, 74–77.
Shklar, G. (1965). *Periodontics* **3**, 239–242.
Shklar, G. and Glickman, I. (1956). *J. Periodont.* **27**, 16–23.
Stahl, S. S. and Joly, O. (1958). *Oral Surg.* **11**, 475–483.
Stahl, S. S., Weinmann, J. P., Schour, I. and Budy, A. M. (1950). *Anat. Rec.* **107**, 21–41.
Steinetz, B. G. and Manning, J. P. (1967). *Proc. Soc. exp. Biol. Med.* **124**, 180–184.
Taubenhaus, M. (1957). *In* "The Healing of Wounds" (M. B. Williamson, ed.), pp. 113–129. McGraw-Hill, New York, U.S.A.
Taylor, A. C. and Butcher, E. O. (1951). *J. exp. Zool.* **117**, 165–188.
Teng, C. T. and Nathan, M. R. (1960). *Am. J. Roentg. Rad. Ther. Nucl. Med.* **83**, 716–731.
Trott, J. R. (1957). *Br. dent. J.* **103**, 421–427.
Wase, A. W., Peterson, A., Rickes, E. and Solewski, J. (1966). *Endocrinology* **79**, 687–691.
Weinmann, J. P. and Schour, I. (1945). *Am. J. Path.* **21**, 857–875.
Weinmann J. P. and Sicher H. (1955). "Bone and Bones", 2nd edn., pp. 235, 240. C. V. Mosby, St. Louis, Mo., U.S.A.
Weiss, M. D., Weinmann, J. P. and Meyer, Julia. (1959). *J. Periodont.* **30**, 208–218.
Weissmann, G. and Thomas, L. (1964). *In* "Recent Progress in Hormone Research" (G. Pincus, ed.), pp. 215–245. Academic Press, New York, U.S.A.
Williams, R. H. (1962). "Textbook of Endocrinology", 3rd edn. Saunders, Philadelphia, U.S.A.
Zachariae, Lis. (1966). *In* "Hormones and Connective Tissue" (G. Asboe-Hansen, ed.), pp. 83, 94. Munksgaard, Copenhagen.
Zipkin, I., Bernick, S. and Menczel, J. (1965). *Periodontics* **3**, 111–127.
Ziskin, D. E. (1947a). *J. dent. Res.* **20**, 243–244.
Ziskin, D. E. (1947b). *J. dent. Res.* **20**, 419–423.
Ziskin, D. E. and Blackberg, S. N. (1946), *J. dent. Res.* **19**, 381–390.
Ziskin, D. E. and Nesse, G. J. (1947). *Am. J. Orthodont.* **32**, 390–432.
Ziskin, D. E. and Stein, G. (1942). *J. dent. Res.* **21**, 296–297.
Ziskin, D. E., Blackberg, S. N. and Slanetz, C. A. (1936). *J. dent. Res.* **15**, 407–428.

Acknowledgement

The help derived from valuable discussions during preparation of this chapter with Professor Hubert R. Catchpole is gratefully acknowledged.

11 | The Gingival Environment

W. H. BOWEN

Department of Dental Science, Royal College of Surgeons, Lincolns Inn Fields, London, England

I. Introduction

There are many factors which comprise the gingival environment. The balance and interaction of these may determine whether the gingiva remains healthy or succumbs to disease. Although it has been known for many years that antibacterial substances are present in saliva, interest in the field sharpened when it was demonstrated that IgA is the predominant immunoglobulin present in this secretion. Indeed a closer study of the interaction of IgA and lysozyme against micro-organisms may elucidate some of the problems related to the defence of mucous membranes. There is an expanding field of interest too in the processes involved in the development of plaque. Although our knowledge of plaque composition has increased, it still has not reached the stage where we can distinguish plaque which is likely to produce disease from that which is harmless. The role of calculus in the etiology of periodontal disease has probably been exaggerated in the past. Nevertheless, its presence on teeth could present a hazard to the healing of inflamed gingiva.

II. Saliva

Since saliva bathes all the mucous membrane surfaces in the mouth it must influence the health and integrity of those surfaces with which it comes in contact. Saliva may help keep mucous membranes healthy simply by its demulcent effect. Although there is little experimental evidence to show that the removal of salivary glands leads to increase gingival disease it is nevertheless a matter of common clinical observation that patients with reduced salivary flow tend to suffer from severe periodontal disease. Gupta *et al.* (1960) have shown that the removal of the major salivary glands in the Syrian hamster leads to severe lesions in both the hard and soft tissues of the periodontium. Saliva may also influence the health of the periodontium by controlling both the types and numbers of micro-organisms in the mouth. This control may be effected not only through substances secreted by the salivary glands, such as lysozyme, but also by micro-organisms present in the mouth.

A. ANTIBACTERIAL SUBSTANCES SECRETED IN SALIVA

1. Lysozyme (Muramidase)

Many human tissues and secretions, including whole saliva were shown by Fleming and Allison (1922) to contain a substance capable of dissolving micro-organisms. They named the substance "lysozyme" because of its enzyme-like properties, although it can survive boiling for 45 minutes in 2% acetic acid.

Lysozyme was found in the saliva of 95% of 336 persons examined by Sktrolskii *et al.* (1937); women were found by Penrose (1930) to have higher levels than men. Pure parotid saliva contains more activity than whole saliva from the same individual (Chauncey *et al.* 1954). This observation suggests that some micro-organisms in the mouth are capable of destroying the activity of lysozyme. Pure sublingual and submandibular saliva have higher levels of lysozyme than parotid saliva; the activity in the latter appears to be dependent on the type of salivary stimulation used (Hoerman *et al.* 1956).

Lysozyme in saliva may well have played a significant role in the evolution of the bacterial flora found in the mouth. Although a large variety of micro-organisms in nature is susceptible to lysozyme, bacteria normally found in the mouth appear resistant to its effect or at least to the concentrations normally found there (Gibbons *et al.* 1966). Lysozyme from human sources has been crystallized. It is a low molecular (14,000) basic protein with an isoelectric point at about pH 10·5. Human and egg-white lysozymes have a similar molecular weight and basicity; they differ however in amino-acid composition, antigenic structure and activity.

The mode of action of lysozyme on bacterial cell walls has been extensively studied by Salton (1952) and Sharon (1967). These investigators have shown that bacterial cell walls are rapidly digested when incubated with lysozyme. Cell walls from *Micrococcus lysodeikticus* are most frequently used to investigate the activity of lysozyme. These walls are believed to be composed of polysaccharide chains built up of alternating N-acetylglucosamine (NAG) and N-acetylmuramic acid residues linked throughout by β 1–4 linkages. The latter linkages are susceptible to the action of lysozyme. Approximately 65% of the resulting digest is not dialysable.

The significance of lysozyme in saliva is not clear. Bartels (1934) suggests that it may play a part as a limiting factor on the bacterial flora of the mouth. It was observed by Wheatcroft and Nemes (1951) that salivary lysozyme levels remained high in dogs moribund from radiation and they concluded that "the question of the actual purpose and importance of this defence mechanism is further complicated". It seems improbable that lysozyme is without function in saliva and possibly further investigation would reveal its purpose (see below).

2. Anti-lactobacillus System

A substance in saliva capable of dissolving certain species of lactobacilli was described by Jay et al. (1932). Its presence in saliva has since been confirmed by a number of workers (Green 1959, Zeldow 1959). Kerr and Wedderburn (1958) demonstrated activity in pure parotid and submandibular saliva from humans. Its presence seems to be dependent to some extent on the age of the person from whom the saliva is collected (Zeldow 1961). This author failed to detect the presence of this substance in the saliva of premature infants or newborn babies during the first few days of life. It was demonstrated by Dogon et al. (1962) and Zeldow (1963) that this antibacterial substance requires thiocyanate as a co-factor for full activity. A substance with similar activity and which also requires thiocyanate has been demonstrated in milk by Reiter and Moller-Madsen (1963).

These substances in saliva and milk contain two components one which is non-dialysable and heat labile, and the other dialysable and heat stable, which has been identified as thiocyanate. There is strong evidence to suggest that the heat labile substance in saliva is peroxidase (Klebanoff and Luebke 1965). These investigators showed that purified peroxidase from milk could replace the heat sensitive substance in saliva and give the same antibacterial activity as whole saliva. Iwamoto et al. (1967) have demonstrated that purified anti-lactobacillus substance in saliva contains peroxidase activity. Purified peroxidase isolated from human parotid saliva, when combined with thiocyanate, was found to match the antibacterial activity of whole saliva.

The peroxidase-thiocyanate system is active, in the absence of an extraneous source of peroxide, against micro-organisms which accumulate peroxide, for example lactobacilli and streptococci. The system appears to operate by preventing accumulation by the cells of amino acids lysine and glutamic acid both of which are essential for growth (Clem and Klebanoff, 1966).

B. ANTIBODIES

The finding of gamma globulin in saliva by Ellison et al. (1960), Mandel and

Ellison (1961), and Kraus and Sirisinha (1962) confirms earlier reports of absorbable antibodies in saliva. Pollaci and Ceraulo (1909) and Wheatcroft (1957) have shown the presence of specific antibodies to *Brucella melitensis* in the saliva of patients infected with brucellosis. The saliva of patients recovering from syphilis was found by Coleman and Appleman (1953) to contain antibodies to *Treponema pallidum*. Using precipitation, haemagglutination, and bacterial agglutination techniques Kraus and Konno (1963) were able to demonstrate antibodies in saliva to various types of bacteria only when similar antibodies were found in serum. The titres were always much lower in saliva than in serum.

Interest heightened in salivary antibodies when it was demonstrated that the main immunoglobulin in saliva is lgA. This immunoglobulin is found in proportionately higher concentrations in saliva than in serum. Tears, tracheobronchial washings and colostrum have lgA as their predominant immune globulin. The lgA in saliva and colostrum are antigenically similar but they differ from that found in serum, that found in saliva and colostrum has an antigenic determinant not present in serum (Tomasi, 1965 and South *et al.* 1966). This extra antigenic determinant is referred to as the transport piece; it travels electrophoretically as gamma globulin. It is not certain whether the salivary glands manufacture lgA *de novo* or secrete it selectively and then attach the transport piece during the process. It was observed by South *et al.* (1966) that when some patients suffering from congenital or acquired agammaglobulinaemia and therefore lacking detectable lgA, were transfused with normal serum, lgA appeared in the saliva.

The concentration of lgA in serum appears to rise with age reaching adult levels at around puberty. The lgA group of antibodies function either alone or with the aid of biologically active substances other than complement. An lgA-specific antigen system in general fixes a small amount of complement only and does not cause lysis. However, lgA with complement and lysozyme will lyse susceptible bacteria (Adinolfi *et al.* 1966). It is of interest as Glynn (1968) points out that lgA antibodies seem to be predominant in situations and secretions that are rich in lysozyme. The lgA-lysozyme system may well represent a defence mechanism specifically associated with mucous membranes. Research into this field could prove rewarding in providing information into the host-plaque (bacteria) interaction at the gingival margin and the role of this interaction in the pathogenesis of periodontal disease. It has been observed by Smith *et al.* (1967) that virus lgA-neutralizing antibodies appear in nasal secretions only after intra-nasal infection; they do not appear in patients, vaccinated through conventional routes. This observation supports strongly the view that mucous membranes have a specialized defence mechanism.

III. Plaque

A. Definition

The terminology used to describe the various deposits that form on tooth surfaces both before and after eruption have been discussed by Dawes and Jenkins (1964). Their classification will be used here for the sake of simplicity and clarity. However, I suggest that, for clarity, any definition of plaque should include information both on the duration between the time of collection and the last intake of food, and the time plaque has been allowed to accumulate on the tooth surface.

B. FORMATION AND STRUCTURE

It is now universally accepted that when a tooth first erupts it is covered by a cuticle which is believed to be the final product of the ameloblasts (Winkler and Dirks 1958). Ussing (1955) however, has shown that its formation takes place in direct continuation with the enamel matrix and she has also identified it at a stage where the enamel had not apparently reached its final maturation. (See also page 157).

The cuticle varies in thickness from 200–500 A (Ussing, 1955, Turner, 1958). It comprises of an inner structureless layer which is non-birefringent and is intimately connected with the enamel lamellae and occasionally an outer cellular unkeratinized layer which may be up to 4 cells in thickness. The inner layer does not stain readily, but is lightly stained with eosin (Turner, 1958) and orange G (Johnson and Bevelander, 1958). The outer cellular layer is stained red with basic fuchsin and occasionally becomes calcified (Meckel, 1968). Shortly after the tooth erupts this cuticle is rapidly worn away except in the most protected areas of the tooth. However, it is rapidly replaced by other cuticles and pellicles presumably derived from the saliva.

The formation of these secondary cuticles has been extensively studied by Vallotton (1945a,b,c). The secondary cuticle seems to be a common factor to all plaques, calculus forming (Voreadis and Zander, 1958) and cariogenic (McDougall, 1963). The secondary cuticle forms rapidly and is fairly free of bacteria. It is thin at first and progressively increases in thickness, and varies from 0·3 to 0·8 microns. The acquired cuticle stains metachromatically with toluidine blue which indicates the presence of acid mucopolysaccharide (Turner, 1958, McDougall, 1963). It also stains p.a.S. positive, showing the presence of mucoproteins. It is stained by amido Schwartz and 1% nile blue which indicates a content of protein and lipid.

This cuticle is insoluble in acids, bases, sodium sulphide, sodium sulphite and urea at room temperature, and its presence on the tooth surface apparently reduces the solubility of enamel in acid *in vitro* (Meckel, 1968). The insolubility of the cuticle has been used to prepare samples of it for chemical analysis. Teeth are immersed in acid and after a short period the cuticle can be floated off (Armstrong, 1966, Leach *et al.*, 1967). Chemical analyses of the acquired pellicle confirm the impression gained from histochemical staining that it contains both protein and carbohydrate. Less than 50% of the pellicle can be accounted for as amino acids with approximately 3% present as hexosamine. The carbohydrate content is 10–15%. The amino acid components of pellicle strongly suggest that sialoprotein derived from saliva secreted from all three glands contributes significantly to its composition (Leach *et al.* 1967). However, on the basis of amino acid composition Armstrong suggests that submandibular saliva contributes more to the protein composition than either of the other two glands. It is however possible that the portion of saliva that forms the pellicle has a relatively constant chemical composition irrespective of the gland of origin.

There are many theories offered to explain the formation of the secondary cuticle. Proteins in solution owe their stability in solution to their hydrophilic groups and will precipitate if the pH of the solution approaches their iso-electric point. It has been suggested that a lowering of pH values on the tooth surface, perhaps following ingestion of carbohydrate, leads to the formation of pH values near the iso-electric point of the mucoproteins, which results in their precipitation (Winkler and Dirks, 1958). There is, however, very little evidence to show that this indeed does occur. Indeed the iso-electric point of mucoproteins is about 3·5, a value which is rarely achieved even in acidogenic plaque. It has frequently been observed that when saliva is collected directly from the ducts of either man (Jenkins, 1968) or monkey (Bowen, 1968) it rapidly becomes cloudy and forms a precipitate which adheres to the walls of the collecting vessel. Presumably a similar mechanism could operate in the mouth, as salivary mucoid by virtue of its physical properties covers every surface in the mouth (Winkler and Dirks, 1958). It appears that neither bacteria nor dietary composition play a prominent part in the development of the secondary cuticle and that its formation is a result of the physico-chemical properties of saliva and can be formed *in vivo* or *in vitro* (Lenz and Muhlemann, 1963).

Following formation of the enamel cuticle a non-bacterial plaque matrix is deposited (McDougall, 1963). This material is paS positive and increases in thickness progressively. It appears amorphous and homogeneous and initially free of bacteria. It is, however, probable that enzymic activities of micro-organisms are responsible for its deposition (Leach, 1963).

Saliva has been shown to contain considerable amounts of glycoprotein which gives saliva its characteristic viscosity. These glycoproteins consist essentially of a protein core to which carbohydrates are attached at various points along its length. The arrangement and type of carbohydrate impart the characteristic properties to glycoprotein; sialic acid and fucose are always found in glycoproteins. However, it has been shown that both sialic acid and fucose are absent from dental plaque (Dawes and Jenkins, 1963; Leach, 1963 and Middleton, 1965). These observations led Leach to propose the theory that oral micro-organisms hydrolyse both sialic acid and fucose from the glyco-proteins leading to a change in their physico-chemical properties; the pH of minimum solubility rises to a value of 7 with an increased tendency for the glycoprotein molecule to precipitate out of solution.

Oral micro-organisms have been demonstrated *in vitro* to have the capacity to hydrolyse sialic acid from glycoproteins (Leach, 1963 and 1964, Thonard *et al.*, 1965). This means that they produce neuraminadase. Sialic acid (N-acetylneuraminic acid) can then be digested by oral micro-organisms into N-acetylmannosamine and pyruvic acid. The presence of glucose or sucrose apparently inhibits the break down of glycoproteins probably because the micro-organisms do not elaborate neuraminadase when a simple source of carbon is available.

There is also a considerable amount of carbohydrate in plaque which is probably not derived from saliva. It appears that a substantial amount of the matrix of plaque is composed of dextran and to a lesser extent levan. (Critchley *et al.*, 1967.) These carbohydrates are polymers of glucose and fructose

TABLE 1

Ca and phosphate concentrations of plaque (ug/mg dry weight)

	Ca	Total P	Inorganic P
2 day pooled plaque			
Dawes and Jenkins (1962)	4·5	16·0	4·3
Schroeder (1963)	14·0	13·9	
Lower lingual incisor plaque	37·1	37·1	
3 day pooled plaque			
Dawes and Jenkins (1962)	5·1	16·1	4·1
Schroeder (1963)	18·2	20·0	—
3 day lower incisor plaque	36·9	30·0	—

respectively, and are formed from sucrose by certain streptococci and some lactobacilli. Dextran was present in all the plaques investigated by Critchley *et al.* and was found to be greatly in excess of the amount of levan. Extracellular polysaccharide represents approximately 10% of the dry weight of plaque; 8–9% of which is dextran and 1–2% levan. Bacteria represent about 70% of the total volume of plaque (Winkler and Dirks, 1958) and 50% of dry weight of plaque (Critchley *et al.*, 1967); it appears therefore that 20% of the matrix of plaque comprises extracellular polysaccharide.

Although formation of plaque seems to be intimately related to its organic composition, the inorganic components are of importance in development of dental caries and formation of calculus. Plaque seems to have the property of concentrating both calcium and phosphorus (Allen and Moore, 1957; Dawes and Jenkins, 1962; Schroeder, 1963 and Luoma, 1964). Plaque formed on foils placed on the lingual surfaces of the lower incisors contained nearly 3 times more calcium and phosphorus than pooled plaque formed elsewhere in the mouth (Schroeder, 1963; Jenkins 1965).

It seems probable that in young plaque the calcium is bound to protein or maybe to other organic constituents (Jenkins 1965). Schroeder (1963, 1964) however suggests that some of the calcium may in fact be bound to phosphate to form apatite in plaque 2–3 days old, and that in some of the types of mineralization form birefringence may be absent.

1. Influence of Diet

The composition of diet has been shown to influence both the rate of formation and bacterial composition of plaque. Carlsson and Egelberg (1965) have shown that humans consuming a diet rich in glucose, form a thin plaque. Sucrose, however, appears to promote the formation of plaque and also influences the bacterial composition (Bowen and Cornick, 1967).

IV. Calculus

Although it has been clearly shown that the chemical composition of plaque from different areas of the mouth varies greatly, the conditions which lead to its calcification and the consequent formation of calculus are not well understood.

A. CHEMICAL COMPOSITION

1. Inorganic

Two types of calculus are recognized, supra-gingival and sub-gingival, depending on its relation to the gingival margin. The sub-gingival type is also frequently referred to as serumnal, based on the assumption that serum is the main source of both organic and inorganic substances present in this variety.

Most investigations into calculus formation have been confined to observations on the supra-gingival type. Calculus has been found to contain up to 80% inorganic material and approximately 20% organic. Young immature calculus contains very much more organic material. The greater proportion of the inorganic faction consists of calcium and phosphorous; traces of other elements such as magnesium, fluorine and sodium are also found (Little et al., 1963, Speirs, 1959). The bulk of the inorganic portion of calculus is probably crystalline. Rowles (1964a,b) has shown that apatite, brushite, whitlochite and octocalcium phosphate are the commonest forms of calcium phosphate present. The significance of the different types of crystals in calculus has not been demonstrated.

2. Organic

The organic content of calculus varies with the age of the deposit. Aged calculus can contain up to 28% organic material (Little, et al., 1961; Mandel *et al.*, 1962). The bulk of the organic material consists of protein (36–40%), some carbohydrate 12–20% (Stanford *et al.*, 1962; Stanford, 1966) and very little fat (0.2%). The source of the protein and carbohydrate has already been discussed. The lipid faction consists of neutral fats, free fatty acids, cholesterol, cholesterol esters, and phospholipids (Mandel and Levy, 1957; Little *et al.*, 1964).

B. MINERALIZATION

There are many theories offered to explain the mineralization of plaque. These can be broadly classified as bacterial and salivary.

1. Bacterial

Many oral micro-organisms have the capacity to become mineralized *in vitro* (Ennever, 1960; Bowen and Gilmour, 1961) and also *in vivo* (Rizzo *et al.*, 1967). Takazoe (1963) has extracted a fraction from *Bacterionema matruchotii* that is capable of being mineralized. Intracellular and extracellular mineralization involving bacteria has been observed in electron microscopic preparations of calculus (Schroeder *et al.*, 1964). These patterns have also been observed in micro-organisms placed in dialysis bags implanted in the peritoneal cavity of rats. The colour of the calculus formed could be associated with particular micro-organisms; deposits formed by *Veillonella* species were always greenish-tan and calcifications formed by *Fusobacterium polymorphum* were yellowish orange. There is little doubt micro-organisms can form a suitable matrix within which mineralization can occur.

Baer and Burstone (1959) have suggested that esterase, particularly associated with micro-organisms may liberate fatty acids from their esters; these acids then form calcium and magnesium soaps. The presence of these compounds, however, has not been demonstrated in calculus.

2. Saliva

Although there is good evidence to suggest bacteria are of importance in calculus formation, germ-free animals can form substantial amounts of calculus (Fitzgerald and McDaniel, 1960, Gustafsson and Krasse 1962). This evidence suggests that saliva itself may have an inherent capacity to form mineralized deposits on the tooth. Indeed Kakehashi *et al.* (1964) have demonstrated that rats which have had their major salivary glands removed failed to develop any calculus.

In vitro investigations have shown that a substance can be extracted from bovine submaxillary glands which causes the formation of a calculus-like material on teeth placed in a calcifying solution. (Draus and Miklos 1963;

Draus *et al.*, 1966). The capacity of the extract to form a deposit was markedly reduced by reducing the number of carboxyl groups present in the extract. The presence of nucleating material associated with amino groups in whole human saliva has been demonstrated by Eilberg *et al.* (1965). Nitrous acid rapidly inactivated the calcifiability of the material, and it could also be inhibited by prior treatment with 1 mmol Cu Cl_2.

The chemical and physical composition of diet too seems to influence calculus formation (Egelberg, 1965; Carlsson and Egelberg, 1965). It is however not known whether this is a direct action, or occurs as a result of altered microbial flora or viscosity of saliva. Baer *et al.* (1961), observed that a diet rich in corn starch enhanced the rate of calculus formation in Sprague-Dawley rats. However, Baer and White (1966) have shown that animals fed a diet containing a high concentration of fat or protein form significantly more calculus than those fed diets rich in sucrose.

V. Gingival Fluid

A. FORMATION AND COMPOSITION

During the past fifteen years particular attention has been paid to the possibility that healthy gingival crevices contain a particular type of exudate which helps to maintain gingival health. The evidence for the existence of such a substance has been gleaned by a number of workers using both animals and man as experimental subjects.

Following intravenous administration of fluorescein, Brill and Krasse (1958) were able to detect an exudate containing this substance on filter paper strips placed either inside or outside the gingival crevice. They suggested that the epithelial lining of gingival pockets in dogs is permeable to the small fluorescein molecules. A correlation was found in humans between the degree of inflammation and the amount of fluorescein occurring on the test strips (Brill & Bjorn, 1959). These groups of workers have also shown that mechanical stimulation such as chewing or tooth brushing increased the flow of gingival fluid and that charcoal particles, or micro-organisms introduced into healthy gingival crevices, are rapidly removed. Indeed, Waerhaug and Steen (1952) suggested that the normal healthy gingival in the dog does not contain micro-organisms

Brill (1959b) concludes that "a health promoting effect may therefore be ascribed to gingival massage enhancing the occurrence of antimicrobial substances in gingival pockets". Using strips of sterile filter paper to collect gingival fluid, Collins and Gavin (1961a) were unable to demonstrate any bactericidal or bacteriostatic effect when the strips were placed on culture plates seeded with micro-organisms. The same investigators (1961b) also demonstrated that the normal healthy gingival crevice appears to contain micro-organisms in the majority of cases, confirming the observation made by Boyd and Rosenthal (1958). These observations would not preclude the possibility that the exudate *in situ* may at least control the numbers of micro-organisms.

This concept of gingival fluid suggests that the epithelium lining the gingival crevice has its own peculiar properties differing significantly from those of epithelia in other parts of the mouth. However, more recent evidence tends to suggest that the "so called" gingival fluid is in fact a simple inflammatory exudate. Using an immunoelectrophoretic technique Brill and Bronnestam (1960) demonstrated the presence of seven different serum protein components including β and α globulin. The proportions of Na^+ and K^+ found in the fluid also suggest that this substance is an inflammatory exudate and not an extracellular fluid. However, Browne-Grant and Browne (1966) have shown that Na^{24} and Na^{131} enter the gingival sulcus of rabbit incisors much more slowly than Na^{131} labelled human serum. Cowley (1968) using a fluorescent protein tracing technique in dogs has shown that the permeability of the crevicular epithelium is greater at the top of the crevice than at the base, which further suggests that the fluid is a result of inflammation. Mann (1963) was able to correlate the amount of gingival fluid collected on strips and the depth of the gingival crevice; this observation was confirmed by Egelberg (1964). Further evidence to correlate the inflammatory nature of the exudate was presented by Browne (1965) who showed that the rate of its formation in rabbits is directly related to the local blood flow.

The different explanations offered for the nature of gingival fluid may be explained by the different species of animals used and also possibly to differences in technique. The rabbit incisor used by Browne-Grant and Browne (1966) is continuously erupting and only occasionally shows the presence of chronic inflammatory cells in the lamina around the bottom of the gingival crevice. In man however, chronic inflammatory cells are invariably found in this site even in clinically normal sites. It is possible as suggested by Browne-Grant and Browne (1966) that inflammatory exudate from the gingival sulcus of man and dogs masks the composition of "normal" gingival fluid. If this is so, it would seem that the presence or absence of "normal" gingival fluid is of academic interest only.

B. Function of the Gingival Exudate

The protective effect of gingival fluid has been suggested by many authors. Charcoal particles introduced in the healthy gingival sulci of young dogs by Brill (1959a) were rapidly removed six to twenty minutes later; a culture of Serratia marcescens was similarly removed. It is also possible that leucocytes present in the gingival crevice may phagocytose micro-organisms. Indeed Sharry and Krasse (1960) and Egelberg (1963) have shown that leucocytes constitute approximately 47% of the somatic cells in scrapings from the gingival sulcus. These observations suggest that the gingival sulcus provides a major site for entrance of leucocytes into the mouth. The presence of immuno-globulins in the gingival sulcus would also contribute to the defence of this area although significant levels of antibody active against micro-organisms present in the mouth have not been demonstrated in gingival exudate. Although much attention has been focused on the buccal sulcus and the nature of the sulcul fluid it must be remembered that there is some evidence that the initial lesion in periodontal disease occurs interdentally (Cohen, 1959) and not in the epithelium of the gingival crevice.

References

Adinolfi, M., Glynn, A. A., Lindsay, M. and Milne, C. M. (1966). *Immunology* **10** 517–525.

Allen, W. I. and Moore, B. W. (1957). *Int. Assoc. dent. Res.* Abstract No. 108.

Armstrong, W. G. (1966). *Nature (Lond.)*, **210**, 197.

Baer, P. M. and Burstone, M. S. (1959). *Oral Surg. Oral Med. Oral Path.* **12**, 1147–1152.

Baer, P. N., Stephan, R. M. and White, C. L. (1961). *J. Periodont.* **32**, 190–192.

Baer, P. N. and White, C. L. (1966). *J. Periodont.* **37**, 113–117.

Bartels, H. A. (1934). *Dent. Stern. Int.* **56**, 8–11.

Bowen, W. H. (1968). Unpublished results.

Bowen, W. H. and Cornick, D. (1967). *Helv. Odont. Acta.* **11**, 27–31.

Bowen, W. H. and Gilmour, M. (1961). *Archs. oral. Biol.* **5**, 145–148.

Boyd, W. S. and Rosenthal, S. L. (1958). *J. dent. Res.* **37**, 288–291.

Brill, N. (1959a). *Acta. odont. Scand.* **17**, 431–438.

Brill, N. (1959b). *Acta. odont. Scand.* **17**, 23–33.

Brill, N. and Bjorn, H. (1959). *Acta. odont. Scand.* **17**, 11–23.

Brill, N. and Bronnestam, R. (1960). *Acta. odont. Scand.* **18**, 95–100.

Brill, N. and Krasse, B. (1958). *Acta. odont. Scand.* **16**, 233–245.

Browne, R. M. (1965). *Dent. Practnr. dent. Rec.* **15**, 240–247.

Browne-Grant, K. and Browne, R. M. (1966). *Archs. oral. Biol.* **11**, 455–471.

Carlsson, J. and Egelberg, J. (1965). *Odont. Revy.* **16**, 42–49.

Carlsson, J. and Egelberg, J. (1965). *Odont. Revy.* **16**, 112–125.

Chauncey, H. H., Lionetti, F., Winar, R. A. and Lisanti, V. F. (1954). *J. dent. Res.* **33**, 321–334.

Clem, W. H. and Klebanoff, S. J. (1966). *J. Bact.* **91**, 1848–1853.

Cohen, B. (1959). *Brit. dent. J.* **107**, 31–39.

Coleman, R. D. and Appleman, M. D. (1953). *J. dent. Res.* **32**, 294–297.

Collins, A. A. and Gavin, J. B. (1961a). *J. Periodont.* **32**, 99–101.

Collins, A. A. and Gavin, J. B. (1961b). *J. Periodont.* **32**, 198–202.

Cowley, G. C. (1968). *J. dent. Res.* **45** (Suppl.), 665–661.

Critchley, P., Wood, J. M., Saxton, C. A. and Leach, S. A. (1967). *Caries Res.* **1**, 122–129.

Dawes, C. and Jenkins, G. N. (1962). *Archs. oral. Biol.* **7**, 161–164.

Dawes, C. and Jenkins, G. N. (1963). Proc. 41st meeting ADR., N. Amer. Div. Abstract 362.

Dawes, C. and Jenkins, G. N. (1964). *Brit. dent. J.* **116**, 433–435.

Dogon, J. L., Kerr, A. C. and Amdur, B. H. (1962). *Archs. oral Biol.* **7**, 81–90.

Draus, F. J. and Miklos, F. L. (1963). *J. dent. Res.* **42**, 1249.

Draus, F. J. and Miklos, F. L. and West, B. (1966). *Archs. oral. Biol.* **II**, 521–525.

Egelberg, J. (1963). *Acta. odont. Scand.* **21**, 283.

Egelberg, J. (1964). *Odont. Revy.* **15**, 381.
Egelberg, J. (1965). *Odont. Revy.* **16**, 50–60.
Eilberg, R. G., Gould, D. and Sobel, A. E. (1965). *Nature (Lond.)*, **207**, 481–483.
Ellison, S. A., Mashimo, P. A. and Mandel, I. D. (1960). *J. dent. Res.* **39**, 892–898.
Ennever, J. (1960). *J. Periodont.* **31**, 304–307.
Fitzgerald, R. J. and McDaniel, E. G. (1960). *Archs. oral. Biol.* **2**, 239–240.
Fleming, A. and Allison, V. D. (1922). *Proc. R. Soc. (London) B.* **94**, 142–151.
Gibbons, R. J., de Stoppelaar, J. D. and Hardens (1966). **45**, 877–881.
Glynn, A. A. (1968). *In* "The Scientific Basis of Medicine Annual Reviews." University of London.
Green, G. E. (1959). *J. dent. Res.* **38**, 262–275.
Gupta, O. P., Blechman, H. and Stahl, S. S. (1960). *Oral. Surg. Oral Med. Oral Path.* **13**, 470–481.
Gustafsson, B. E. and Krasse, B. (1962). *Acta. odont. Scand.* **20**, 135–142.
Hoerman, K. C., Englander, H. R. and Shklair, I. L. (1956). *Proc. Soc. exp. Biol. Med.* **92**, 875–878.
Iwamoto, G., Inoue M., Tsunemitsu, A. and Matsumura, T. (1967). *Archs. oral Biol.* **12**, 1009–1012.
Jay, P., Crowley, Mary, Hadley Faith, P. and Bunting, R. W. (1932). *J. Am. dent. Assoc.* **20**, 2130–2148.
Jenkins, G. N. (1965). *Ann. New York Acad. Sci.* **131**, 786–794.
Jenkins, G. N. (1968). *Caries Res.* **2**, 130–138.
Johnson, P. L., Bevelander, G. (1958). *Oral. Surg.* **11**, 1055–1063.
Kakehashi, S. and Baer, P. N. and White, C. L. (1964). *J. Periodont.* **35**, 467–489.
Kerr, A. C. and Wedderburn, Doreen (1958). *Brit. dent. J.* **105**, 321–326.
Klebanoff, S. J. and Luebke, R. G. (1965). *Proc. Soc. exp. Biol.* **118**, 483–487.
Krasse, B. and Egelberg, J. (1962). *Acta. odont. Scand.* **20**, 143–152.
Kraus, F. W. and Sirisinha, S. (1962). *Archs. oral Biol.* **7**, 221–233.
Kraus, F. W. and Konno, J. (1963). *Ann. N.Y. Acad. Sci.* **106**, 311–329.
Leach, S. A. (1963). *Nature (Lond.)*, **199**, 486–487.
Leach, S. A. (1964). *Archs. oral Biol.* **9**, 461–467.
Leach, S. A., Critchley, P., Kolendo, A. B. and Saxton, C. A. (1967). *Caries Res.* **1**, 104–111.
Lenz, H. and Muhlemann, H. R. (1963). *Helv. Odont. Acta.* **7**, 30–38.
Little, M. F., Bowman, L. M. and Dirkson, T. R. (1964). *J. dent. Res.* **43**, 836–840.
Little, M. F., Casciani, C. and Lensky, S. (1961). *Int. Ass. dent. Res.* Preprinted abstract, **39**, 311.
Little, M. F., Casciani, C. and Rowley, J. (1963). *J. dent. Res.* **42**, 78–84.
Luoma, H. (1964). *Acta. odont. Scand.* **22**, suppl. 41.
Mandel, I. D. and Ellison, S. A. (1961). *Archs. oral Biol.* **3**, 77–85.
Mandel, I. D., Hampar, B. and Ellison, S. A. (1962). *Proc. Soc. exp. Biol. (N.Y.)*, **110**, 301–303.
Mandel, I. D. and Levy, B. M. (1957). *Oral Surg.* **10**, 874–878.
Mann, W. V. (1963). *J. Periodont.* **34**, 379–387.
McDougall, W. A. (1963). *Aust. dent. J.* **8**, 261–273.
Mechel, A. H. (1968). *Caries Res.* **2**, 104–114
Middleton, J. D. (1965). *Archs. Oral Biol.* **10**, 227–236.
Penrose, L. S. (1930). *Lancet (London)*, **219**, 689–690.
Pollaci, G. and Ceraulo, S. (1909). *Centrabl. f. Bakteriol*, **52**, 268–275.
Reiter, B. and Moller-Madsen, A. (1963). *J. dairy Res.* **30**, 419–423.
Rizzo, A. A., Mitchell, C. T., Lifsehis, J. M. and Frazier, P. B. (1967). *Archs. Oral Biol.* **12**, 79–83.

Rowles, S. L. (1964a). Bone and Tooth, Proceedings of the First European Symposium. Oxford, 1963. H. J. J. Blackwood (ed.). Pergamon Press, London.

Rowles, S. L. (1964b). *Dent. Practnr. dent. Rec.* **15**, 2–6.

Salton, M. R. J. (1952). *Nature (Lond.)* **170**, 746.

Schroeder, H. E. (1963). *Helv. odont. Acta.* **7**, 17–24.

Schroeder, H. E. (1964). *Helv. odont. Acta.* **8**, 117–125.

Schroeder, H. E., Lenz, H. and Mühlemann, H. R. (1964). *Helv. odont. Acta.* **8,** 1–7.

Sharon, N. (1967). *Proc. R. Soc.* B. **167**, 402–415.

Sharry, J. J. and Krasse, B. (1960). *Acta. odont. Scand.* **18**, 347–353.

Sktrotskii, E. V., Makhlinorskii, L. I. and Slutskoia, G. (1937). *Ann. Mechnikov. Inst.* **6**, 91–96.

Smith, C. B., Bellante, S. A. and Channock, R. M. (1967). *J. Immunol.* **99**, 133–141.

South, Mary Ann, Cooper, M. D., Wollheim, H. R. and Good, R. A. (1966). *J. exp. Med.* **123**, 615–627.

Speins, R. L. (1959). *Brit. dent. J.* **107**, 209–211.

Stanford, J. W. (1966). *J. dent. Res.* **45**, 128–136.

Stanford, J. W., Forziati, A. F. and Paffenbarger, G. C. (1962). *Int. Ass. dent. Res.* Preprinted abstracts, **40**, 61.

Takazoe, I. (1966). *Paradontolagie*, **20**, 22–28.

Thonard, J. C., Heflin, C. H. and Steinberg, A. (1965). *J. Bact.* **89**, 924–925.

Tomasi, T. B. (1965). *J. exp. Med.* **121**, 101–124.

Turner, E. P. (1958). *Dent. Practnr. dent. Rec.* **8**, 373–382.

Ussing, M. J. (1955). *Acta odont. Scand.* **13**, 123–154.

Vallotton, C. F. (1945a). *J. dent. Res.* **24**, 161–169.

Vallotton, C. F. (1945b). *J. dent. Res.* **24**, 171–181.

Vallotton, C. F. (1945c). *J. dent. Res.* **24**, 183–187.

Voreadis, E. G. and Zander, H. A. (1958). *Oral Surg. Oral Med. Oral Path.* **11**, 1120–1125.

Waerhaug, J. and Steen, E. (1952). *Odont. Tidskr.* **60**, 1–32.

Wheatcroft, M. G. (1957). *J. dent. Res.* **36**, 112–117.

Wheatcroft, M. G. and Neames, J. L. (1951). *J. dent. Res.* **30**, 494–496.

Winkler, K. E. and Dirks, O. B. (1958). *Internat. dent. J.* **8**, 561–585.

Zeldow, B. J. (1959). *J. dent. Res.* **38**, 798–804.

Zeldow, B. J. (1961). *J. dent. Res.* **40**, 446–453.

Zeldow, B. J. (1963). *J. Immunol.* **90**, 12–16.

12 Healing of Wounds in the Periodontium

*A. H. MELCHER

Department of Dental Science, Royal College of Surgeons of England, London, England

I. Introduction

The relationships between the epithelia, the soft, and the hard connective tissues of the periodontium are unique; for this organ comprises not only hard and soft connective tissues and epithelium, but also diverse types of each of these tissues. This means that some aspects of the organization and synchronization of the processes involved in repair of wounds in the organ must differ from those elsewhere in the body. Nevertheless, it is important to realize that these differences are in respect of detail only, and that the basic principles of tissue repair apply here as elsewhere. In all areas of the body fundamental processes of tissue repair are modified by environment and structure, but a thorough grasp of the means by which each constituent tissue is repaired is essential if the significance of local adaption is to be appreciated.

Descriptions of wound healing use the terms *regeneration* and *repair* to describe the processes by which defects in tissues or organs are "made good". Gillman (1961) has underlined the importance of understanding that restoration of lost tissue may be achieved by two distinct processes. In the one, the

*Present address: Faculty of Dentistry, University of Toronto, Toronto, Canada.

architecture and function of the lost tissue is completely renewed, and for this process he reserves the term *regeneration*. In the other, continuity of the disrupted tissues is restored by new tissues which do not replicate the structure and function of the lost tissue. He calls this process *repair*. This distinction is important, for it implies that not all tissues can regenerate themselves after injury, and that their capacity to do so varies with the type of injury, and from tissue to tissue. There is also variations between species. To quote two extreme examples; following amputation, the salamander will regenerate a new limb with all its complicated arrangement of tissues; by contrast, man cannot replace even a small amount of lost central nervous tissue. So, in considering the healing of a wound, it is not only necessary to assess the capacity of the organism to fill the defect with new tissue, but it is also important to observe how this is done, to what extent the new tissue is able to carry out the functions of the old, and finally whether, with the passage of time, repair may be followed by regeneration as may occur to some extent in wounds of muscle.

The material in this chapter will embrace two main topics; the principles of healing of soft tissues and bone, and healing of wounds in the periodontium. No attempt will be made to cover the first topic exhaustively, as this has been done admirably by a number of workers. For example, the healing of soft tissues has been described fully by Gillman *et al.* (1955), Allgower (1956), Edwards and Dunphy (1958), Johnson and McMinn (1960), Douglas (1963), Ordman and Gillman (1966), McMinn (1967), and Gillman (1968). Instead, an endeavour will be made to describe the essential histogenetic manoeuvres which result in the filling of a defect in injured tissues. Attention will not be paid to the details of all of these however, as fibrogenesis and osteogenesis, remodelling, and the origin of the involved cells, have been dealt with in Chapter 6, and the effect of nutrition and endocrine secretions on some of the processes in Chapters 9 and 10.

II. Principles of Repair

A. SOFT TISSUES

Most of our knowledge about healing of soft tissues stems from observations on wounded skin. The reasons for this are apparent. Firstly, the clinical implications are of prime importance, and secondly, skin offers a readily exploitable experimental system. Wounding of soft tissues is followed by shedding of blood and lymph, which subsequently forms a clot in and over the wound. The clot, together with altered collagen fibres from the dermis, subsequently constitutes the scab, which is demarcated from the underlying dermis by a zone of leucocytes (Buntine, 1967). The scab provides surface protection, initially for the damaged tissues, and later for the delicate new epithelium which comes to cover the wound. Haemorrhage is followed by inflammation of the part. This reaction is succeeded by biological debridement; that is, removal by macrophages of both damaged tissue and the constituents of shed blood.

A number of processes effect replacement of the destroyed tissue. An essential requirement is a supply of cells. These move into the affected area, which they gradually fill either themselves or by producing extracellular material. Finally, the new tissue is usually remodelled to meet the demands of function.

1. Mobilization of Cells

Mobilization of cells to colonize the damaged area is achieved by two distinct processes. These are the movement of epithelial and connective tissue cells into the part, and the provision of a sufficient number of cells for the purpose by local mitotic division. These occurrences may be due to one or both of two consequences of injury; a deficiency of tissue or damage to cells (Abercrombie, 1964).

The mechanisms which allow or stimulate epithelial or connective tissue cells to migrate to an area where they are needed will be considered first. A great deal of insight into this process has been provided by study of the behaviour of cells in tissue culture, and much of the knowledge has come from the work of Abercrombie and of Weiss (see the reviews by Abercrombie, 1964 and 1966, and by Weiss, 1958, 1959 and 1961.) The ability to move across a solid substrate appears to be an inherent property of both epithelial and connective tissue cells. Locomotion is apparently effected by the attachment of the peripheral fringe of the cell to a substrate which, *in vivo*, may be viable or damaged tissue. When cells are completely surrounded by like-cells, their movement is apparently inhibited. Abercrombie has called this phenomenon *contact inhibition*. It possibly arises from adhesion between the surfaces of like-cells, or perhaps due to some special property of their micro-environment. When contact between like-cells is broken, an inevitable consequence of wounding, the cells at the free margin tend to move across the surface of the substrate into the space so created. If the substrate is orientated, as for example are strands of fibrin, the cells will be provided with routes to follow, and so may move in a predetermined direction. Weiss, who has termed this phenomenon *contact guidance*, believes that the orientation of the fibrin strands *in vivo* may depend on the stresses exerted upon them. Cells will continue to move until contact is made with other cells. If colliding cells are alike, then movement in the direction which was being followed will stop. Contact may be maintained, or else the cells will part, moving off in new directions, but never moving *over* each other. If contact occurs between unlike cells, for example between cells of different epithelia, or between malignant fibroblasts, then the moving cells

17

will treat each other as substrate. After a short period of contact they will move on in the same direction, moving over each other to do so. The process of making and breaking contact between like-cells continues until contact is made on all sides, when further movement is inhibited. Once this has been accomplished, the cells will settle down, and the pattern of the new tissue will be established.

This explanation of cell movement appears to apply in principle equally well to epithelial and connective tissue cells, but there are differences between them. Epithelial cells *in vivo* are surrounded on all sides by other epithelial cells. The exception to this rule is provided by the deep aspect of the basal cells. However, it is tempting to think that, in this context, the lamina densa which separates them from the connective tissue fulfils the role of an adjacent cell membrane. (See Chapter 2). *In vivo*, contact between fibroblasts appears to be limited to small areas of their processes. It is conceivable that their movement is inhibited not only by this, but also by the extracellular substance which envelopes them (Glücksmann, 1964). A further difference between epithelial and connective tissue cells is evident in the way the two populations move. Epithelial cells tend to move as a sheet with a free edge, whereas connective tissue cells seem to move individually.

New cells are provided by mitotic division to replace those that are lost through trauma. Control of cell division in intact tissue has been discussed in Chapter 5. The reason why mitotic activity is stimulated following wounding is unclear. A strong case has been made out to support the belief that the deficiency of tissue which follows trauma leads to a reduction in the stimuli which normally inhibit mitotic activity of tissue cells (Bullough, 1966; see also Chapter 5). However, Abercrombie (1964 and 1966) maintains that we should not discount the older concept that a product of damaged and dead cells stimulates mitotic division of neighbouring viable cells. Evidence has been adduced to support both views. Although, at present, there is still argument about which of these mechanisms is responsible, there is some strong evidence against the latter (Calnan *et al.*, 1964) and in favour of the former.

2. Restoration of Epithelium

Continuity of the epithelium is established before continuity of the connective tissue, in healing of both incised and shallow excised cutaneous wounds (Gillman *et al.*, 1955; Ordman and Gillman, 1966a). Mobilization of cells from the margin of the wound, and their centripetal migration into the defect, is the first step in restoring continuity of epithelium.

Regeneration of micro-wounds of the epidermis may be achieved by mobilization and migration of adjacent epithelial cells without the necessity of providing new cells (Johnson and McMinn, 1960). In contrast to this, as discussed above, larger wounds require in addition, a supply of new cells. Evidence of mitotic division is not obtained until after active migration has started.

Abercrombie (1966) has pointed out that tissue cells in the intact adult are probably immobile. This means that cells migrating into a tissue defect following wounding must start to move from a standstill. The cells of the epithelium bordering the wound tend to become hypertrophied and to exhibit large vesicular nuclei. Migration is largely restricted to the cells of the middle layers (Johnson and McMinn, 1960). The classical belief that sheets of epithelial cells migrate across the surface of the clot has been disputed by Gillman et al. (1955) and again by Ordman and Gillman (1966a). Independent observations on healing wounds in skin have corroborated their description of the behaviour of the epithelium (Calnan et al., 1964 and Buntine, 1967). Epithelial coverage of the wound begins usually within 24 hours of operation. Incised wounds may be covered by a layer of epithelial cells in 24 to 48 hours, whereas the time taken for an excised wound to be fully epithelialized will depend on its surface area. The migrating sheets of cells move across the surface of the cut dermis and *beneath* the clot, apparently digesting fibrin and damaged extracellular substance of connective tissue in the process. It follows that damaged collagen fibres are included in the clot or scab, which subsequently comes to lie superficial to the immigrant epidermal cells. Support for the belief that epithelial cells may possess lytic properties has come from Grillo and Gross (1964), who have shown that a collagenase is produced in healing wounds, possibly by the epithelial cells. Of particular interest in relation to the main subject of this chapter is the finding of Winter (1964) that epithelial migration is much more superficial and rapid in experimental wounds that have been kept wet, than in those which have been dried. Possibly relevant to this is Block et al's (1963) observation that a tongue wound closes much more rapidly than a similar incision in skin. The path followed by the converging epithelial sheets results in their lining the walls of the defect. Consequently, particularly in incised wounds, they may penetrate quite deeply into the dermis before making contact with each other, slicing through the clot to do so. It is important to emphasize that they do not cross the wound at the level of the pre-existing epithelium and as a result, when the scab is shed about a week or so after wounding, the surface of the healing defect is found to be depressed below the level of the adjacent epithelium. Migration does not appear to stop completely when contact is made between the covering sheets of cells, as further small epithelial spurs are intruded into the underlying connective tissue.

Mitotic figures are not usually seen in the epithelium until about 24 to 36 hours after wounding. These are mostly restricted to a zone of cells (Bullough and Laurence, 1960 and 1961) that have remained stationary in the wall of the wound. The zone extends for about 1 mm from the edge of the wound.

Mitotic activity appears to occur in waves, probably due to initial synchronization of the mitotic cycles of the reacting cells (Bullough, 1966). Periodic bursts of activity have also been described by Hell and Cruickshank (1963) and by Epstein and Sullivan (1964). Bullough has found that activity in epithelial cells adjacent to a skin wound is raised about 20 times above the resting rate, and that the duration of the mitotic cycle is greatly reduced. Epstein and Sullivan (1964) have shown that although, in resting tissues, mitoses are usually restricted to the deeper layers of the epidermis (see Chapter 5), following wounding they occur at all levels including those cells immediately beneath the granular layer. The cells of all the injured skin appendages can also contribute new epithelial cells to the healing defect (Gillman et al., 1955; Ordman and Gillman, 1966a). It has been pointed out above that cells migrating over the wound surface rarely exhibit mitotic figures. It may be that, in general, cells are able to perform one function only at a time, as has been suggested by Bullough and Rytömaa (1965).

When the wound surface has been covered by a layer of epithelial cells, these also begin to divide, so providing new cells to thicken the scar epithelium. In the case of a large excised wound, mitotic activity is seen in epithelial cells covering the peripheral part of the wound before its central part is epithelialized (Johnson and McMinn, 1960). The mitotic activity leads to thickening of both the pre-existing epithelium at the margin of the wound and the new epithelium in the wound. Later, remodelling occurs and, whereas the former is returned to normal, the latter is reduced to a thin epithelium.

Before leaving the subject of epithelial proliferation, it is necessary to discuss the influence that sutures may have on this process. Gillman et al. (1955) and Ordman and Gillman (1966b) have shown that epithelium proliferates along the sutures, surrounding them and making epithelial tracts down the suture tracks in to the dermis, and even the subcutaneous tissues. These epithelial tracts, together with the epithelial spurs described above, are eventually remodelled and removed. It is evident that sutures complicate healing but to what extent they delay healing in practical terms it is not possible to say. However, these investigators have shown that early removal of sutures reduces epithelial invasion of the connective tissue.

3. Restoration of the Connective Tissue

Restoration of continuity of the connective tissue involves four processes; production of new fibroblasts; migration of these cells into the wounded zone; formation of new extracellular substance; remodelling of the extracellular material in the wound. Formerly it was believed that formation of connective tissue occurs early in the healing process, and that the migrating epithelium would cross only this newly formed young connective tissue. However, Gillman and his group have shown that the onset of fibrogenesis occurs after migration of epithelial cells has been initiated in healing of incised and shallow excised wounds. Furthermore, Bullough and Laurence (1961) have found that the onset of mitotic activity in connective tissue cells occurs after that in the cells of the epithelium. In incised wounds, light microscopic evidence of fibrogenesis cannot be obtained before the wound has been epithelialized. However, Gillman *et al.* (1955) point out that the healing of deep excised wounds involving the loss of most of the dermis follows a totally different course. "Granulation tissue" (that is, highly vascular young connective tissue) is built up from the base of the wound (Hadfield, 1963a,b,c; Gillman, 1968), and the epithelium extends slowly across the surface of this new connective tissue. Nevertheless even here, thickening of the epithelium at the wound edges and its migration over the walls of cut dermis and beneath the blood clot is seen in the first 3–4 days, although new connective tissue cannot be detected until the 5–6th day (Gillman, 1968).

The above investigators have also shown quite clearly that, in skin, new fibroblasts do not originate from the densely fibrous dermal stratum reticularis constituting the walls of the wound. This tissue is remarkably unreactive following wounding and, as has been confirmed by Bullough and Laurence (1961) and Glücksmann (1964), mitotic figures are rarely seen in the fibrocytes of the transected fibrous connective tissue. They have found that, in skin wounds, mitotic activity is maximal in the cells of loose areolar tissue transected by the wound, and in the fat at the wound base. Loose areolar connective tissue is found in the papillary layer, in the perivascular and periappendigeal connective tissue of the dermis, and in the septa of the adipose tissue. Perivascular activity has also been described by Glücksmann (1964), who points out that, in healing of excised wounds, the main bulk of cells stems from the hypodermis. Grillo (1964) has found it impossible to separate the proliferative response of the capillaries from that of the fibroblasts. He suggests that, in mammals, the fibroblast-capillary system may represent a primary reparative response.

The provision of new blood vessels for the deficient area is necessary for the early stages of healing. These are provided by mitotic division of the endothelial cells of pre-existing capillaries which, as a result, produce new sprouts (Cliff, 1963 and 1965; Schoefl and Majno, 1964). In this connection, it is of interest to note that according to Edwards and Dunphy (1958) it is only in healing of the cornea that normal fibroplasia occurs in the absence of an intimate blood supply.

Once the denuded connective tissue of a shallow excised wound has been covered by epithelium, the two become separated by exudate (Gillman *et al.*, 1955; Gillman and Penn, 1956). It is this sub-epithelial exudate that seems to become colonized by the new connective tissue. The recently wounded connective tissue is characterized by the presence of strands of fibrin which, at least in incised wounds of skin, become orientated perpendicularly to the wound surface (Ordman and Gillman, 1966a). Organization of the wound contents occurs from about the second to the fifth day after wounding, and this is accompanied by the proliferation of fibroblast-like cells and thin-walled vessels into the area. These cells and vessels, as well as the argyrophilic fibres that the former produce, also appear to be orientated at right angles to the surface of the wound rather than across it (Glücksmann, 1964; Ordman and Gillman, 1966a); an observation which is consistent with the concept of *contact guidance*. According to the latter authors, it is from the sixth day on-wards that the newly secreted collagen fibres tend to become orientated parallel to the surface. Glücksmann has noted that mitosis of fibroblast-like cells tends to cease as fibrogenesis begins. This is again consistent with Bullough and Rytömaa's (1965) view, mentioned above, that cells can possibly perform only one function at a time.

About fourteen days post-operatively the wound is filled with fibres that run in all directions, whereafter remodelling (which Howes (1959) has called *differentiation*) begins. In Howes' view, remodelling consists of two distinct processes; resorption and/or changing of the orientation of these first-deposited fibres, and enlarging or increasing the number of orientated fibres present. A particular aspect of remodelling is the re-arrangement of the fibres that occurs at the periphery of the wound, establishing continuity between new fibres and pre-existing fibres in the wound wall. Two to three weeks after tenotomy, the cut ends of pre-existing collagen fibres appear frayed, and new connective tissue originating from the wound, is laid down between them (Skoog and Persson, 1954; Wassermann, 1954). In wounded connective tissue of skin, changes in the appearance of the cut ends of dermal fibres are seen 5-7 days post-operatively (Gillman, 1968). Before leaving fibrogenesis, it should be mentioned that Gillman et al. (1955) and Gillman (1968) postulate an inter-relationship between the roles of epithelium and connective tissue in wound healing. They suggest that the connective tissue response is stimulated by epithelial proliferation and that, in due course, the new young connective tissue, in its turn, inhibits the proliferation of epithelium, especially intradermally.

In animals where the skin is loose, excised wounds are only partly restored by new connective tissue. Healing is largely due to reduction in the size of the wound by contraction of the surrounding connective tissue. This means that the final scar has an area considerably smaller than that of the original wound. *Contraction* starts early in healing, from about the third to the fifth day (see Abercrombie et al., 1961), and continues for a number of weeks. It should not be confused with *contracture*, the onset of which occurs much later, and which is responsible for the cicatrization that occurs after healing of wounds in the soft tissues covering the flexor aspect of joints. Van Winkle (1967), who has recently reviewed the topic, has defined contraction as the diminution in size of an open wound as a result of centripetal movement of the whole thickness of the surrounding skin. A number of theories have been advanced to explain this phenomenon. However, the available evidence suggests that only those of Grillo and Potsaid (1961) or of Abercrombie *et al.* (1961) are tenable. The former workers believe that traction is exerted on wound margins by the centripetal migration of fibroblasts resident in the "picture-frame" area comprising the narrow band of connective tissue surrounding the wound. The latter authors, on the other hand, have produced considerable evidence to support their contention that the wound margins are pulled inwards by the contractile faculty of fibroblasts resident within the newly synthesized healing connective tissue. In the light of current knowledge, the arguments of Abercrombie's group appear to be more convincing (see, for example, Van Winkle, 1967). Following contraction, a repaired square or oblong excised wound may appear as a forked, linear scar, which is densely collagenous and poor in cells and blood vessels (Billingham and Russell, 1956; Luccioli *et al.*, 1964). It is not clear whether contraction plays a significant role in the repair of human wounds. Edwards and Dunphy (1958) regard it as a major factor in the closure of large defects in tissues that are not splinted to underlying structures; however Johnson and McMinn (1960) suggest that the process is restricted in human beings because they do not possess skin as loose as that found in some animals. Van Winkle concludes that contraction does occur in man, but to a lesser extent than in animals. By contrast Abercrombie *et al.* (1961) think that contraction is not limited only to loose skin in man, and point out that it occurs in the healing of wounds in the back of the neck where the skin is firmly adherent to the underlying tissues. The effect of contraction on the connective tissue of the surrounding skin should also be considered. For contraction to occur, it is conceivable that the surrounding skin needs to be extensively stretched; Billingham and Medawar (1955) do not think that this is so. They have suggested that as contraction takes place, new connective tissue is deposited on, or within, the framework provided by the existing connective tissue. They have called this phenomenon *intussusceptive growth*.

Before leaving soft tissues, mention must be made of the oft repeated dictum that re-entry wounds and remote secondary wounds heal quicker than primary wounds by virtue of a circulating "wound hormone". There is little evidence to substantiate the existence of such a "wound hormone", and what evidence there is appears suspect on the grounds of poor experimental design (Johnson and McMinn, 1960). The issue has been clarified by Douglas (1963) who points out that second wounds in the environment of, and especially in the line of, the first incision heal well because of the local changes that have already taken place in the primary wound. In other words, the day of secondary wounding cannot be regarded as day O, but must be considered to correspond to whatever post-operative day is compatible with the stage of healing reached by the primary wound. That is, the machinery for repair has already been assembled in the latter, hence, healing of the second injury is considerably expedited.

B. BONE

Much of present day understanding of the mechanisms involved in the healing of a wound in bone has been derived from observations made on experimental fractures and osteotomies of long bones. A detailed description of the healing of this type of wound is not relevant to the problems being dealt with in this book, and the reader requiring such knowledge is referred to the many excellent papers which are available, for example those by Ham and Harris (1956), Urist (1956) and Pritchard (1964). As in the foregoing section, only the principles of the mechanisms which effect healing of bone wounds will be discussed.

The responses which follow fracture of a bone or disruption of its substance, and which lead to healing, are in some ways similar to those which effect healing of soft connective tissue wounds. But, because of the specialized nature of bone, there are some very important differences. As in soft connective tissues, wounding is followed by outpouring of blood which eventually forms a clot. This fills the defect, and may extend into the marrow and the surrounding soft tissue. If the soft tissues are also wounded, they will be repaired in the normal way. The clot is removed by macrophages, and replaced by loose connective tissue, the fibrous callus. Unless cartilage or bone is then laid down in the fibrous callus, this soft tissue will mature into dense-fibred connective tissue which will then constitute the tissue by which the bone defect is repaired. This means that there are two distinct requirements for effective healing of bone to occur. The first of these demands provision of an adequate supply of cells possessing the potential to synthesize cartilage (which subsequently will be replaced by bone) or bone. The second demands that these cells are also able to induce the cells of the fibrous callus to produce cartilage or bone.

Urist and McLean (1952) have indicated that bone can be produced by two types of connective tissue cells. The first type, the osteogenic cell, has an inherent potential for producing bone. The natural potential of the second type is to produce soft connective tissue, but it will produce bone if induced to do so by an osteogenic stimulus—a process known as *induction*. Cells possessing inherent osteogenic potential are confined to tissues surrounded by the fibrous periosteum. These cells will produce bone even when transplanted to soft tissues (Urist and McLean, 1952; Cohen and Lacroix, 1955; Williams, 1957), or explanted and cultured *in vitro* (Fell, 1932 and 1933). The cells in question include those of the endosteum and the bone marrow, and of the cambium layer of the periosteum of young bones. Urist and Mc-Lean have found that cells of the cambium layer of old bone are dormant unless stimulated first by trauma. This finding has received some support from the work of Tonna (1965). In a radioautographic study he noticed that although old periosteal cells do not appear to retain the capacity to synthesize proteins for export, they are stimulated by trauma to proliferate. In so doing, they produce a new population of cells which, by contrast, are capable of intense protein synthesis. Finally, perivascular cells, both periosteal and in Haversian canals, appear to have osteogenic potential (Bassett et al., 1961; Trueta, 1963; see also Chapter 6); but, comparable with the fibrocytes in the wall of a soft tissue wound, the osteocytes have not yet been proved to play a part in bone repair.

There is a belief that active osteoblasts, whether derived from potentially osteogenic or induced osteogenic cells, can induce cells normally resident in, or originating from, soft connective tissue to produce bone (Ham and Harris, 1956; Bridges and Pritchard, 1958; Bassett and Ruedi, 1966). Goldhaber (1961) has provided elegant proof of this capacity by implanting, subcutaneously, diffusion chambers containing young developing bone. The cells of the subcutaneous connective tissue were induced, through the Millipore filter, to produce new bone by the young bone being synthesized inside the implanted chamber. The two deposits of new bone were found to lie opposite one another on different sides of the presumably, cell-excluding Millipore filter of the chamber, across which Goldhaber believes osteogenic inductors are able to diffuse.

Osteoblasts are not the only cells possessing the capacity to induce non-osteogenic cells to produce bone. Transitional urinary tract epithelium which is proliferating, either after transplantation or in situ after interference with the blood supply to the kidney, can induce formation of ectopic bone (see Beresford and Hancox, 1967, and Bridges, 1958, respectively, for reviews of the subject). A number of tissues from which viable cells have been excluded appear to have a similar capacity (see, for example, Bridges and Pritchard, 1958; Bassett, 1962, and Urist, 1965). However, as originally pointed out by Urist and McLean in 1952, no substance has yet been isolated from these tissues that can be shown convincingly to have bone-inducing properties.

There is therefore no doubt that stimuli exist which induce connective tissue cells that normally do not produce bone to take on the function of active osteoblasts, or possibly chondroblasts. This implies that at least some of the cells in soft connective tissues possess the genetic apparatus which controls formation of the extracellular substance of bone (and possibly cartilage), but that this function is dormant unless activated by a specifically osteogenic stimulus. The nature of this stimulus (or perhaps stimuli, because it is by no means certain that there are not a number of different mechanisms capable of producing the same result) is of more than academic interest. As will be seen below, there are bones in which even relatively small defects are rarely wholly repaired by new bone, and where repair is effected largely by

17*

fibrous connective tissue. In these situations, control of the mechanisms of induction could lead to development of clinical techniques whereby a weak and inadequately repaired bone could be transformed into a regenerated and fully functional one.

Following wounding, flattened resting cells of the cambium layer of intact periosteum and, even in a closed fracture of a long bone, connective tissue cells peripheral to the fibrous layer of the periosteum, show evidence of DNA synthesis (Tonna and Cronkite, 1961; Tonna, 1965). This activity is usually a prelude to cell division, and numerous mitotic figures can be recognized among these cell populations as well as those of the endosteum and bone marrow. The periosteum, as a result, becomes markedly cellular and thickened, and the fibrous layer is lifted away from the bone surface. This possibly involves dissolution of the fibres of Sharpey. The response of periosteal and endosteal cells is accompanied by a similar proliferation of vascular cells. There is evidence of a close link between the proliferation of vascular and perivascular cells and the development of new blood vessels and new bone trabeculae of similar orientation (Trueta and Cavadias, 1955; Trueta, 1963; Cavadias and Trueta, 1965; and see also Chapter 6 for origin of osteoblasts). This relationship between vascularization and osteogenesis has a counterpart in the association between vascularization and fibrogenesis discussed in Section A above. The proliferating cells rapidly differentiate into osteoblasts and lay down new bone. In a long bone the subperiosteal trabeculae are first deposited on the surface of the cortex at a distance from the wound. The cells form collars of new bone around the wound. In the case of a fracture, these encircle each fragment. If the medullary cavity is involved, the endosteal trabeculae are distributed similarly on the medullary surface of the bone.

In long bones, cartilage is frequently found to be associated with the subperiosteal callus, even in the repair of a small wound, but rarely with the endosteal callus. This cartilage is laid down by the periosteal cells, which have the capacity to produce either bone or cartilage. There is general belief that the cells modulate to chondroblasts where the blood supply is poor (Ham, 1930; Pritchard and Ruzicka, 1946; Cavadias and Trueta, 1965); both *in vivo* (Girgis and Pritchard, 1958) and *in vitro* (Bassett and Herrmann, 1961) studies provide some support for this concept. Other factors, such as species, age and stress, may also influence cartilage formation (McLean and Urist, 1955; Pritchard, 1964). Cartilage produced in repair is eventually replaced by bone in a manner similar to that seen in sites of embryonic endochondral ossification.

Concurrent with proliferation and differentiation of periosteal and endosteal osteoblasts, cells in the loose connective tissue overlying the wounded bone, and cells in the marrow, proliferate, differentiate, and migrate into the wound. These cells subsequently produce the fibrous callus. Those originating from marrow have inherent osteogenic potential (Urist and McLean, 1952).

In contrast to this, the extra-periosteal cells have a natural potential to synthesize soft connective tissue, but they seem to have a latent capacity for chondrogenesis and osteogenesis. One of the great problems of bone repair is the understanding of when and how these powers are invoked (Pritchard, 1964).

A fracture of a long bone is usually well healed by bone. This is effected primarily by the osteogenic cells of the periosteum and endosteum, and secondly by cells of the fibrous callus that have been induced to osteogenesis. Cavadias and Trueta (1965) have shown that the major role in healing of this type of wound is played by the subperiosteal callus, but that the endosteal callus alone can effect union of the fragments, although less efficiently. On the other hand, there is some evidence that in healing of a deep excised-type wound of a long bone, it is the endosteal cells that play the critical role (Bassett et al., 1961; Melcher and Irving, 1962 and 1964). The work of the latter authors suggests that, at least in this type of wound in the rat, the cells of the endosteum and marrow are responsible for most of the osteogenesis in the fibrous callus. Furthermore, they have also found that in healing of this type of defect, bridging of the wound by subperiosteal callus is dependent on the antecedent synthesis of endosteal callus. This contrasts strongly with the proliferative capacity of the periosteal callus in healing of a fracture, as shown so clearly by Cavadias and Trueta (1965) in the rabbit. It is possible that investigation of this variation in periosteal response may elucidate the stimuli responsible for reactivation of resting osteogenic cells. An understanding of the nature of these stimuli is of paramount importance in the clinical approach to healing of bones developed in membrane, as will be discussed below.

The early trabeculae of healing callus consist of woven bone. These are soon remodelled. Remodelling of the pre-existing bone also takes place, especially at the margins of the wound and elsewhere where bone has died. Necrosis of bone occurs particularly beneath damaged and stripped periosteum. The outer one-third of the cortex of long bones is supplied by periosteal vessels (Trueta, 1963), so damage to the overlying periosteum may result in interference with its nutrition, and its consequent death. This also appears to be true of flat bones (Beresford and Hancox, 1967). Bony callus is laid down in excess, so this must also be removed by remodelling and the junction between the bony callus and pre-existing bone must be obliterated. Remodelling may result in the site of damage in a long bone becoming unrecognizable; true regeneration would then have occurred.

Repair of wounds in flat bones, particularly those developed in membrane, appears to be much less efficient. For example, it has frequently been shown that most defects in parietal skull bones, particularly of the rat, are not healed by bone (Pritchard, 1946; Ham and Harris, 1956; Burger et al., 1962; Beresford and Hancox, 1967). These wounds are usually largely occluded by fibrous connective tissue. It is therefore clear that here the mechanisms that induce osteogenesis in fibrous callus are largely lacking. Alternatively, or perhaps in addition, the contribution made to the fibrous callus from cells normally resident in and around endosteum may be minimal. This stands in strong contrast to the remarkable feats of regeneration that can be achieved by long bones, particularly if attention is paid to conservation of the periosteum (McClements et al., 1961). The reasons for this apparent difference in behaviour between bones developed originally in cartilage and those developed originally in membrane is obscure, but are most relevant to the problem being dealt with in the second part of this chapter, healing of tissues in the periodontium. As far as is known, little attempt has been made to elucidate the difference in reaction to wounding between cells in bones of the former type and those of the latter.

Exclusion of mature soft connective tissue from the bone wound is essential for successful healing. It seems apparent that osteogenesis is inhibited by the presence of this tissue (Mulholland and Pritchard, 1959; Melcher and Irving, 1964). Furthermore, where osteogenesis is active, new bone will occupy areas from which normally resident soft connective tissue has been excluded (Murray et al., 1957; Hurley et al., 1959; Melcher and Dreyer, 1962). This finding also has potential application to the clinical treatment of wounds of the periodontium.

III. Healing of the Periodontium

There have been numerous investigations into healing of wounds of the periodontium (see below). Not unnaturally, the aim of most of these has been elucidation of the features of healing following clinical procedures, and very few have been concerned with explaining basic phenomena. Perhaps the most notable fact to emerge is the relative rapidity with which wounds in the gingiva heal, compared, for example, with wounds of the skin.

A. Incised Wounds

1. Gingiva and Periosteum

Surprisingly few investigations into healing of a simple incised wound of the gingiva have been reported. Cohen (1963) and Mittelman et al. (1964) have described respectively the healing of linear incised wounds in marginal gingiva of monkeys and attached gingiva of humans. Both have been impressed by the rapidity with which healing processes proceed, the latter authors having found fibrogenesis to be well advanced 72 hours post-operatively. In general, the sequence of events that takes place in gingiva appears similar to that which has been described to occur in comparable wounds in skin. Although Mittelman et al. describe the epithelium as proliferating from the wound margins over the surface of the clot, Cohen's photomicrographs suggest that vestibular gingival epithelium migrates deep to the overlying clot, and down the cut surfaces of the lamina propria before fusing. The former authors have found that connective tissue proliferates subsequent to epithelial closure and that cellular division of connective tissue cells is first seen in the perivascular connective tissue.

Healing of the more complicated incision produced by raising and replacing a flap of gingival soft tissue has also been studied. Two different types of wounds appear to have been examined. In the first, a flap is prepared by making two vertical incisions which are carried into the lamina propria but not down to the periosteum, and these are joined by a third incision which penetrates the crevicular epithelium and the lamina propria of the marginal and attached gingiva and the alveolar mucosa. This "split-thickness flap" leaves the attached epithelial cuff adhering to the teeth, and the central part of the lamina propria and the periosteum adhering to the teeth and alveolar bone respectively. In the second type of wound, the two vertical incisions are carried down to bone, and the third incision is placed between the soft tissues and tooth or bone, so that the hard tissues are denuded of all overlying soft tissues, that is of epithelium, lamina propria and periosteum.

Staffileno et al. (1962) have described healing in dogs of the first type of wound. Again, the general sequence of events appears similar to that seen in repair of a cutaneous incised wound, but there are some important differences. They report that the incisions are nearly bridged by epithelium at 48 hours. Although they do not specifically discuss the relationship between the new epithelium and the blood clot, there is some evidence to be seen in their photomicrographs that the epithelium advances a short distance down the cut connective tissue walls before fusing. At the same time period, there is evidence of fibrogenesis in the parts of the wound from which blood clot has been removed by macrophages. The new connective tissue grows in from the sides of the wound, and there is accompanying cellular and vascular activity in the periosteum. Of particular interest is the fact that, although apparently not directly traumatized, the underlying bone responds to wounding of the overlying soft tissues; for, as early as 2 days post-operatively, there is evidence of resorption of the internal surfaces of the vestibular alveolar plate. This is not accompanied by any evidence of osteitis. Resorption of bone reaches a peak at 6 days, by which time the vestibular aspect and crest of the alveolar process is also involved. Thereafter, bone resorption gradually gives way to osteogenesis, which leads to restoration of lost bone. The collagen fibres that colonize the wound are at first orientated vertically. However, by 2 months post-operatively they seem to have been remodelled, as they are now orientated similarly to those in control gingiva. Two months post-operatively the alveolar process has also been restored to its former height and contour, and Staffileno et al., state that there is "functional repair" of the wound with no anatomical deformity. That is, true gingival regeneration is achieved two months after incision—a result profoundly different from that described for cutaneous incisions, but one which seems to compare with split-thickness skin-graft donor sites.

In a subsequent investigation, Giblin *et al.* (1966) repeated the work of Staffileno *et al.* but re-prepared a second flap along the site of the original incisions 21 days post-operatively. They found that epithelialization was achieved a little more quickly in the re-entry wound than in the original, but that connective tissue repair was not enhanced. It is of particular interest that they observed fusion of epithelium to take place within the incision below the surface of the tissues.

Healing of the second type of flap wound has been investigated in man by Dedolph and Clark (1958) and Kohler and Ramfjord (1960). Their work indicates that restoration of connective tissue continuity, and re-attachment of the epithelial cuff to enamel and cementum, is completed in 3–4 weeks. Pfeiffer (1965), in a comparative study of healing "split-thickness" and "gingivo-mucoperiosteal" flaps in man, found less osteoclastic activity in biopsies taken from the former, provided that a sufficiently thick layer of connective tissue is left covering the bone. These investigations on healing of gingivo-mucoperiosteal flaps were not as detailed as those reported above on "split-thickness" flaps, and as they were also carried out in a different species, no direct comparison can be made between the results. Kohler and Ramfjord found that a thin layer of new cementum may be deposited on the surface of the root during healing. Similarly, Morris (1957), investigating healing in a smaller, but similar type of incision in human subjects, observed that re-attachment of connective tissue to the surface of a root from which cementum had been removed, was achieved by laying down new cementum.

The controversy concerning the natural relationship between the epithelium of the gingival cuff and the hard tissues has raged long and wide. Recent evidence has shown that there is a union between the two (see Chapter 5). There is now also some evidence to show that this union is reconstituted by the processes of healing that follow wounding (Cimasoni *et al.*, 1963; Listgarten, 1967). Epithelium can apparently re-attach to enamel, dentine or cementum, but not, according to Wilderman *et al.* (1960), to precementum.

2. Periodontal Ligament

Procedures in which teeth are extracted and then replanted, without deliberately interfering with the vitality of the separated parts of the perio-dontal ligament adhering to tooth and bone, may be considered to constitute an incised wound of the the periodontal ligament. Löe and Waerhaug (1961) experimented with dogs and monkeys. They found that the fibres of the healing periodontal ligament are still partly disorganized 30–80 days post-operatively, but after healing for 3 years, the ligament resembles that associated with normally functioning teeth. The attached epithelial cuff does not appear to be displaced apically as a result of the procedure. Auto-transplantation of teeth with partly developed roots in young monkeys has produced similar results, except that the appearance of the periodontium returns to normal between 3 weeks and 3 months post-operatively. (Fong *et al.*, 1967). These results, together with those of Edwards (1966) from dogs, and Andreasen and Hjørting-Hansen (1966) from man, suggest that the cells of the periodontal ligament can heal breaches in the continuity of its fibres but, as will be discussed below, they seem less able to replace large quantities of its substance.

3. Cementum

An incised-type wound of cementum may occur as a result of fracture of the root of the tooth. The nature of the ensuing healing process depends on the degree of displacement of the fragments. When the fragments are well aligned they may be reunited by calcified tissue, including cementum, which may also be found on the pulpal aspect of the dentine (Andreasen and Hjørting-Hansen, 1967). If the fragments are displaced (Boulger, 1928; Coolidge, 1938; Bevelander, 1942; Omnell, 1953; Andreasen and Hjørting-Hansen, 1967), they are frequently covered by cementum, and reunited by cementum or by fibrous connective tissue continuous with the periodontal ligament. If widely separated, bone may be interposed between them, and connected to each by collagen fibres and cementum. In the presence of infection, the space between the fragments may be filled by granulation tissue. A fragment of cementum torn from an intact root may have its continuity with the root restored in a manner similar to those described above (Aisenberg, 1947). Thus, the cells of the periodontal ligament participate in repair of wounds in the cementum in particular, and of the root in general, by laying down new cementum or new soft connective tissue. It is evident too, that these cells can be induced to produce new bone in certain circumstances.

B. Excised Wounds

1. Gingiva and Periosteum

Small partial thickness excised wounds made in the epithelium of human gingiva are healed within 18 hours (Kollar *et al.*, 1955). In contrast to this, removal of a relatively large area of epithelium only from the palatal gingiva and mucosa of rats has more severe consequences (Klingsberg and Butcher, 1963). The underlying lamina propria and periosteum rapidly become the seat of inflammatory change. There is active resorption of the crest of the alveolar process during the first four days post-operatively. However, by the eighth day, reconstruction of soft and hard connective tissues is evident. Healing is completed by the twenty-fifth day, but the alveolar process is not restored to its pre-operative dimensions. Re-epithelialization is achieved by proliferation of epithelium from the periphery of the wound over the pre-existing lamina propria, but Klingsberg and Butcher do not say how long this takes. They point out that this type of wound constitutes almost as severe an insult to the periodontium as excision of a gingivo-mucoperiosteal flap of similar dimensions, and that the two types of wound take similar periods to heal. This finding underlines the significant role that the integrity of the epithelium plays in maintaining the health of the underlying soft connective tissue and bone.

The size of an excised wound involving the epithelium and connective tissue of gingiva, has been shown to influence directly the rate of healing (Stahl, 1965). Healing of the excised wound that results from classical gingivectomy has been studied widely. The process of epithelialization has been well described by Ramfjord and Costich (1963) in man, and particularly by Engler et al. (1966) in monkeys. In a manner similar to that which occurs in skin wounds, the epithelium migrates as a wedge-shaped sheet beneath a layer of clot and necrotic connective tissue. In monkeys it reaches the vicinity of the tooth on about the fifth day and, in humans, may gain attachment to the tooth a day later, forming a rudimentary epithelial cuff and crevice. Synthesis of DNA, probably a prelude to mitotic division, reaches a peak in monkey gingival epithelium 24 hours post-operatively. The ^{3}H-thymidine-labelled cells are initially restricted to the basal and spinous layers within about 2 mm of the wound margin. McHugh and Persson (1958) have found that, in dogs, new epithelial cells originate from a ring of enlarged rete pegs surrounding the wound, but Engler et al. report no evidence of such a situation in monkeys. When present, cells in remnants of the attached epithelial cuff are also labelled at 24 hours, and are seen to migrate towards the wound surface. Presumably, they are also able to contribute to epithelialization. Further evidence of the reactivity, after wounding, of the cells of the attached epithelial cuff has been provided by Stone et al. (1966) and Staffileno et al. (1966). As the epithelial sheet advances, there is evidence that migrant cells, located near the wound margin, prepare to divide, presumably as a prelude to forming a stratified epithelium. Twelve to fourteen days after wounding, the vestibular aspect of the new marginal gingiva is covered by a keratinized stratified squamous epithelium. It is believed that the new marginal gingiva is formed by upgrowth of connective tissue newly synthesized in the base of the wound; a process similar to that which occurs in repair of a deep excised wound of skin. In monkeys, the process starts between the fifth and seventh day after wounding. That this proliferation of connective tissue produces a free cuff of gingiva is quite a remarkable accomplishment, and a study of the factors that govern its initiation and spread could be most rewarding. Thirty-five days after wounding, the crevicular aspect of the marginal gingiva is covered by well organized epithelium. Engler et al. have drawn attention to the clinical implications arising from the differences in time taken for complete epithelialization of the vestibular and crevicular aspects of the marginal gingiva.

A detailed account of the reactions of the connective tissue to gingivectomy has been provided by Ramfjord et al. (1966), in monkeys which had been injected with ^{3}H-thymidine. As happens in healing of other wounds, migration of connective tissue cells lags behind that of epithelial cells. The first sign of increased incorporation of ^{3}H-thymidine into the nuclei of connective tissue cells is evident 24 hours after wounding. The affected cells are located in and around the walls of blood vessels situated just beneath the wound surface, in the superficial part of the periodontal ligament and in the adjacent marrow spaces. It would seem that these are the only sites from which new cells can be culled for repair of gingival connective tissue, whereas in skin, for example, other sites are available. Shortly after wounding there may be loss of superficial cementoblasts, and of osteoblasts covering the alveolar crest. Three days after wounding, ^{3}H-thymidine-labelled connective tissue cells are present superficially under new epithelium, an area now occupied by new, young vascular connective tissue. Some osteoblasts also show evidence of mitotic activity, as do epithelial rests in the connective tissue superficial to the alveolar crest. As maturation of the newly formed connective tissue proceeds, osteoclasts may be found in association with the alveolar bone crest, but by fourteen days the bone is once again covered by a well-defined layer of osteoblasts. After observing the effect of gingivectomy upon the alveolar bone crest in humans, Ramjford and Costich (1963) found it difficult to decide whether resorption was a sequel to pre-operative periodontal disease or to wounding. Thirty-five days after wounding the appearance of the connective tissue of the marginal gingiva is indistinguishable from that of unoperated controls.

Reconstruction of the gingiva after gingivectomy has been observed by a number of investigators (Hagerman and Arnim, 1954; Waerhaug, 1955; Tonna and Stahl, 1967). However, the new attachment of the reformed epithelial cuff may be located slightly apical to its position before wounding (Ramfjord and Costich, 1963). Stahl (1964) has made some interesting observations on the position of the newly-formed attached epithelial cuff after healing of full-thickness excised wounds in rats. He has found that the position of the healed, attached epithelial cuff is frequently not maintained and that, with the passage of time, it may move apically. This change is not accompanied by a reduction in the distance between the base of the epithelial cuff and the crest of the alveolar process, which suggests an associated resorption of bone. The factors that control the relationship between the epithelial cuff and the crest of the alveolar process have not been elucidated. Stahl has also noticed that dentine, adjacent to the cervical margin of the tooth, which is exposed by removal of cementum during wounding, is covered by proliferating cuff epithelium and not by a layer of new cementum. This is a significant observation and warrants confirmation, as it may not be the case in man (Morris 1957).

Another interesting feature pertaining to the restoration of excised marginal gingiva has emerged from healing of resected interdental gingival septa. Contrary to the finding of Holmes (1965) in humans, Kohl and Zander (1961) and Stahl (1963) have reported that the new interdental gingival septa which develop after resection in monkeys and humans, are restored to the same height and outline as the old. Kohl and Zander, and also Stahl, believe that the shape of the new tissue is governed by the morphology of the adjacent teeth. This conclusion is supported by the alteration in contour of healing marginal gingiva that occurs in rats after the shape of the adjacent tooth has been changed (Stahl, 1962). Thus, there is considerable evidence that, for all practical purposes, the tissues of the marginal gingiva are regenerated after excision.

It is apparent that the excised wound which results from gingivectomy has only a limited effect on the crest of the alveolar process. However, the bone reacts more severely when the extent of the excision is increased so that the attached as well as the marginal gingiva is removed, even if the periosteum is left intact. The changes occurring in soft and hard tissues of dogs have been described by Glickman et al. (1963), Wilderman (1963) and Staffileno et al. (1966). Shortly after wounding, the periosteum may become oedematous, and there may be evidence of superficial necrosis of the external plate of the alveolar process. Bone of the external plate of the alveolar process and, to a lesser extent, of the alveolar crest and its vicinity, are resorbed within 4–6 days after wounding. The number of osteoclasts in the periodontal ligament and marrow spaces is increased when the layer of lamina propria left covering the periosteum is inadequate. Resorption of bone leads to thinning of the alveolar process and widening of the periodontal ligament. Osteogenesis increases as healing progresses, and reaches a peak about three weeks after wounding, new bone being laid down both by apposition and the formation of new trabeculae. Wilderman has found that most of the resorbed bone has been replaced 6 months after wounding, but that the alveolar process rarely attains its former height, and that frequently it is thinner than that in unwounded controls. In contrast to the behaviour of bone cells, the early disappearance of cementoblasts following excision of soft tissue does not seem to be followed by a speedy reversal of the process, and a return to active deposition of cementum. Although Glickman et al. claim to have seen new cementum deposited 4 weeks post-operatively, Wilderman reports obtaining the first evidence of cementogenesis only 90 days after wounding.

Epithelialization of this type of excised wound starts early in the healing period. The epithelium grows in centripetally from the margins of the wound, remnants of crevicular epithelium and attached epithelial cuff making an active contribution. Staffileno et al. spared part of the attached epithelial cuff in their experiment, and found that the attached epithelial cuff shows functional repair after 7 days' healing, but that 21 days after wounding the depth of the gingival sulcus is only half of that occurring in unoperated animals.

Proliferation of new connective tissue in these excised wounds reaches a peak at 6 days. The new cells apparently arise from perivascular tissue in the walls of the wound and, in addition, according to Wilderman, from similar tissues in the periodontal ligament and alveolar process when these are exposed by bone resorption. Staffileno *et al.* have found that 14 days after wounding the attachment of lamina propria to tooth appears to be normal. However, Glickman *et al.* have found a long, dense collagenous scar running vertically in the attached gingiva, and Wilderman reports that, even 6 months after wounding, the lamina propria appears to be narrower than it was postoperatively. The last author concludes that healing of this type of large excised wound results in functional repair with anatomical deformity.

Excision of the periosteum in addition to the overlying soft tissue complicates the repair process (Wilderman *et al.*, 1960; Glickman *et al.* 1963; Pfeiffer, 1963). Shortly after wounding there is evidence of necrosis of the denuded external plate of the alveolar process to a depth of about 1 mm. Wilderman *et al.* have found that, in dogs, necrosis is rapidly followed by resorption, which reaches a peak of activity 4–6 days after operation. Osteoclasts are seen in the marrow spaces, in the connective tissue at the wound margins, and in the periodontal ligament. Resorption leads to removal of the crestal bone and external plate of the alveolar process. Despite the extensive resorption of bone that occurs in these wounds, sequestra are rarely seen, and involucra have never been reported (Grant, 1967). The resorptive phase is followed by osteogenesis which, in dogs, reaches a peak 3–4 weeks postoperatively. Although the interdental bone septa appear to be regenerated completely 3–6 months after wounding, the vestibular alveolar bone reaches only about half to two-thirds the pre-operative level.

Two days after wounding there is evidence of new proliferating connective tissue. This originates at the wound edge and in the periodontal ligament. There is need for detailed observation on the source of this new connective tissue. Later, connective tissue has been observed in dogs to proliferate from the marrow spaces exposed by resorption of bone. Glickman *et al.* have found that after maturation, the new lamina propria is scarred in the same way as when the periosteum is left intact, but Wilderman *et al.* have reported the interdental connective tissue to be fully restored. The periodontal ligament is also restored to normal width, but the height of lamina propria between the crest of the alveolar process and the base of the attached epithelial cuff may be increased. Epithelialization appears to be delayed (Arnold and Hatchett, 1962; Carranza *et al.*, 1966). This is consistent with the basic principles described in Section I. It is evident that a migrating sheet of epithelium requires a base of relatively healthy tissue along which to proliferate. To achieve this the epithelial cells cleave a path beneath the necrotic connective tissue and blood clot. In the type of wound under discussion it would be necessary for the epithelium to resorb bone in order to find a healthy base. This, apparently, is not possible; epithelialization of the wound must await the covering of its base by a carpet of new, young connective tissue (Arnold and Hatchett, 1962). As far as can be ascertained, a detailed description of these processes is not available. This is unfortunate, as comprehensive observations on the problem could elucidate some aspects of interaction between different types of proliferating tissue in the adult animal. Two to three weeks after excision, the wound is re-epithelialized and a new dento-gingival junction is formed, but this is located in a more apical position than formerly.

Experiments aimed at comparing healing of excised wounds in which the periosteum has been retained with those in which it has been resected (Carranza and Carraro, 1963; Glickman et al., 1963) have shown that repair of the latter results in the loss of greater amounts of hard and soft connective tissues. A functional restitution of tissue occurs, but not regeneration of the periodontium.

Carranza et al. (1966) have shown that if the alveolar mucosa adjacent to the attached gingiva is excised with the underlying periosteum, the new lamina propria will be fibrous and firmly attached to the adjacent bone. This results in extension of the width of the attached gingiva at the expense of the alveolar mucosa. It would appear that little attention has been paid to contraction of the attached gingiva during healing. The author has found that excision of the attached gingiva and its associated periosteum in monkeys is not followed by contraction. In contrast to this, the adjacent alveolar mucosa does contract to some degree during repair of an excised wound in which the periosteum has been spared. The effect of trauma from occlusion on healing of periodontal wounds has received scant attention. Hypofunction and hyperfunction of associated teeth does not have any noticeable effect on healing gingiva, but does seem to influence the bone associated with the healing wound (Glickman et al., 1966).

2. Alveolar Bone

Few studies, explicitly aimed at assessing the reparative powers of alveolar bone, appear to have been carried out. In dogs, it has been reported that some regeneration of the alveolar process over maxillary canines appears possible, but, surprisingly, little over mandibular canines (Linghorne and O'Connel, 1950). These investigators removed alveolar process and periodontal ligament, but conserved the overlying periosteum. Periodontal ligament regenerates where there is restoration of alveolar bone, and fibres of lamina propria become re-attached to part of the root surface. However, epithelium comes to cover appreciable areas of root surface to which connective tissue was attached pre-operatively. Differences between the response of alveolar bone in the maxilla and mandible appear not to have been confirmed independently. This problem merits further investigation.

Although dealing with mandibular jaw bone rather than alveolar bone, Retief and Dreyer (1967) have found that excised wounds in rats are first filled with endosteal callus which forms a scaffolding over which periosteal callus subsequently proliferates. This sequence of events is comparable with that which takes place in the repair of an excised defect in the rat femur. These investigators remark on the comparatively slow reaction of the periosteal bone. Excised defects involving bone and periodontal ligament covering the "root" of the continuously erupting rat incisor also exhibit a comparatively sluggish periosteal reaction, and heal incompletely (Melcher, 1967a). In this situation there is a small contribution of new bone by osteoblasts on the endosteal surface of the bone bordering the defect, and that produced by the periosteal osteoblasts does not bridge the defect. Cartilage is not formed during healing of either of these defects in rat mandibles. There appears to be little understanding of the factors which either inhibit healing of alveolar bone, or which might promote its repair. This problem is closely linked with that of the difference between the reparative capacities of bone originally formed in cartilage and bone originally developed in membrane. Conceivably there are in addition, other factors operating, which are governed by the unique anatomy and physiology of the alveolar process.

3. Periodontal Ligament

In the experiment described above, Linghorne and O'Connel found that when periodontal ligament and bone are excised from the alveolar margin, new periodontal ligament will be constructed adjacent to newly formed bone. Despite deficient bone repair of the excised defect over the "root" of the rat incisor, also described above, the periodontal ligament is repaired, and attached to a "limiting membrane" of collagen fibres formed across the osseous defect. Although it is believed that the fibres of the cemental aspect of the ligament are carried on the advancing tooth (Melcher, 1967b), the arrangement of the peripheral fibres, which also extend partly into the unrepaired defect, is such that they appear to have been laid down after wounding.

Another situation in which partial excision of the periodontal ligament has been studied is in experimental reimplantation of teeth. Löe and Waerhaug (1961) have found in their experiments with monkeys, that, ankylosis will result if the remnants of periodontal ligament adhering to the extracted tooth are removed prior to reimplantation. Hammer (1955) has come to a similar conclusion. In contrast to the clear-cut results of Löe and Waerhaug (1955), Butcher and Vidair (1955), in a similar experiment carried out on monkeys, found that the same treatment produced a variable outcome. The teeth they reimplanted not only showed areas of ankylosis, but also areas in which the periodontal ligament was repaired, and areas of root resorption. It is possible that the reactivity of the osteoblasts on the periodontal surface of the alveolar bone is controlled to some extent by the integrity of the periodontal ligament, and this topic will be raised again in Section 5. If this is the case, then ankylosis could follow failure of repair of the periodontal ligament. In the two experiments described above, the extent and vitality of the part of the periodontal ligament left adhering to the alveolar bone appears to have been overlooked. If an experiment were designed which took account of the behaviour of the remnant of periodontal ligament left adhering to alveolar bone, it might be possible to gain some further insight into the circumstances that favour ankylosis.

Shklar et al. (1966) have implanted polymethacrylate replicas of extracted teeth into sockets of baboons. Although difficulties arose out of histological technique they have found that 3–5 years after operation, the roots of the plastic teeth are separated from bone by soft connective tissue, which they strongly suspect is firmly attached to the plastic. The fibres of the connective tissue are dense and appear to be orientated parallel to the long axis of the teeth. It seems possible that this connective tissue is more in the nature of a capsule than a functioning periodontal ligament, as it appears to resemble the connective tissue which has been found to surround polytetrafluorethylene implants placed in long bones of rats (Melcher and Dreyer, 1961).

4. Cementum

It has long been known that excised wounds in cementum can be repaired by deposition of new cementum, which may be acellular, cellular, or a mixture of both (Orban 1928; Gottlieb 1943; Henry and Weinmann, 1951). It is apparent that differentiation of functioning cementoblasts occurs much more slowly than differentiation of functioning osteoblasts (Wilderman et al., 1960; Morris and Thompson, 1963). The nature of the factors that control differentiation of cementoblasts is obscure. Although it is evident that cementoblasts are derived from cells of the periodontal ligament, it is by no means certain which are their precursors.

5. Periodontal Ligament and Cementum

Excision of periodontal ligament and cementum occurs following extraction of teeth. Healing of these wounds has been studied in a number of animals, as well as in man, and it is of interest that the process is apparently faster in the former than in the latter (Mangos, 1941; Pietrokovsky and Massler, 1967).

Classical descriptions of the sequence of events that lead to repair of a socket following tooth extraction have been provided by Claflin (1936) in dogs and Mangos (1941) in man. As in bone wounds elsewhere, the socket is immediately filled with shed blood, which coagulates to form a clot. The wound is covered by epithelium after 7 days in dogs and 10 days in man. It is said that the clot is gradually replaced by connective tissue which originates peripherally, the central part enduring longest. There is resorption of bone at the crests of the alveolar process. Deposition of new bone is initiated in the fundus, and this is later augmented by formation of bone on the walls of the socket. The connective tissue of the new lamina propria matures and, in monkeys, new transseptal fibres regenerate within 3 weeks of extraction (Simpson, 1960). It is of interest that, in dogs, Claflin found that newly-deposited bone reaches the crestal bone by 19 days post-operatively, when remnants of blood clot are still present in the centre of the socket. Final healing is achieved by development of keratinized stratified squamous epithelium over the wound, and remodelling of the new bone and soft connective tissue which has recently been laid down in the socket.

The processes which are believed to bring about repair of tissues after tooth extraction will now be examined in greater detail. Although Huebsch et al. (1952) and Simpson (1960) pay some attention to the route taken by the emigrating sheet of epithelial cells, as far as can be determined no studies aimed specifically at elucidating which epithelial cells are concerned in the process, where they proliferate in relation to the clot occupying the socket, and the relationship between the onset of mobilization of epithelial and connective tissue cells, have been undertaken. Some photomicrographs, such those in the papers of Claflin, Huebsch et al. and Pietrokovsky and Massler, suggest that, as elsewhere, the new epithelium proliferates in a plane below the level of the pre-existing epithelium. If the point of origin of the new epithelium is the base of the remnant of the attached epithelial cuff, it would be natural for it to migrate along a plane deeper than that occupied by the pre-existing gingival epithelium. However, it is not clear whether the new epithelium proliferates horizontally at the level of the attached epithelial cuff, or penetrates more deeply into the clot. It would also be interesting to know precisely what tissue provides the base along which these epithelial cells move.

There appears to be evidence which shows that fibrous callus is produced at least in part, by cells derived from the remnants of the periodontal ligament adhering to the walls of the socket (Alling and Kerr, 1957). Schulte (1967) has also suggested that cells in the remnants of the periodontal ligament may also be responsible for initiating osteogenesis but states that there is no direct proof of this. It was conjectured in Section 3 that the periodontal ligament or some of its constituents, may in some way control osteogenesis in the periodontal space. Some of the observations on healing sockets tend to support this concept. In healing mandibular first molar sockets of rats, Huebsch *et al.* have observed the first indications of new bone in the socket itself five days after extraction. They also point out that, after the same time period, the organized periodontal ligament has disappeared completely and that the connective tissue in the area has the same appearance as that in the rest of the socket. Similarly, Radden (1959) has stated that, in wounds ten days after extraction of teeth in monkeys, osteoblasts are absent where remnants of periodontal ligament persist. No definite conclusions can be drawn from these observations, but they suggest that the problem could profitably be investigated further.

Finally, it is evident that new endosteal bone is laid down in marrow spaces surrounding the socket before new bone appears in the socket itself (Huebsch *et al.*, 1952; Boyne, 1966). Furthermore, Boyne has found that, in humans, the first new bone laid down in the socket may appear on the lateral walls and not in the fundus.

C. Conclusions

Perusal of the literature shows that healing processes in the periodontium have attracted a great deal of attention. It is apparent however, that most of this interest has been focused on the sequelae of clinical procedures rather than on the biological processes which bring about healing. It would be unfortunate if sight was lost of the biological implications of healing in the periodontium, for when thoroughly understood, the correct application of this new knowledge could provide great clinical benefit. For example, it is not really known how important is the presence of a blood clot. It has been shown that, in repair of excised wounds of skin and of gingiva, the epithelium must burrow beneath the clot to cover the defect. Perhaps repair would be hastened if the clot was removed. On the other hand, its retention may be beneficial, because it may play an important part in protecting the vitality of the underlying connective tissue, which itself must be undermined by the epithelium if necrosed.

Through differences in anatomy, it seems that there are many more sites in skin from which connective tissue cells can be mobilized for wound repair than there are in gingiva. Little attention has been paid to the precise tissues from which cells can be recruited to repair large connective tissue defects in gingiva. For instance, will cells that have migrated from cut edges of the loose connective tissue of alveolar mucosa produce the dense fibrous connective tissue required for the formation of a new attached gingiva? If they will, what then are the factors that influence fibroblasts to produce different qualities of connective tissue?

Attention has been paid to the ability of the periodontium to regenerate itself after wounding. What has emerged is the remarkable capacity of the gingiva, and particularly the marginal gingiva, to regenerate after resection. What are the factors which stimulate the generous formation of new connective tissue developing as a free structure, and what are the forces that limit its growth? If these were clearly understood, could the knowledge be applied to improving repair processes elsewhere in the body?

Mention has been made of the possible relationship between the maintenance of the periodontal space and the interaction between the periodontal ligament and the alveolar bone. Clarification of this problem, may come from the type of investigations discussed in Chapter 12. It is evident, however, that carefully designed healing experiments could also throw some light on the influence of one upon the other, and in addition, contribute to our knowledge of the behaviour of the bone of the alveolar process. Experiments of this type could also help to illuminate some features of the remodelling of collagen fibres that takes place in the periodontal ligament.

In concluding this chapter, it is necessary to admit that our knowledge of healing processes in the periodontium is meagre. A feature of interest, as yet unexplored, is the comparatively rapid reaction to wounding, particularly as exemplified by the early onset of fibrogenesis. An understanding of the mechanisms that mediate this response would be useful. We have in the periodontium a potentially rewarding system for experiment: a system that can provide information of value to clinicians and, in addition, one that can provide information of a fundamental nature about the interaction between epithelia and connective tissues, and between different types of connective tissues.

References

Abercrombie, M. (1964). *In* "Advances in Biology of the Skin. Vol. V. Wound Healing" (W. Montagna and R. E. Billingham, eds), pp. 95–112. Pergamon Press, Oxford.

Abercrombie, M. (1966). *In* "Wound Healing" (Sir Charles Illingworth, ed.), pp. 61–68. J. and A. Churchill, London.

Abercrombie, M., James, D. W. and Newcombe, J. F. (1961). *In* "Wound Healing" (D. Slome, ed.), pp. 10–25. Pergamon Press, Oxford.

Aisenberg, M. S. (1947). *J. dent. Res.* **26**, 421–425.

Allgower, M. (1956). "The cellular basis of wound repair." Charles C. Thomas, Springfield, Illinois, U.S.A.

Alling, C. C. and Kerr, D. A. (1957). *J. Oral Surg.* **15**, 3–11.

Andreasen, J. O. and Hjørting–Hansen, E. (1966). *Acta odont. Scand.* **24**, 287–306.

Andreasen, J. O. and Hjørting–Hansen, E. (1967). *J. Oral Surg.* **25**, 414–426.

Arnold, N. R. and Hatchett, C. M. Jr. (1962). *J. Periodont.* **33**, 129–139.

Bassett, C. A. L. (1962). *J. Bone Jt. Surg.* **44A**, 1217–1244.

Bassett, C. A. L. and Herrmann, I. (1961). *Nature, Lond.* **190**, 460–461.

Basset, C. A. L. and Ruedi, T. P. (1966). *Nature, Lond.* **209**, 988–989.

Bassett, C. A. L., Creighton, D. K. and Stinchfield, F. E. (1961). *Surg. Gynec. Obst.* **112**, 145–152.

Beresford, W. A. and Hancox, N. M. (1967). *Acta Anat.* **66**, 78–117.
Bevelander, G. (1942). *J. dent. Res.* **21**, 481–487.
Billingham, R. E. and Medawar, P. B. (1955). *J. Anat. Lond.* **89**, 114–123.
Billingham, R. E. and Russell, P. S. (1956). *Ann. Surg.* **144**, 961–981.
Block, P., Seiter, I. and Oehlert, W. (1963). *Expt. Cell Res.* **30**, 311–321.
Boulger, E. P. (1928). *J. Am. dent. Assoc.* **15**, 1778–1779.
Boyne, P. J. (1966). *Oral. Surg. Oral Med. Oral Path.* **21**, 805–813.
Bridges, J. B. (1958). *J. Urol.* **79**, 903–910.
Bridges, J. B. and Pritchard, J. J. (1958). *J. Anat., Lond.* **92**, 28–38.
Bullough, W. S. (1966). *In* "Wound Healing" (Sir Charles Illingworth, ed.), pp. 43–59. J. and A. Churchill, London.
Bullough, W. S. and Laurence, Edna B. (1960). *Proc. R. Soc.* Ser. B. **151**, 517–536.
Bullough, W. S. and Laurence, Edna B. (1961). *In* "Wound Healing" (D. Slome, ed.), pp. 1–9. Pergamon Press, Oxford.
Bullough, W. S. and Rytömaa, T. (1965). *Nature, Lond.* **205**, 573–578.
Buntine, J. A. (1967). *Brit. J. Surg.* **54**, 699–700.
Burger, M., Sherman, B. S. and Sobel, A. E. (1962). *J. Bone Jt. Surg.* **44B**, 675–687.
Butcher, E. O. and Vidair, R. V. (1955). *J. dent. Res.* **34**, 569–576.
Calnan, J., Fry. H. J. H. and Saad, N. (1964). *Brit. J. Surg.* **51**, 448–456.
Carranza, F. A. Jr. and Carraro, J. J. (1963). *J. Periodont.* **34**, 223–226.
Carranza, F. A. Jr., Carraro, J. J., Dotto, C. A. and Cabrini, R. L. (1966). *J. Periodont.* **37**, 335–340.
Cavadias, A. X. and Trueta, J. (1965). *Surg. Gynec. Obst.* **120**, 731–747.
Cimasoni, G., Fiore-Donno, G. and Held, A-J. (1963). *Helv. odont. Acta.* **7**, 60–67
Claflin, R. S. (1936). *J. Am. dent. Assoc.* **23**, 945–959.
Cliff, W. J. (1963). *Philosoph. Trans. R. Soc. (London).* Ser. B. **246**, 305–325.
Cliff, W. J. (1965). *Quart. J. exp. Physiol.* **50**, 79–89.
Cohen, B. (1963). *Les Paradontopathies.* Georg and Co., Geneva. **59**.
Cohen, J. and Lacroix, P. (1955). *J. Bone and Jt. Surg.* **37A**, 717–730.
Coolidge, E. D., (1938). *J. Am. dent. Ass. dent. Cosmos.* **25**, 343–357.
Dedolph, T. H., Jr. and Clark, H. B., Jr. (1958). *J. Oral Surg.* **16**, 367–376.
Douglas, D. L. (1963). "Wound Healing and Management" E. and S. Livingstone Ltd., Edinburgh.
Edwards, L. C. and Dunphy, J. E. (1958). *New Eng. J. Med.* **259**, 224–233.
Edwards, T. S. F. (1966). *Brit. dent. J.* **121**, 159–166.
Engler, W. O., Ramfjord, S. P. and Hiniker, J. J. (1966). *J. Periodont.* **37**, 298–308.
Epstein, W. L. and Sullivan, D. J. (1964). *In* "Advances in Biology of Skin. Vol. V. Wound Healing" (W. Montagna and R. E. Billingham, eds), pp. 68–75. Pergamon Press. Oxford.
Fell, H. B. (1932). *J. Anat. Lond.* **66**, 157–180.
Fell, H. B. (1933). *Proc. R. Soc.* Ser. B, **112**, 417–427.
Fong, C., Morris, Merle, Grant, T. and Berger, J. (1967). *J. dent. Res.* **46**, 492–496.
Giblin, J. M., Levy, S., Staffileno, H. and Gargiulo, A. W. (1966). *J. Periodont.* **37**, 238–253.
Gillman, T. (1961). *In* "Structural aspects of ageing" (G. H. Bourne, ed.), pp. 143–176. Pitman Medical Publishing Co. Ltd., London.
Gillman, T. (1968). *In* "Treatise on Collagen, Volume 2, Part B" (G. N. Rama-chandran and B. S. Gould, eds), pp. 331–407. Academic Press Inc., New York.
Gillman, T. and Penn, J. (1956). *Med. Proc.* **2**, 150–186.
Gillman, T., Penn, J., Bronks, D. and Roux, M. (1955). *Brit. J. Surg.* **43**, 141–153
Girgis, F. G. and Pritchard, J. J. (1958). *J. Bone Jt. Surg.* **40B**, 274–281.
Glickman, I., Smulow, J. B., O'Brien, T. and Tannen, R. (1963). *Oral. Surg. Oral. Med. Oral. Path.* **16**, 530–538.

Glickman, I., Smulow, J. B., Vogel, G. and Passamonti, G. (1966). *J. Periodont.* **37,** 319–325.

Glücksmann, A. (1964). *In* "Advances in Biology of Skin, Vol. V. Wound Healing" (W. Montagna and R. E. Billingham, eds), pp. 76–94. Pergamon Press, Oxford.

Goldhaber, P. (1961). *Science, N.Y.* **133,** 2065–2067.

Gottlieb, B. (1943). *J. Am. dent. Assoc.* **30,** 1872–1883.

Grant, D. A. (1967). *J. Periodont.* **38,** 409–425.

Grillo, H. C. (1964). *Arch. Surg.* **88,** 218–224.

Grillo, H. C. and Gross, J. (1964). *J. Cell. Biol.* **23,** 39A.

Grillo, H. C. and Potsaid, M. S. (1961). *Ann. Surg.* **154,** 741–750.

Hadfield, G. (1963a). *Brit. J. Surg.* **50,** 649–661.

Hadfield, G. (1963b). *Brit. J. Surg.* **50,** 751–764.

Hadfield, G. (1963c). *Brit. J. Surg.* **50,** 870–881.

Hagerman, D. A. and Arnim, S. S. (1954). *J. Am. dent. Assoc.* **48,** 158–165.

Ham, A. W. (1930). *J. Bone Jt. Surg.* **12,** 827–844.

Ham, A. W. and Harris, W. R. (1956). *In* "The Biochemistry and Physiology of Bone" (G. H. Bourne, ed.), pp. 475–505. Academic Press Inc., New York.

Hammer, H. (1955). *Int. dent. J.* **5,** 439–457.

Hell, E. A. and Cruickshank, C. N. D. (1963). *Exp. Cell. Res.* **31,** 128–139.

Henry, J. L. and Weinmann, J. P. (1951). *J. Am. dent. Assoc.* **42,** 271–290.

Holmes, C. H. (1965). *J. Periodont.* **36,** 455–460.

Howes, E. L. (1959). *In* "Wound Healing & Tissue Repair" (W. Bradford Patterson, ed.), pp. 18–21. University of Chicago Press, Chicago, Ill.

Huebsch, R., Coleman, R. D., Frandsen, A. M. and Becks, H. (1952). *Oral. Surg. Oral. Med. Oral. Path.* **5,** 864–876.

Hurley, L. A., Stinchfield, F. E., Bassett, C. A. L. and Lyon, W. H. (1959). *J. Bone Jt. Surg.* **41A,** 1243–1254.

Johnson, F. R. and McMinn, R. M. H. (1960). *Biol. Rev.* (Cambridge Philosophical Society), **35,** 364–412.

Klingsberg, J. and Butcher, E. O. (1963). *J. Periodont.* **34,** 315–321.

Kohl, J. and Zander, H. (1961). *Oral. Surg. Oral. Med. Oral. Path.* **14,** 287–295.

Kohler, C. A. and Ramfjord, S. P. (1960). *Oral. Surg. Oral. Med. Oral. Path.* **13,** 89–103.

Kollar, J. A., Wentz, F. M. and Orban, B. (1955). *J. Periodont.* **26,** 95–98.

Linghorne, W. J. and O'Connel, D. C. (1950). *J. dent. Res.* **29,** 419–428.

Listgarten, M. A. (1967). *J. Periodont. Res.* **2,** 46–52.

Löe, H. and Waerhaug, J. (1961). *Archs. Oral Biol.* **3,** 176–184.

Luccioli, G. M., Kahn, D. S. and Robertson, H. R. (1964). *Ann. Surg.* **160,** 1030–1040.

Mangos, J. F. (1941). *New Zealand dent. J.* **37,** 4–23.

McClements, P., Templeton, R. W. and Pritchard, J. J. (1961). *J. Anat. Lond.* **95,** 616 (Abstract).

McHugh, W. D. and Persson, P. A. (1958). *Acta odont. Scand.* **16,** 205–231.

McLean, F. C. and Urist, M. R. (1955). "Bone. An Introduction to the Physiology of Skeletal Tissue." The University of Chicago Press, Chicago.

McMinn, R. H. H. (1967). *In* "International Reviews of Cytology", Vol. 22 (G. H. Bourne and J. F. Danielli, eds), pp. 64–145. Academic Press, London.

Melcher, A. H. (1967a). *Archs. Oral Biol.* **12,** 1645–1647.

Melcher, A. H. (1967b). *Archs. Oral Biol.* **12,** 1649–1651.

Melcher, A. H. and Dreyer, C. J. (1961). *S. Afr. J. Med. Sci.* **26,** 125–128.

Melcher, A. H. and Dreyer, C. J. (1962). *J. Bone Jt. Surg.* **44B,** 424–340.

Melcher, A. H. and Irving, J. T. (1962). *J. Bone Jt. Surg.* **44B,** 928–936.

Melcher, A. H. and Irving, J. T. (1964). *In* "Bone and Tooth" (H. J. J. Blackwood, ed.), pp. 337–341. Pergamon Press, Oxford.

Mittleman, H. R., Toto, P. D., Sicher, H. and Wentz, F. M. (1964). *Periodontics* **2**, 106–114.

Morris, M. L. (1957). *J. Periodont.* **28**, 222–238.

Morris, M. L. and Thompson, R. H. (1963). *Periodontics* **1**, 189–195.

Mulholland, H. C. and Pritchard, J. J. (1959). *J. Anat. Lond.* **93**, 590 (Abstract).

Murray, G., Holden, R. and Roschlau, W. (1957). *Am. J. Surg.* **93**, 385–387.

Omnell, K-A. (1953). *Brit. dent. J.* **95**, 181–185.

Orban, B. (1928). *J. Am. dent. Assoc.* **15**, 1768–1777.

Ordman, L. J. and Gillman, T. (1966a). *Arch. Surg.* **93**, 857–882.

Ordman, L. J. and Gillman, T. (1966b). *Arch. Surg.* **93**, 883–910.

Pfeiffer, J. S. (1963). *J. Periodont.* **34**, 10–16.

Pfeiffer, J. S. (1965). *Periodontology.* **3**, 135–140.

Pietrokovsky, J. and Massler, M. (1967). *J. dent. Res.* **46**, 222–231.

Pritchard, J. J. (1946). *J. Anat. Lond.* **80**, 55–60.

Pritchard, J. J. (1964). *In* "Modern Trends in Orthopaedics. Vol. 4, Science of Fractures" (J. M. P. Clark, ed.), pp. 69–90. Butterworths, London.

Pritchard, J. J. and Ruzicka, A. J. (1946). *J. Anat., Lond.* **84**, 236–261.

Radden, H. G. (1959). *Ann. R. Coll. Surg. Eng.* **24**, 366–387.

Ramfjord, S. P. and Costich, E. R. (1963). *J. Periodont.* **34**, 401–415.

Ramfjord, S. P., Engler, W. O. and Hiniker, J. J. (1966). *J. Periodont.* **37**, 179–189.

Retief, D. H. and Dreyer, C. J. (1967). *Archs. Oral Biol.* **12**, 1035–1039.

Schoefl, G. I. and Majno, G. (1964). *In* "Advances in Biology of Skin. Vol. V, Wound Healing" (W. Montagna and R. E. Billingham, eds), pp. 173–193. Pergamon Press, Oxford.

Schulte, W. C. (1967). *J. dent. Res.* **46**, 656–660.

Shklar, G., Hodosh, M. and Povar, M. (1966). *Oral. Surg. Oral. Med. Oral. Path.* **22**, 349–357.

Simpson, H. E. (1960). *J. Oral Surg.* **18**, 391–399.

Skoog, T. and Persson, B. H. (1954). *Plastic Reconstruc. Surg.* **13**, 384–399.

Staffileno, H., Wentz, F. M. and Orban, B. (1962). *J. Periodont.* **33**, 56–69.

Staffileno, H., Levy, S. and Garguilo, A. W. (1966). *J. Periodont.* **37**, 117–131.

Stahl, S. S. (1962). *Oral. Surg. Oral. Med. Oral. Path.* **15**, 1172–1177.

Stahl, S. S. (1963). *J. Am. dent. Assoc.* **67**, 48–53.

Stahl, S. S. (1964). *Periodontics.* **2**, 97–105.

Stahl, S. S. (1965). *J. Periodont.* **36**, 471–473.

Stone, S., Ramfjord, S. P. and Waldron, J. (1966). *J. Periodont.* **37**, 415–430.

Tonna, E. A. (1965). *In* "The Use of Radioautography in Investigating Protein Synthesis" (C. P. LeBlond and Katherine B. Warren, eds), pp. 215–245. Academic Press, London.

Tonna, E. A. and Cronkite, E. P. (1961). *J. Bone Jt. Surg.* **43A**, 352–362.

Tonna, E. A. and Stahl, S. S. (1967). *Acta. Odont. Helv.* **11**, 90–104.

Trueta, J. (1963). *J. Bone Jt. Surg.* **45B**, 402–418.

Trueta, J. and Cavadias, A. X. (1955). *J. Bone Jt. Surg.* **37B**, 492–505.

Urist, M. R. (1956). *In* "Wound Healing and Tissue Repair" (W. Bradford Patterson, ed.), pp. 65–74. The University of Chicago Press, Chicago.

Urist, M. R. (1965). *Science, N.Y.* **150**, 893–899.

Urist, M. R. and McLean, F. C. (1952). *J. Bone Jt. Surg.* **34A**, 443–476.

Van Winkle, W. Jr. (1967). *Surg. Gynec. Obst.* **125**, 131–142.

Waerhaug, J. (1955). *Oral. Surg. Oral. Med. Oral. Path.* **8**, 707–718.

Wassermann, F. (1954). *Am. J. Anat.* **94**, 399–437.

Weiss, P. (1958). *In* "International Review of Cytology", Vol. 7 (G. H. Bourne and J. F. Danielli, eds), pp. 391–423. Academic Press, New York.

Weiss, P. (1959). *In* "Wound Healing and Tissue Repair" (W. Bradford Patterson, ed.), pp. 1–9. University of Chicago Press, Chicago, Ill.

Weiss, P. (1961). *Exptl. Cell Res. Suppl.* **8**, 260–281.

Wilderman, M. (1963). *J. Periodont.* **34**, 487–503.

Wilderman, M., Wentz, F. M. and Orban, B. J. (1960). *J. Periodont.* **31**, 283–299.

Williams, R. G. (1957). *Anat. Rec.* **129**, 187–210.

Winter, G. D. (1964). *In* "Advances in Biology of Skin. Vol. 5, Wound Healing" (W. Montagna and R. E. Billingham, eds), pp. 113–127. Pergamon Press, Oxford.

Author Index

18*

Subject Index

Numbers in italics refer to pages where the Subject is mentioned in a figure.

551